LAW RELATING TO
HOSPITALS

SPELLER'S LAW RELATING

TO

HOSPITALS

AND KINDRED INSTITUTIONS

Sixth Edition

edited by JOE JACOB

of Gray's Inn, Barrister-at-Law
Lecturer in Law, London School of Economics

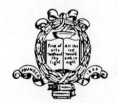

LONDON

H. K. LEWIS & Co. Ltd.

1978

First Edition	.	.	.	1947
Second Edition	.	.	.	1949
Third Edition	.	.	.	1956
Fourth Edition	.	.	.	1965
Reprinted	.	.	.	1966
Fifth Edition	.	.	.	1971
Sixth Edition	.	.	.	1978

©

H. K. LEWIS & Co. Ltd.
1978

SBN 0 7186 0438 5

*Made and Printed in Great Britain by
Robert MacLehose and Company Limited
Printers to the University of Glasgow*

PREFACE TO SIXTH EDITION

In the Preface to the previous edition of this book Dr. Speller wrote:

'I have sought to provide something useful for legal practitioners who may be concerned with any matter touching the hospital field, whilst at the same time providing a reference book for hospital administrators.'

In this edition I have endeavoured to follow that purpose. Previous editions were enhanced by Dr. Speller's knowledge and experience. This edition could not have been written at all except that it is based on that sure foundation. Further, although I am responsible for the whole of this edition, a considerable part of the editing work on it was done by Dr. Speller himself. It is probably true that it would not have appeared without the effort that he put into it. Certainly I could not have done it. In particular, he provided the drafts of the changes necessitated by the re-organisation of the health service, including much of the text of Chapters 3 (Hospitals under the National Health Service) and 17 (Complaints Machinery). He also provided other draft changes too numerous to mention.

The pace of and extent of change in the law relating to hospitals in the past seven years more than justifies this new edition of Dr. Speller's work. Among the major changes are: the re-organisation of the health service; the phasing in of the separation of the public and private sectors of medicine; the bringing into force of further sections of the 1968 Medicines Act; the creation of the Health Service Commissioners; and the passage and repeal of the Industrial Relations Act 1971 and the great changes made in the structure of the law relating to safety at work. These, and other changes, are recorded in this edition. Further, since the last edition the Law Commission's programme of consolidation of statutes has gathered momentum. When the text was in page proof Parliament enacted the National Health Service Act of 1977. This consolidates much, but not all, of the previous statutory law relating to the structure and working of the health service. Publication of this edition was delayed in order that account could be taken of this consolidation. Also noted are the consolidation of the Nursing Homes legislation (in the 1975 Act) and the Poison legislation (in the 1972 Act). This last statute, as will be seen, is to come into force with the making of regulations under the Medicines Act. Unfortunately the 1978 Poisons Rules (S.I. 1978 No. 1) have been published after the text had gone to press. They too will come into force at the same time. Although the Congenital

Disabilities (Civil Liability) Act 1976 came too late to be properly included in Chapter 14 (Injury to Patient), I have been able to include a
note about it in an Appendix. I hope I have correctly stated the law up
to September 1977.

In all, this edition notes about fifty new statutes, one hundred and
twenty new statutory instruments and one hundred and thirty new cases.
I have throughout been mindful of the need to maintain brevity and
despite all this extra material, this edition is only some seventy odd
pages longer than its predecessor. This has however only been achieved
by some extensive but, I hope, not damaging pruning, especially among
the Appendices. Gone from these, apart from spent matters, are the
statutory instruments relating to changing powers of health authorities,
and the Appendices on the liability of a supplier or manufacturer of
dangerous articles, cinematographs in hospital and simple wills. The
reason is that increasingly nothing in the law is simple. In the midst of
all this new material and having regard to the fact that Parliament has
found time to re-organise the health service, I have taken the opportunity
to re-arrange the contents of the work.

I am hopeful that major changes will not be made in any of the fields
covered for some time. I do not, however, expect this. Not merely is the
Government already consolidating the law relating to the individual
contract of employment, but more ominously we still await the revision
of the Whitley machinery in the light of Lord McCarthy's Report and
further off there lies the prospect of further re-organisation which might
follow the Report of the Royal Commission on the Health Service. So
also any new edition will need to take account of any legislation which
follows the Royal Commission on Compensation for Personal Injuries
and of the final outcome of the Department of Health's Review of the
1959 Mental Health Act.

In the Preface to the First Edition, Dr. Speller wrote:

> 'In a work covering such a wide field as the present one —
> although the fruit of ten years' close study of hospital legal
> problems — some subjects may be dealt with less fully than
> their importance merits and some inaccuracies may have crept
> in, such imperfections revealing themselves to the critical
> reader. Respecting such imperfections the writer asks not
> indulgence but help, and hopes that readers will draw his
> attention to any errors or omissions they may notice.'

Dr. Speller is not responsible for any such imperfections in this
edition. I alone must shoulder that burden. However I too ask not for
indulgence but help and I too hope that readers will draw my attention
to any errors and any omissions they may notice.

It is customary in a Preface to mention those who have helped a writer. It is not however custom but gratitude that leads me first to repeat my acknowledgement to Dr. Speller for his contribution. I must also thank my friend and colleague Mr. Roy Lewis, Lecturer in the Industrial Relations Department at the London School of Economics for reading the first draft of the Chapters that became 22 (Labour Law) and 23 (Injury at Work). He made some fundamental suggestions for improvement and many other suggestions and corrections. Also deserving my sincere thanks is Mrs. Shirley Harden whose cheerful and willing manner especially in sorting and deciphering scarcely legible pieces of paper made my task so much easier. Finally, but by no means least, my thanks are also due to my wife, Miriam, for rendering my years of editing this edition less painful than they would otherwise have been.

JOE JACOB

London School of Economics,
Houghton Street,
Aldwych,
London W.C.2.
January 1978

EXTRACT FROM PREFACE TO
FIRST EDITION

THIS book has been in contemplation since . . . 1940. . . . The delay in giving form to the project was due partly to wartime difficulties and partly to the passing of the Nurses Act, 1943, which rendered it desirable to wait on the issue of the statutory rules and orders to be made thereunder and the fixing of the prescribed dates for the various purposes so as to present a practical summary. Whilst the writer was waiting on these developments successive Ministers of Health have had under consideration measures of social security on the lines of the *Beveridge Report*, but only last year did Mr. Aneurin Bevan achieve the distinction of being the first Minister of Health to embody provisions for a comprehensive health service in a Bill which has now become law as the National Health Service Act, 1946.

S. R. SPELLER

January, 1947

TABLE OF CHAPTERS

TABLE OF CONTENTS

INDEX TO CASES CITED

TABLE OF STATUTES

TABLE OF STATUTES

STATUTORY INSTRUMENTS

LAW RELATING TO HOSPITALS

CHAPTER 1

HOSPITALS — DEFINITION AND CLASSIFICATION

A. HOSPITAL, DEFINITION OF

TO-DAY the term *hospital* usually means any institution maintained for the reception, care and treatment[1] of those in need of medical or surgical[2] attention, being an institution which is not carried on for private gain,[3] and it is in this general sense that the term is used throughout this book except where otherwise indicated. The use of the expression *those in need of medical or surgical attention* in the definition instead of the more elegant term *sick persons* is necessary because the former — but not the latter — is apt to include women in childbirth,[4] the mentally afflicted and also persons suffering from bodily disablement or disability, not popularly regarded as sick persons. The word *attention* to *treatment* is preferred because the former, but not the latter, is apt to include hospitals and homes for the incurable and the dying where the patients need nursing care under medical supervision rather than active medical treatment.[5] Hence, by definition, are included hospitals popularly so called, maternity homes and psychiatric hospitals, including hospitals for the mentally sub-normal, as well as homes for the dying, provided always that they are not carried on for private gain. Equally, by definition, are excluded nursing homes because they are conducted for private gain, and also charitable institutions otherwise than for the care and treatment of those in need of medical or surgical attention, such as Christ's Hospital, the famous bluecoat school, mention of which takes us back to an earlier and more extensive definition of the word hospital than the modern one. Still it must be emphasised that at the present time there is nothing in law restricting the use of the term *hospital* either to institutions for medical care or to charitable institutions in the older sense. Seemingly, the only risk a nursing home would run in adopting a name including the word hospital would be

---

[1] For a full discussion of the justification of the statement that hospitals provide treatment reference should be made to Chapter 14 dealing with liability for injuries to patients.

[2] Including dental.

[3] Following *re Smith (deceased)* [1962[1 W.L.R. 763. See further p. 71

[4] Strictly, a woman in normal childbirth may not need medical attention and, even in hospital, she may for her delivery, be in the care of a midwife; but even then she will ordinarily have been attended by a medical practitioner both before and after birth.

[5] See *Minister of Health* v. *General Committee of the Royal Midland Counties Home for Incurables* [1954] Ch. 530, referred to on p. 2.

that a patient with whom, or in respect of whom, no express contract has been made, might refuse to pay his account on the ground that he thought he had entered a public or charitable institution.[1] The expression *private hospital* is sometimes used as part of the name of a nursing home, to distinguish it from a public or charitable hospital. Hospitals as here defined may be classified either as being voluntary or public authority hospitals, or according to their function.

In the National Health Service Act 1977 the term *hospital* is given a wider connotation so as to include institutions such as nursing homes which are carried on for profit, the definition in s 128[2] of the 1977 Act reading as follows:

'hospital' means —
  (a) any institution for the reception and treatment of persons suffering from illness,
  (b) any maternity home, and
  (c) any institution for the reception and treatment of persons during convalescence or persons requiring medical rehabilitation,
and includes clinics, dispensaries and out-patient departments maintained in connection with any such institution or home as aforesaid, and 'hospital accommodation' shall be construed accordingly.

In *Minister of Health* v. *General Committee of the Royal Midland Counties Home for Incurables*[3] the Court of Appeal held that an institution for incurables, where no active treatment was given, was a hospital within that definition and so properly transferred to the Minister under s. 6 (1) of the 1946 Act. The basis of the decision was that the patients required nursing and that nursing is treatment for the purpose of the definition of *hospital* even though the nursing is not associated with active medical or surgical treatment.

For the purposes of the Mental Health Act 1959, the definition of *hospital* is much more restricted,[4] viz.:

  (a) any hospital vested in the Minister under the National Health Service Act 1977;
  (b) any accommodation provided by a local authority and used as a hospital by or on behalf of the Secretary of State under the National Health Service Act 1977;
  (c) any special hospital.[5]

---

[1] That such a defence would avail the patient were the claim for payment pursued in Court seems most unlikely unless the patient had been in any way misled.
[2] Formerly s. 79 of the 1946 Act.
[3] [1954] Ch. 530.
[4] S. 147 as amended.
[5] S. 147. *Special hospitals* in the Mental Health Act 1959 and in the N.H.S. Act 1977 means establishments provided and maintained by the Secretary of State for persons subject to detention under the Mental Health Act 1959 who in his opinion require treatment under conditions of special security on account of their dangerous, violent or criminal propensities (S. 4 of the 1977 Act formerly s. 40 of the N.H.S. Reorganisation Act 1973.)

This definition excludes all private institutions whether conducted for profit or not. Non-profit or charitable hospitals or institutions receiving mentally disordered patients for treatment are, for the purposes of the Nursing Homes Act 1975 relating to registration *etc.*, within the definition of *mental nursing home*, being premises used for the reception of and the provision of nursing or other medical treatment for one or more mentally disordered patients (whether exclusively or in common with other persons) not being (*a*) a hospital as defined in the 1959 Act;[1] (*b*) any other premises managed by a Government department or provided by a local authority.[2] Nevertheless, Part IV of that Act, in which are set out rules relating to the detention of mentally disordered persons in hospital, applies also to mental nursing homes, registered for the reception of patients liable to be detained, except where otherwise expressly provided.[3]

From what has been said it will be apparent that no one definition of *hospital* will suffice for all purposes. The broad definition in the opening paragraph can, therefore, do no more than serve as a pointer to the limits of the scope of this book. Hence, in so far as the law relating to them is different, residential homes are excluded, even though for disabled, mentally disordered or old persons and registerable under the National Assistance Act 1948.[4] It may, however, be observed that, broadly, apart from rules as to registration and inspection, there are no significant differences in law between hospitals and residential homes or between hospitals and nursing homes.

B. VOLUNTARY AND PUBLIC AUTHORITY HOSPITALS DISTINGUISHED

1. Voluntary Hospitals

For our present purpose, a voluntary hospital may conveniently be defined as a hospital not carried on for private gain and having the legal status of a charity, being supported — partly at least — out of endowments and voluntary contributions.

The charitable status of voluntary hospitals within that definition is founded on the spirit and intention of the now repealed preamble to the Statute of Elizabeth I,[5] now surviving only in the broad guiding principles laid down by Lord Macnaghten in his judgment in *Commissioners of Inland Revenue* v. *Pemsel*,[6] when he said — ' "Charity" in its

---

[1] S. 147 as amended.   [2] S. 14 (2).   [3] S. 59 (2), as amended.
[4] Ss. 37 to 40 as extended by s. 19 of the Mental Health Act 1959.
[5] 43 Eliz. I, c. 4. (Charities).
[6] [1891] A.C. at p. 583. In the Charities Act 1960 there is no attempt at a statutory definition of 'charity' or of 'charitable purpose', 'charity' being defined in s. 45 as 'any institution whether corporate or not established for charitable purposes . . .' and 'charitable purposes' as 'purposes which are exclusively charitable according to the law of England and Wales'. Hence *Pemsel's* case is still authoritative although based on a statute now repealed.

legal sense comprises four main divisions; trusts for the relief of poverty; trusts for the advancement of education; trusts for the advancement of religion; and trusts for other purposes beneficial to the community not falling under any of the preceding heads. The trusts last referred to are not the less charitable in the eye of the law because incidentally they benefit the rich as well as the poor . . . !' It must be appreciated, however, that the fourth head of Lord Macnaghten's definition does not embrace every object of public utility,[1] though it is now settled that it does include a hospital owned by the Secretary of State for the purposes of the National Health Service.[2]

The older voluntary hospitals which were founded exclusively for the relief of the sick poor are clearly charities within Lord Macnaghten's first division 'trusts for the relief of poverty'. That non-profit voluntary hospitals established later on the lines of the earlier ones, save that they had power to admit paying patients as well as the sick poor, were also charities was put beyond doubt with the passing of the Voluntary Hospitals (Paying Patients) Act 1936[3] which authorised the Charity Commissioners, by Order, to modify the trusts of any voluntary hospital not having power to admit paying patients to permit it to do so, such modification being subject to conditions giving assurance that the original objects of the charity are not thereby prejudiced. Since that time there has been no question but that a non-profit hospital providing care for rich and poor alike is a charity falling within the fourth of Lord Macnaghten's divisions of charity, *viz.*, 'trusts for other purposes beneficial to the community . . .' and it seems that, today, even a non-profit nursing home for paying patients will be accepted by the charity commissioners for registration as a charity under s. 4 of the Charities Act 1960, always providing its constitution is otherwise acceptable.[4] Furthermore, it has been held by the Court of Appeal in *re Adams, deceased; Gee and Another* v. *Barnet Group Hospital Management Committee*[5] that, *inter alia*, the endowment of beds for paying patients is a good charitable bequest. Hence it seems that, today, the broad test of whether a hospital is a charity is whether it is a non-profit institution for

---

[1] Benevolent objects are not necessary charitable. See further *Diplock's* case, discussed briefly on p. 73 *et seq.*
[2] *re Frere* (deceased) [1950] 2 All E.R. 513.
[3] See Chapter 6, p. 103.
[4] The Charity Commissioners have registered as a charity the Nuffield Nursing Homes Trust which itself provides or assists financially in providing non-profit nursing homes, mainly intended to meet the need for pay-bed accommodation for persons subscribing to provident associations, such as the British United Provident Association, as an 'insurance' against cost of treatment in a hospital or nursing home as a private patient. Such nursing homes would therefore fall within our broad definition of voluntary hospitals. Significantly, the B.U.P.A. played a major part, financially and otherwise, in floating the above Trust, and, it is understood continues to give it financial backing. The word *insurance* is in inverted commas because it is used only in a colloquial sense. Subscribers to a provident association do receive the benefits offered but not, strictly, on an insurance basis.
[5] [1968] Ch. 80; [1967] 3 All E.R. 285.

the relief of sickness — whether or not all the patients are able to pay full cost seems only marginally relevant, if at all.

Many of the voluntary hospitals in existence today — excluding non-profit nursing homes — are voluntary hospitals receiving mainly patients not able to pay full cost of treatment, which were disclaimed by the Minister of Health in 1948 under the provisions of ss. 6 and 7 of the National Health Service Act 1946. They are, in the main religious foundations, mostly Roman Catholic, the patients — except paying patients—being mostly admitted under contract with the health authority for the area which the hospital serves. The admission of patients under such contractual arrangements would not in itself have brought their status as charities into question. There might be instances in which the trusts of the charity have to be modified to permit it.

2. Public Authority Hospitals

A public authority hospital may be conveniently defined as one which is established or carried on directly by the Central government or by some other public authority. This definition includes national health service hospitals[1] as well as hospitals run by the military, naval or air force authorities and the special hospitals owned and administered by the Secretary of State for Social Services under s. 4 of the National Health Service Act 1977.[2] However, the hospitals administered by health authorities in England on behalf of the Secretary of State for Social Services and, in Wales (including Monmouthshire) on behalf of the Secretary of State for Wales[3] under the National Health Service Acts are administered by statutory corporations and it is accordingly convenient to reserve them for separate treatment. It may be mentioned at this point that the statutory corporations are charities.[4]

C. FUNCTIONAL CLASSIFICATION OF HOSPITALS

1. General and Special Hospitals Distinguished

In medical and hospital parlance, a general hospital is one where treatment of a substantial range of diseases and injuries is provided, but not necessarily for certain rare conditions such as leprosy or conditions requiring neuro-surgery. Deep X-ray therapy and radium treatment are also being restricted to hospitals properly equipped and

[1] The Radioactive Substances (Thorium X) Exemption (Amendment) Order[51] S.I, 1974 No. 500 provides (Reg. 2) 'A National Health Service hospital means a hospital with respect to the management and control thereof any functions are exercised by an Area Health Authority or a Board of Governors specified in an order made under s. 15 of the Reorganisation Act.
[2] Formerly s. 40 of the Reorganisation Act and s. 97 of the Mental Health Act 1959.
[3] See p. 13.
[4] See re Frere (deceased): Kidd and Another v. Farnham Group H.M.C. [1950] 2 All E.R. 513 and other cases mentioned at p. 82 et seq.

staffed for the purpose. A general hospital serving the needs of a particular area within the national health service is referred to as a district general hospital.

The expression *special hospital* is generally used as referring to (i) a hospital for treatment of patients suffering from a particular type of illness, *e.g.*, cancer, or from conditions requiring a particular range of treatment, *e.g.*, orthopædic hospitals; or (ii) a hospital for treatment of patients suffering from diseases of a particular organ or group of organs, *e.g.*, diseases of the eyes or chest or diseases peculiar to women; or (iii) a hospital for treatment of patients of a particular class, *e.g.*, children or women. Any particular special hospital may fall wholly or partly into one or more of these classes. Such having been for many years the accepted use of the term, it is somewhat unfortunate that for the purposes of the Mental Health Act 1959 and of the National Health Service Act 1977, an altogether different statutory meaning has been given it, *viz.*, 'an establishment provided by the Secretary of State for Social Services for persons subject to detention under the 1959 Act who, in his opinion, require treatment under conditions of special security on account of their dangerous, violent or criminal propensities'.[1]

Also it may be noted that a patient suffering from mental disorder,[2] even one liable to detention may be treated at *any* hospital — not necessarily a so-called psychiatric hospital — administered under the National Health Service Act 1977 which is willing to receive him. But any voluntary hospital, private hospital or private nursing home which receives a mentally disordered patient, whether the patient be liable to detention or not, must be registered as a mental nursing home under the provisions of the Mental Health Act 1959. Consequently, so far as the voluntary and private sectors are concerned, psychiatric hospitals or, to use the words of the Act, 'mental nursing homes' are still to be distinguished from other hospitals and nursing homes.[3]

2. Specialist and General Practitioner Staffed Hospitals

Possibly the distinction most likely to be of importance, especially in relation to the question of liability for injuries to patients, is between a hospital — whether general or special — where the treatment of patients is the immediate responsibility of specialists of consultant[4] rank and a small general hospital — sometimes called a cottage hospital — the regular staff of which consists of visiting local general practitioners but which may be visited either more or less regularly, or on request only, by specialists.

[1] Formerly N.H.S. Reorganisation Act 1973, s. 40 (1).
[2] For definition of mental disorder see s. 4 of the Mental Health Act 1959.
[3] For further information on the definition of hospitals and mental nursing homes under the Mental Health Act 1959, see pages 475–477.
[4] See p. 257 *et seq.* as to meaning of consultant.

3. Hospitals, Changes in User of

Whether there can be a change in the nature of the work carried on at a voluntary hospital depends on the terms of the trust and on whether that trust can, if necessary, be altered.[1] In the case of hospitals within the national health service there are other considerations and in 1949 the Minister of Health drew the attention of regional hospital boards[2] to the fact that any alteration of the user of hospitals under their control should only be made with due regard to the provisions of s. 6 (4) of the Act of 1946 and is also subject to his powers of direction. Under s. 6 (4), which substantially has been re-enacted as s. 88 of the N.H.S. Act 1977, he is bound in using hospitals transferred under the Act of 1946 'so far as practicable' to 'secure that the objects for which it was used immediately before the appointed day are not prejudiced by the provisions of this section' (*i.e.*, for transfer to the Minister). He cannot, therefore (states the circular quoted), ignore representations made to him by members of the public and the profession (*sic*, presumably the medical profession).

The circular then goes on to examine in detail the general questions involved in decision on changes in the user of hospitals and, presumably, therefore the considerations that will weigh with the Secretary of State in deciding whether to issue a directive to a health authority on the subject if appealed to by members of the public or of the medical profession. The circular continues 'The principal factors are, of course, (1) the possible loss of service to patients; (2) the disturbance of medical staff', and in the light of those 'principal factors' discusses the things to be taken into account in (*a*) changing over the use of the hospital from one specialty to another or from a special to a general hospital; (*b*) changing it from being a general practitioner (cottage) hospital to specialist hospital and (*c*) changes in method of staffing general practitioner maternity hospitals.

Whilst it must be agreed that it was appropriate for the attention of boards to be drawn to the provisions of s. 6 (4) and also to the kind of consideration that will influence the Secretary of State in giving directions to health authorities it may be suggested that the circular tends to confuse issues that are separate and distinct. There is almost more than a suggestion that 'the disturbance of medical staff' might amount to an infringement of the obligation 'so far as practicable' to 'secure that the objects for which any such property[3] was used immediately before the appointed day are not prejudiced'. This point of view seems completely

---

[1] See further pp. 67–68.

[2] Circular R. H. B. (49) 132. The Minister's views were somewhat modified — and expanded — in H.M. (58) 29, issued in the light of the decision in *Adams* v. *Maclay* (*The Secretary of State*) discussed below, p. 8. Regional hospital boards have now been abolished, and their functions taken over by health authorities constituted under N.H.S. Act 1977. See also HSC (15) 207.

[3] *i.e.*, a hospital and its contents transferred in 1948 under the N.H.S. Act 1946.

C

untenable in relation to what were charitable hospitals and suggests a vested interest of medical staff therein. The hospital was surely used for the treatment of patients, the method of staffing being wholly incidental to the attainment of that object. The circular sought to give the quite unjustifiable impression that 'the disturbance of medical staff' is a factor co-equal under s. 6 (4) with 'the possible loss of service to patients'.

A Scottish case, *Adams and others* v. *Maclay* (*Secretary of State*) *and the South Eastern Regional Hospital Board*,[1] turned on the meaning of the word *practicable* in s. 6 (4) of the National Health Service (Scotland) Act 1947, which sub-section is in terms substantially identical with those of s. 6 (4) the National Health Service Act 1946, and has brought seriously into question whether the Secretary of State has quite the freedom to deal with transferred hospitals that it had been thought that he had.

S. 6 (4) of the Act of 1946 read:

'All property transferred to the Minister under this section shall vest in him free of any trust existing immediately before the appointed day,[2] and the Minister may use any such property for the purpose of any of his functions under this Act, but shall so far as practicable secure that the objects for which any such property was used immediately before the appointed day are not prejudiced by the provisions of this section.'

The corresponding sub-section of the Scottish Act differs from the above only by the substitution of 'Secretary of State' for 'Minister' and of 'exercise of the power hereby conferred' for 'provisions of this section'.

The circumstances of the case were that the Bruntsfield and Elsie Inglis Hospitals had been founded for the treatment of women and children by women medical practitioners and that on the retirement of a woman consultant some years after the hospitals had been transferred, the regional board proposed to throw open the appointment to men as well as to women. Although the board of management of the hospitals had objected the Secretary of State had declined to intervene. Thereupon ten women raised an action, in effect seeking a declaration that by virtue of the latter part of s. 6 (4) of the Scottish Act the appointment should be restricted to women.

Lord Walker, giving judgment in favour of the pursuers, held that under s. 6 (4) it was the duty of the Secretary of State to secure, if practicable, the continued use of the hospitals for the objects for which they had been used before the appointed day. He did not consider it possible to determine by hearing evidence whether the appointment of a woman consultant was or was not practicable. He therefore ordered that it was the duty of the Secretary of State to secure that a male medical practitioner be not appointed consulting physician at the two

[1] [1958] S. C. 279.   [2] 'appointed day' here means 5th July 1948.

hospitals unless and until, after the advertisement of the post as being open to women medical practitioners only, it should appear that no women suitable for appointment had applied. He also interdicted the regional board from appointing a male medical practitioner to the post.

It seems clear from the judgment that, in Scotland, if a transferred hospital *can* be used for the objects for which it was used immediately before the appointed day,[1] it must be. In other words 'practicable' is equated with 'possible'. And it is difficult to avoid the conclusion that in England and Wales, under s. 88 of the Act of 1977 the law is the same, the more particularly as in *re Hayes' Will Trusts*[2] an English court had already, though not on the interpretation of the National Health Service Act, 1946, decided that 'impracticable' meant 'not able to be done'.

All that can be said on the other side is that as the Scottish decision is not binding on English courts, an English court might — in different circumstances — be disposed to apply s. 88 more liberally and to be satisfied if the objects for which the property had been being used immediately before the appointed day were in fact being satisfactorily provided at another hospital reasonably available to the patients for whose benefit the charity had been established. There are so many possibilities that to say more than that would be idle speculation. It will, however, be appreciated that the Scottish case has raised very serious issues as, presumably, the use to which the Secretary of State may put any former voluntary hospital can seemingly be challenged in the courts at any length of time after its being taken over on 5th July, 1948.[3]

There were two other points from Lord Walker's judgment in the *Bruntsfield and Elsie Inglis Hospitals* case which might be of great persuasive force in an English Court. First, the objects for which the property must be used 'if practicable' are those for which it was used immediately before the appointed day, not those for which it might have been used under the trust deed, if any. Indeed, a strict interpretation of s. 88 of the 1977 Act or the Scottish Act suggests that the objects within the protection of the 'if practicable' requirement, are those for which the property was used immediately before the appointed day, even though so used in contravention of the terms of an express trust.

The other point was that the duty of complying with the requirement that the property be used as far as practicable for the pre-appointed day objects fell on the Secretary of State who was, therefore, properly made a co-defendant. Seemingly, under the 1946 Act, the Secretary of State for Social Services or the Secretary of State for Wales would likewise be a co-defendant.

[1] See footnote 2, previous page.
[2] See p. 84.
[3] There is no statutory restriction on change of user of any voluntary hospital which might be taken over by the Minister otherwise than under s. 88 of the Act of 1977.

After the decision in the Scottish case the Minister of Health issued fresh instructions to hospital authorities on the procedure to be adopted when it is proposed to close or change the use of a hospital, the new procedure being designed to take particular account of the duty to secure as far as practicable that the objects for which a hospital was used immediately before transfer in 1948 are not prejudiced by the change.[1]

[1] Circular H.M. (58) 29.

CHAPTER 2

STATE HOSPITALS

STATE hospitals are to be broadly divided into two classes: (i) those controlled directly by a department of State such as special hospitals under s. 4(1) of the National Health Service Act 1977,[1] owned by the Secretary of State for Social Servies[2] and administered directly by his department and also naval, military and air force hospials and prison hospitals administered by other Government departments and (ii) hospitals owned by the Secretary of State[2] under the National Health Service Act 1977 and administered on his behalf by one of the corporate health authorities established under the National Health Service Act 1977. These two classes must be treated separately not only on grounds of convenience but because the legal liabilities of the Secretary of State and of officials and the rules regarding proceedings in respect of the two classes still differ.

In this chapter we shall confine our attention to those hospitals controlled directly by the central government, leaving hospitals administered by statutory authorities established under the 1977 Act for treatment in the next chapter.

Detailed consideration of the nature and extent of the liability of the Crown, or of Ministers and of subordinate officers, whether for their own acts or the acts of others, in respect of the administration of directly controlled State hospitals is rather beyond the scope of this work, being but an application of the general principles of constitutional law, coupled with particular relevant statutes, e.g., the Army Act as to rights and duties in respect of military hospitals. It must be observed, however, that by virtue of the Crown Proceedings Act 1947, the Crown is not generally immune from liability in tort in respect of loss or damage suffered by a subject as a result of the wrongful act or omission of a public servant or other agent of the Crown. Generally speaking, as a result of the passing of that Act, anyone injured in person, property or reputation by a servant of the Crown will have the same recourse against the Crown as against any other principal or employer in like circumstances. But there are certain exceptions, the most important for our present purpose being injury suffered by a person in the armed forces of the Crown caused by some other person also so serving and certified by the Secretary of State for Social Services to have been treated or which will be treated as attributable to service for the pur-

[1] See p. 476.   [2] See p. 2.

poses of entitlement under the Royal Warrant, Order in Council or order relating to the disablement or death of members of the force of which he is a member.[1] And where this exception operates the member of the forces causing the injury is exempt from personal liability in tort unless the Court is satisfied that the act or omission was not connected with his duties as a member of those forces.[2] Unless the certificate as to entitlement under Royal Warrant, etc., is given by the Secretary of State the Crown is liable to an action in tort even by a member of the armed forces when the circumstances justify.

It follows from what has been said that:

(a) The Crown will not ordinarily be liable in tort for injury done to a member of the Navy, Army or Air Force at a service hospital by reason of the negligence or incompetence of another person in the forces of the Crown (e.g., a doctor or a ward orderly in the R.A.M.C.). And as the definition of armed forces is apt to include the women's nursing and auxiliary services under control of service departments[2] the Crown immunity will extend to members of such women's services. In the cases here dealt with the person responsible for the injury would also be exempt from liability in tort within the limits already indicated.

(b) If a service patient in a service hospital is injured by someone who is a servant or agent of the Crown but not a member of the armed forces (e.g., a civilian doctor or nurse) within the extended meaning of armed forces in s. 38 (5) of the Act, in circumstances which would give rise to a claim in tort against a private individual then, seemingly, the injured person will have a claim in tort both against the Crown and against the tortfeasor.

(c) If a person were injured whilst a patient in a hospital administered by the Secretary of State,[3] if he were then still technically in the armed forces of the Crown and the person causing his injury was likewise in the forces — a most unlikely state of affairs in time of peace — the position would be as in (a) supra. Otherwise the rules as to vicarious liability in tort would be the same as in respect of any other employer and employee or principal and agent.

Subject to what has been said in respect of persons in the armed forces, to prerogative powers[4] and to statutory exceptions, whether under the Crown Proceedings Act 1947, or otherwise, superior civil servants will seemingly be responsible in law for the acts and omissions of their subordinates in like manner and to the like extent as if they were superior and subordinate in the service of a private employer. That is, they will, in effect, be liable only for such wrongful acts and omissions of their subordinates as they have expressly authorised.

---

[1] Crown Proceedings Act 1947, s. 10.
[3] See p. 4.
[2] Crown Proceedings Act 1947, s. 38 (5).
[4] Crown Proceedings Act 1947, s. 11.

CHAPTER 3

HOSPITALS ADMINISTERED UNDER THE
NATIONAL HEALTH SERVICE ACT 1977

A. OUTLINE OF ADMINISTRATIVE PATTERN OF
THE NATIONAL HEALTH SERVICE
(With Special Reference to Hospitals)

1. Introductory

THE intention of the National Health Service Act 1977 is to maintain
the establishment in England and Wales of a comprehensive health
service available to all in need of hospital, specialist or general practitioner or dental or optical services or of those public health services
such as maternity and child welfare clinics, midwifery, health visitors or
home nursing formerly sometimes provided by local authorities. The
services provided are free of any charge[1] either to the patients or to their
relatives except in respect of private or part-paying hospital patients as
noted elsewhere; in respect — with certain exceptions — of supply of
dentures, glasses and other appliances and drugs; in respect of maintenance of in-patients engaged in remunerative employment during the
day; in respect (should the Secretary of State by regulation prescribe,
as he has not so far done) of treatment of persons not ordinarily resident
in Great Britain; in respect of dental treatment under Part II of the Act.

The 1946 Act established the basis of the scheme. It came into force,
for all practical purposes, on 5th July 1948. The National Health Service
Reorganisation Act 1973 made considerable modifications to the administration of the health service. In particular under the old arrangements, although the Minister (and later the Secretary of State[1]) was
responsible for both the hospital service and general medical, ophthalmic and dental services they were administered by separate agencies. So
also local authorities had a considerable jurisdiction in the health field.
The 1973 Act has abolished this last and with it brought the other health
services under the same administrative regime. The 1977 Act has consolidated the bulk of the legislation into one statute. Administrative problems may still arise at the boundary of health and social services.

The duty of the Secretary of State[2] in respect of the provision of

[1] See 1977 Act s. 1 (2).
[2] By the Secretary of State for Social Services Order S.I 1968 No. 729, the functions of
the Minister of Health under the National Health Services Acts 1946 to 1968 became the
responsibility of the Secretary of State. Under the Transfer of Functions (Wales) Order
S.I. 1969 No. 358 the functions of the Secretary of State for the Social Services under the

health services is now laid down in s. 1 (1) of the National Health Service Act 1977 which reads:

'1 (1) It is the Secretary of State's duty to continue the promotion in England and Wales of a comprehensive health service designed to secure improvement:

(a) in the physical and mental health of the people of England and Wales and

(b) in the prevention, diagnosis and treatment of illness,

and for that purpose to provide or secure the effective provision of services in accordance with this Act.'

S. 1 (1) of the Act of 1977 must be read with sections 2, 3, and 4. S. 2, which relates to the general powers and duties of the Secretary of State in respect of the National Health Service says:

2 (1) Without prejudice to his powers apart from this sub-section, the Secretary of State shall have power:

(a) to provide such services as he considers appropriate for the purpose of discharging any duty imposed on him by this Act; and

(b) to do any other thing whatsoever which is calculated to facilitate, or is conducive or incidental to, the discharge of such a duty.

This section is subject to section 3 (3) below.

Section 3 says

3 (1) It is the Secretary of State's duty to provide throughout England and Wales, to such extent as he considers necessary to meet all reasonable requirements:

(a) hospital accommodation;

(b) other accommodation for the purposes of any service provided under this Act;

(c) medical, dental, nursing and ambulance services;

(d) such other facilities for the care of expectant and nursing mothers and young children as he considers are appropriate as part of the health service[1];

(e) such facilities for the prevention of illness, the care of persons suffering from illness and the after-care of persons who have suffered from illness as he considers are appropriate as part of the health service.

(f) such other services as are required for the diagnosis and treatment of illness.

(2) Where any hospital provided by the Secretary of State in accordance with this Act was a voluntary hospital transferred by virtue of the National Health Service Act 1946, and —

(a) the character and associations of that hospital before its transfer were such as to link it with a particular religious denomination, then

above-mentioned Acts in respect of Wales, including Monmouthshire, passed to the Secretary of State for Wales. When used in this book in relation to functions under the National Health Service Act 1977 the expression Secretary of State must be read accordingly. Functions under the Mental Health Act 1959 in respect of Wales were not transferred to the Secretary of State for Wales.

[1] See s. 21 and Schedule 8 on distribution of these functions between the Secretary of State and the local Social Services authority.

(*b*) regard shall be had in the general administration of the hospital to the preservation of that character and those associations.

(3) Nothing in section 2 above or in this section affects the provisions of Part II of this Act (which relates to arrangements with practitioners for the provision of medical, dental, ophthalmic and pharmaceutical services).

Section 5(1) confers on the Secretary of State powers and duties in respect of the provision of medical and dental inspection and the treatment of pupils in schools and establishments of further education maintained by local education authorities or receiving primary or secondary education otherwise than at a school or in a non-maintained school. Under s. 5(2) he has the duty of providing a family planning service and supplying contraceptive substances and appliances to the extent which in his opinion it is necessary to meet all reasonable requirements and may make charges for substances and appliances so supplied.

In substance, the effect of the 1973 Act, which came fully into force on 1st April 1974 was to impose upon the Secretary of State the duties formerly carried out by regional hospital boards, boards of governors of teaching hospitals and hospital management committees, as well as those of former local health authorities[1] and to provide for the discharge of those functions on his behalf and subject to his directions by Regional and Area Health Authorities and by Area Health Authorities (Teaching).[2] Special hospitals for persons subject to detention under the Mental Health Act 1959 who in his opinion require treatment under conditions of special security on account of their dangerous, violent or criminal propensities are still administered directly by the Secretary of State.[3] Exceptionally, the twelve London postgraduate teaching hospitals named in Schedule 2 of the Act continue as yet to be administered by Boards of Governors appointed in accordance with the provisions of the 1946 Act.[4] Their Boards of Governors are known as 'preserved Boards'.

2. The Constitutional Position of Health Authorities

The provisions relating to the administration of health and hospital services provided by the Secretary of State under the National Health Service Act 1977 (at least so far as they relate to hospital activities) are set out below. Since all the authorities so constituted are administering a Crown service it seems that they are not bound by any statutory

[1] S. 2 (2) and (3) of the 1973 Act.
[2] Ss. 5–7. Now ss. 8 and 9 of the 1977 Act.
[3] As to the administration of *special hospitals* under s. 4 of the 1977 Act, replacing s. 97 of the Mental Health Act 1959, and s. 40 of the 1973 Act.
[4] N.H.S. (Preserved Boards of Governors) Order S.I. 1974 No. 281 made under s. 15 of the 1973 Act. This section is not repealed by the 1977 Act. Unless revoked earlier the Order expires at the expiration of five years beginning with the date at which it was made, 22nd February 1974.

provision which does not bind the Crown[1] unless by necessary implication or expressly by the terms of the statute they are. It is to be noted, however, that a number of Statutes which the Secretary of State has not regarded as legally binding on health and hospital authorities, have been substantially applied by administrative action.

3. Effect of National Health Service Reorganisation Act 1973 on the Administration of Hospitals

On 1st April 1974, the main appointed day for the purposes of the Reorganisation Act 1973, the responsibility for the administration of virtually the whole of the hospital and specialist services, until then provided on behalf of the Secretary of State by boards and committees established under the provisions of the 1946 Act, became the responsibility of the Secretary of State.[2] However, by delegation by him, they are to be carried on by Regional Health Authorities, Area Health Authorities and Area Health Authorities (Teaching) constituted under ss. 8 and 9 of the 1977 Act.[3] Similarly, these same Authorities are, again by delegation, responsible for the administration of those health services which were formerly the responsibility of local health authorities, unless any such services were transferred to a local authority social services committee under s. 2 of the Local Authority Social Services Act 1970. The responsibility for social services to hospital patients, such as has in the past been undertaken by medical social workers employed by hospital boards and committees, is now likewise the responsibility of the appropriate local authority under the 1970 Act, though medical social workers and others concerned may still be carrying out their duties at hospitals.[4]

It is now necessary to consider in greater detail the constitution and functions of Regional and Area Health Authorities under the 1977 Act, particularly in respect of hospital and closely related services. Later in this Chapter, so far as is relevant to our central topic — the hospital service — other matters are touched upon, e.g. the constitution and functions of certain other bodies constituted under the 1977 Act, e.g. Community Health Councils[5] and local professional advisory committees.[6] Since this book is concerned with the Law, it does not discuss the administrative flesh that covers the legal bones of the reorganised health

---

[1] *Pfizer Corporation* v. *Minister of Health* [1965] A.C. 512; *Hills (Patents) Ltd.* v. *University College Hospital* [1956] 1 Q.B. 90; and, *Wood* v. *Leeds A.H.A.(T)* [1974] I. C.R. 535. This view is taken throughout this book, and for convenience it is repeated elsewhere as appropriate.

[2] S. 2. By the Isles of Scilly (N.H.S.) Order S.I. 1973 No. 1935 the reorganisation is applied to the Isles of Scilly. The local authority is the Council of the Isles.

[3] And see generally the National Health Service Functions (Directions to Authorities) Regulations, S.I. No. 1974 No. 24 and circular HRC (74) 18.

[4] As to transferred hospital social workers, see s. 18 (5) of the 1973 Act.

[5] S. 20 and Schedule 7. Formerly s. 9 of the 1973 Act

[6] S. 19 and Schedule 6. Formerly s. 8 of the 1973 Act.

service. Thus maybe somewhat surprisingly no mention is made of the functions of the health districts, nor the organization of the management teams.[1]

B. EXECUTIVE BODIES

1. Regional Health Authorities

(a) Introductory

A Regional Health Authority appointed by the Secretary of State under the provisions of s. 8 and Part I of Schedule 5 of the 1977 Act is a body corporate with perpetual succession and a common seal.[2] Paragraph 1(2) of Part I of the Schedule imposes on the Secretary of State the duty of consulting with bodies there named when appointing members: he is not, however, bound by the advice he receives.[3]

The regions for which Regional Health Authorities are established are determined by the Secretary of State in the N.H.S. (Determination of Regions) Order 1973[4] and the names of the authorities in the N.H.S. (Constitution of Regional Health Authorities) Order 1975.[5] No specific numbers of members are now laid down by statute or statutory instrument.[6] The regions covered by the Regional Health Authorities broadly correspond to those which formerly were covered by the Regional Hospital Boards. Dealt with in the N.H.S. (Regional and Area Health Authorities: Membership and Procedure) Regulations 1973[7] as amended by the N.H.S. (Health Authorities: Membership) Regulations 1977[8] are: the term of office of members (Reg. 3 1977 Regs.[9]); variation of membership of authorities (Reg. 4 of 1977 Regs.); eligibility for reappointment (Reg. 6 of 1977 Regs.); disqualification (Regs. 8 and 9 of 1977 Regs.); termination of membership (Reg. 5 of 1977 Regs.). The rest of the 1973 regulations are unamended and relate to constitution and proceedings — election of vice-chairman (Reg. 10); appointment of committees and sub-committees (Reg. 11). Arrangements for exercise of functions is dealt with in Reg. 12 which, subject to restrictions and conditions, allows delegation not only to a committee or sub-committee appointed under

---

[1] The *district* is the 'basic operational unit of the integrated health service' HRC (73) 3.

[2] S. 8 and Schedule 5 Part III. Formerly 1973 Act s. 5 and Schedule 1, Part III.

[3] Under the N.H.S. (Health Authorities: Membership) Regs. S.I. 1975 No. 1101 certain appointments could be made without consultation between the 1st August 1975 and 1st July 1976. Reg. 2. The effect is now spent.

[4] S.I. 1973 No. 1191 as amended by the Isles of Scilly (N.H.S. Administration) S.I. 1973 No. 2192 (which affects Cornwall and the Isles of Scilly) and as further amended by N.H.S. (Constitution of Regional Health Authorities) Order S.I. 1975 No. 1100.

[5] S.I. 1975 No. 1100.

[6] S.I. 1975 No. 1100 having revoked the earlier S.I. 1973 No. 1192 of the same name.

[7] S.I. 1973 No. 1286. HRC (73) 24 suggests that members of the R.H.A. should not also be members of an A.H.A. in the region.

[8] S.I. 1977 No. 1103 replacing S.I. 1975 No. 1101 which they also revoke.

[9] Transitional provisions are contained in the Schedules to the 1977 Regs.

Reg. 11 but also to an officer.[1] Exercise of functions by one Regional Health Authority on behalf of another, is provided for in the N.H.S. Functions (Administration Arrangements) Regulations 1974.[2] Reg. 13 of the Membership and Procedure Regulations requires that meetings be conducted in accordance with the rules set out in the schedule to the regulations and of standing orders made in accordance with that regulation. Disability of members in proceedings on account of pecuniary interests is the subject of Reg. 14.

(b) Admission of Press and Public to Meetings

Regional (and Area Health) Authorities are public bodies to which the provisions of the Public Bodies (Admission to Meetings) Act 1960 apply. The effect of the Act was summarised in a departmental circular to regional hospital boards, a copy of that summary having since been made available to Regional (and Area Health) Authorities under cover of a later circular.[3] It reads as follows:

4. Subject to what is said below, any meeting of a *Board* will be open to the public and if during a meeting the *Board* resolves itself into committee, the proceedings in committee will be treated as if they were proceedings of the *Board* (s. 1 (1) and 1 (6)).

5. The *Board* may by resolution exclude the public from the whole or part of a meeting "whenever publicity would be prejudicial to the public interest by reason of the confidential nature of the business to be transacted, or for other special reasons stated in the resolution and arising from the nature of that business or of proceedings"; and these special reasons may include "the need to receive or consider recommendations or advice from sources other than members, committees or sub-committees" of the *Board* "without regard to the subject or purport of the recommendations or advice" (s.1 (2) and 1 (3)).

6. Where a meeting is required by the Act to be open to the public in whole or in part, the *Board* has a duty under s. 1 (4):

(a) to give public notice of the time and place of the meeting by posting it at the *Board's* offices at least three clear days before the meeting or, if the meeting is convened at shorter notice, then at the time it is convened;

(b) to supply, on request and on payment of postage or other necessary charge for transmission, for the benefit of any newspaper, a copy of the agenda as supplied to members of the *Board* but excluding, if thought fit, any item during which the meeting is likely not to be open to the public), together with such further statements or particulars, if any, as are necessary to indicate the nature of the items included or, if thought fit, copies of any reports or other documents supplied to *Board* members.

---

[1] The intention of the Secretary of State concerning the nature and extent of delegation to officers and also, in general terms, the functions to be performed by health authorities and, on their behalf, by chairman or other member or members is set out in a departmental circular HRC (73) 22, Appendix I.

[2] S.I. 1974 No. 36. Reg. 3. See p. 688.

[3] Appendix II of HRC(73)22 quoting from HM(61)59.

(In so far as the supply of this material to the Press or to a member of the public is "publication" of any defamatory matter contained therein, then that publication is privileged, unless it is proved to be made with malice — s. 1 (5).)

(c) to afford so far as practicable to accredited representatives of newspapers, attending for the purpose of reporting the proceedings for those newspapers, reasonable facilities for taking their report and, unless the meeting is held in premises not belonging to the *Board* or not on the telephone, for telephoning the report at their own expense.

7. The above references to a newspaper apply also to a news agency whether it serves the Press or the broadcasting services. But the *Board* is not required to permit the taking of photographs of any proceedings, or the making of a visual or aural broadcast or recording, or the making of a running commentary (s. 1 (7)).

8. The above provisions are without prejudice to the *Board's* power of exclusion to suppress or prevent disorderly conduct or other misbehaviour at a meeting (s. 1 (8)).[1]

In *R.* v. *Liverpool City Council ex. p. Liverpool Taxi Fleet Operators Association*[2] it was held that there must be reasonable but not unlimited accommodation for members of the public.

(c) Functions of Regional Health Authorities

The functions of Regional Health Authorities are imposed on them by the National Health Service Functions (Directions to Authorities) Regulations 1974,[3] wherein those authorities are directed to carry out on behalf of the Secretary of State specific functions[4] under particular sections of the National Health Service Act 1977, subject to such restrictions and limitations as are laid down in the Regulations.[5] In general terms, the effect of the Regulations is to delegate to each Regional Authority in respect of its own region all the powers and duties of the former regional hospital boards, boards of governors and hospital management committees and of the former local health authorities. But this all over delegation is coupled with a direction to the Regional Health Authorities themselves by direction to delegate almost all those same functions to Area Health Authorities,[6] also subject to certain restrictions.[7]

It would be wrong to draw the conclusion from what has been said that a Regional Health Authority is no more than a conduit pipe for transmitting functions from the Secretary of State to Area Health Authorities since subject to the guidance and directions of the Secretary of

---

[1] In the above extract from HM(61)59 for 'Board' should now be read *Regional or Area Area Health Authority*. The provisions of the Public Bodies (Admission to Meetings) are also applicable to special health authorities, *e.g.* the Prescription Pricing Authority, the Welsh Health Technical Services Organisation, and Community Health Councils (HRC(74)4).

[2] [1975] 1 W.L.R. 701; [1975] 1 All E.R. 379.

[3] S.I. 1974 No. 24 made under s. 7 of the 1973 Act. Now see s. 13 of the 1977 Act.

[4] Reg. 3.   [5] Reg. 4.   [6] Reg. 5.   [7] Regs. 5 and 6.

State, it is responsible for policy, planning and allocation of resources in its region. It also has supervisory functions. Its intended role was indicated in general terms in the White Paper on National Health Service Reorganisation[1] in a passage which, since the 1973 Act was passed, has been brought to the notice of Health Authorities for their guidance in a departmental circular.[2] It reads as follows:

2.27. The RHA has to delegate major executive responsibilities to its AHAs and to its Regional officers (for Regionally-deployed services), and focus the limited time of its Members on the important issues of policy, planning and resource allocation. The Authority can, therefore, be expected to review proposals on policies and priorities submitted to it by AHAs and by the RTO and decide on Regional policies and priorities within the framework of national policy. The Authority will establish planning guidelines for AHAs on priorities and available resources. Subsequently, it will review objectives, plans and budgets submitted to it annually by AHAs and by the RTO (for Regional services), resolve competing claims for resources between AHAs and agree targets with AHAs against which their performance can be assessed. In making planning decisions the Authority will call upon the advice of the Regional advisory committees.

2.28 In addition the RHA must control the performance of its AHAs and its Regional officers. To do so it will receive reports on AHA performance from each AHA, ensure that progress is according to plan and that services are being provided throughout the Region with efficiency and economy, challenge the performance of AHAs if necessary and ensure that appropriate remedial action is taken. It will also receive performance reports on Regionally-deployed services from its principal Regional officers. RHA Members, and the RHA Chairman in particular, will be expected to meet individual AHA Chairmen regularly to discuss the problems and opportunities of their Areas. The Authority will be responsible for appointing AHA Members [with exceptions noted], and for appointing consultants and senior medical staff, with the exception of those employed by AHA(T)s.

2.29. A further important responsibility of the RHA will be to assist the Secretary of State to establish realistic national policies and priorities by providing him with information and advice on developments in the field. Thus RHA Chairmen will be expected to meet regularly with the Secretary of State and with senior officers of the DHSS.

(d) *Wales*

In Wales, there is no regional health authority and the functions of the regional authorities are left with the Secretary of State. In order, however, that he may have assistance the Welsh Health Technical Services Organisation has been established.[3] This organisation is given extra powers relating to (a) capital works, the procurement of supplies and the provision of computer services; (b) the checking and passing

[1] Cmnd. 5055.
[2] HRC(73)22 — 'Membership and Procedure of Regional and Area Health Authorities'. In the same appendix there is also a passage summarising the role of the Area Health Authorities.
[3] Welsh Health Technical Services Organisation (Establishment and Constitution) Order S.I. 1973 No. 1624 made under s. 5 (6) of the Act. Now see s. 11 of the 1977 Act.

of prescriptions for drugs, medicines and appliances supplied as pharmaceutical services on behalf of Family Practitioner Committees and (c) some other functions to be performed on behalf of himself, an Area Health Authority or a Family Practitioner Committee.[1] Provision is made for: the appointment of the chairman and members and the election of a vice-chairman;[2] the term of office of members and disqualification and termination of membership;[3] the appointment of committees and sub-committees, the arrangements for the exercise of its functions and the conduct of its proceedings;[4] the disability of members on account of a pecuniary interest;[5] and the appointment, functions and procedure of the Welsh Pricing Committee.[6]

2. Area Health Authorities

(a) Introductory

By sections 8 and 9 of the National Health Service Act 1977[7] Area Health Authorities constituted in accordance with the provisions of paragraphs 2 to 5 of Schedule 5 of the Act have been formed to cover in aggregate the whole of England and Wales.[8] Every such authority is a body corporate with perpetual succession and a common seal.[9]

S. 9 (1) provides that where the Secretary of State is satisfied that an area authority is to provide for a university or universities substantial facilities for undergraduate or postgraduate clinical teaching he may by order add the word *Teaching* in brackets after its name. He was allowed to do so in the original orders establishing the Area Health Authorities and the sub-section maintains a reserve power for him to add the word *Teaching* in brackets to the Area Authority if he is satisfied the facilities are provided or conversely for him to remove the word from Area Health Authority (Teaching) if they cease to be provided. S. 9 (3) goes on to provide that before the Secretary of State makes either of such orders he shall consult with the university or universities in question.

For the sake of both clarity and simplicity, in this book s. 8 (1) is followed since it provides that normally references to an Area Health Authority include references to an Area Health Authority (Teaching).

The areas for which Area Health Authorities are constituted are set out in the N.H.S. (Determination of Areas) Order 1973 and the N.H.S. (Constitution of Area Health Authorities) Order[10] 1975 and their con-

---

[1] Art. 3. [2] Arts. 4 and 8. [3] Arts. 5–7.
[4] Arts. 9–11, 14. [5] Art. 12. [6] Art. 13.
[7] Formerly ss. 5 and 6 of the 1973 Act.
[8] N.H.S. (Determination of Areas) Order S.I. 1973 No. 1275 as amended by Isles of Scilly (N.H.S. Administration) Order S.I. 1973 No. 2192. Now see N.H.S. (Constitution of AHAs) Order S.I. 1975 No. 1099.
[9] 1977 Act, Sched. 5, para. 8.
[10] S.I. 1973 No. 1275 and S.I. 1975 No. 1099.

stitution in the Constitution Order of 1975.[1] By the last-mentioned order each Authority is given a name broadly indicative of the location for which it is to be responsible. The Order also determines the total number of members of each Authority, the number of members to be appointed thereto on the nomination of named universities and by local authorities as well as, in the case of Area Health Authorities (Teaching), the number of additional members under paragraph 4 of Schedule 5 of the Act.[2] The following matters are subject to the provisions of the N.H.S. (Regional and Area Health Authorities: Membership and Procedure) Regulations 1973[3] as amended by N.H.S. (Health Authorities: Membership) Regulations 1977[4]: term of office of members; variation of membership of authorities; eligibility of members for re-appointment; disqualification for membership; termination of membership; election of vice-chairman;[5] appointment of committees and sub-committees;[6] arrangements for exercising functions;[7] meetings and proceedings;[8] disability of members in proceedings on account of pecuniary interest, direct or indirect, including interest of spouse;[9] rules as to meetings.[10]

(b) Functions of Area Health Authorities

The functions of Area Health Authorities are, in effect, broadly those of the former hospital management committees coupled with those of the former local health authorities under the National Health Service Acts 1946 to 1968. In the case of Area Health Authorities (Teaching) the correspondence is with the functions of the former Boards of Governors or, in some cases, those of university hospital management committees together with those of local health authorities under the above Acts. Additional functions were given under the 1973 Act, e.g. in relation to the giving of advice on contraception and the supply of contraceptive substances and appliances.[11] The Area Health Authorities are therefore in law the main operational units within the re-organised health service. The functions have been imposed on Area Health Authorities in England by directions given by the Regional Health Authorities to the Area Health Authorities in their regions in accordance with the direction given to them by the Secretary of State in the National Health Service Functions (Directions to Authorities) Regulations 1974[12] and their

---

[1] S.I. 1975 No. 1099. This revokes the S.I. 1973 No. 1305 of the same name and its amendment orders.

[2] See p. 618.   [3] S.I. 1973 No. 1286.   [4] S.I. 1977 No. 1103.

[5] Reg. 10 of the 1973 Regs.   [6] Reg. 11.

[7] Reg. 12 covers delegation to committees and to officers. As to exercise of functions by one Regional Health Authority or one Area Health Authority on behalf of another, or by an officer of an Authority on behalf of another Authority, reference should be made to the N.H.S. Functions (Administration Arrangements) Regulations S.I. 1974 No. 36. As to Family Practitioner Committees see Section F of this chapter.

[8] Reg. 13.   [9] Reg. 14.

[10] Reg. 13(1) and Schedule.

[11] Now 1977 Act s. 5(1) (a). 1973 Act, s. 4.   [12] S.I. 1974 No. 24. For text, see p. 678.

exercise is subject to certain express restrictions,[1] besides being subject to any directions which might from time to time be given by the Secretary of State or by the Regional Health Authority.[2]

There being no Regional Health Authority in Wales, delegation of functions to Welsh Area Health Authorities is by direction from the Secretary of State for Wales.[3]

3. Preserved Boards of Governors —
London Postgraduate Teaching Hospitals

The effect of the N.H.S. (Preservation of Boards of Governors) Order 1974,[4] made by the Secretary of State in exercise of the power conferred on him in s. 15 of the 1973 Act is to preserve to Boards of Governors of the twelve London postgraduate teaching hospitals,[5] *viz.* the Hospitals for Sick Children;[6] the National Hospitals for Nervous Diseases;[6] the Royal National Ear Nose and Throat Hospital; the Moorfields Eye Hospital, the Bethlem Royal Hospital and the Maudsley Hospital;[6] St. John's Hospital for Diseases of the Skin; the Royal National Orthopaedic Hospitals;[6] the National Heart and Chest Hospitals;[6] St. Peter's Hospitals;[6] the Royal Marsden Hospital; Queen Charlotte's Hospital for Women; and the Eastman Dental Hospital. They are therefore still administered by Boards of Governors constituted in accordance with Part III of Schedule 3 of the National Health Service Act 1946, save that governors who, under Part III, would have been appointed by the regional board for the region in which the hospital is situated are now appointed by the Regional Health Authority for the region.[7] The Order, which was made on 22nd February 1974 came into operation on 31st March 1974 and, unless previously revoked, is operative until 21st February 1979 (i.e. for five years from the date on which it was made).[8] It keeps in effect, as relating to the preserved Boards only,

---

[1] Reg. 6.   [2] Reg. 5 (1).

[3] Reg. 7 and, as to restrictions on exercise of functions, Reg. 8.   [4] S.I. 1974 No. 281.

[5] Under s. 11 (8) of the 1946 Act, which is still operative in respect of preserved Boards only, teaching hospitals are hospitals or groups of hospitals so designated by the Secretary of State after consultation with the university or universities concerned, being hospitals which appear to him to provide any university facilities for postgraduate clinical teaching. Other teaching hospitals are now managed by Area Health Authorities (Teaching).

[6] It is not beyond doubt whether the two named hospitals are in law two separate institutions under a single board of governors or, notionally and more likely, one hospital. In *Re Bawden's Settlement* ([1954] 1 W.L.R. 33; [1953] 2 All E.R. 1235) as to which see further p. 99 in so far as it concerned gifts to teaching hospitals was decided on the footing that, under the N.H.S. (Designation of Teaching Hospitals (No. 2)) Order 1948, all institutions under a single Board of Governors had become a single hospital. It does not, however, follow that by a different form of order the Secretary of State could not preserve or revive the identity of two or more teaching hospitals administered by the same preserved board.

[7] See N.H.S. (Designation of London Teaching Hospitals) Amendment Order 1974 No. 341 amending S.I. 1974 No. 32.

[8] Art. 1(2). No order under s. 15 may be made for any longer period than five years from the date it was made: but before the expiry of any such order another may be made securing that a preserved Board continues for a further period (s. 15 (2)).

repealed sections of the National Health Service Acts 1946 to 1968 as to the powers, constitution, legal status of Boards of Governors of teaching hospitals and such like matters, as well as sections 7 (1), (2), (3), (7), (8) (*a*), (9) and 60 of the 1946 Act relating to endowments and to gifts from trust funds. But s. 59 of the 1946 Act (relating to gifts) does not remain applicable, being expressly replaced now by s. 95 of the 1977[1] Act. The Order also makes such other *ad hoc* modifications of legislation relevant to health authorities for the full integration into the reorganised National Health Service of the hospitals administered by the preserved Boards.[2]

C. INTERNAL ARRANGEMENTS

1. Contracts

Regional Health Authorities, Area Health Authorities, Special Health Authorities and Family Practitioner Committees as well as preserved Boards of Governors being bodies corporate with perpetual succession and a common seal[3] fall within the provisions of the Corporate Bodies' Contracts Act 1960, as follows:

1. (1) Contracts may be made on behalf of any body corporate, wherever incorporated, as follows:

(*a*) a contract which if made between private persons would be by law required to be in writing, signed by the parties to be charged therewith, may be made on behalf of the body corporate in writing signed by any person acting under its authority, express or implied, and

(*b*) a contract which if made between private persons would by law be valid although made by parol only, and not reduced into writing, may be made by parol on behalf of the body corporate by any person acting under its authority, express or implied.

(2) A contract made according to this section shall be effectual in law, and shall bind the body corporate and its successors and all other parties thereto.

(3) A contract made according to this section may be varied or discharged in the same manner in which it is authorised by this section to be made.

(4) Nothing in this section shall be taken as preventing a contract under seal from being made by or on behalf of a body corporate.

(5) This section shall not apply to the making, variation or discharge of a contract before the commencement of this Act but shall apply whether the body corporate gave its authority before or after the commencement of this Act.

[1] Formerly s. 29 (2) of the 1973 Act.
[2] For the text of the Order see p. 693. The otherwise repealed sections of the N.H.S. Acts 1946 to 1968 which remain applicable to preserved Boards are not set out *in extenso* in this book.
[3] National Health Service Act 1977 s. 8 and Schedule 5. replacing National Health Service Reorganisation Act 1973 s. 5 and Schedule I Part III Paragraph 8 and National Health Service Act 1946, s. 11 and Third Schedule, Part II.

The Act does not apply to any company formed and registered under the Companies Act 1948[1] (*e.g.* some voluntary hospitals and private nursing homes), though, in fact, the rules in respect of the making of contracts by such a company are substantially the same as for a corporate body to which the provisions of the Corporate Bodies Contracts Act 1960, apply.[2]

2. Legal Proceedings

An authority shall, notwithstanding that it is exercising any function on behalf of the Secretary of State or another authority, be entitled to enforce any rights so acquired and be liable in respect of any liabilities incurred (including liabilities in tort) in the exercise of that function, in all respects as if it were acting as a principal and all proceedings for the enforcement of such rights and liabilities are to be brought by or against the authority, and only the authority, in its own name.[3] This is of course without prejudice to the provisions in the Rules of Court relating to the correction or substitution of a party's name.

A Health Authority is not entitled in any proceedings to claim any privilege of the Crown in respect of the discovery or production of documents, but this is without prejudice to any right of the Crown to withhold or procure the withholding from production of any document on the ground that its disclosure would be contrary to the public interest.[4] This is a curious provision since it has been held in *Rogers* v. *The Secretary of State for the Home Department*[5] that it is not only the Crown that may make a valid claim for Crown privilege. In that case a claim made by the Gaming Board was allowed. Although it is probable that in any proper case the Court of its own motion can refuse to order discovery or to admit evidence where it considers it would be contrary to the public interest (and thus the matter does not fully depend on a party to the litigation making a claim), it appears that this provision is designed to secure a measure of uniformity of practice between the various Health Authorities; any claim they might wish to make has to be done by the Secretary of State.

All charges recoverable under the Act by the Secretary of State, a local Social Services Authority or any body constituted under the Act may, without prejudice to any other method of recovery, be recovered summarily as a civil debt.[6] As to hospital charges generally see Chapter 7.

The text of departmental circulars[7] to Health Authorities on arrange-

[1] S. 2. [2] Companies Act 1948, s. 36.
[3] National Health Service Act 1977 s. 8 and 5th Sch. Part III para. 15 (1). National Health Service Reorganisation Act 1973 s. 5 and 1st Sch. Part III para. 15 (1) and s. 13 (1) of the 1946 Act.
[4] See now *D* v. *N.S.P.C.C.* [1977] 1 All E.R. 589.
[5] [1973] A.C. 388.
[6] 1977 Act s. 122 (1). Formerly National Health Service Act 1946 s. 71 as amended.
[7] R.H.B. (49) 128; H.M. (54) 32, 43; H.M. (54) 73.

ments in connection with claims and legal proceedings given in an appendix at p. 721 may be helpful to those called on to advise Health Authorities and others involved in proceedings by or against them. The circulars have no binding force in themselves but serve a useful purpose by drawing attention as to the appropriate authority to sue or be sued. They also indicate the measure of consultation desirable between a Health Authority and the Department regarding actions at law. However, by Reg. 8 of the National Health Service Financial (No. 2) Regulations 1974[1] it is provided that where a loss occurs or a claim for damages or compensation is made against a Health Authority it shall follow such procedures, maintain such records and make such reports in relation thereto as the Secretary of State may require.

Attention is drawn to part 6 of departmental circular R.H.B. (49) 128 as to the defence of a nurse[2] against whom negligence is alleged. If the hospital authority alone is sued it will not ordinarily join the nurse[2] as co-defendant. The special arrangements made by the Secretary of State with the medical and dental defence societies for defence of actions in which medical negligence is alleged and for payment of any damages awarded and set out in H.M. (54) 32, those arrangements having been extended to dentists by H.M. (54) 43.

3. Applicability of Prevention of Corruption Acts

The reasoning in the judgment in *R. v. Newbould*[3] in which it was held that the National Coal Board was not a public authority for the purposes of the Prevention of Corruption Acts 1889 to 1916, left in doubt the question whether a Health Authority established by virtue of the National Health Service Act, is a public authority for the purposes of the Acts. The test laid down by Winn, J., by application of the *ejusdem generis* rule, was whether the body for which the status of a public authority under the Prevention of Corruption Acts 1889 to 1916, was sought was a local or public authority of the general kind, character, or genus referred to in s. 7 of the Public Bodies Corrupt Practices Act 1889, *viz.*, 'any council of a county or council of a city or town, any council of a municipal borough, also any board, commissioners, selected vestry, or other body which has power to act under and for the purposes of any Act relating to local government'.

R. v. Newbould has now been overruled and a Health Authority is a public authority for the purposes of the Prevention of Corruption Acts 1889 to 1916. *R. v. Newbould* was not followed by Judge Rigg in *R. v. Joy and Emmony*[4] where he he held that the Gas Board was a 'public

---

[1] S.I. 1974 No. 541.

[2] *Nurse* here presumably includes *midwife* and also any analogous officer of similar standing, *e.g.* a physiotherapist.

[3] [1962] 2 Q.B. 102.   [4] (1974) 60 Cr. App. Rep. 132.

authority' for the purposes of the Acts. In *D.P.P.* v. *Holley, D.P.P.* v. *Manners*[1] the House of Lords adopted Judge Rigg's reasoning. The importance of the matter is where the burden of proof will fall in case of an offence being charged under the Acts.

4. Conditions of Employment and the Appointment of Officers

Officers may be appointed directly by Regional and Area Health Authorities on such terms as the Authority may determine.[2] The word *officer* includes *servant*[3] and accordingly employees of all grades. The Secretary of State has power by regulation or discretion to place limits on the scope of the Authority's discretion. The Schedule goes on to provide that the regulations made under this power shall not require that all consultants employed by an Authority are to be employed whole-time.

Under the National Health Services (Remuneration and Conditions of Service) Regulations 1974,[4] officers whose remuneration is the subject of negotiations by a negotiating body are to receive by way of remuneration no more and no less than has been approved by the Secretary of State whether or not it is paid out of monies provided by Parliament.

So far as medical practitioners are concerned, it is expressly laid down in s. 40 of the Act of 1977[5] that any power conferred by the 1946 Act to prescribe qualifications includes a power to prescribe a requirement that the practitioners or optician shall show, to the satisfaction of a committee recognised by the Secretary of State for the purpose, that he possesses such qualifications, including qualifications as to experience, as may be mentioned in the regulations.

Special regulations have been issued with respect to the appointment of consultants. Under the National Health Service (Appointment of Consultants) Regulations 1974[6] provision is made for the appointment of the more senior hospital medical and dental officers including such matters as when and how advertisement for vacancies shall be made and the constitution of the appointments committees for the filling of every such vacancy.

---

[1] [1977] 2 W.C.R. 178.
[2] 1977 Act s. 8 and 5th Sch. para. 10 replacing 1973 National Health Service Reorganisation Act, s. 5 and 1st Sch. Part III para. 10 and s. 66 of the 1946 Act.
[3] 1977 Act s. 128 replacing 1946 Act, s. 79.
[4] S.I. 1974 No. 296 set out on p. 698, replacing the 1951 Regulations.
[5] Replacing s. 21 of the 1949 Act as amended.
[6] S.I. 1974 No. 361 and in Wales see the N.H.S. (Appointment of Consultants) (Wales) Regs. S.I. 1974 No. 477.

5. Finance

(a) Financial Provisions for Health Authorities

S. 97[1] of the N.H.S. Act 1977 provides that every Regional Health Authority (and every Health Authority in Wales) is to receive from the Secretary of State,[2] the sums needed to defray its approved expenditure. Every Regional Authority shall pay to every Area Authority in its region such sums as are needed to meet the expenditure of the Area Authority as the Regional Authority approves.[3] special Health Authorities are to receive their monies from first a Regional or Area Health Authority as provided in the order establishing the special Health Authority (or if the order provided there should be two or more such Authorities, in such proportions as the order determined) and secondly, for the balance of their expenditure, from the Secretary of State.[4] Each of the sums due under s. 97 shall be payable subject to compliance with such conditions as to records, certificates or otherwise as the Secretary of State may determine.[5]

The National Health Service Financial (No. 2) Regs. 1974[6] amplify these provisions. Each Regional and Area Health Authority must appoint a Treasurer[7] whose tasks include the giving of financial advice, supervision of implementation of the Health Authority's financial policies, the design etc. of systems of financial control and the maintenance of such records etc. as are required by the Authority for the purpose of carrying out its duties.[8] Each Regional Health Authority has to submit estimates of its expenditure and income to the Secretary of State and he may approve or vary them (which he may do at any time).[9] Similarly the Area Authorities submit their estimates to their Regional Health Authority.[10] Each Health Authority shall issue Standing Financial Instructions for the regulation of the conduct of its members and officers in relation to all financial matters and it shall incorporate in them such requirements as the Secretary of State may direct.[11]

Each Health Authority and body of Special Trustees[12] is to submit its accounts to the Secretary of State in such form as he, with the approval of the Treasury, may direct.[13] They are subject to audit by auditors of the Department of Health and Social Security and the Comptroller and Auditor-General may examine all such accounts etc.

S. 8 of the Charities Act 1960 requires the accounts of a charity with

---

[1] Formerly, s. 47 of the 1973 Act and s. 54 of the 1946 Act.
[2] Out of monies provided by Parliament s. 48.
[3] S. 97 (2).   [4] S. 97 (3) and 1 (c).   [5] S. 97 (4).   [6] S.I. 1974 No. 541.
[7] Reg. 9 (1). In the Welsh Health Technical Services Organisation the Chief Administrator is its Chief Financial Officer Reg. 12 (1). See Reg. 12 (2) and (3) for the other amendments to the Regs. in Wales.
[8] Reg. 9 (2).   [9] Reg. 3 (1) and (2).   [10] Reg. 3 (3).   [11] Reg. 5.
[12] See below, p. 92.   [13] Reg. 6. See Reg. 7 for further provisions as to audit.

a permanent endowment to be transmitted annually to the Charity Commissioners unless the charity is excepted by order or regulation. Hospital authorities under the 1946 Act were so exempted,[1] and the exemption is now extended to the new Health Authorities.[2]

(b) Travelling Allowances etc., of Members of Health Authorities

Travelling and other allowances of and payments to Health Authorities including compensation in respect of loss of remunerative time, are subject to determination by the Secretary of State with the approval of the Treasury.[3]

(c) Travelling Expenses of Officers

In practice scales and conditions of allowances for travelling expenses, including subsistence, for officers generally are subject of agreement in the General Council of the Whitley Councils for the Health Services (Great Britain). On any such agreement being approved by the Secretary of State under the N.H.S. (Remuneration and Conditions of Service) Regulations 1974,[4] the agreed scales and conditions become binding on authorities and officers alike. For the Secretary of State's power of variation and for his other powers under the regulations see Reg. 3 (3).

(d) Travelling Expenses of Patients etc.

Payment of a patient's travelling expenses out of Exchequer funds and of the expenses of a companion when the patient needs one on his journey to or from hospital is permitted only in accordance with the provisions of the N.H.S. (Expenses of Attending Hospitals) Regulations 1950.[5] The regulations do not prevent non-Exchequer funds being used to help with payment of a patient's travelling expenses or with the expenses of an escort, should the hospital authority be satisfied that there would otherwise be hardship,[6] this even though on the means test, the patient does not qualify for payment out of Exchequer funds.

Travelling expenses of long-stay patients returning home for short periods, when such patients are sent home for therapeutic reasons or to meet the hospital's convenience, may be paid direct by the Health Authority out of Exchequer funds and without any means test. If a patient takes leave at his own request, but with the hospital's permission,

---

[1] Charities (Exempted Accounts) Regs. S.I. 1963 No. 210.

[2] Charities (Exempted Accounts) Regs. S.I. 1976 No. 929.

[3] 1977 Act s. 8 and 5th Sch. Part III para. 9 National Health Service Reorganisation Act 1973 s. 5 and 1st Sch. Part III para. 9 and s. 36 of the 1968 Act.

[4] S.I. 1974 No. 296.

[5] S.I. 1950 No. 1222. The text of the regulations is given on p. 677. For an explanation of the occasions for application to the Supplementary Benefits Commission and generally as to the application of the regulations, reference should be made to the Supplementary Benefits Handbook and H.M. (73) 20.

[6] The responsibility of deciding whether hardship would be caused is usually delegated to an officer. It could be the medical–social worker who investigated the circumstances or it could be some other officer on consideration of the report of the medical–social worker.

travelling expenses are not payable out of Exchequer funds either by the Health Authority or through the Department of Health and Social Security. Such expenses may, however, be paid by the Health Authority out of non-Exchequer funds provided that the Authority is satisfied that the patient, or his relatives or friends, would otherwise suffer some hardship or that there is some good reason for recourse to *free moneys* for the purpose. Travelling expenses of visitors to patients detained in special hospitals may be paid out of Exchequer funds in accordance with arrangements made by the Secretary of State with the approval of the Treasury under s. 66 (1) of the Health Services and Public Health Act 1968.[1]

(e) Free Moneys: Position of Health Authorities as Trustees of

The limitations above-mentioned as to authorised expenditure do not extend to *free moneys* as to which see p. 82 *et seq.* Property and income held under s. 90 of the 1977[2] Act, also constitute *free moneys* for the expenditure of which the Minister's consent is not required. There is, however, the over-riding limitation that gifts may be accepted under that section for all or any of the purposes relating to the health service.

It may here be observed that the expression *free moneys* is not a term of art but an expression first used in departmental circulars as a convenient way of distinguishing non-Treasury funds from moneys provided by the Treasury, the former being free of Departmental and Treasury control unless, maybe, it is argued that the Secretary of State might exercise control over them by using his powers of direction under s. 13 of the 1977 Act.[3] Also the Charity Commissioners[4] and the Court have their normal powers under the Charities Act 1960, in respect of charity funds controlled by a Health Authority. The position of Health Authorities under that Act has been summarised in departmental circular H.M. (61) 74. In effect, Health Authorities, in respect of capital and income, as distinct from land, buildings equipment and money taken over by the Secretary of State for hospital purposes under s. 6 of the National Health Service Act 1946 are not exempt from any of the provisions of the Charities Act 1960. Nor, incidentally, are they exempt from the provisions of the Trustee Act 1925, nor of the Trustee Investments Act 1961. It is here observed, however, that the Charity Commissioners have undertaken that some of their powers, particularly those of inquiry, or of dismissal of trustees or officers under ss. 6 and 20 of the Act of 1960, will not be exercised without consultation with the Department of Health and Social Security 'so as'. they said 'not to duplicate the powers of the Secretary of State'.

[1] The section is *not* affected by the consolidation.   [2] Formerly s. 21 of the 1973 Act.
[3] See also ss. 14–18. These sections replace s. 7 of the 1973 Act and s. 12 of the 1946 Act.
[4] Or, in the case of an educational charity, the Secretary of State for Education

What is said in Chapters 4 and 5 about the position of voluntary hospital boards and committees as charity trustees and their position in respect of investments broadly, also applies to Health Authorities under the National Health Service Act in so far as they are charity trustees. In particular, Health Authorities are not exempt from registration as charities if their capital or income brings them within the definition of a charity obliged to register. A charity not obliged to register may nevertheless do so.[1]

Further as to non-Treasury funds see Chapter 5. The disposal of alms collected at religious offices and at services conducted by chaplains on hospital premises is dealt with in Chapter 11.

6. Default and Emergency Powers of the Secretary of State

The Secretary of State, after such enquiry as he thinks fit, may make an order declaring any of certain authorities established under the 1977 Act, including a Regional Health Authority, Area Health Authority or special Health Authority is in default. In the case of any of the authorities there named the effect of such order is that the members forthwith vacate their office, the order shall provide for the appointment of new members and, if expedient, authorise any person to act in place of the body in question, pending appointment of new members.

Provision is also made for transfer to the Secretary of State in case of need of the property and liabilities of a body in default and of transfer back to the body together with any additional rights and liabilities, acquired or incurred by the Secretary of State on its behalf.[2]

The 1977 Act also makes provision for the Secretary of State, in an emergency, to direct that any function which should be carried out by any body or person under the Health Service Acts be carried out by another body or person.[3]

7. Land

(a) Transfer to the Minister

S. 6 of the 1946 Act transferred to and vested in the Minister all interests in or attaching to premises forming part of a voluntary hospital or a local authority hospital.[4] Although the section was repealed[5] on the reorganisation; naturally the property remains vested in the Minister. Space prevents a discussion of the full effect of the 1946 rationalisation.[6]

---

[1] Charities Act 1960, s. 4 (2).
[2] National Health Service Act 1977 s. 85 (Formerly 1946 Act, s. 57 as amended).
[3] S. 86. Formerly 1973 Act s. 54 (1).
[4] It will be noted that the section covered moveable property as well as land.
[5] With the exception of sub-section 6 (4). See now s. 88 of the 1977 Act.
[6] The reader who needs to know more about it is referred to the 5th Edition of this book at pp. 514–16 and to re Majoribanks [1952] Ch. 181, Minister of Health v. Fox [1950] 1 All E.R. 1050, Minister of Health v. General Committee of the Royal Midland Counties Home for Incurables [1954] Ch. 530 and re Roberts and re Perkins The Times May 23 1957 and to the Scottish case Royal Victoria Hospital Dundee v. Lord Advocate [1950] S.C. 511.

S. 7 of the 1946 Act dealt with the transfer of endowments of the voluntary hospitals. Again space prevents a discussion of this issue.[1] It suffices here to note that s. 24[2] of the Reorganisation Act 1973 specified the re-distribution of these (and other endowments) from the pre- to the post-1973 authorities.

Also worthy of mention is s. 16[2] of the 1973 Act which transferred all local authority property held or used mainly for its pre-reorganisation health functions.

(b) Acquisition

Health Authorities may hold land received by way of gift and also accept gifts of personal property to be laid out in the purchase of land[3] but, except so far as might be authorised by the terms of the particular trust, may not hold land by way of investment, since they may only hold trustee securities including legal mortgages on land authorised by the Trustee Act 1925, and the Trustee Investments Act 1961 for this purpose.[4] But land may properly be purchased for use for health service purposes either in the name of the health authority or of the Secretary of State.[5] Unless, however, land to be purchased will be needed for health purposes within a reasonably short time, the consent of the Charity Commissioners to the purchase should be obtained. Land held by way of permanent endowment may not be mortgaged or charged by way of security for money borrowed, nor sold, leased or otherwise disposed of without an order of the court or of the Charity Commissioners.[6]

A departmental booklet issued under cover of circular H.M. (55) 72[7] should be referred to for official guidance to Health Authorities and their legal advisers on departmental policy and also the procedure relating to dealings with land for health service purposes both by the Secretary of State and by Health Authorities, including compulsory and other purchases, leases, licences and sales[8] as well as exchanges, grants of easements and other rights. The instructions on compulsory acquisition of land contained in the departmental booklet have since

---

[1] The reader who needs to know more is referred to the 5th Edition of this book at pp. 516–19 and to the cases cited in the previous footnote.

[2] These sections have not been affected by the Consolidation.

[3] National Health Service Act 1977, s. 90 replacing s. 59 of the 1946 Act and s. 21 of the 1973 Act.

[4] Under its private Act, Guy's Hospital, before the appointed day, had power to invest in land. The new board of Governors, being advised that under the 1946 Act they had no such power, it is understood that an application was made to the Chancery Division, and such investment was approved on the same conditions as under the former Acts.

[5] 1977 Act s. 87 (1) formerly 1973 Act, s. 53 (1).

[6] Charities Act 1960, s. 29.

[7] As amended. It is understood that an updated version is to be published in Autumn 1977.

[8] As to disposal of surplus, see H.M. (62) 46 and H.M.G. (50) 96, R.H.B. (50) 99 and, as to transactions for hospital purposes, H.M. (55) 72, H.M. (58) 37 and (58) 40.

been amended to take account of the recommendations of the Committee on Administration Tribunals and Inquiries.[1]

In an appendix to the booklet formal authorisation was given to secretaries of regional hospital boards and boards of governors and hospital management committees to sign certain documents on the Minister's behalf and as his duly authorised agents,[2] including leases granted to or by the Secetarry of State where not required to be under seal (*i.e.*, for a period not exceeding three years); licenses or other rights not amounting to an easement over hospital property to a public utility authority; tenancies for not more than 364 days or licences to occupy land for use as agricultural land and licences for use for grazing or mowing during some specific period of the year. In the case of a hospital management committee the authority given is subject to the consent of the appropriate regional hospital board. The advice of the District Valuer is available to hospital authorities.

If land, including buildings, is held on lease for hospital purposes, advantage may, in appropriate cases, be taken of the Landlord and Tenant Act 1954, to obtain a renewal of the lease or, alternatively, compensation for disturbance.[3]

(c) Hospital Land, Building and Development

Land which vested in the Secretary of State under s. 6 of the National Health Service Act 1946 (*i.e.*, transferred hospitals) or which vested in him under s. 16 of the National Health Service Reorganisation Act 1973 (*i.e.* transferred local authority land) acquired by him for hospital purposes otherwise, as well as land included in endowments transferred to the Secretary of State is generally[4] exempt from the provisions of the Town and Country Planning Act 1971 and the Community Land Act 1975. The land may be subject to a development plan but interests of the Secretary of State in land (or in land held on his behalf) are not subject to compulsory purchase.[5] The consent of the Secretary of State for Health and Social Security is, however, required where Crown land (*i.e.*, land in which *any* interest belongs to the Secretary of State) is concerned, whether the Crown interest is affected or not, before any action of the following kinds is taken under the 1971 Act:

   (i) the service of an enforcement notice under s. 87;
  (ii) the making of an order for the discontinuance of a use or the alteration or removal of a building under s. 51;
 (iii) the making of a tree preservation order under s. 60;

[1] H.M. (58) 37.
[2] Now presumably Regional and Area Health Authorities.
[3] The necessary procedure, as well as the Minister's policy are outlined in H.M. (56) 68.
[4] See Town and Country Planning Act 1971, s. 266.
[5] *Private interests* in land are. Community Land Act 1975, s. 39.

   (iv) the making of a building preservation order under s. 51;

   (v) the service of a notice requiring proper maintenance of waste land under s. 65;

   (vi) the compulsory acquisition of any interest in the land.

Land or any interest in land held directly by any Health Authority constituted under the National Health Service Act is privately held and as such subject to the provisions of the Town and Country Planning Act 1971 and the Community Land Act 1975.

For fuller information readers are referred to the departmental booklet issued with Circular H.M. (55) 72,[1] which also outlines the steps which should be taken by hospital authorities in consultation with the local planning authority for reservation of land for hospital purposes and stresses that regional boards and boards of governors should watch for advertisements of proposals by the local planning authority and take the appropriate steps to obtain any requisite variation.

(d) Land, not Required for Hospital Purposes — Disposal of

Except in the case of endowment properties all land held for national hospital purposes being owned by the Secretary of State, any conveyance must be over his official seal. The practical procedure is outlined in the departmental booklet referred to above.[2]

(e) Land not Required for Hospital Purposes — Grant of Lease of

Health Authorities have been authorised to grant leases on behalf of the Secretary of State, but leases, except for a term of not more than three years, for which a letting under seal is not necessary, must be forwarded to the Secretary of State's solicitor for execution. For a term not exceeding three years the secretary to an Authority is authorised to sign as his duly authorised agent. It seems that a Health Authority can effectively bind the Secretary of State by an agreement in writing on his behalf to grant a lease, even though the agreement may turn out to be one the terms of which he would not have approved and, seemingly, damages could be claimed against the Secretary of State if he refused to execute the lease.

If a lease has been granted for business, professional or other purposes so as to bring the property within the Landlord and Tenant Act 1954, the Secretary of State may, nevertheless, under ss. 57 and 58 of the Act refuse a new tenancy on the expiry of the old one on grounds of departmental necessity or national security. If the Secretary of State grants a certificate under s. 57, the tenant may be entitled to compensation under ss. 59 and 37. For further information reference should be made to

---

[1] As amended, see footnote 7 on p. 32 above.

[2] And see H.S.C. (15) 207. However the Secretary of State has devolved disposal powers to R.H.A.s.

departmental Circular H.M. (56) 68 which should be read in conjunction with the earlier Circular H.M. (55) 72 and the booklet enclosed therewith.

(f) Service and Other Tenancies

If a house is occupied on a service tenancy, possession can generally be obtained when the officer ceases to be employed, there being no question of protection under the Rent Act 1977[1]; as to this see further p. 419 *et seq*. In the case of other than service tenancies different considerations apply. If the tenancy is of property belonging to the Crown, again the Rent Act does not apply; but if it is of endowment property the Act in appropriate cases, will apply. In the case of Crown property the Secretary of State indicated that he does not wish authorities to shelter behind exclusion from the Rent Act except for urgent need and without undue hardship to the tenant or his family.[2]

(g) Compulsory Purchase of Land

Under s. 113 of the Town and Country Planning Act 1971, the Secretary of State for the Environment may compulsorily purchase land required for 'the public service'. Under s. 37 of the Community Land Act 1975 this power is extended to cover any other land which ought also to be acquired together with the public service land in the interests of proper planning for the area or where it can be used with the public service land in the best or the most economic way. Further, the section provides that where the Secretary of State for the Environment is disposing of land owned by him, he may compulsorily purchase any adjoining land in order to facilitate the sale. It appears that the Secretary of State for the Environment may use these powers for the benefit not only of his own department but quite generally for any public authority including therefore the Secretary of State for Health and Social Security.

8. Hospital Farms — Milk Production

In a circular to hospital authorities it has been indicated that whilst in general the various Acts and Regulations concerned with methods and standards of milk production and treatment are not binding on hospitals vested in the Secretary of State, it is desirable that the conditions under which milk is produced and the health of the herds at the hospital dairy farms should be of the highest standard, and subject to the same degree of surveillance by the Ministry of Agriculture, Fisheries and Food as is given to commercial dairy farms. The Secretary of State,

[1] This Act, together with the Protection from Eviction Act 1977 consolidate the previous Rent Acts.
[2] See also Ministry circular R.H.B. (50) 43.

therefore, desires hospital dairy farms to comply with the Acts and Regulations concerned.[1]

9. Motor Vehicles used for Hospital Purposes

(a) Registration and Licensing

All health service vehicles used solely for such purposes and solely by members and employees of Health Authority committees have operated under a certificate of Crown ownership and no Excise licence duty is payable. Vehicles must, however, still be registered and a registration mark assigned but no registration documents are issued.[2]

(b) Insurance

In accordance with Government policy, health service vehicles being Crown property are not insured[3] and, in departmental Circular R.H.B. (50) 121, particulars are given of arrangements for handling claims and of certain 'Forbearance and Sharing Agreements' with insurers of other vehicles. Detailed treatment of these matters is rather beyond the scope of the present work. It will be noted that privately owned vehicles, even though the expenses of their owners may (or must) be paid when they are travelling on official health service business, must still be insured.

(c) Petroleum Spirit: Safety Precautions

The Secretary of State has advised authorities established under the Health Service Acts, that as the hospitals are Crown property, they are not bound by the provisions of the Petroleum (Consolidation) Act 1928,[4] and the regulations made thereunder laying down safety precautions in respect of storage of petroleum spirit.[5] He has, however, intimated that authorities should voluntarily comply with the regulations and, in the same memorandum, set out the precautions to be taken.[6] Voluntary hospitals and institutions owned by local authorities, not being Crown property, are not exempt.

10. Protection of Members and Officers of Health Authorities, etc.

By s. 125 of the N.H.S. Act 1977,[7] s. 265 of the Public Health Act 1875 is extended to Regional and Area Health Authorities, special Health Authorities (including therefore the Welsh Health Technical Services Organisation). Section 265 of the Public Health Act 1875, reads:

[1] For a full explanation of the position see R.H.B. (52) 28.
[2] For full particulars see R.H.B. (50) 123.
[3] See the N.H.S. (Vehicles) Order S. I. 1974 No. 168.
[4] As amended.
[5] The provisions are however too detailed to be set out in this book.
[6] Circular H.M. (58) 30.
[7] Formerly s. 72 of the 1946 Act.

'No matter or thing done, and no contract entered into by any local authority or joint board or port sanitary authority, and no matter or thing done by any member of such authority or by any officer of such authority or other person whomsoever acting under the direction of such authority, shall if the matter or thing were done or the contract were entered into *bona fide* for the purpose of executing this Act subject them or any of them personally to any action, liability, claim or demand whatsoever; and any expense incurred by any such authority, member, officer or other person acting as last aforesaid shall be borne and repaid out of the fund or rate applicable by such authority to the general purposes of this Act.

'Provided that nothing in this section shall exempt any member of any such authority from any liability to be surcharged with the amount of any payment which may be disallowed by the auditor in accounts of such authority, and which such member authorised or joined in authorising.'

The proviso does not apply to members of Health Authorities under the National Health Service Act, since no power of surcharge is anywhere conferred on the departmental auditors. But it must be appreciated that the section does not protect a Health Authority in its corporate capacity against any action in respect of any contract or other matter referred to in the section, nor does it protect officers against actions in tort based on negligence, etc.

In *McGinty* v. *Glasgow Victoria Hospitals Board*[1] in which a workman claimed damages at common law and under the Factories Act 1937, against a hospital board established under the National Health Service (Scotland) Act 1947, in respect of injury in a hospital laundry due to an unfenced machine, it was held by the Second Division of the Court of Session (Lord Mackay dissenting) that s. 70 of the National Health Service (Scotland) Act 1947, corresponding with s. 125 of the National Health Service Act 1977, did not bar such a claim against the authority as the present one, being based on negligence. Further it was said that the breach of common law and statutory duty in this case arose out of the private relationship of the contract of employment, and not from the duties imposed by Parliament on the board to provide health services for the public at large. (Reference should be made to the judgments in this case for an examination of the extent of the duties and liabilities of statutory corporations and of earlier authorities, *Mersey Docks Trustees* v. *Gibbs*[2] and *Sanitary Commissioners of Gibraltar* v. *Orfila*[3] being cited.)

Similarly, in Scotland, in *Walker* v. *Greenock and District Combination Hospital Board*,[4] on appeal to the First Division of the Court of Session, it has been held that a hospital authority could not escape the consequences of a breach of contract by reliance on s. 70.

In *Bullard* v. *Croydon Group H.M.C.*[5] it was held that s. 72 of the

[1] 1951 S.C. 200; 1951 S.L.T. 92.
[2] [1866] L.R. 1 E. and I. 91
[3] (1890) App. Cas. 400, 411.
[4] 1951 S.C. 464; 1951 S.L.T. 329.
[5] [1953] 1 Q.B. 511.

National Health Service Act 1946, applying s. 265 of the Public Health Act 1875, to hospital authorities did not protect a hospital management committee in its corporate capacity in respect of actions for negligence.

D. RELATIONS OF HEALTH AUTHORITIES WITH OTHER STATUTORY BODIES UNDER THE NATIONAL HEALTH SERVICE ACT

The relationship of Regional and Area Health Authorities to the Secretary of State and of those Authorities one to another and similar matters have already been dealth with. In this part of the chapter will be examined their relations with other statutory bodies and with persons having statutory duties, this in so far as those relationships and duties have any significant bearing on the functions of Health Authorities in respect of hospital services. The position of the Health Service Commissioner is discussed in Chapter 17.

1. Central Administration

(a) Central Health Services Council

The Secretary of State is aided in an advisory capacity by a Central Health Services Council constituted in accordance with Schedule 4[1] to the 1977 Act and appointed in accordance with the Regulations.[2] It will there be observed that the Secretary of State is under a duty to consult with certain representative organisations before making appointments to the Council though he is under no obligation to accept the advice of those organisations he may consult and, even when he does, the persons appointed do not serve in a representative capacity. The Secretary of State may, after consultation with the Central Council, by order vary the constitution of the Council (s. 6 (2)).

The provisions as to tenure of office, rules of procedure, etc., are contained in paragraphs 2–6 of Schedule 4 to the 1977 Act.

(b) Standing Advisory Committees

Standing Advisory Committees may by order be set up by the Secretary of State to advise him and the Central Council and paragraphs 2–6 of Schedule 4 of the 1977 Act applies to any such committee to the extent indicated. Any Standing Advisory Committee must consist partly (but to no specified extent) of members of the Central Council appointed and partly of persons (whether members of the Central Council or not)

[1] 1977 Act, s. 6. The N.H.S. (Central Health Service Council and Standing Advisory Committees) Regs. S.I. 1974 No. 187 contain provisions for the staggering of the retirement of members of the Council (and the Standing Advisory Committees).

[2] The provisions of Art. 3 of the Central Health Services Council (Variation of Constitution) Order S.I. 1974 No. 186 substituted those previously contained in para. 1 of 1st Sch. of the 1946 Act. It now appears as para.1 of the Sch. 4 to the 1977 Act.

appointed after consultation with such representative organisations as the Secretary of State may recognise for the purpose, but such persons are not appointed in a representative capacity.[1]

The Standing Advisory Committees currently established and their terms of references are set out in the Schedule to the 1974 N.H.S. (Standing Advisory Committees) (Amendment) Order.[2] They are the Standing Medical Advisory Committee, the Standing Dental Advisory Committee, the Standing Pharmaceutical Advisory Committee, the Standing Ophthalmic Advisory Committee and the Standing Nursing and Midwifery Advisory Committee.

2. Local Advisory Committees

(a) Regional Advisory Committees: Recognition and Functions[3]

Provision is made in s. 19 (1) for the recognition by the Secretary of State of committees formed for the region of a Regional Health Authority as representative of (a) the medical practitioners of the region; (b) the dental practitioners of the region; (c) the nurses and midwives of the region; (d) the registered pharmacists of the region; and (e) the ophthalmic and dispensing opticians of the region. These committees are called the Regional Medical, Dental, Nursing and Midwifery, Pharmaceutical or Optical Committees as the case might be.[4] Provision is also made for the recognition by the Secretary of State of committees representative of any category of persons (other than a category mentioned above) who provide services forming part of the health service and also for the recognition of committees representative of any two or more of the categories of persons mentioned or referred to above.[5] The section also provides that the Secretary of State may withdraw recognition from a committee, recognising in its place another committee established within the above provisions of the section.[6]

(b) Duties of Advisory Committees: Obligation of Regional Health Authority

Schedule 6 paragraph (3) provides as follows:

'It shall be the duty of a committee duly recognised by reference to the region of a Regional Health Authority area of an Area Health Authority:

(a) to advise the Authority on the provision by the Authority of services of the kind provided by the categories of persons of whom the committee is representative; and

(b) to perform such other functions as may be prescribed;

and it shall be the duty of the Authority to consult the committee with respect to such matters and on such occasions as may be prescribed.'

---

[1] See p. 38 above.   [2] S.I. 1974 No. 196.   [3] See H.R.C. (74) 9.
[4] S. 19 (2) formerly s. 8 (1).   [5] Sch. 6 para. 1 (1).   [6] Sch. 6 para. 1 (2).

D

(c) Welsh Advisory Committees: Recognition and Functions[7]

There being no Regional Health Authority for Wales, provision was made in the 1973 Act adapting the provisions of S. 8[1]. Under the Consolidation, the special provisions for Wales are to be found in s. 19 (2) (a) and Schedule 6 paragraph 3. The other provisions of s. 19 (1) and Schedule 6 paragraphs 1, 2 and 5 are applicable.

The effect of all this is that there are Welsh Medical, Dental, Nursing and Midwifery, Pharmaceutical and Optical Committees operating under the same terms as in the Regions in England.

(d) Expenses of Advisory Committees

Regional Health Authorities are authorised — but not obliged unless so directed — to pay expenses etc. of members of local advisory committees within the limits laid down in Schedule 6 paragraph 5 which reads as follows:

An Authority may defray such expenses incurred by such a committee in performing the duty imposed on the committee by paragraphs 3 and 4 above and those expenses may as the Authority considers reasonable include travelling and other allowances and compensation for loss of remunerative time for members of the committee at such rates as the Secretary of State may determine with the approval of the Minister for the Civil Service.

An Authority in the paragraph means, in Wales the Secretary of State and, in England, the Regional or Area Health Authority as the case may be.

(e) Area Advisory Committees: Recognition and Functions

Area advisory committees in all respects corresponding with regional advisory committees under s. 19 and Schedule 6 save that their functions relate to the Area Health Authority and not the Regional Health Authority shall be recognised both in England and Wales under the provisions of s. 19 (3) reading as follows:

19.—(3) Where the Secretary of State is satisfied that a committee formed for the area of an Area Health Authority is representative of persons of any of the categories mentioned in paragraphs (a) to (e) in subsection (1) it shall be his duty to recognise the committee.

A committee recognised in pursuance of this subsection shall be called the Area Medical, Dental, Nursing and Midwifery, Pharmaceutical or Optical Committee, as the case may be, for the area in question.

Accordingly, the same pattern of functional advisory committees is reproduced in the areas. They have the same tasks to perform.

[7] See circular in H.R.C. (74) 1.

3. Community Health Councils

(a) *Introductory*

It was the duty of the Secretary of State under s. 9 of the Act of 1973 to establish a Community Health Council for the area of each Area Health Authority or separate Councils for separate parts of an area or, possibly, for a district comprising parts of more than one Area Health Authority.[1] They are now constituted under s. 20 and Schedule 7 of the 1977 Act. At least half of the members of such a Council are local authority representatives and at least a third are appointed by bodies (other than public or local authorities) of which the activities are carried on otherwise than for profit.[2] The remaining members are appointed by the establishing Authority after consultation with local authorities in accordance with the requirements of Reg. 6 of the N.H.S. (Community Health Councils) Regulations 1973. The regulations also provide for under paragraph 2 of Schedule 7 other matters relating to the Councils which, are to be so prescribed.

(b) *Functions etc. of Community Health Councils*

Schedule 7 paragraph 1 of the 1977 Act provides that it shall be the duty of a Community Health Council — (a) to represent the interests in the health service of the public in its district; and (b) to perform such other functions as may be conferred on it by virtue of the following paragraph (i.e. paragraph 2). This gives the Secretary of State power to provide by regulation for various matters relating to Community Health Councils including *inter alia*, consultation of Councils by Area Health Authorities;[3] the furnishing of information to Councils by Area Health Authorities[4] and entry and inspection by Council members of premises controlled by Area Health Authorities;[5] consideration by Councils of any matters relating to the health service within their districts that they think fit and the giving of advice on such matters to Area Health Authorities;[6] the preparation and publication of reports by Councils;[7] and any additional functions.

The regulations also set out in detail the duties of the establishing authority — in England by delegation from the Secretary of State and the Regional Health Authority and in Wales, the Secretary of State for Wales[8] — relating to the provision of staff, premises and other facilities for the Councils and for their finance. What concerns this book mostly is not these matters[9] but rather the powers and duties of a Council in

---

[1] Sch. 7 para. 3. See also H.R.C. (73) 4 and H.R.C. (74) 4.
[2] Provision for appointment of members of voluntary bodies is made in Reg. 4 (5) and Reg. 7 of the N.H.S. (Community Health Council) Reg. S.I. 1973 No. 2217. See also N.H.S. (Community Health Council) Amendment Regs. S.I. 1976 No. 791.
[3] See Reg. 20 below, p. 42.   [4] See Reg. 21.   [5] See Reg. 22 below, pp. 43–44.
[6] See Reg. 19 below.   [7] See Reg. 18.
[8] Reg. 2.   [9] But see H.R.C. (74) 4.

relation to the hospitals in its district and the degree of co-operation it is the duty of the relevant Area Health Authority[1] to afford.

Although it is the duty of a Council to represent the interests in the health service of the public in its district[2] that does not give it any rights of management of the hospital and other health services for which the Area Health Authority is responsible. Its strictly advisory function[3] is clearly brought out in Reg. 19 reading as follows:

It shall be the duty of each Council to keep under review the operation of the health service in its district and make recommendations for the improvement of such service or otherwise advise any relevant Area Authority upon such matters relating to the operation of the health service within its district as the Council thinks fit.

(c) Consultation of Councils by relevant Area Authority

Consultation is required in respect of matters within Reg. 20[4] and subject to the provisions of that regulation, which reads as follows:

(1) It shall be the duty of each relevant Area Authority to consult a Council on any proposals which the authority may have under consideration for any substantial development of the health service in the Council's district and on any such proposals to make any substantial variation in the provision of such service:

Provided that this regulation shall not apply to any proposal on which the Area Authority is satisfied that, in the interest of the health service, a decision has to be taken without allowing time for consultation; but, in any such case, the Area Authority shall notify the Council immediately of the decision taken and the reason why no consultation has taken place.

(2) An Area Authority may specify a date by which comments on any such proposals as are referred to in the foregoing paragraph of this regulation should be made by the Council to be taken into consideration by the Area Authority and in any case where a Council is not satisfied that sufficient time has been allowed or that consultation on any such proposal has been adequate, the establishing authority shall have power to require the Area Authority to carry out such further consultations with the Council as the establishing authority considers appropriate and the Area Authority shall reconsider any decision taken on the proposals having regard to such further consultations.

(d) Information to be furnished by relevant Area Authority

Reg. 21 lays down the duty of the relevant Area Authority to provide a Community Health Council with such information about the planning and operation of the services as it may reasonably require in order to carry out its duties, but this is subject to the right to withhold confidential

---

[1] Ordinarily, the 'relevant Area Authority' will mean the Area Health Authority within whose area the district covered by the Community Health Council is wholly situated but, more strictly, it is as defined in Reg. 2, that definition providing for anomalous cases.

[2] Para. 1 of Sch. 7.

[3] See also H.R.C. (74) 4 Appendix 5. Matters to which CHCs might wish to direct AHAs attention.

[4] *Ibid.* paras 32–36.

information. Information which relates to the diagnosis and treatment of individual patients or any personnel matter relating to the individual officers should be regarded as confidential. So too may other information be withheld on this basis unless (apparently) it is reasonably required by the Council in order to carry out its duties. In the event of a dispute between a Council and an Area Authority the decision of the establishing authority as to whether the information is so necessary for the Council is normally final. Reg. 21 provides:

(1) It shall be the duty of a relevant Area Authority to provide the Council with such information about the planning and operation of health services in the area of that Authority as the Council may reasonably require in order to carry out its duties:
Provided that confidential information about the diagnosis and treatment of individual patients or any personnel matters relating to individual officers employed by a health authority should not be given to any Council or member or officer of such Council and, subject to the provisions of the next following paragraph of this regulation, an Area Authority may refuse to disclose to a Council any other information which the Authority regards as confidential.
(2) In the event of a relevant Area Authority refusing to disclose to a Council information requested, the Council may appeal to the establishing authority by which the Council was established and a decision of the establishing authority as to whether the information is reasonably required by the Council in order to carry out its duties or as to whether the Area Authority may regard the information as confidential shall be final for the purposes of this regulation.

(e) Inspection of premises by Councils

Regulation 22 provides as follows:

A Council shall have the right to enter and inspect any premises controlled by a relevant Area Authority at such times and subject to such conditions as may be agreed between the Council and the Area Authority or, in default of such agreement, as may be determined by the establishing authority:
Provided that:

(a) premises or parts of premises used as residential accommodation for officers employed by any health authority may not be entered by members of a Council without their having first obtained the consent of the officers residing in such accommodation; and
(b) premises or parts of premises made available to persons providing general medical services, general dental services, general ophthalmic services or pharmaceutical services may not be entered by members of a Council without their having first obtained the consent of the persons providing such services.

That the right of a Community Health Council to enter and inspect premises controlled by an Area Health Authority is to be 'at such times and subject to such conditions as may be agreed . . .' or as 'determined by the establishing authority'[1] is important. If necessary through the

[1] See H.R.C. (74) 4 para 37.

imposition of conditions that uncontrolled entry (by perhaps the full Council) can be prevented so as to save, at the very least, embarrassment and, at worst, danger to the lives of patients.[1] However, it appears that neither the Area nor the establishing authority can use this power to totally frustrate the right of inspection. If need be, a balance must be found.

(f) Meetings between Council and Area Authority

Regulation 23 provides as follows:

It shall be the duty of each relevant Area Authority to arrange, not less than once every year, a meeting between members of that Authority, being not less than one-third of the whole number of such members, and the members of the Council to discuss such matters relating to the functions of the Council as may be raised by the Council or the relevant Area Authority.

(g) Advice and assistance to Community Health Councils

It is also worth noting that Schedule 7 paragraph 5[2] of the Act provides:

The Secretary of State may:[3]

(a) provide for the establishment of a body—

    (i) to advise Councils with respect to the performance of their functions and to assist Councils in the performance of their functions; and

    (ii) to perform such other functions as may be prescribed.

(h) The Importance of Community Health Councils

It can be readily seen from the foregoing that the *legal* position of the Councils as regards their Area Authorities is very weak. They have no management functions and only circumscribed rights to information and of inspection. Nevertheless, it would be wrong to conclude that they are an anomolous and irrelevant creation of the N.H.S. Act. As the Davis Committee on Hospital Complaints Procedure[4] remarked, this is the age of the consumer. These Councils are intended to be the place in which the consumer's voice is heard in the re-organised health service.

---

[1] A possible condition might be that the Council should exercise its functions of entry and inspection of a hospital or particular parts of a hospital through a small committee appointed for the purpose, such condition in no way conflicting with the opening words of Reg. 22 'A Council shall have the right to enter and inspect . . .' since Reg. 13 expressly provides that a Council may appoint committees of the Council to exercise . . . functions, and that such committees may include persons who are not members of the Council, though, ordinarily, at least two-thirds of the members must be members of the Council. That non-members may be appointed to a committee of a Council would leave open the possibility of the inclusion of an expert or experts or, say, of the Secretary to the appointing Council.

[2] Formerly 1973 Act s. 9 (6).

[3] See now N.H.S. (Association of Community Health Councils) Regs. S.I. 1977 No. 874 and the N.H.S. (Association of Community Health Councils — Establishment) Order S.I. 1977 No. 1204.

[4] Published in 1973 by the Department of Health and Social Services.

Used wisely they enable the Area Authorities to respond to consumer demand and so improve the efficiency and public acceptance of the service they administer.

In the modern world, it is wrong to departmentalise things so that law cannot be considered as a wholly separate subject from administration. It is not however the task of this book to discuss in any detail administrative as opposed to legal practices. It suffices to say that merely because the legal position of a body is weak, it does not follow that it has little administrative importance.

E. CO-OPERATION AND ASSISTANCE BETWEEN HEALTH AUTHORITIES

1. Local Authorities, Voluntary Bodies etc.

(a) *Health Authorities and local authorities — establishment of consultative committees*

Section 22 (1) of the Act of 1977 provides as follows:

In exercising their respective functions Health Authorities and local authorities shall co-operate with one another in order to secure and advance the health and welfare of the people of England and Wales.[1]

S. 22 (2) specifically requires the establishment of joint consultative committees who shall advise Area Health Authorities and the corresponding local authorities[2] there indicated on the performance of their duties under s. 22 (1) and on the planning and operation of services of common concern to those authorities. The Secretary of State has power by Order under s. 22 (4)[2] to deal with various matters relating to the composition and functioning of such joint consultative committees. This has been done by the Health Authorities and Local Authorities Joint Consultative Committees Order 1974.[3]

(b) *Supply of goods and services etc. by or on behalf of the Secretary of State*

The supply of goods and services and the provision of other facilities of a kind used or available in the health service to local authorities and other public bodies is dealt with in s. 26, the two main subsections reading as follows:

26 (1) The Secretary of State may:

(a) supply to local authorities, and to such public bodies or classes of

---

[1] The functions of local Social Services authorities are set out in s. 21 and Sch. 8.

[2] Formerly s. 10 (4) of the 1973 Act.

[3] S.I. 1974 No. 190. Practical guidance is given to health authorities on the setting up of joint consultative committees in circular H.R.C. (74) 19. The circular also commends the second report of the working party on collaboration.

public bodies as may be determined by the Secretary of State, any goods or materials of a kind used in the health service;[1]

(b) make available to local authorities, and to such bodies or classes of bodies, any facilities (including the use of any premises and the use of any vehicle, plant or apparatus) provided by him for any service under this Act and the services of persons employed by the Secretary of State or by a health authority;

(c) carry out maintenance work[2] in connection with any land or building for the maintenance of which a local authority is responsible.

Section 26 (3) provides as follows:

(3) The Secretary of State shall make available to local authorities:

(a) any services or other facilities (excluding the services of any person but including goods or materials, the use of any premises and the use of any vehicle, plant or apparatus) provided under this Act;

(b) the services provided as part of the health service by any person employed by the Secretary of State or a Health Authority; and

(c) the services of any medical practitioner, dental practitioner or nurse employed by the Secretary of State or a Health Authority otherwise than to provide services which are part of the health service,

so far as is reasonably necessary and practicable to enable local authorities to discharge their functions relating to social services, education and public health.

It will be observed that under s. 26 (1) the Secretary of State has discretion whether or not to do any of the things he is there permitted to do. Under s. 26 (3) he is under a duty to make available to local authorities the services and facilities there referred to *so far as is reasonably necessary and practicable* to enable local authorities to discharge their functions relating to social services, education and public health.

For the purposes of s. 26 (1) (b) or (3) (b) or (c), the Secretary of State may give such directions to health authorities[3] to make the services of their officers available as he considers appropriate and it shall be the duty of a health authority[4] to comply with any such direction.[5] Terms for supply of goods and services etc., under s. 26 (1) and (3)[6] including financial terms are to be as may be agreed. In default

---

[1] Power to supply goods and materials includes necessary incidental powers of purchase, storage, arrangements with third parties etc. s. 27 (6). *Public bodies* includes public bodies in Northern Ireland s. 26 (1).

[2] '*Maintenance work*' includes minor renewals, minor improvements and minor extensions, s. 11 (9).

[3] See p. 45 footnote 2. *Health Authority* in ss. 23, 26, 27 and 28 does not include a preserved Board of Governors.

[4] Except in case of emergency, the Secretary of State before making the services of a person available under s. 26 (1) (b) or under s. 26 (3) (b) or (c) is under a duty of consultation with the officer or with a body recognised as representing the officer (S. 27 (1) and (2))

[5] S. 27 (3).

[6] And also under s. 26 (2) — supply of goods, materials and other facilities to persons providing general medical, dental or ophthalmic services or pharmaceutical services.

of agreement between the Secretary of State and the local authority as to charges to be made by the Secretary of State for services or facilities under s. 26 (3), i.e. services and facilities he is under a duty to provide, the matter will be determined by arbitration.[1]

The effect of the N.H.S. (Vehicles) Order 1974[2] is to make provision for N.H.S. vehicles made available for the use of any person, body or local authority to be exempted from the statutory requirements in respect of vehicle excise duty and third party insurance, provided that they are used in accordance with the terms under which they are made available.

(c) Supply etc. of goods, materials etc. to persons providing general medical, dental, ophthalmic or pharmaceutical services

Such goods, materials and other facilities as may be prescribed[3] may be provided for persons in the above categories.[4] The supply of goods, materials and other facilities under s. 26 (2), like provision under s. 26 (1) or (3) may be subject to charges under s. 27 (4) and to s. 27 (5) in respect of vehicles.

(d) Supply of goods and services by local authorities

Section 28 (1) of the 1977[5] Act allows local authorities to supply goods or services to any Health Authority and, so far as relates to his functions under the Health Service Acts to the Secretary of State. The section also provides for the variation or revocation of that authorisation by an order under s. 1 (5) of the Local Authorities (Goods and Services) Act 1970.

The making of services available to Health Authorities by local authorities is obligatory to the extent laid down in s. 12 (2) which reads:

(2) Every local authority shall make available to Health Authorities acting in the area of the local authority the services of persons employed by the local authority for the purposes of the authority's functions under the Local Authorities Social Services Act 1970 so far as is reasonably necessary and practicable to enable Health Authorities to discharge their functions under this Act.

The purpose of the sub-section is in the main to secure to the health service, particularly to hospitals, the continued availability of medical social workers and others who have been transferred to the employment of local authorities under the Act of 1970.

---

[1] S. 27 (4).
[2] S.I. 1974 No. 168, and see above, this chapter, section C.9
[3] *Prescribed* means prescribed by regulations (s. 128 (1)).
[4] See N.H.S. (Family Practitioner Committees: Supply of Goods) Regulations S.I. 1974 No. 191.
[5] Formerly s. 12 of the 1973 Act.

2. Voluntary Organisations and Other Bodies

(a) *Services under the National Health Service Act, provision of by voluntary and other bodies and persons*

Section 23 (1) of the 1977 Act[1] provides as follows:

23 (1) The Secretary of State may, where he considers it appropriate, arrange with any person or body (including a voluntary organisation)[2] for that person or body to provide, or assist in providing, any service under this Act.

(b) *Provision of facilities, including goods or materials, premises, vehicles etc., to persons and bodies providing services under s. 23 (1).*[3]

Section 23 (2) to (5) of the 1977 Act in effect authorises the provision of facilities, including goods or materials, or the use of any premises and of any vehicle, plant or apparatus and of persons in connection with anything made available, substantially, as to conditions on the lines of ss. 26–27.

3. Ancillary Services Provided on Behalf of the Secretary of State

Microbiological services, supplies of human blood and provision of other substances or preparations not readily obtainable may be provided by Health Authorities on behalf of the Secretary of State under ss. 5 (2) and 25 of the 1977 Act[4].

F. GENERAL MEDICAL, DENTAL, PHARMACEUTICAL AND GENERAL OPHTHALMIC SERVICES

It has been remarked above that the Area Health Authorities are the principal executive bodies in the reorganised health service. However, each of them is required[5] to establish a body to be called a Family Practitioner Committee. Subject to any special circumstances,[6] these Committees have 30 members[7] drawn from the Area Authority, the local authority and the local professional committees.[8] Like the Regional and Area Health Authorities, the Committees are corporations with perpetual succession and a common seal.[9]

By s. 15 (1) of the 1977 Act and Regulations each Family Practitioner Committee administers on behalf of the Area Authority the general

[1] Formerly s. 13 of the 1973 Act.
[2] *Voluntary organisation* in s. 23 means a body the activities of which are carried on otherwise than for profit, but does not include any public or local authority. (S. 23 (1).)
[3] S. 23 (3) to (5) also applies to any voluntary organisation eligible for assistance under s. 64 or s. 65 of the Health Services and Public Health Act 1968. (S. 23 (2) (b).)
[4] Formerly ss. 12 and 18 of the 1946 Act as amended.
[5] S. 10 of the 1977 Act. Formerly 1973 Act, s. 5 (5).
[6] 1977 Act, Sch. 5, Part II, para. 7.   [7] 1977 Act, Sch. 5, Part II, para. 6.
[8] See 1946 Act s. 32 as amended   [9] 1977 Act. Sch. 5. para. 8.

medical services, the general dental services, the general ophthalmic services and the pharmaceutical services for the area. Thus the Family Practitioner Committees have largely replaced the former Executive Councils. The 1946 Act dealt with the services in question in Part IV. Except to note that there have been minor amendments to Part IV[1] and that it is now to be found as Part II of the 1977 Act, further treatment of these matters are outside the scope of this book. It will also be noted that although the legal constitution has not been radically changed on the reorganisation, the total integration has caused substantial administrative changes to the work done in this field. Such matters are, however, even further beyond the scope of this book.

[1] See 1973 Act, Sch. 4.

CHAPTER 4

VOLUNTARY HOSPITALS

A. GOVERNING BODIES AND THEIR POWERS AND DUTIES

THE powers of a voluntary hospital governing body as well as the effect of acts apparently *ultra vires* depend on the constitution of the hospital, *e.g.*, Charter, memorandum and articles of association or trust deed. It is therefore proposed briefly to draw attention to the different types of constitution and their general effect but for a full exposition of the law relating to companies, statutory bodies, charitable trusts, etc., the reader must refer to standard works on these several subjects. Reference will, however, be made where relevant to the more important provisions of the Charities Act 1960.

Subject to what is said elsewhere in this book on the problem of responsibility for injuries to patients, it may be observed that a voluntary hospital authority, if a corporate body, is ordinarily responsible in law for loss or damage suffered by a third party as a result of the wrongful acts and omissions of its officers, employees or other persons acting on its behalf and with its authority. As to the position of the trustees or committee of an unincorporated voluntary hospital see sections A 5 and B 2 of this chapter.[1]

1. Chartered Hospitals

The general effect of the grant of a Royal Charter is to confer on the hospital the status of a corporate body which may hold land and other property and investments,[2] enter into contracts and sue and be sued in its corporate name. The members of the governing body of the hospital are under no personal liability otherwise than for any breach of trust to which they may be parties or for their own personal acts and omissions (*e.g.*, a surgeon who, being on the governing body, is negligent when operating on a patient in hospital).

A Royal Charter may be granted on petition to the Privy Council and usually provides for the making of bye-laws, also subject to the sanction of the Privy Council, the first bye-laws usually being annexed as a schedule to the Charter. Roughly, the Charter may be compared to the memorandum of association of a hospital incorporated under the

[1] P. 53 and p. 56.
[2] Apart from special powers, charity trustees cannot invest in land though under Charities Act 1960, the law of mortmain has disappeared. For range of authorised investments *see* Trustee Investments Act 1961.

Companies Act 1948, and the bye-laws to the articles of association, though it must be emphasised that the correspondence is not exact.

2. Hospitals Incorporated by Private Act of Parliament

The constitution, powers and functions of a hospital incorporated by Act of Parliament are all entirely governed by the relevant Act together with any bye-laws or rules properly made thereunder. A hospital so incorporated can hold land, investments and other property, make contracts and sue and be sued in its corporate name subject only to restrictions contained in the Act. The members of the governing body are usually free of any personal liability whatever in respect of the affairs of the corporation except as regards any breach of trust to which they may be parties, including any loss of trust property due to their personal negligence.

A few of the older hospitals, such as St. Bartholomew's and St. George's in London, had been incorporated by way of Act of Parliament for a very long time before being taken over by the Minister of Health in 1948, but these older statutes do not form very satisfactory precedents. More recent private Acts to which reference might usefully be made by anyone in search of precedents are the Birmingham United Hospitals Act 1934, the Liverpool United Hospital Act 1937, and the Royal Sheffield Infirmary and Hospital Act 1938.[1]

In any modern Act incorporating a charity the powers of the High Court and of the Charity Commissioners in respect of the charity are usually expressly preserved and power is also usually conferred on them to authorise amendments in the sanctioned scheme and bye-laws subject only to the over-riding provisions of the Act. Hence it should seldom be necessary to go back to Parliament for an amending Act. Further powers in relation to alteration of provisions of a private Act relating to an incorporated charity are conferred on the Charity Commissioners by s. 19 of the Charities Act 1960, which provides for amending schemes to be approved by resolution of both Houses of Parliament, this without going through the troublesome and expensive private bill procedure.

3. Hospitals Incorporated under the Companies Act 1948

Application under the Companies Act 1948, is now the simplest, cheapest and most expeditious way of obtaining the advantages of incorporation with limitation of the liability of the members and the most frequently adopted. A hospital so incorporated may take and hold land,[2] investments and other property, make contracts and sue

---

[1] As to repeal of these Acts see s. 77 of the National Health Service Act 1946. But see *re Kellner's Will Trusts* referred to on p. 86.

[2] Normally only for use — not for investment. See p. 77.

and be sued in its corporate name in the same manner as hospitals incorporated by Royal Charter or by special Act of Parliament.

Formation of a company limited by guarantee rather than one limited by shares is the method appropriate to a hospital or other charitable organisation, the subscribers to the memorandum, *i.e.*, those co-operating in the formation of the company, and all subsequent members of the company — often called 'governors' in the case of a voluntary hospital — undertaking to find a nominal amount, usually one pound, towards meeting any outstanding liabilities of the company on its being wound up.

It is desirable that the objects clause of the memorandum should be in the widest possible terms but there are certain limitations. For example, if it is an existing hospital which is being incorporated, the Charity Commissioners will have to be satisfied that the objects as set out do not allow the possibility of existing endowments and other trust funds being diverted from the purposes for which they were given or subscribed unless the circumstances are such that the commissioners authorise application *cy-près* under ss. 13 or 14 of the Charities Act 1960.[1] Moreover, if, as would ordinarily be the case, it were desired to obtain a Department of Trade licence to omit the word *limited* from the name of the incorporated body, a paragraph in terms approved by the Department would almost invariably have to be incorporated in the memorandum expressly forbidding the payment of dividends to members or fees or emoluments to members of governing bodies[2] and providing for the handing over of any surplus assets on liquidation to a similar charity or, if that is impossible, to some other charity selected by the members or by the Court. Such provisos would probably in any event be required by the Charity Commissioners who would need to be consulted in the preliminary stages. As regards the name used, it may be observed that even when — by licence of the Department of Trade — the word *limited* is omitted there is no obligation to substitute the word *incorporated* and so in the case of an unincorporated hospital that becomes incorporated the old name may be adopted unchanged, this subject only to s. 17 of the Companies Act 1948, which prevents the adoption of any name which, in the opinion of the Department of Trade, is undesirable.

4. Incorporation under the Charitable Trustees Incorporation Act 1872

So far as is known to the editor no hospital is incorporated by the Charity Commissioners under the Act of 1872. In fact the powers given

---

[1] See pp. 67–69.

[2] Payments to members of the governing body of an incorporated charity with licence to omit the word 'limited' from its title, are occasionally authorised for special reason and within strict limits.

by the Act are apparently never used since the benefits of such incorporation, without its disadvantages, are secured by vesting the charity property in the Official Custodian for Charities. The trustees of a charity, notwithstanding their incorporation under the Act of 1872 continue personally answerable for such property of the charity as comes into their hands and also for their own acts, receipts, neglects and defaults and for the due administration of the charity.[1]

5. Unincorporated Hospitals

Such unincorporated hospitals and similar institutions as may still exist will generally be carried on under the provisions of a trust deed providing for the responsibility of administering the trust to be exercised by a committee or board of management. The method of appointment of the committee, except in the case of certain hospitals carried on by religious orders, was at one time almost invariably by election by and from amongst the subscribers either generally or on a franchise restricted to, say, annual subscribers of a certain minimum amount who might be designated 'governors'. In the years immediately prior to the taking over of most of the voluntary hospitals by the Minister of Health in 1948, representatives of the medical staff, of contributory scheme subscribers, of local authorities and of other interests may be found to have been added. There cannot be said to be any prevailing pattern among surviving voluntary hospitals or among any which may have been established since 1948.

Unless transferred into the name of the Official Custodian for Charities as custodian trustee,[2] the real property and investments of an unincorporated hospital must ordinarily be held in the names of a small number of trustees, usually elected by the subscribers or governors unless the trust deed vests the powers of appointment in the committee of management or there are other provisions for their nomination. The trustees may themselves have discretionary power as to selection of investments within the limits laid down in the Trustee Investments Act 1961, or may be mere custodian trustees obliged to carry out the instructions of the committee of management so long as those instructions are in accordance with the provisions of the trust deed and are not otherwise contrary to law.

The essential disadvantages of an unincorporated hospital even with a well drawn trust deed are (i) that there is considerable trouble and expense when a trustee dies or resigns or when the removal of a trustee is imperative and a new trustee or trustees have to be appointed, (ii) that the absence from England or the illness of a trustee may create difficulties, (iii) that the extent of the personal liability of the members of

---

[1] Charitable Trustees Incorporation Act 1872, s. 5 and see also Tudor on Charities (6th Edn. 1967), p. 439.
[2] See p. 61.

the committee of management in respect of hospital affairs and even of members of the general body of subscribers who take an active interest by attending meetings for the election of members of the committee, etc., is by no means clear and could well be extremely onerous.

The first two disadvantages mentioned in the preceding paragraph are not absolutely inevitable, for it is possible to arrange both for real property and investments to be held by the official custodian for charities as custodian trustee. But the third disadvantage is one that can by no means be avoided, and it is not possible to say dogmatically that the personal liability of the members of the committee of management would in all circumstances be limited to the amount of the charity funds under their control. For example, if the committee were sued in respect of negligence in their management of hospital affairs leading to loss or injury to a patient, *e.g.*, negligent appointment of an incompetent or unqualified medical practitioner to the staff, they might be personally liable in damages.

There have in the past been in existence a few unincorporated charitable hospitals not having a constitution embodied in a trust deed. Probably none survived the coming into operation of the National Health Service Act 1946. In such cases there may have been a set of rules, possibly adopted at a meeting of subscribers or by a meeting of local residents. The rules will certainly have provided for some sort of committee of management and there must have been trustees of property and investments.

6. Hospitals administered under a Scheme established by the Court or the Charity Commissioners

In any of the circumstances set out in ss. 13 and 14 of the Charities Act 1960, the Court or the Charity Commissioners or, in the case of an educational charity, the Secretary of State for Education and Science may make a scheme for the administration of a charity. This matter is more fully discussed on pp. 67 *et seq.*

7. Effect of Health Service Acts on Voluntary Hospitals

As from July 5th, 1948,[1] all existing voluntary hospitals other than such as may have been excluded by the Minister of Health under s. 6 (3) of the 1946 Act, were transferred to the Minister and placed under the control of governing bodies constituted in accordance with the provisions of the Act. By s. 78 (1) (c) of the Act, the governing bodies of the voluntary hospitals so transferred, *whose functions wholly ceased in consequence of the passing of the Act*, were dissolved as from the appointed day, the Minister being empowered to make any necessary regula-

---

[1] N.H.S. (Appointed Day) Order S.I. 1948 No. 112.

tions for the winding up of their affairs.[1] The N.H.S. Act 1977 Schedule 14 paragraph 6[2] provides for the case of a hospital constituted or whose affairs are regulated under a private Act or charter, the Secretary of State being given power by order to alter, amend or repeal such provisions of the private Act or charter as may be inconsistent with those of the National Health Service Act 1946.

Any voluntary hospitals not taken over under the Act on the appointed day retained their existing constitution. The law relating to such hospitals and to any new voluntary hospitals is unaffected by the Acts.

A transferred hospital still remains a charity, as to which see p. 86 *et seq.* For a discussion of the position of charitable corporations which formerly owned hospitals transferred to the Secretary of State under the Act of 1946, reference may be made to *re Kellner's Will Trusts.*[3]

B. POWERS OF VOLUNTARY HOSPITALS[4]

1. Limits of Powers of Incorporated Hospitals

The general outline of the powers of voluntary hospital governing bodies has already of necessity been given above in outlining the various possible constitutions of such hospitals. The general powers of a hospital incorporated by Royal Charter or by Act of Parliament are to be found in the Charter or Act and detailed rules of procedure in bye-laws, rules or regulations made thereunder. In the case of a hospital incorporated under the Companies Acts, the memorandum of association indicates the limits of the powers of the incorporated body by defining its objects and the articles of association the detailed rules of procedure. The Companies Acts contain provisions regarding meetings, audit and also as to annual and other returns to the registrar of companies.[5]

(a) Acts in Excess of Powers

If a chartered hospital does anything which is outside the objects of powers specified in its Charter, such acts would not apparently, *ipso facto*, be invalid, but would constitute grounds for revocation of the Charter. Futhermore, if such abuse of power amounted to a use or trust funds for objects other than those for which they had been provided, members of the governing body would seemingly be personally liable to make restitution.

Generally speaking, if the board of a hospital incorporated otherwise than by Royal Charter acts outside the limits of the objects of the

[1] See also N.H.S. (Dissolved Authorities) Regulations S.I. 1948 No. 1292.
[2] Formerly 1946 Act s. 77.   [3] [1949] 2 All E. R. 774; 65 T. L. R. 695. See further p. 86.
[4] See separate heads as to loans and overdrafts, dealings with land and investments.
[5] For further information on the various types of incorporation see Part A of this chapter.

incorporated body as set out in the special Act or in the memorandum of association, the wrongful act is invalid and is incapable of ratification. If, however, an act done is not *ultra vires* the corporation or company but exceeds the powers delegated to the board it is still invalid but is usually capable of ratification by a general meeting of governors or other body to which the board is responsible.

(b) Indemnity for Board Members

If the members of the board of an incorporated hospital exceed their powers and a third party suffers loss thereby they may find themselves personally liable on the ground of breach of warranty of authority, though with exercise of ordinary prudence this risk is far more remote than the risk of personal liability for a possibly technical breach of trust. However, in the case of modern incorporations by special Act the scheduled scheme usually gives blanket cover against personal liability for purely technical breaches of trust as in the case of the paragraph 30 of the scheme annexed as a schedule to the Royal Sheffield Infirmary and Hospital Act 1938,[1] which read as follows:

No matter or thing done and no contract entered into by the court and no matter or thing done by any member of the court acting under the direction of the court shall if the matter or thing be done or the contract be entered into *bona fide* for the purposes of the Hospital subject any member of the court personally to any action liability claim or demand whatsoever and any expense incurred *bona fide* for the purposes of the Hospital by the court shall be borne and repaid out of the funds of the Hospital.

Similar cover for reasonable actions in the course of carrying out their duties is usually given by the articles to members of the board of a hospital incorporated under the Companies Acts. Such cover does not confer the same immunity as when embodied in a special Act for there is always inserted a clause in the memorandum of association saving the jurisdiction of the Court and of the Charity Commissioners and reserving the personal liability of the managers and trustees of the hospital as answerable for their own acts, receipts, neglects and defaults, *and for the due administration of its property* in the same manner and to the same extent as they would have been had there been no incorporation. The words in italics apparently preserve the full liability of the board as trustees subject always to the power of the Court to excuse a breach of trust under s. 61 of the Trustee Act 1925.

2. Powers of Unincorporated Hospitals

(a) Limits on the Powers

The powers of the trustees or committee of management of an unincorporated hospital are strictly limited by the terms of the trust

---

[1] Now repealed.

deed,[1] if any, and except so far as expressly therein duly varied, under the provisions of the Charities Act 1960.

(b) Indemnity for Trustees and Committee

Trustees of unincorporated charities as well as persons concerned with administration of an incorporated charity may in respect of any breach of trust apply to the Court to be relieved of personal liability under the provisions of s. 61 of the Trustee Act 1925, on the grounds that they have acted honestly reasonably and ought fairly to be excused and the Court may make an order relieving them wholly or partly of personal liability. If, however, charity trustees[2] have doubt of the lawfulness of any action they propose to take and they act on the advice of the Charity Commissioners given under s. 24 of the Charities Act, 1960, they are protected against any personal liability.[3]

C. LOANS AND OVERDRAFTS

The borrowing power of voluntary hospitals varies according to the constitution. Voluntary hospitals incorporated by Act of Parliament in modern times frequently had unrestricted borrowing powers coupled with correspondingly wide powers of pledging hospital property as security e.g., Birmingham United Hospital Act, 1934, s. 8 (9).[4]

Similarly wide powers were apparently contained in modern charters as in that of the General Infirmary at Leeds,[5] though in that case it may possibly be implied that funds raised by mortgage or sale of real property or other capital assets could be used only for capital expenditure. This view is borne out by the additional power expressly conferred to 'Borrow temporarily from the Corporation's bankers or otherwise as the Board may think expedient for the purpose of meeting current expenses'.

Apparently unlimited borrowing powers including the right to secure the loan on hospital property or investments is usually taken in the memorandum of a hospital incorporated under the Companies Act 1948, but these apparently unlimited powers will ordinarily be found of be limited by a standard proviso on the following lines:

Provided that in case the Hospital shall take or hold any property subject to the jurisdiction of the Charity Commissioners for England and Wales or the Secretary of State for Education and Science, the Hospital shall not sell,

---

[1] It is beyond the scope of this work to discuss the position where there is no trust deed nor other written constitution; reference may be made, however, to pp. 67–69 as to the powers of the Charity Commissioners to make a scheme for such a charity.

[2] For definition of expression *charity trustees* see p. 62.

[3] See further p. 67 where also is mentioned the power of the commissioners under s. 23 to sanction action otherwise outside the powers of the trustees.

[4] Now repealed.

[5] No longer operative.

mortgage, charge or lease the same without such authority, approval or consent as may be required by law, and as regards any such property the Managers or Trustees of the Hospital shall be chargeable for such property as may come into their hands, and shall be answerable and accountable for their own acts, receipts, neglects and defaults, and for the due administration of such property in the same manner and to the same extent as they would as such Managers and Trustees have been if no incorporation had been effected and the incorporation of the Hospital shall not diminish or impair any control or authority exercisable by the Chancery Division, the Charity Commissioners or the Secretary of State for Education and Science over such Managers or Trustees, but they shall as regards such property, be subject jointly and severally to such control or authority as if the Hospital were not incorporated. In case the Hospital shall take or hold any property which may be subject to any trusts, the Hospital shall only deal with the same in such manner as allowed by law, having regard to such trusts.

The general effect of such a proviso, apart from preserving the personal responsibility of members of the board and others dealing with the hospital property, is to make dealings, whether by way of sale, mortgage, exchange or otherwise, with real property (*i.e.*, land and buildings) being *permanent endowments*[1] of the hospital subject to consent of the Charity Commissioners or of the Court or, in the case of an educational charity (*e.g.*, a medical school or, possibly, a nurses' training school), of the Secretary of State for Education and Science.

Furthermore, the powers of any charity other than an exempt or an excepted charity[2] to borrow money against property forming part of the permanent endowment,[1] or to deal with land, whether part of its permanent endowment or not, are subject to the provisions of s. 29 of the Charities Act 1960, reading as follows:

(1) Subject to the exceptions provided for by this section, no property forming part of the permanent endowment of a charity shall, without an order of the court or of the Commissioners, be mortgaged or charged by way of security for the repayment of money borrowed, nor, in the case of land in England or Wales, be sold, leased or otherwise disposed of.

(2) Subsection (1) above shall apply to any land which is held by or in trust for a charity and is or has at any time been occupied for the purposes of the charity, as it applies to land forming part of the permanent endowment of a charity; but a transaction for which the sanction of an order under subsection (1) above is required by virtue only of this subsection shall, notwithstanding that it is entered into without such an order, be valid in favour of a person who (then or afterwards) in good faith acquires an interest in or charge on the land for money or money's worth.

(3) This section shall apply notwithstanding anything in the trusts of a charity, but shall not require the sanction of an order —

(a) for any transaction for which general or special authority is expressly given (without the authority being made subject to the sanction of

[1] For the definition of *permanent endowment* see p. 64 and p. 94.
[2] See Charities Act 1960 s, 4 and s. 29 (4).

an order) by any statutory provision contained in or having effect under an Act of Parliament or by any scheme legally established; or

(b) for the granting of a lease for a term ending not more than twenty-two years after it is granted, not being a lease granted wholly or partly in consideration of a fine; or

(c) for any disposition of an advowson.

(4) This section shall not apply to an exempt charity, nor to any charity which is excepted by order or regulations.

Unless specifically authorised by the terms of the trust the use as income of a loan raised on the security of permanent endowments is invalid no less than similar use of the proceeds of realisation of investments comprising part of such endowments.

If there is any doubt as to the validity of borrowing powers which it is desired to exercise, the advice of the Charity Commissioners under s. 24 of the Charities Act 1960 should be sought.[1]

[1] As to the measure of cover afforded to trustees acting on such advice, see p. 67.

CHAPTER 5

THE CHARITY COMMISSIONERS AND CHARITY TRUSTEES

In previous chapters reference has been made to specific duties of charity trustees and to particular powers of the Charity Commissioners. In this chapter it is proposed to outline other duties and powers of both so far as is of immediate importance and not dealt with elsewhere.

This outline has been prepared primarily from the point of view of trustees and governing bodies of voluntary hospitals and of authorities constituted under the National Health Service Act 1977, administering property for charitable purposes. But, subject to any statutory exemption, the same rules apply to all charity trustees, including for example, leagues of hospitals friends established for helping local hospitals and also the National League of Hospital Friends to which most local leagues are affiliated, though they are quite independent of it.[1]

A. THE CHARITY COMMISSIONERS

1. Constitution and General Powers

The Charity Commissioners were first constituted under the Charitable Trusts Act 1853, now repealed. By s. 1 and the First Schedule of the Charities Act 1960 they now exercise the wider powers given to them under that Act, and have the general function of promoting the effective use of charitable resources by encouraging the development of better methods of administration, by giving charity trustees information or advice on any matter affecting the charity and by investigating and checking abuses.[2] They have also been vested with ample powers to appoint and remove charity trustees in case of need but are expressly prohibited from themselves administering a charity.[3]

The Secretary of State for Education and Science has powers concurrent with those of the Charity Commissioners for use particularly in respect of educational charities.[4]

---

[1] Another example is that of the student's union at a medical school. In *London Hospital Medical College* v. I.R.C. [1976] 2 All E.R. 113 it was held that the union was charitable because its purpose was to advance the purposes of the medical school which was itself charitable.

[2] S. 1 (3) of the 1960 Act.

[3] S. 1 (4).

[4] S. 2.

2. Relations generally between the Charity Commissioners and Charities: Registration

A distinction is to be made between charities obliged to be registered by the Charity Commissioners under s. 4 of the Charities Act 1960 and those not so obliged. Whilst it is true that exempt charities[1] are not subject to inquiry[2] or audit[3] at the instance of the Commissioners, all other charities, even charities excepted from registration,[4] are subject to the jurisdiction of the Commissioners. All charities, including exempt charities,[1] may have recourse to the help of the Commissioners, e.g. by seeking the protection of their advice under s. 24 of the Act.

In some matters the powers of the Court and the Charity Commissioners or the Secretary of State for Education and Science are concurrent and, generally, any order of the Commissioners or of the Secretary of State may be subject of appeal to the High Court, as specifically provided for in various sections of the Act.

Neither voluntary hospitals as a class, nor N.H.S. hospitals[5] are exempt charities,[1] nor are they excepted from registration under s. 4 of the Act. To voluntary hospitals in particular registration is, in fact, an advantage, for so long as a charity is registered, it is recognised for all purposes as a charity.[6] Appeal to the High Court against any decision of the Commissioners to enter or not to enter an institution on the register of charities or to remove or not to remove it therefrom, is provided for in s. 5 (2).

3. The Official Custodian for Charities

The responsibility for acting on request as custodian trustee of charity property, real and personal, subject to the provisions of the Charities Act 1960, is placed on the official custodian for charities, a corporation sole with perpetual succession[7] who replaces the official trustee of charity lands and the official trustee of charity funds. Ss. 16 and 17 of the Act of 1960 deal with matters relating to the entrusting of property to the official custodian for charities.

[1] S. 4 (4) (a) and 2nd Schedule.　　　　　　　[2] S. 6.
[3] S.8.
[4] S.4 (2) (4) (b) (c).
[5] But N.H.S. hospitals do not have to send their accounts to the charity commissioners annually under s. 8 (1), being excepted therefrom, as to which see p. 29. For the position of N.H.S. hospitals generally under the Charities Act 1960, reference may be made to departmental circular H.M. (61) 74. In that circular it is also indicated that an understanding has been reached between the Secretary of State for Social Services and the Charity Commissioners to avoid any clash of jurisdiction where there are concurrent powers, e.g. of inquiry and of dismissal.
[6] An unregistered but registrable charity whose objects do not change is a charity for the purpose of s. 5 of the 1960 Act and is accordingly eligible to receive a gift made before it registers re Murawski's W. T., Lloyds Bank Ltd. v. R.S.P.C.A. [1971] 1 W.L.R. 707; [1971] 2 All E.R. 328.
[7] Charities Act 1960 s. 3.

B. VISITORS

In the case of an endowed, incorporated charity the founder and his heirs or the person nominated by him became *visitor* with the right to regulate all the internal affairs of the charity, *e.g.*, disputes as to elections, appointment of officers, etc., but this did not oust the jurisdiction of the court and the Charity Commissioners in respect of proper application of trust property. When there is no other visitor of a charitable corporation the jurisdiction is vested in the Crown either through the Lord Chancellor, the court or the Charity Commissioners. The rules regarding extent and exercise of visitorial jurisdiction are complex and obscure but, fortunately, are not likely to be of great practical importance except possibly in the case of a few old foundations, and even in some of those cases visitorial jurisdiction other than of the court or of the Charity Commissioners may be excluded by virtue of a Charter or special Act of Parliament.

C. CHARITY TRUSTEES

1. Who are Charity Trustees?

By s. 46 of the Charities Act 1960, the expression *charity trustee* is defined as meaning 'the person having the general control and management of the administration of a charity' which in turn is defined so as to include a corporate body. The Act is in such terms as generally to make such trustees personally responsible for any breach of trust. Consequently, the responsibilities and liabilities of a trustee generally fall upon any person undertaking the administration of charity funds by whatever name he may be called though, particularly in the case of some older hospitals incorporated by special Act or Charter, there may have been some modifications or exceptions.[1] Generally, however, it is prudent to assume that even in the case of an incorporated hospital the full liabilities of trustees in respect of the administration of its property fall upon the members of the governing body. Indeed, in the case of hospitals incorporated under the Companies Act 1948, the personal responsibility of members of the board is now invariably expressly preserved in the memorandum of association.[2] Also, when, as frequently happens in the case of an unincorporated hospital, there are trustees so-called in whose name investments are made and there is also a committee of management, the members of the latter body, no less than the trustees so-called, have the full responsibilities and liabilities of trustees in respect of the functions entrusted to them.

In some pre-1974 trust instruments, reference is made to bodies which

---

[1] As to such exceptions see Chapter 4.
[2] See p. 56.

were abolished by the 1973 N.H.S. Re-organisation Act. In particular some charity trustees of charities which were not incorporated under the Companies Acts (or by charter) or were defined by reference to offices held on Regional Hospital Boards or a Board of Governors.

Under the N.H.S. (Amendment of Trust Instruments) Order 1974[1] such references are now to the Regional Health Authority, the Area Health Authority etc. The Order does not affect the preserved Boards.[2] Nor does it affect the trusts themselves so that although the trustees may now be defined by reference to the region or area, the trusts remain as they were affecting only the same purposes as they did before the re-organisation.

2. General Duties of Trustees

In general terms it may be said that a person in the position of a trustee or member of a health authority or the board of management of a hospital avoids all personal liability if he attends with due diligence to the affairs of the trust he has undertaken; if he approves only investments authorised by or under the Trustee Investments Act 1961 or expressly authorised by the trust instrument; if he sees that trust property is not left unreasonably under the control of any fellow trustee or any agent; if he sees that trust funds are spent only on authorised objects,[3] any necessary consents being duly obtained; if he accepts no personal remuneration or profit out of trust funds except as expressly authorised by the trust instrument;[4] and, above all, if he sees to it scrupulously that he does not allow himself to get into a position in which his own interests and those of the trust are, or may be, at variance.

3. Accounts and Inquiries

In s. 32 of the Charities Act 1960, it is provided that charity trustees must keep proper books of account with respect to the affairs of the charity, and if not required by or under the authority of any other Act to prepare periodical statements of account must prepare consecutive statements of account consisting on each occasion of an income and expenditure account relating to a period of not more than fifteen months, and a balance sheet to the end of that period.

A hospital incorporated under the Companies Act 1948, is required to keep proper books and prepare accounts under the provisions of that Act. Similarly, health and hospital authorities under the National Health

---

[1] S.I. 1974 No. 63. See also the 1977 Act ss. 91 and 93 (formerly 1973 Act ss. 22 and 27) and H.R.C. (74) 10.
[2] See pp. 15–16.
[3] As to variation of trusts under ss. 13 and 14 of the Charities Act 1960, when the original terms of the trust cannot be carried out or, for good reason, it is desired to vary them, see pp. 67–69.
[4] See further, pp. 77–78.

Service Act 1977, are under a like obligation by s. 98 (1) of the 1977 Act, and of directions given thereunder.[1]

The books of account and statements of account relating to any charity must be preserved for a period of seven years at least, unless the charity ceases to exist and the Charity Commissioners permit them to be destroyed or otherwise disposed of.[2] It must be appreciated however that records and accounts of authorities under the National Health Service Act 1977 may be destroyed or disposed of only in accordance with the provisions of the Public Records Act 1958.[3]

Statements of account giving the prescribed information about the affairs of a charity must be transmitted to the Commissioners by the charity trustees on request; and in the case of a charity having a permanent endowment such a statement relating to the permanent endowment is to be transmitted yearly without any request, unless the charity is excepted by order or regulations.[4] Subject to s. 22 (9) relating to common investment funds, a charity is deemed for the purposes of the Charities Act 1960, to have a permanent endowment unless all property held for the purposes of the charity may be expended for those purposes without distinction between capital and income, and, in the Act, 'permanent endowment' means, in relation to any charity, property held subject to a restriction on its being so expended.[5]

It seems most unlikely that any voluntary hospital would not have permanent endowments as so defined and hardly more likely that any health or hospital authority under the National Health Service Act 1977 would escape that net if not an excepted charity.[6] Most, if not all voluntary hospitals, are therefore, under the duty of making annual returns to the Commissioners. Those returns will be open to public inspection so long as retained by the Commissioners.[7]

The Commissioners under s. 8 (3) of the Charities Act 1960, may by order require that the condition and accounts of any charity for such period as they think fit be investigated and audited by an auditor possessing one of the qualifications laid down in the Act and appointed by them.

Under s. 7 the Commissioners may by order require any person having in his possession or control any books, records, deeds or papers relating to a charity — other than an exempt charity[8] — to furnish them with copies of or extracts from any of those documents or, unless the document forms part of the records or other documents of a court or

---

[1] Formerly s. 55 (2) of the 1946 Act N.H.S. Financial (No. 2) Regs. S.I. 1974 No. 541 and Direction accompanying circular H.M. (69) 93.

[2] Charities Act 1960, s. 32 (2).

[3] See further p. 340 et seq.

[4] S. 8 (1). By the Charities (Excepted Accounts) Regulations S.I. 1976 No. 929 and S.I. 1963 No. 210 Charities administered by the new health authorities preserved Boards are exempted charities for the purpose of s. 8 (8).

[5] Ss. 45 (3) and 46.

[6] See p. 61, footnote 5.   [7] S. 8 (2).

[8] S. 7 (3). Exempt means exempt from registration under s. 4 (4) (a).

of a public or local authority, require him to transmit the document itself to them for their inspection.

By s. 6 the Commissioners may from time to time institute inquiries with regard to charities or a particular charity or class of charities, either generally or for particular purposes. Ample provision is made for the effectiveness of any such inquiry including compulsory attendance of persons whose evidence is required and for the taking of evidence on oath.

4. Notice of Charity Meetings

S. 33 of the Charities Act 1960, provides:

(1) All notices which are required or authorised by the trustees of a charity to be given to a charity trustee, member or subscriber may be sent by post and, if sent by post, may be addressed to any address given as his in the list of charity trustees, members or subscribers for the time being in use at the office or principal office of the charity.

(2) Where any such notice required to be given as aforesaid is given by post, it shall be deemed to have been given by the time at which the letter containing it would be delivered in the ordinary course of post.

(3) No notice required to be given as aforesaid of any meeting or election need be given to any charity trustee, member or subscriber, if in the list above-mentioned he has no address in the United Kingdom.

These provisions would presumably not apply to an incorporated charity whether by Royal Charter, Act of Parliament or under the Companies Act 1948. Nor are they relevant to a health or hospital authority under the National Health Service Act 1977.

5. Manner of Executing Instruments

S. 34 of the Charities Act 1960, provides as follows:

34.—(1) Charity trustees may, subject to the trusts of the charity, confer on any of their body (not being less than two in number) a general authority, or an authority limited in such manner as the trustees think fit, to execute in the names and on behalf of the trustees assurances or other deeds or instruments for giving effect to transactions to which the trustees are a party; and any deed or instrument executed in pursuance of an authority so given shall be of the same effect as if executed by the whole body.

(2) An authority under subsection (1) above —
    (a) shall suffice for any deed or instrument if it is given in writing or by resolution of a meeting of the trustees, notwithstanding the want of any formality that would be required in giving an authority apart from that subsection;
    (b) may be given so as to make the powers conferred exercisable by any of the trustees, or may be restricted to named persons or in any other way;
    (c) subject to any such restriction, and until it is revoked, shall, notwithstanding any change in the charity trustees, have effect as a continuing authority given by and to the persons who from time to time are of their body.

(3) In any authority under this section to execute a deed or instrument in the names and on behalf of charity trustees there shall, unless the contrary intention appears, be implied authority also to execute it for them in the name and on behalf of the official custodian for charities or of any other person, in any case in which the charity trustees could do so.

(4) Where a deed or instrument purports to be executed in pursuance of this section, then in favour of a person who (then or afterwards) in good faith acquires for money or money's worth an interest in or charge on property or the benefit of any covenant or agreement expressed to be entered into by the charity trustees, it shall be conclusively presumed to have been duly executed by virtue of this section.

(5) The powers conferred by this section shall be in addition to and not in derogation of any other powers.

It would appear that this section has no relevance to incorporated charities.

6. Employment of Agents

The greatest safeguard charity trustees have against being held liable for financial loss to the trust due to unauthorised or ill-advised investment, or to misappropriation or mismanagement of the trust property is by employing suitably qualified agents and advisers — solicitors, bankers, surveyors, stockbrokers and others — according to the needs of the case, though it must be remembered that the employment of agents in no degree excuses them from personal attention to the affairs of the charity.[1] Furthermore if an agent, other than a banker, is allowed to retain under his control for an unreasonable time trust property, such as the proceeds of the sale of investments, the trustees or board members may be held personally responsible for any loss due to the agent's fraud or bankruptcy. The occasions when advice should be obtained in respect of investments, and from whom it should be obtained, are matters dealt with in the Trustee Investments Act 1961.

7. Precautions against Misapplication of Trust Funds

Perhaps the gravest risk run by charity trustees is in respect of innocent misapplication of trust funds to objects not within the terms of the trust, and in this connection it must be remembered that rarely, if ever, can the terms of a trust be varied except for good cause and then with the consent either of the Court or of the Charity Commissioners.[2] If, therefore, the governing body of a hospital is not absolutely certain that a proposed use of trust funds or other property is strictly within the terms of the trust they should not embark on such course of action without legal advice. And unless that advice is clearly in favour of or

---

[1] As to the personal obligations of a trustee and, in particular, the degree of diligence he is expected to exercise, see Snell's *Principles of Equity*, 26th Edition, pp. 221 *et seq.* and cases there referred to.

[2] Or, in the case of an educational charity, the Secretary of State for Education and Science.

against the course proposed, the governing body should seek the advice of the Charity Commissioners under s. 24 of the Charities Act 1960, for upon such advice being given any charity trustee or trustee for the charity acting upon it is deemed to have acted in accordance with the terms of the trust and is relieved from any personal liability should a breach of trust in fact have been committed unless he knew or had reasonable cause to suspect that the opinion or advice was given in ignorance of material facts; or the decision of the Court had been obtained on the matter or proceedings were pending to obtain one.[1]

Under s. 23 the Charity Commissioners also have power to sanction action proposed by the trustees, being action expedient in the interests of the charity, although that action would not otherwise be within the powers of the trustees.

8. Application of Property cy-près

The Court or the Charity Commissioners or the Secretary of State may, on application, make a scheme superseding to the extent stated the trust deed or other instrument under which a charity has been carried on. The grounds on which this may be done are now set out in ss. 13 and 14 of the Charities Act 1960. Ss. 15 and 19 provide a simplified procedure for altering charitable trusts established by Royal Charter or Act of Parliament. Ss. 16 to 21 also refer. Ss. 13 and 14 of the Act provide:

13.—(1) Subject to subsection (2) below, the circumstances in which the original purposes of a charitable gift can be altered to allow the property given or part of it to be applied cy-près shall be as follows:
    (*a*) where the original purposes, in whole or in part,
        (i) have been as far as may be fulfilled; or
        (ii) cannot be carried out, or not according to the directions given and to the spirit of the gift; or
    (*b*) where the original purposes provide a use for part only of the property available by virtue of the gift; or
    (*c*) where the property available by virtue of the gift and other property applicable for similar purposes can be more effectively used in conjunction, and to that end can suitably, regard being had to the spirit of the gift, be made applicable to common purposes; or
    (*d*) where the original purposes were laid down by reference to an area which then was but has since ceased to be a unit for some other purpose, or by reference to a class of persons or to an area which has for any reason since ceased to be suitable, regard being had to the spirit of the gift, or to be practical in administering the gift; or
    (*e*) where the original purposes, in whole or in part, have, since they were laid down,
        (i) been adequately provided for by other means; or
        (ii) ceased, as being useless or harmful to the community or for other reasons, to be in law charitable; or

[1] S. 24 (2).

(iii) ceased in any other way to provide a suitable and effective method of using the property available by virtue of the gift, regard being had to the spirit of the gift.

(2) Subsection (1) above shall not affect the conditions which must be satisfied in order that property given for charitable purposes may be applied cy-près, except in so far as those conditions require a failure of the original purposes.

(3) References in the foregoing subsections to the original purposes of a gift shall be construed, where the application of the property given has been altered or regulated by a scheme or otherwise, as referring to the purposes for which the property is for the time being applicable.

(4) Without prejudice to the power to make schemes in circumstances falling within subsection (1) above, the court may by scheme made under the court's jurisdiction with respect to charities, in any case where the purposes for which the property is held are laid down by reference to any such area as is mentioned in the first column in the Third Schedule to this Act, provide for enlarging the area to any such area as is mentioned in the second column in the same entry in that Schedule.

(5) It is hereby declared that a trust for charitable purposes places a trustee under a duty, where the case permits and requires the property or some part of it to be applied *cy-près*, to secure its effective use for charity by taking steps to enable it to be so applied.

14.—(1) Property given for specific charitable purposes which fail shall be applicable cy-près as if given for charitable purposes generally, where it belongs —

(*a*) to a donor who, after such advertisements and inquiries as are reasonable, cannot be identified or cannot be found; or

(*b*) to a donor who has executed a written disclaimer of his right to have the property returned.

(2) For the purposes of this section property shall be conclusively presumed (without any advertisement or inquiry) to belong to donors who cannot be identified, in so far as it consists —

(*a*) of the proceeds of cash collections made by means of collecting boxes or by other means not adapted for distinguishing one gift from another; or

(*b*) of the proceeds of any lottery, competition, entertainment, sale or similar money-raising activity, after allowing for property given to provide prizes or articles for sale or otherwise to enable the activity to be undertaken.

(3) The court may by order direct that property not falling within subsection (2) above shall for the purposes of this section be treated (without any advertisement or inquiry) as belonging to donors who cannot be identified, where it appears to the court either —

(*a*) that it would be unreasonable, having regard to the amounts likely to be returned to the donors, to incur expense with a view to returning the property; or

(*b*) that it would be unreasonable, having regard to the nature, circumstances and amounts of the gifts, and to the lapse of time since the gifts were made, for the donors to expect the property to be returned.

(4) Where property is applied cy-près by virtue of this section, the donor

shall be deemed to have parted with all his interest at the time when the gift was made; but where property is so applied as belonging to donors who cannot be identified or cannot be found, and is not so applied by virtue of subsection (2) or (3) above —

    (*a*) the scheme shall specify the total amount of that property; and

    (*b*) the donor of any part of that amount shall be entitled, if he makes a claim not later than twelve months after the date on which the scheme is made, to recover from the charity for which the property is applied a sum equal to that part, less any expenses properly incurred by the charity trustees after that date in connection with claims relating to his gift; and

    (*c*) the scheme may include directions as to the provision to be made for meeting any such claim.

(5) For the purposes of this section, charitable purposes shall be deemed to 'fail' where any difficulty in applying property to those purposes makes that property or the part not applicable cy-près available to be returned to the donors.

(6) In this section, except in so far as the context otherwise requires, references to a donor include persons claiming through or under the original donor, and references to property given include the property for the time being representing the property originally given or property derived from it.

(7) This section shall apply to property given for charitable purposes, notwithstanding that it was so given before the commencement of this Act.

S. 14 provides for the kind of difficulties which arose in *re Hillier's Trusts, Hillier and Another* v. *Attorney-General and Another*,[1] and in *re Ulverston District New Hospital Building Fund*.[2]

If application for variation of a trust has to be made, it is generally advisable on grounds of economy and expedition to make such application to the Charity Commissioners rather than to the Court unless there is special reason to the contrary.

The proper person to make application to the Charity Commissioners for a scheme is the charity itself as defined in s. 45.[3] But as to application to the Court reference should be had to s. 28 under which proceedings may be commenced by the charity, by any of the charity trustees, or by any person interested in the charity, or by any two or more inhabitants of the area of the charity, if it is a local charity, but not by any other person[4] other than the Attorney-General with or without a relator.[5] Except when proceedings are brought by the Attorney-General the consent of the Charity Commissioners is required.[6]

Further reference is made at pp. 80 and 82 *et seq.* and also in Chapter 3 to the position of authorities established by the National Health Service Act 1977 as charity trustees.

---

[1] [1954] 1 W.L.R. 700.

[2] [1956] Ch. 622; [1956] 3 All E.R. 164. It does not however cover the difficulties found in *re Gillingham Bus Disaster Fund* [1959] Ch. 62; [1958] 2 All E.R. 749 where money was collected from a benevolent public for what were eventually held to be non-charitable purposes.

[3] S. 18 (4).   [4] S. 28 (1).   [5] S. 28 (6).   [6] S. 28 (2).

9. Gifts to Hospitals by Will or from a Trust Fund

Our purpose here is not to explore in any detail the law of wills, nor even the law generally relating to charitable bequests and kindred matters, but simply to discuss difficulties which have arisen in respect of testamentary gifts to charitable hospitals and gifts from discretionary funds established by will, this in light of the relevant decisions of the courts.

(a) Gifts by Will
(i) Misdescription

In spite of the great pains charitable hospitals are at to acquaint would-be benefactors with their proper names and to suggest a convenient form of words for a legacy, misdescription is still a serious source of trouble. One of the most notable instances was that in which a testator left a legacy to 'Westminster Hospital, Charing Cross' when it was decided on the particular facts of the case that the gift should go to Charing Cross Hospital.[1] Similarly, 'King's Cross Hospital' has been taken to mean 'Great Northern Hospital, King's Cross'.[2] Generally, in such cases, the court will take into account any reliable evidence which may be available to indicate the testator's interest in a particular hospital. If as between two hospitals doubt cannot be removed, the legacy may be divided — not necessarily in equal shares — or one may take the whole if the other assent. Reference may also be made to re Nesbitt deceased, Dr. Barnardo's Home v. Board of Governors of United Newcastle on Tyne Hospital,[3] in which case an earlier will was admitted to identify a hospital which had been misdescribed.

(ii) Vague description or expression of charitable intention — Application of cy près doctrine

Sometimes the testator's mode of expressing himself may be so vague or his bequest in such general terms that it is not practicable to identify the particular institution he intends to benefit; or, even if the testator's intention is certain, it may be manifestly impossible to carry it out; or the institution he names may have ceased to exist, or it may have amalgamated with another before the testator's death. In these and certain analogous cases, if there is a general over-riding charitable intention, the court will give effect as nearly as possible (cy près) to the testator's wishes and, if necessary, will order a scheme to be prepared.[4]

---

[1] *Bradshaw* v. *Thompson* (1843), 2 Y & C. C. C. 295.
[2] *Re Lycett* (1897), 13 T. L. R. 373.
[3] [1953] 1 W.L.R. 595.
[4] Thus is *Ballingall's Judicial Factor* v. *Hamilton* 1973 S.L.T. 236 (Ct. of Sess.) the residue of the deceased's estate was to be divided equally between 'heart diseases and cancer research'. It was held that there was an intention to benefit charitable organisations dealing with treatment and research in the fields and that accordingly a scheme could be drawn up.

In *re Smith (deceased)*; *Barclays Bank Limited* v. *Mercantile Bank Limited*[1] the testator, who made his will in 1931 and died in 1938, left residue after the death of his widow, which occurred in 1958, 'upon trust to pay and apply the same and the income thereof to or for the benefit of such hospital and/or hospitals and/or charitable institutions as the chairman for the time being of Barclays Bank Ltd., shall, in his absolute and uncontrolled discretion, think fit'. On appeal from Wilberforce, J., who had held that the expression 'hospital or hospitals' included profit-making nursing homes and that, therefore the gift, not being exclusively charitable, failed for uncertainty, the Court of Appeal reversed that judgment, holding that in the context of the will the word 'hospital' had to be given what would have been its ordinary meaning in the context at the time the will was made, *viz.*, a charitable voluntary hospital. As Lord Denning put it, 'In short, when people spoke of giving money to a "hospital" or "hospitals" in 1931, they meant, as of course, voluntary hospitals . . .' or, somewhat differently, Upjohn, L.J., 'But, in my judgment (and it is a very short point) in a will such as this the word "hospital" is apt and appropriate to describe what used to be called a voluntary hospital and is not appropriate to describe an institution, however expert medical and surgical services may be available therein, which is run for profit and which is normally and ordinarily described as a nursing home'.

(iii) *Testamentary gifts to discontinued charities — Application of cy près doctrine*

This situation must be distinguished from those cases where the testator designates the object of his bounty but for one reason or another it does not exist at the time the gift comes into effect. If the object used to exist (*e.g.* at the time when the will was made) and there is no *general* charitable intention the gift will fail.[2] If however, although the object is specifically described in the will, it never existed, the Court has held, in order to give the words describing the object some meaning, that there is a general charitable intent and accordingly room for the *cy près* doctrine to apply.[2]

Where the gift was made contingently on some other event happening then so long as the will had taken effect, it was held in *re Faraken*[3] that a general charitable intention had been demonstrated.

The question remains: what is required to evidence the general charitable intent? The answer the Court has given (and one may be forgiven for agreeing with Goff, J., that it is a surprising answer) is that where the gift is to an unincorporated body which has ceased to

---

[1] [1962] 1 W.L.R. 763.   [2] *Re Harwood* [1936] Ch. 285.
[3] [1912] 2 Ch. 488. The converse applies in Scotland *Fergusson's Trustees* v. *Buchmann* [1973] S.L.T. 41 (O.H.).

E

exist but its purposes are still being carried out, effect would be given to the gift by way of a scheme, but where it was incorporated and although its purposes were still being carried out but it had ceased to exist then other and indeed strong evidence was required to show the general charitable intent.[1]

(iv) *Conditional gifts and gifts in perpetuity for non-charitable objects*[2]

A testator will sometimes attempt to achieve some such object as the permanent maintenance of a family grave by linking the maintenance of the grave with a gift to a charity, such as a hospital. Provided no obligation to maintain the grave is laid on the charitable trustees it is lawful to direct a trustee to pay the income of a trust fund to the governing body of a hospital for so long as the grave is in good condition, with a gift over to another charity should the grave cease to be in good condition. On the other side of the fence is *re Elliott, Lloyds Bank* v. *Burton on Trent Hospital Management Committee and Others*[3] in which case £100 was left to the hospital to be invested 'for the purpose of maintaining my grave and headstone' and subject to the hospital accepting that legacy and the condition attached to it, he bequeathed the residue of his estate to be applied for the purposes of the hospital. It was held that the condition was void as infringing the rule against perpetuities but being a *malum prohibitum* which could be disregarded, the gift of the residue therefore passed to the hospital authority unfettered by the condition.

The whole subject, however, bristles with difficulties in application of legal principles and a full examination of the effect of different versions of grave maintenance clauses coupled with a charitable bequest is beyond the scope of a work of this nature.

(b) *Discretionary Distribution by Executors or Trustees*[2]

Frequently executors or trustees are instructed to distribute either a certain sum or the residue of an estate at their discretion among charities generally or among charities of a particular kind such as hospitals and, perhaps, in a particular locality. If the distribution is limited to hospitals either generally or of a particular locality the definition of hospital becomes important. In *re Alchin's Trusts*[4] it was laid down that there is a presumption that 'hospital' means a general hospital whilst in another case it was decided that a free dispensary dealing with out-patients only could not share in a bequest to the

---

[1] In *re Finger's W.T., Turner* v. *Ministry of Health* [1972] Ch. 286 applying *re Vernon's W.T., Lloyds Bank Ltd.* v. *Group 20 H.M.C. (Coventry)* (Note) [1972] Ch. 300. Both cases are somewhat further confused by misdescription of the name of the intended donee.

[2] See also p. 82 *et qse.* as to discretionary and conditional gifts for charitable purposes to authorities within the National Health Service.

[3] [1952] 1 Ch., 217.   [4] (1872) 14 Eq. 230.

hospitals of Birmingham. Also, in *re Davis's Trusts*,[1] decided in 1871, the principle was adopted that unless the context of the will indicated an intention to benefit institutions supported out of rates a hospital supported by voluntary contributions will be preferred. But it may be suggested that that ruling became obsolete with the transfer of most hospitals to the Secretary of State for Health and Social Security under the National Health Service Act 1946, and the express power given to governing bodies of such transferred hospitals to receive and administer charitable gifts, as to which see ss. 59 and 60 of the 1946 Act.[2] Moreover, hospitals will not in future be supported out of the rates. An expression such as 'the hospitals of London' is for such purpose ordinarily construed in a popular sense and without definite boundaries. One can speculate, however, whether, in the case of London, the creation of the enlarged London administrative area under the Greater London Council might lead the courts, where there was no indication in the will to the contrary, to regard London as comprising the whole of the administrative area of the Greater London Council, always assuming that the will had been made after the coming into force of the London Government Act 1963.[3]

Yet another class of case of exceptional difficulty is illustrated by the facts in *Chichester Diocesan Fund and Board of Finance* v. *Simpson and Ors*.[4] in which a testator named Diplock had left the residue of his estate to his executors upon trust for sale and conversion and he directed them to apply the proceeds of sale 'for such charitable institution or institutions or other charitable or benevolent object or objects as my acting executors in their or his absolute discretion select and to be paid to or for such institutions or objects if more than one in such proportion as my executor or executors may think proper'.

A distribution amounting to some quarter of a million pounds was made by the executors under that residuary bequest, many hospitals participating. Then the validity of the bequest was challenged by relatives of the deceased who would have benefited on an intestacy. The grounds for the action were that a testamentary gift of this kind to unascertained objects is valid only if there is expressed in the will an over-riding charitable intention and that the residuary bequest in Caleb

---

[1] 21 W. R. 154. But see now *re Smith deceased*; *Barclays Bank Ltd.* v. *Mercantile Bank Ltd.* [1962] 1 W. L. R. 763 discussed on p. 71.

[2] See pp. 86–87.

[3] It is interesting to observe that King Edwards Hospital Fund for London, a charitable trust for the benefit of hospitals of the metropolis, now extends its activities to cover the whole area of the four Regional Health Authorities, an area very substantially larger than even the Metropolitan Police District. Incidentally the four metropolitan regions *are* very specially linked with London because their services are, in a sense, based on the London teaching hospitals. The point is, of course, not now confined to London. See also Tudor on Charities, 6th Edition (1967), p. 204 and cases there cited.

[4] [1944] A. C. 341. Also *Minister of Health* v. *Simpson and Others* [1950] 2 All E. R. 1137; [1951] A. C. 251; 66 T. L. R. 1015.

Diplock's will, which permitted an unascertained proportion of the residue to be distributed to *benevolent objects* — as distinguished from *charitable* objects in the legal sense of the term — was therefore invalid.

A decision[1] of Farwell, J., in favour of the validity of the residuary bequest as a good charitable gift was subsequently reversed in the Court of Appeal[2] and in the House of Lords[3] the judgment of the Court of Appeal was affirmed, the Lord Chancellor (Viscount Simon) in his judgment saying that the phrase 'charitable or benevolent' in a will must in its ordinary context be regarded as too vague to give the certainty necessary before such a provision could be supported or enforced. There was no context in the will under consideration to justify a different interpretation: the use of the conjunction 'or' in the will appeared to him to indicate a variation rather than an identity between the coupled conceptions. The clause in question was not a valid testamentary disposition and the appeal failed.

That the House of Lords has thus affirmed a considerably earlier interpretation of the expression 'charitable or benevolent' when used in a will, and one which is apt to prevent charities from benefiting under loosely drawn wills and to rejoice the hearts of the next of kin of the deceased, was perhaps the least serious feature of the Diplock will case. What was more serious was that a substantial distribution having been made and the sums distributed used in various ways, there arose the possibility of the charitable institutions which had received gifts under the invalid bequest being called upon to refund to the estate. An action by the next of kin of the deceased was later brought to that end and is reported as *re Diplock's Estate; Diplock and Ors.* v. *Wintle and Ors.*[4] and in the House of Lords as *Minister of Health* v. *Simpson and Others.*[5] Judgment was given by Wynn-Parry, J., substantially in favour of the defendant charities. Subsequently, the Court of Appeal,[6] the judgment of which was upheld in the House of Lords, did permit the recovery of some of the money received by the charities, the decision in respect of each charity depending on a consideration of the rules of equity relating to the recovery of money from an innocent trustee who received it in good faith and also as to tracing orders, the application of the rule in *Clayton's Case*[7] and of several other leading cases. That there had been

---

[1] [1940] Ch. 988, *sub nom. In re Diplock; Wintle* v. *Diplock.*
[2] [1941] Ch. 253, *sub nom. In re Diplock; Wintle* v. *Diplock.*
[3] [1944] A. C. 341.   [4] [1947] 1 All E. R. 522.
[5] [1951] A. C. 251; 66 T. L. R. (Pt. 2) 1015; [1950] 2 All E. R. 1137; see also *in re Woolton, deceased* ([1968] 1 W. L. R. 681).
[6] [1948] 2 All E. R. 318–367 and 429–432.
[7] *Devaynes* v. *Noble, (Clayton's Case)* (1816) 1 Mar. 529, 572 Dig. 483, 3961. The effect of *Clayton's* case is that if moneys are mixed in an active banking account the first paid in is the first drawn out. But the rule is not without exception. If a trustee has mixed trust funds with his own moneys in a banking account he will be presumed to have drawn out his own moneys first unless the drawings were for the purposes of the trust. Such is the effect of *re Hallett's Estate* (1879) 13 Ch. D. 696 (C. A.).

a mistake of law on the part of the executor-trustees was held not to bar the right of the next of kin of the deceased testator to recovery — in accordance with the rules of equity — from innocent recipients from the executor-trustees of money belonging to the estate.

The substantial effect of the decision of the Court of Appeal as affirmed in the House of Lords is that whenever under the provisions of a will (*e.g.*, in the present case a discretionary distribution to charities) a wrongful distribution is made by the executors, the sums wrongly paid may be recovered from the recipient by the person or persons who have suffered thereby (*e.g.*, next of kin, beneficiaries or creditors), subject only to action being brought within 12 years of the expiry of the 'executor's year', this period of limitation being in accordance with s. 20 of the Limitation Act 1939. It appears, too, that the fact that a charity may have received a monetary gift — as in the Diplock case — in complete good faith and may have spent it before any claim is made by, say, the next of kin for repayment on grounds of invalidity of the particular provisions of the will under which the gift was made, is no defence to the claim.

It follows from what is said above that hospitals offered substantial benefits under a will — particularly under discretionary trusts — should, when circumstances suggest that it is expedient, take all practicable steps to assure themselves of the validity of the gift and, if in real doubt, not dispose of the fund, even if accepted, until either the doubt is cleared up or the possibility of a claim statute-barred. Apparently even the absence of grounds for suspicion will not protect in all circumstances the innocent recipient, as might have been thought from the decision in the Court of Appeal.

In light of *Diplock* it seems unlikely that the decision of the Privy Council in *re Resch's Will Trusts Le Cras* v. *Perpetual Trustee Ltd*[1] on appeal from New South Wales would be followed in this country. The essential facts were that a bequest had been made to the Sisters of Charity for the general purposes of St. Vincent's private hospital for paying patients, the validity of the bequest depending on whether the hospital was a charity. The Privy Council decided that it was, this notwithstanding that surpluses from the private hospital had been used not only to contribute to the maintenance of an ordinary general hospital nearby, which was also run by the Sisters of Charity, but also for the general purposes of the Order, which latter purposes were not all necessarily charitable.

(c) Charitable Trusts (Validation) Act 1954

The Charitable Trusts (Validation) Act 1954, makes it very improbable that further claims on the lines of the *Diplock* case would

[1] [1969] 1 A.C. 514; [1967] 3 All E.R. 915 (P. C.).

succeed, in respect of any trust instrument taking effect before December 16th, 1952. That Act validated any imperfect trust instrument which took effect before December 16th, 1952, being an instrument under which the trust property could be used for exclusively charitable objects but could nevertheless be used for purposes that were not charitable. Broadly any such trust instrument was validated provided it would have been valid if the declared objects had been restricted to charitable objects and provided that the trust had not before December 16th, 1952, been treated as invalid on the ground that its objects were not exclusively charitable. From the commencement of the Act, the objects of any trust validated under the provisions of the Act are limited to such of its purposes as are charitable. The reader is referred to the Act for saving of adverse claims, etc.

In passing it may be noticed that the *Gillingham Bus Disaster Fund*[1] case illustrates both the limits of the Charitable Trusts (Validation) Act, 1954, and, quite apart from the provisions of that Act, the importance of there being a clear statement of the objects of any public appeal or, for that matter, of any trust instrument. The facts of the case were that, following an accident in which several cadets were killed by a bus, the mayors of three towns, in a letter to the editor of the *Daily Telegraph*, appealed for contributions to a fund 'to be devoted among other things to defraying the funeral expenses, caring for the boys who may be disabled, and then to such worthy cause or causes in memory of the boys who lost their lives as the mayors may determine . . . '. It was decided by Harman, J.,[2] that the trusts were void for uncertainty and that the Act of 1954 did not apply to validate them. This decision was upheld in the Court of Appeal by Lord Evershed, M.R., and Romer, L.J. (Ormerod, L.J., dissenting) but as regards the non-applicability of the Act of 1954 on somewhat narrower grounds than in the court of first instance.

10. Dealings with Land

The law of mortmain has been repealed by s. 38 (1) and Part II of the 7th Schedule of the Charities Act 1960. Consequently, charity trustees, whether incorporated or not, are now free to hold land for the purposes of the charity subject only to the same rules as other persons, provided that the holding of land is in accordance with the terms of the trust. But it must be appreciated that land is not ordinarily an authorised investment under the Trustee Investment Act 1961, though, subject to proper advice, mortgages on land are authorised.[3]

S. 38 (2) of the Charities Act 1960, cures any defect of title to land by reason of any breach of the now repealed law of mortmain, provided

---

[1] [1958] Ch. 300; [1958] 1 All E.R. 37; [1959] Ch. 62; [1958] 2 All E.R. 749 (C. A.).
[2] [1958] Ch. 300; [1958] 1 All E. R. 37.
[3] See further Trustee Investment Act 1961, s. 1 and 1st Schedule, para. 12.

that no step had been taken before the passing of the Act to assert an adverse claim by virtue of any of the repealed enactments. By s. 49 (3), of the Charities Act 1960, s. 38 of that Act and also Part II of the 7th Schedule containing further repeals of Acts and of Church Assembly Measures relating to mortmain, as well as s. 1 and the 1st Schedule (which relates to the constitution of the Charity Commissioners), came into force on the date on which the Act was passed, *viz.*, July 29th, 1960, although the rest of the Act did not take effect until January 1st, 1961.

11. Investments

Within the limits and subject to the safeguards laid down in the Trustee Investments Act 1961, trustees, including charity trustees, who have not been given wider powers of investment by their trust instrument, may invest part of their trust fund in first class equities, 'wider range securities' as defined in the Act, the remainder still having to be invested in gilt-edged and similar 'narrower range' fixed interest securities, etc., somewhat more liberally defined than were trustee securities in s. 1 of the Trustee Act 1925.[1]

Charity trustees may also invest in the Charities Official Investment Fund established by the Charity Commissioners by virtue of the authority given in s. 22 of the Charities Act 1960. Participation in the Fund, which takes full advantage of the wider investment powers given by the 1961 Act,[2] relieves charity trustees of all responsibility regarding the suitability and legality of their investments.[3]

12. Payments to Trustees and Board Members

Unless the conditions of the trust clearly provide otherwise, trustees, including members of the board or committee of a hospital, may properly be reimbursed all reasonable expenses, including travelling expenses, actually incurred by them in respect of their duties, but equally surely, unless the terms of the trust so provide, they are not entitled to any remuneration for their time and trouble nor, whilst trustees or members of the board, can they properly accept any office or undertake any work for the hospital remunerated in any way whether by salary or fees.[4] The effect of this general rule is not avoided by any form of

[1] For the provisions of the Trustee Investments Act 1961, *see* Lewin on Trusts, 16th Edn. (1964).

[2] In fact, it is understood that the Fund has been given authority to invest a greater proportion of its capital in wider range securities than have trustees generally.

[3] In departmental circular H.M. (62) 80 attention of N.H.S. authorities was drawn to the possibility of investing endowment capital in the Charities Official Investment Fund.

[4] *Re The French Protestant Hospital* [1951] 1 Ch. 567. In this case it was held that although the directors of a charitable hospital established by Royal Charter in 1718 were not technically trustees, they were in the same fiduciary position as trustees and that it was therefore improper for them, of their own motion, to introduce a revised bye-law removing the ban on their receiving any payment from the charity for professional services, such a provision

words, as by calling the payment made an *honorarium*, and it applies to medical practitioners no less than to others. It is no justification for payments made in contravention of the rule to show that the trustee or member of the board has undertaken work for the hospital far in excess of that undertaken by his fellow trustees, *e.g.*, as solicitor or accountant or as a medical member of the staff of the hospital; nor that he has undertaken a peculiarly onerous office, *e.g.*, as chairman of the board or as organiser of an appeal. Equally, it is no justification that the payment is small in relation to the work done, and that anyone else would have required substantially higher payment. The general rule against payment for time and trouble would also prevent payment of board members for loss of earnings whilst attending board meetings.[1]

(a) Unincorporated hospitals

In the case of unincorporated hospitals there is only the application of the general principle stated above to be considered, and it seems clear that the board itself could not vote remuneration to any of its members unless the trust deed expressly conferred that power. Nor does it seem that an annual meeting of subscribers could regularise the position without the sanction of the Court or of the Charity Commissioners, which would be given only if the course proposed were manifestly in the interests of the charity and there were no reasonable alternative.

(b) Incorporated hospitals

Whether in the case of an incorporated hospital the authority must be embodied in the principal instrument of incorporation or whether it suffices if it is contained in the bye-laws or articles is not a problem capable of a conclusive answer in general terms and each case must be considered separately. The *French Protestant Hospital* case[2] does, however, illustrate the obstacles in the way of alteration of bye-laws or articles to permit remuneration being paid to directors of an incorporated charity. The approval of the Court or of the Charity Commissioners to any provision to that effect in bye-laws or articles or to any amendment to that effect in the principal instrument of incorporation is almost invariably necessary. What happens in practice is illustrated in the following paragraphs.

---

being *prima facie* repugnant to law. In the course of his judgment, Dankwerts, J., said 'It is plain that, in the administration of charitable trusts by the Court. it has always been the practice in settling schemes, to exclude the administering trustees from any power to make a profit or to obtain remuneration'. This has only limited application to health or hospital authorities within the N.H.S. as to which see p. 82 *et seq.*

[1] As to loss of remunerative time by members of authorities under the National Health Service Act 1977, see pp. 80–82.

[2] [1951] 1 Ch. 567. See footnote 4 on p. 77.

(i) *Hospitals incorporated under the Companies Acts*

In every case examined of a hospital incorporated under the Companies Acts, the hospital, in order to obtain permission to omit the word 'limited' from the title, has been required by the Department of Trade to insert in its memorandum of association a clause categorically forbidding any payment to members of the board or governing body in respect of services rendered. In some few cases, however, a special exception has been made in favour of representatives of the medical staff, but subject to very stringent safeguards so that such medical members of the board should, with the other doctors, receive no more than their due share of any amount allocated to the medical staff, as, for example, from a contributory scheme pool. No instance comes to mind of any medical member of the board of such a hospital being permitted to receive payment for services rendered otherwise than within the narrow limits indicated, nor of any other member of the board being permitted to receive any payment whatsoever.[1]

(ii) *Hospitals incorporated by Royal Charter*

There are wide variations in the terms of the Royal Charters incorporating different hospitals[2] but in not one of several Charters examined was payment for services rendered by members of the board expressly or by necessary implication authorised, nor does it seem that authority for such payment could properly be inferred. Furthermore, where the detailed constitution of the board was contained in bye-laws annexed as a schedule to the Charter, there was generally in those bye-laws a provision to the effect that no paid officer of the hospital and no governor supplying any article to the hospital (*i.e.*, for which he received some consideration) was eligible to serve on the board. Almost invariably, if not in every case, in modern times the Charter contained a stipulation that the original bye-laws contained in the schedule could not be altered except with the approval of the Privy Council. It is difficult to imagine circumstances in which such approval would be given to any amendment authorising the payment of board members either for their services as such or otherwise. It would certainly have to be demonstrated that the unorthodox proposal was necessary in the interests of the charity.

An older Charter which provided in detail for the constitution of a 'Council' including the patron, etc., and representative 'Governors' made no provision for their payment and it is difficult to assume any intention that they should be paid. The same Charter authorised bye-laws to be made (this without the usual modern proviso as to approval

[1] See also p. 77.
[2] Most of these charters were revoked, consequent on the coming into operation of the National Health Service Act 1946.

by the Privy Council), *inter alia* as regards appointment, removal, stipends and emoluments of officers, but it is clear from the context that the power to fix emoluments did not refer to or contemplate payment of members of the Council. It also expressly provided that any such bye-laws should not be repugnant to the general design and *spirit* of the Charter, which stipulation alone would raise an interesting argument against payment of Council members.

(iii) *Hospitals incorporated by Act of Parliament*

Since even the most generally recognised rule of law or equity may be over-ridden by express provisions of an Act of Parliament, and since the special Acts obtained by various hospitals over a long period vary greatly in their form and content, following no single pattern, it is impossible to generalise about them.

In some modern private Acts relating to hospitals[1] it was found that the detailed constitution was embodied in a scheme set out in a schedule to the Act and that alterations to the scheme might be made only with sanction of the Charity Commissioners or of the Court. In the specimens examined by Dr. Speller not only was no provision made for payment of members of the board but there was an express prohibition against any board member being concerned in any bargain or contract with the hospital to any greater extent than as a shareholder in a company. It does not appear likely that in such circumstances either the Court or the Charity Commissioners would sanction alterations of the scheme to allow remuneration or personal profit to any members of the governing body. Although other private Acts are not so explicit it is difficult to avoid the conclusion that authority to pay members of the board was neither sought nor desired by those who promoted those Acts and that they would have repudiated any such suggestion. It may be suggested that the Court would not readily accept an interpretation of a private Act which ran counter to a generally recognised principle if any other reasonable interpretation were possible.

(iv) *Hospital authorities under the National Health Service Act*

There is in the National Health Service Act 1977, no prohibition on appointment to membership of any health or hospital authority of a person who is receiving payment for services to that authority and, indeed under the Re-organisation, places on the Health Authorities are reserved for medical practitioners, and in effect other employees. It

---

[1] Probably all the private Acts in mind at the time this section was written were repealed by s. 77 of the National Health Service Act 1946, or are practically ineffective, but the principles discussed remain valid as regards any hospitals or kindred institutions such as convalescent homes or orphanages which are or may later be incorporated by special Act. The section is now to be found in the 1977 Act Sch. 14 para. 6.

should, however, here be mentioned that the model standing orders proposed to authorities by the Department[1] and almost certainly adopted by all such authorities, includes a limitation on any member's taking part in a decision on any matter in which he has a personal interest. The model standing order is in the following terms:

'(e) Interest of members in contracts and other matters

15. If any member of the Board/H.M.C. has any pecuniary interest, direct or indirect, in any contract or proposed contract or other matter and is present at a meeting of the Board/H.M.C. at which the contract or other matter is the subject of consideration, he shall at the meeting, as soon as practicable after the commencement thereof, disclose the fact, and shall not take any part in the consideration or discussion of, or vote on any question with respect to, the contract or proposed contract or other matter and shall retire from such meeting unless the Board/H.M.C. invite him to remain.

If any question should arise as to what in any circumstances amounts to a direct or indirect pecuniary interest, the Chairman shall adjudicate on the issue and his decision shall be final.'

As guidance on the meaning of 'indirect pecuniary interest', there was a footnote[2] to the model standing order in which is set out a summary of the rules applicable to members of local authorities under s. 76 of the Local Government Act 1933 as amended.[3] The summary reads as follows:

1. A member of an authority who has any pecuniary interest, direct or indirect, in any contract or proposed contract or any other matter, and is present at a meeting of the authority or of a committee or sub-committee of the authority at which the contract or other matter is the subject of consideration, must disclose the fact at the meeting as soon as practicable after its commencement, and must not take any part in the consideration or discussion of, or vote on any question with respect to, the contract or other matter.

This disqualification does not extend to —

(a) an interest in a contract or other matter which a member may have as a rate-payer or inhabitant of the area or as an ordinary consumer of gas, electricity or water;
(b) an interest in any matter relating to the terms on which the right to participate in any service, including the supply of goods, is offered to the public;
(c) an interest of a member in a contract or other matter which is so remote or insignificant that it cannot reasonably be regarded as likely to influence a member in the consideration or discussion of, or in voting on, any question with respect to that contract or matter;

and in these cases disclosure of the interest is not required.

2. A person is to be treated as having indirectly a pecuniary interest in a contract or other matter if —

---

[1] Under cover of circular H.M. (56) 67. See also H.M. (65) 67. Presumably since these circulars have not been replaced the reference to *Board/H.M.C.* should now be taken to refer to R.H.A. or A.H.A.
[2] As substituted by circular H.M. (65) 67.
[3] Now see Local Government Act 1972, ss. 94–98.

(*a*) he or any nominee of his is a member of a company or other body with which the contract is made or proposed to be made or which has a direct pecuniary interest in the other matter under consideration; or

(*b*) he is a partner, or in the employment, of a person with whom the contract is made or is proposed to be made or who has a direct pecuniary interest in the other matter under consideration.

But a person is not disqualified —

(i) by reason of his being a member of a public body;* or

(ii) by reason of his being a member of a company or other body, if he has no beneficial interest in any shares of the company or other body; or

(iii) by reason of a pecuniary interest in a contract or other matter arising by virtue of a connection mentioned in (*a*) or (*b*) of this paragraph, if the interest of the body or person connected with him is so remote or insignificant that it cannot reasonably be regarded as likely to influence a member in the consideration or discussion of, or in voting on, any question with respect to the contract or matter.

Nor is a person who is a member of a company or other body disqualified for taking part in consideration or discussion or for voting (though in this case he is required to disclose the interest) if the total nominal value of shares therein in which he has a beneficial interest does not exceed £500 or one-hundredth of the total nominal value of the issued share capital of the company or body, whichever is the less.†

For the purposes of the foregoing 'shares' includes stock, and 'share capital' is to be construed accordingly.

3. In the case of married persons living together, the interest of one spouse, if known to the other, is to be deemed to be also an interest of the other spouse.

* 'Public body' includes a body established for carrying on under national ownership any industry or part of an industry or undertaking the governing body of any university, university college, college in a university or college of advanced technology; and the National Trust.

† If the company or other body issues more than one class of shares, the member is disqualified if the total nominal value of all the shares of any one class in which he has a beneficial interest exceeds one-hundredth part of the total issued share capital of that class of the company or body.

Although the above summary of what is meant by 'indirect pecuniary interest' would doubtless carry great weight in any legal proceedings concerning the conduct of a member of a Health Authority, it has not the statutory force it would have in relation to a member of a local authority.

D. HEALTH AND HOSPITAL AUTHORITIES UNDER THE NATIONAL HEALTH SERVICE ACT, AS CHARITY TRUSTEES

1. Introductory

In *re Frere (deceased). Kidd and Another* v. *Farnham Group Hospital Management Committee*,[1] Wynn-Parry, J., said that a hospital did not

[1] [1950] 2 All E. R. 513.

cease to be a charity merely because of the coming into effect of the National Health Service Act 1946. Reference may also be made to *re Morgan's Will Trusts*[1] and *re Dean's Will Trusts*[2] which were followed in this case. Subsequently, *re Hillier's Trusts, Hillier and Another* v. *Attorney-General and Another*[3] was also decided on the basis that hospitals in the National Health Service are legal charities. Other cases which may be mentioned are *re Hunter; Lloyds Bank* v. *Girton College*[4] and *re White's Will Trusts; Tindall* v. *Board of Governors of Sheffield United Hospitals and Others*.[5] In the last-mentioned case a gift for the purpose of providing a home of rest for the nurses at a particular hospital was held to be charitable since the purpose of the gift was to increase the efficiency of the hospital for the healing of the sick. Consequently the income passed to the new hospital authority under s. 60 (1) of the 1946 Act. It appears that the re-organisation of the health service has not affected the charitable status of health service authorities.[6]

2. Power of Health Authorities to accept Gifts

S. 90[7] of the National Health Service Act 1977 provides as follows:

A Health Authority[8] shall have power to accept, hold and administer any property on trust for all or any purposes relating to the health service. Accordingly charitable gifts may be accepted, held and administered by a Health Authority for any health service purpose.

Such gifts, like any other charitable gifts, are accepted to any conditions laid down by the donor or testator, if such that the Courts will ordinarily enforce, that being a matter beyond the scope of this work. They can be freed from such conditions, or the conditions relaxed, only by order of the Court or, in appropriate cases, of the Charity Commissioners.

All such gifts will be subject to the Trustee Investments Act 1961 as to authorised investments.[9]

3. Private Trusts for Hospitals: Payments to Health Authorities

Section 91[9] of the 1977 Act provides:

91 (1) Where —
(a) the terms of a trust instrument authorise or require the trustees, whether

---

[1] [1950] Ch. 637; 1 All E. R. 109.   [2] [1950] 1 All E. R. 882; [1950] 66 T. L. R. 728.
[3] [1954] 1 W. L. R. 700.   [4] [1950] Ch. 190.
[5] [1951] 1 All E.R. 528. See also *re Bernstein's Will Trusts, National Westminster Bank* v. *Board of Governors of the United Liverpool Hospitals* (1971) 115 Sol. Jo. 808 (Extra comforts for the nursing staff — held charitable) and *London Hospital Medical College* v. *I.R.C.* [1976] 2 All E.R. 113.
[6] See above p. 31, and the N.H.S. (Amendment of Trust Instruments) Order S.I. 1974 No. 63 and 1973 Act ss. 22 and 27 and now 1977 Act ss. 91 and 93.
[7] The section replaces s. 21 of the 1973 Act and s. 59 of the 1946 Act.
[8] Defined in s. 128 (1).   [9] Formerly s. 22 of the 1973 Act.

immediately or in the future, to apply any part of the capital or income of the trust property for the purposes of any health service hospital vested,

(b) the trust instrument shall be construed as authorising or (as the case may be) requiring the trustees to apply the trust property to the like extent, and at the like times, for the purpose of making payments, whether of capital or income, to the appropriate hospital authority.[1]

By s. 96 (1), any provision made in ss. 90 to 95 for the transfer of property to the appropriate hospital authority[1] includes provision for the transfer of any rights or liabilities arising from that property. Seemingly, however, s. 96 (1) will not apply to what is authorised by s. 91, i.e. payments of money. If, however, when offering a payment, trustees of a private trust sought to impose on the authority some liability beyond the requirements of s. 91 (2), it could refuse to receive the payment on such terms and should indeed do so, if, in its opinion, it was not in the interests of the charity to accept. S. 91 (2) provides:

Any sum so paid to the appropriate hospital authority shall, so far as practicable, be applied by them for the purpose specified in the trust instrument.

S. 91 (2) must be read subject to s. 96 (2) which provides that nothing in sections 90 to 95 shall affect the power of Her Majesty, the Court (as defined in the Charities Act 1960) or any other person to alter the trusts of any charity.[2] The only problem of interpretation posed by this subsection is the meaning to be attributed to the word *practicable*, a word previously used in sub-section (2) of the corresponding sections of the Acts of 1946 and 1973. Its use in s. 60 (2) of the 1946 Act was not, however, the subject of judicial interpretation. Although in *Hayes' Will Trusts, Dobie and Others* v. *Board of Governors of the National Hospital and Others*,[3] which concerned a gift to a hospital, the word *impracticable* was held equivalent to *not able to be done* and from that it might be argued that *practicable* in s. 60 (2) meant *able to be done* or *possible*, thus to interpret *practicable* in that context would imply a rigidity in the inter-

---

[1] S. 91 (3) provides:
In this section *the appropriate hospital authority* means —
(a) where Special Trustees are appointed for the hospital, those trustees,
(b) in any other case, the Area Health Authority exercising functions on behalf of the Secretary of State in respect of the hospital.
Special Trustees here means those trustees appointed under s. 95 as to which see pp. 92–93.
Where in respect of a hospital administered by an Area Health Authority (Teaching) special trustees have not been appointed, that Authority will be in exactly the same position as any other Area Health Authority both in respect of transfer of existing trusts on reorganisation and allocation to it of a share of the Hospital Endowments Fund. It will also be free to accept any new trusts falling within s. 90, including trusts which, had special trustees been appointed, it would have been debarred from accepting, by virtue of s. 95 (2).
S. 91 (4) says:
Nothing in this section shall apply to a trust for a special hospital or to a property transferred under section 24 of the National Health Service Reorganisation Act 1973.
[2] See p. 67.
[3] [1954] 1 W.L.R. 22; [1953] 2 All E.R. 1243.

pretation of the section which the use of the word *practicable* instead of *possible* seemed designed to avoid. There is the same objection to giving the word that meaning in s. 91 (2) of the 1977 Act.

For the necessarily fine distinctions between the meanings of *practicable* and *possible* and between *practicable* and *reasonably practicable* when used in a statute reference may be made to *Jayne* v. *National Coal Board*,[1] an industrial injury case in which the two expressions *practicable precautions* and *reasonably practicable*[2] *precautions* used in s. 157 of the Factories Act 1937 were considered. Giving judgment in that case, Veale, J., quoting Holroyd Pearce, L. J., in *Brown* v. *National Coal Board*,[3] said 'It is slightly more difficult to show that avoidance of the breach was impracticable than that it was not reasonably practicable'.

He continued:

The difference in meaning between the two expressions is hard to define and further definition of words that in themselves express a shade of meaning is not helpful. But the difference, though hard to define, exists and in a borderline case it might produce a difference in result. The word 'reasonably' has a slight tendency to modify the word 'practicable'. But in my judgment there may well be precautions which it is 'practicable' but not 'reasonably practicable' to take. . . . The distinction therefore exists but it is slight.

He then turned to distinguish *practicable* from *possible*. There was, he said, in his view clearly a difference between those two words. Had the legislature intended to lay down possibility as a test, it would have been simple to have used the word *impossible* in s. 157, but they did not do so. In his view *impracticability* as a conception was different from that of *impossibility*; the latter was absolute, the former introduced at all events some degree of reason and involved at all events some regard for practice. To interpret these words and expressions in the National Health Service Act in the same way as did Veale, J., in *Jayne's* case would see fairly to represent the intentions of the legislature.

The meaning of *practicable* in s. 6 (4) of the National Health Service (Scotland) Act 1947[4] was considered in *Adams and Others* v. *Maclay (Secretary of State) and the South Eastern Regional Hospital Board*.[5] This was a case in which it was proposed to open to male practitioners a post for a consultant at two former voluntary hospitals which had been established *inter alia* to provide for the treatment of women and children by female practitioners. The hospitals having been taken over under s. 6 of the 1947 Act the Secretary of State was bound under s. 6 (4) 'so far as practicable to secure that the objects for which any

[1] [1963] 2 All E.R. 221.
[2] The expression 'reasonably practicable' is used in s. 93 of the National Health Service Act 1977 with reference to property transferred under s. 23 of the 1973 Act, being trust property originally acquired for the N.H.S. under s. 7 of the Act of 1946.
[3] [1961] 1 Q.B. 303; [1960] 3 All E.R. 599.
[4] Corresponding with s. 6 (4) of the 1946 Act in England. Now s. 88 of the 1977 Act.
[5] [1958] S.C. 279.

such property was used immediately before the appointed day are not prejudiced by the provisions of this section'. It was held that because of that requirement, it was the duty of the Secretary of State to secure that a male medical practitioner was not appointed consulting physician at the two hospitals unless and until, after the advertisement of the post as being open to women medical practitioners only, it should appear that no women suitable for the appointment had applied.

This decision, like that in *Jayne's* case, leaves room for a distinction between the meaning of *possible* and *practicable* since, although under the trust instrument relating to the former voluntary hospitals the board administering those hospitals might have been under an obligation to appoint none but women to the medical staff even though the best they could find at any particular time — although on the medical register — might lack such higher qualification and experience as might nowadays be regarded as necessary to the post to be filled, the Secretary of State or the Board acting for him having considered women applicants and decided that none was suitable, could appoint a man. Thus in the case of the two former voluntary hospitals the governing condition would have been a possibility; after transfer to the Secretary of State it was a practicability. After the decision in the Scottish case, the Minister of Health issued fresh instructions to hospital authorities in England and Wales on the procedure to be adopted when it was proposed to close or change the use of a hospital, the new procedure being designed to take particular account of the duty to secure that, as far as practicable, the objects for which a hospital was used immediately before transfer in 1948 would not be prejudiced by the proposed change.[1]

It may also be convenient to note at this stage although s. 78 of the 1946 Act abolished many of the governing bodies of hospitals and the Act brought them, and in particular the trusts they controlled, within the new health service, it has been doubted whether corporations created by Royal Charter or Act of Parliament were similarly dissolved.[2] Thus gifts by will expressed to be to the former trustees may still be valid even though the gift goes directly to the new authority. Power still exists now under Schedule 14 paragraph 6 of the 1977 Act[3] to abolish these authorities where they are redundant or are inconsistent with the legislation under s. 77 of the 1946 Act.

4. Some Cases decided on ss. 59 and 60 of the 1946 Act

These sections were repealed by the 1973 Act. They are now substantially to be found in ss. 90 and 91 of the 1977 Act[4]. It appears that the

[1] Circular H.M. (58) 29.
[2] *Re Kellner's Will Trusts* [1949] 2 All E.R. 774 (concerning funds passing under the 1946 Act, s. 60); *Re Meyers* [1951] 1 All E.R. 538 (concerning funds passing under s. 59 of the 1946 Act).
[3] Formerly s. 77 of the 1946 Act.   [4] Formerly ss. 21 and 22 of the 1973 Act.

following decisions are relevant to the interpretation of the new sections although decided under the 1946 Act.

Charitable purpose — In a number of cases, mentioned on page 83 of which *re Frere (deceased), Kidd and Another* v. *Farnham Group Hospital Management Committee*[1] and *re Hillier's Trusts*[2] are the most significant, the decision turned on whether a transferred hospital is still a charity. In *re Frere* Wynn-Parry, J., said that a hospital did not cease to be a charity merely because of the coming into effect of the 1946 Act and so a gift to such a hospital for purposes specified in s. 59 of that Act, after the transfer of the hospital to the Minister, is none the less a charitable gift. The following are the facts of reported cases.

Re Hunter: Lloyds Bank v. *Girton College.*[3] A testator who died before July 5th, 1948, left a share of his estate to the trustees of Ingham Infirmary, a voluntary hospital, expressing himself as being desirous of commemorating his deceased father in conjunction with a place where such beneficient work was carried on. The trustees distributing after the transfer of the hospital to the Minister sought directions. Vaisey, J., said:

Although from an administrative point of view and from the point of view of ownership of the property of these charities, great differences have been pointed out, I do not think that, from the point of view of a testator making a gift of this kind, there is really sufficient difference to justify me in saying that there is no object of his bounty or that the gift has failed.

Re Dean's Will Trusts — Cowan v. *Board of Governors of St. Mary's Hospital, Paddington.*[4] The testator, who made his will in 1947 and died in April 1948, bequeathed the residue to the hospital to be applied in providing accommodation for the use of relatives who came from a distance of patients who were critically ill, and secondly for the assistance of the work of the hospital almoners. Held by Harman, J.: that finding accommodation for patients' relatives was one of the purposes of the hospital which had been frequently carried out by the hospital almoner so that it constituted a valid charitable gift to the hospital. Incidentally, it may be observed that the testator had foreseen the effect of the Act for he had said if the that hospital had been transferred the money was to be paid to the new management committee — an inaccurate expression as used of a teaching hospital which nevertheless served to underline his general charitable intention.

Re Morgan's Will Trusts — Lewarne v. *Minister of Health.*[5] A testatrix who made her will in 1944 died on September 28th, 1948. She directed her trustees to hold certain property 'for the benefit of Liskeard Cottage Hospital'. It was not disputed that this was the 'Passmore

---

[1] [1950] 2 All E.R. 513.   [2] [1954] 1 W.L.R. 700.
[3] [1950] Ch. 190.   [4] [1950] 66 T.L.R. 728.
[5] [1950] 2 Ch. 637; [1950] 1 All E.R. 1097; 66 T.L.R. 1037.

Edwards Cottage Hospital at Liskeard', a voluntary hospital which had been transferred to the Minister on the appointed day. The former committee of management and trustees having been dissolved, from July 5th, 1948, the hospital had been managed by the Plymouth, South Devon and East Cornwall Hospital Management Committee. Held (by Roxburgh, J.): That the vesting provisions of the Act did not cause the gift to lapse. On a true construction of the will, the gift was for the general purposes of the hospital which was still being carried on. Consequently, the sums due should be paid to the hospital management committee under s. 59.

Re Glass (*deceased*). *Public Trustee* v. *South-West Middlesex Hospital Management Committee*.[1] In this case a testator whose will was made on July 2nd, 1948, and who died on January 21st, 1949, left a bequest 'to the King Edward VII Memorial Hospital, Ealing'. Vaisey, J., held this case to be indistinguishable from *re Morgan's Will Trusts* (*supra*) where the words were 'for the benefit of' and accordingly ordered that the gift should be paid to the hospital management committee under s. 59.

Re Frere (*deceased*). *Kidd and Another* v. *Farnham Group Hospital Management Committee*.[2] In this case the testator who made his will in March 1941 and died after July 5th, 1948, left a cash legacy of £6,000 to the Fleet and District Hospital 'if still at my death run on voluntary system and not taken over by the State'. After other provisions of his will had been fulfilled he gave the residue of his estate 'to the Fleet and District Hospital for endowment purposes'. It was conceded that the condition had come into operation to prevent the gift of £6,000 taking effect. Wynn-Parry, J., held that, there being no similar condition attached to the gift of the residue, that took effect as a good charitable gift. Referring to the submission on behalf of the next-of-kin that the hospital had ceased to be a charity his Lordship said that the force of the submission lay in that the gift of the residue was for endowment purposes, that it was a gift of a capital sum on trust to apply the income in perpetuity, and was therefore a gift which could be good only if it was charitable. He found that the work of the Fleet and District Hospital was still being carried on; also that having regard to the provisions of s. 59 of the Act of 1946 and to *re Morgan's Will Trusts*[3] and *re Dean's Will Trusts*[4] it was not open to hold that there had not been a good charitable disposition of the residuary estate. In *re Dean's Will Trusts*, Harman, J., had, in effect, held that a hospital does not cease to be a charity merely because of the coming into effect of the National Health Service Act 1946. Accordingly the gift passed under s. 59.

[1] [1950] Ch. 643.   [2] [1950] 2 All E.R. 513.
[3] [1950] Ch. 637; 66 T.L.R. 1037; [1950] 1 All E.R. 1097.
[4] [1950] 66 T.L.R. 728.

Re White's Will Trusts. Tindell v. *Board of Governors of the United Sheffield Hospitals and Others.*[1] A testator who died in 1920 had left residuary estate subject to a life interest to be transferred to the Royal Infirmary, Sheffield, to be invested and the income applied for the purpose of a home of rest for nurses of that institution in perpetuity. The life interest ceased in 1949, *i.e.*, after transfer of the hospital to the Minister. It was held by Harman, J., that the purpose of the gift being to increase the efficiency of the hospital it was charitable and as it was for a specific purpose the board of governors must under s. 60 (1) so far as practicable apply it to that purpose.

There was a somewhat different situation in *re Gartside, Coote and Eyre-Kaye* v. *Lees and Others.*[2] In this case recourse was had to s. 60 to save benefactions to two hospitals. Under a family settlement by will, the Manchester Children's Hospital and St. Mary's Hospital, Manchester, were to benefit on the death of B. G., a daughter of the settlor, who died in 1946. It was held that the right of the trustees of the will to receive from the settlement trustees — who were, in fact, the same persons — the whole of the settlement funds was a right enforceable by action. The right was therefore 'property' within s. 60 (1) and the income should accordingly be used to make payments to the committee of the non-teaching hospital and to the board of the teaching hospital which, respectively, had administered the hospitals since July 5th, 1948.

Reference should also be made to *re Kellner's Will Trusts*[3] and to *re Meyers (deceased)*[4] where the question of whether a former voluntary hospital governing body had been dissolved was discussed and the effect of continuing existence of the old corporation on the operation of s. 60 and of s. 59 of the Act respectively considered.

Re Little (deceased). Barclays Bank v. *Bournemouth and East Dorset Hospital Management Committee and Others.*[5] By his will made in 1945 the testator, who died in 1951, left residuary estate to 'the trustees for the time being of the . . . Cornelia and East Dorset Hospital and by them to be appropriated for or towards the building funds of the said hospital'. Following *re Morgan's Will Trusts*[6] and *re Glass*,[7] Vaisey, J., ordered the residuary estate to be handed over to the hospital management committee on their undertaking to use it for building fund purposes, which might be not only erection of new buildings but also maintenance and improvement of existing buildings. This gift fell under s. 59.

[1] [1951] 1 All E.R. 528.
[2] [1949] 2 All E.R. 546.
[3] [1949] 2 All E.R. 774; 65 T.L.R. 695. See p. 80.
[4] [1951] 1 All E.R. 536.
[5] [1953] 1 W.L.R. 1932.
[6] [1950] Ch. 637; 66 T.L.R. 1037; [1950] 1 All E.R. 1097.
[7] [1950] Ch. 643 n.

5. The Hospital Endowments Fund
Distribution on Winding-up

The Hospital Endowments Fund was established under the 1946 Act and to it were transferred the endowments of all hospitals transferred to the Minister of Health except those which were designated as teaching hospitals. S. 23 of the 1973 Act required the Secretary of State to wind-up the Fund and to provide by order for the distribution of its assets to Regional and Area Health Authorities and Special Trustees. This has now been done by N.H.S. (Hospital Endowments Fund — Distribution of Assets) Order 1974.[1] Broadly, the Order provided for the distribution of the Fund in accordance with the responsibility for hospitals as at 1st April 1974. The distribution was based upon the average number of occupied beds during the year 1973 in non-teaching hospitals (with beds used for *e.g.* long-stay patients being counted twice).[2] Subject to this, in England 10 per cent of the apportioned assets were distributed to the Regional Health Authorities and 90 per cent to Area Health Authorities and Special Trustees[3] and in Wales (where there are no Regional Health Authorities or Special Trustees) all the apportioned assets are distributed to Area Health Authorities.[4]

Under s. 7 (2) of the 1946 Act it had been the duty of the Secretary of State to secure, so far as had been reasonably practicable, that pre-nationalisation objects and conditions were not prejudiced by transfer to the Fund. S. 7 is now repealed but s. 93 of the 1977[5] Act imposes a similar obligation. It provides:

(2) The person holding the property after the transfer or last transfer shall secure, so far as is reasonably practicable, that the objects of any original endowment and the observance of any conditions attached thereto, including in particular conditions intended to preserve the memory of any person or class of persons, are not prejudiced by the provisions of this Part of this Act or Part II of that Act of 1973.

In this subsection 'original endowment' means a hospital endowment which was transferred under section 7 of that Act of 1946 and from which the property in question is derived.

The section continues:

(3) Subject to the preceding subsection, the property shall be held on trust for such purposes relating to hospital services (including research), or to any other part of the health service associated with any hospital, as the person holding the property thinks fit.

(4) Where the person holding the property is a body of special trustees, the power conferred by the preceding subsection shall be exercised as respects the hospitals for which they are appointed.

---

[1] S.I. 1974 No. 1915.
[2] There were two now relatively unimportant exceptions.
[3] Art. 6.   [4] Art. 7.
[5] Formerly s. 27 of the 1973 Act. It is not repealed but is re-enacted.

6. Trust Property held by Abolished Hospital Authorities

All trust property held by a hospital authority abolished on re-organisation of the National Health Service under the 1973 Act, was at that time transferred to the corresponding Health Authority or to Special Trustees, in accordance with the provisions of s. 24 of that Act, provision for apportionment, if necessary, being made in s. 30. The uses to which such transferred trust property may be put, the discretion exercisable by the person to whom the property has been transferred etc., are set out in s. 94.[1] If, however, the trust property was first acquired as an *endowment* under s. 7 of the Act of 1946, the stricter provisions of s. 93 apply.

7. Endowments acquired Directly or Indirectly under s. 7 of the 1946 Act, transferred to new Health Authorities or to Special Trustees under s. 20 of the 1973 Act

If any trust property transferred under s. 24 from an abolished hospital authority to a Health Authority or to Special Trustees had in origin been received by a hospital authority as an endowment then under the now repealed provisions of s. 7 of the Act of 1946, and now as with the assets of the old Hospital Endowments Fund under s. 27 (2) of the Act of 1973 there is an obligation to secure, so far as is reasonably practicable that the objects of the endowment and the observance of any conditions are not prejudiced by the transfer. Subject thereto, Health Authorities may hold such 'original endowments' for purposes within s. 93 (3) and special trustees for purposes within s. 93 (4). S. 93 begins by saying

(1) This section applies:

    (*a*) to property which is transferred under section 23 of the National Health Service Re-organisation Act 1973 (winding up of hospital endowments funds); and

    (*b*) to property which is transferred under section 24 of that Act (transfer of trust property from abolished authorities) and which immediately before the appointed day was, in accordance with any provision contained in or made under section 7 of the National Health Service Act 1946, applicable for purposes relating to hospital services or relating to some form of research, and this section shall continue to apply to the property after any further transfer under the preceding section.

The objects and conditions referred to in s. 93 (2) are those to which the trust property was subject at the time it was transferred to a hospital authority under s. 7 of the 1946 Act. Like other property transferred under s. 24 of the 1973 Act, original endowments may, if necessary have been subject to apportionment under s. 92 of the 1977 Act[2] or may

---

[1] Formerly s. 28 of the 1973 Act.   [2] Formerly s. 30 of the 1973 Act.

in future be subject to transfer to another Authority or other Special under s. 92 on any change being made of a kind mentioned in s. 92 (1).

8. Trust Property formerly held by Local Health Authorities

Provision was made in s. 25 of the 1973 Act for trust property held by the former local health authorities to be transferred to and vest in such Health Authorities may be specified by an order made by the Secretary of State.[1] Such transfers in some cases were made subject to apportionment under s. 92 of the 1977 Act. Property transferred under s. 25 of the 1973 Act may also be subject to subsequent transfer under s. 92 of the 1977 Act.

9. Power of Secretary of State to make further transfers of Trust Property

Power to make further transfers of trust property between Health Authorities and Special Trustees and *vice versa* and between one Health Authority and another and between Special Trustees is conferred by s. 92 of the 1977 Act[2], reading as follows:

(1) The Secretary of State may, having regard to any change or proposed change in the arrangements for the administration of a hospital or in the area or functions of any Health Authority, by order provide for the transfer of any trust property from any Health Authority or Special Trustees to any other Health Authority or Special Trustees.

(2) If it appears to the Secretary of State at any time that all the functions of any Special Trustees should be discharged by one or more Health Authorities then, whether or not there has been any such change as is mentioned in the preceding subsection, he may by order provide for the transfer of all trust property from the Special Trustees to the Health Authority or, in such proportions as he may specify in the order, to those Health Authorities.

(3) Before acting under this section the Secretary of State shall consult the Health Authorities and Special Trustees concerned.

10. Special Trustees

Under s. 29 (1) of the 1973 Act Special Trustees were to be appointed for those hospitals which immediately before 1st April 1974 were controlled and managed by any University Hospital Management Committee or Board of Governors (except the preserved Boards under s. 15) and anybody on whose request an order was made under s. 24 (2). These Special Trustees who now operate under s. 95 of the 1977 Act hold and administer the property transferred to them. Thus Special Trustees handle property which would otherwise have become the responsibility of the Area Health Authority (Teaching). Likewise the Special Trustees took a share of the Hospital Endowments Fund. By s. 95 (2) the Special

---

[1] The N.H.S. (Transfer of Local Authority Trust Property) Order S.I. 1974 No. 246.
[2] Formerly s. 26 of the 1973 Act. The section is not repealed but is re-enacted.

Trustees have the power to accept further gifts relating to hospital services. The subsection reads:

95—(2) Special Trustees shall have power to accept, hold and administer any property on trust for all or any purposes relating to hospital services (including research), or to any other part of the health service associated with hospitals, being a trust which is wholly or mainly for hospitals for which the Special Trustees are appointed.

As will be seen from a comparison of s. 90 and 95 (2) the trusts on which Special Trustees may hold property are more strictly circumscribed than those on which property may be held by an Area Health Authority. Consequently, where Special Trustees have been appointed, the Area Health Authority (Teaching) may nonetheless accept any trust, the purpose of which falls outside s. 95 (2) but within s. 90.

11. Endowment of Beds

A bed (or cot) may be endowed in a hospital within the health service by payment of such conventional sum as the Area Health Authority is prepared to accept. It normally now means 'naming' a bed according to the donor's wishes and investing the sum paid as capital, the income to be expended for the purposes of the hospital or perhaps the health service generally. Such is the general effect of re Ginger (deceased). Wood Roberts and Another v. Westminster Hospital Board of Governors and Others[1] and of re Mills and Mills (deceased). Midland Bank Executor & Trustee Co. Ltd. v. Board of Governors of United Birmingham Hospitals.[2] In the former case, a gift to endow a cot at Westminster Hospital was left by a will made in 1940, the testator dying in November 1948. The continuity of the work of the hospital was not disputed but the governors although they could still agree to name a cot could not, as had formerly been the custom, give a right to nominate patients to occupy it. It was held that nomination was not a condition of the bequest and therefore the fact that the trustees could not nominate did not invalidate the gift and that it was accordingly payable to the board of governors on their undertaking to name in perpetuity a cot in memory of the testatrix's uncle in Westminster Hospital, St. John's Gardens or such other building to which the hospital might be removed and on their undertaking to invest the sum in investments for the time being authorised by law and to apply the income for the purposes of the hospital. This gift fell within s. 59.

In re Mills and Mills (deceased)[2] the bequest was 'of such sum as shall be necessary to endow a bed in the Children's Hospital Birmingham . . . to be known at all times as the "Mills" bed, in memory of my father, mother and brother'. The testator had died in 1929 but as the bequest

[1] [1951] Ch. 458; [1951] 1 T. L. R. 750.   [2] [1953] 1 W. L. R. 554.

had been subject to a life interest which expired only in 1950, the question had to be settled whether the board of governors could take the gift.

The board of governors said that for thirty years before 1948 the sum of £1,000 had been accepted to endow a bed, that they had not considered the matter since nationalisation but were still willing to name a bed for that sum. They conceded that it was a purely conventional amount, having no reference to the sum required to maintain a bed. On the other side it was contended that testatrix had had in contemplation that there would be a recognised scheme and recognised sum for endowing a bed. Held: That such a scheme was not essential, and that the sum necessary to endow a bed was a conventional sum acceptable to the hospital. The hospital would therefore receive £1,000 on undertaking to name a bed as desired by the testatrix. This gift, presumably, fell within s. 60.

If a sum received by an Authority in return for naming a bed is accepted as capital only the income of which can be spent otherwise than for capital purposes, it constitutes a *permanent endowment* as defined in s. 45 of the Charities Act 1960. Also it must be observed that if the Authority itself resolves that, say, some other amount received be treated as capital, that too will constitute a *permanent endowment*.

12. Endowment of Beds for Private Patients in N.H.S. Hospitals[1]

The question of endowment of beds for private patients came before the court in re *Adams, deceased; Gee and Another* v. *Barnet Group Hospital Management Committee and Another*.[2] Mrs. Adams in her will had made bequests for the endowment of beds for paying patients at Barnet General Hospital and at Finchley Memorial Hospital, both hospitals being within the N.H.S. Cross, J. held that the gift to Barnet General Hospital was good as there was a need at that hospital for beds for paying patients but that the gift to Finchley Memorial Hospital, which already had sufficient pay beds, failed because the words 'endowing beds for paying patients' could not be construed so as to allow the gift to be used to provide a higher standard of maintenance for paying patients than the hospital was already able to provide out of the payments made by paying patients.

On appeal, the judgment in re *Adams, decd.*, so far as it related to Finchley Memorial Hospital was reversed. In the course of his judgment, Dankwerts, L. J., said:

'Mr. Kelly's affidavit which I earlier mentioned suggests a number of ways in which the income of such a fund given by a testator would be used and I think I ought to read them — "The following improvements are desirable (*a*) the provision of better beds, bedding, furniture, crockery, cutlery, floor

---

[1] This class of patient will continue despite the passage of the Health Services Act 1976, see Chapter 6.

[2] [1968] Ch. 80; [1967] 3 All E. R. 285.

coverings, curtains and other furnishings and the better maintenance of all such things; (b) the more frequent redecoration of the accommodation; (c) the sound-proofing of rooms; (d) the provision of telephones and television sets for the use of patients; (e) the provision of better food and a wider choice of food; (f) the provision for patients (who are not required to remain in bed) of a day or sitting room and also a dining room." '

Having quoted that list of things which might be done, he continued:

'It appears to me perfectly proper to apply the income of the fund given to Finchley Memorial Hospital for any of those purposes. As regards the idea that paying patients will not have these amenities, there is nothing unlawful in making provision for them in that way. In view of the heavy payments which they have to make, they may well benefit from any provision which may be made for their comfort and welfare in that hospital. Moreover, it is to be remembered that charity in certain respects is not confined to absolute poverty. In the Statute of Elizabeth, which I suppose may be thought of as the fount and origin of most of the law on this subject, there is, I think, a reference to "poor and infirm" persons.[1] That does not mean that such persons must be both poor and infirm or both infirm and poor. Such infirm persons may be any people suffering from sickness or injury and so such as to fall within the ambit of the term "charity".'

The rather unattractive conclusion which it appears that one has to draw from re Adams is that it is charitable to provide funds not only for providing pay-bed accommodation in a national health service hospital but also for maintaining that accommodation and for providing better food and a wider choice of food, as well as other amenities, presumably without these things being taken into account in determining the charge to be made to patients in that accommodation, this without regard to the patient's means and beyond what is reasonably necessary. If that be so, it would seem to follow that an Authority would commit no breach of trust if it used endowment funds held for the general purposes of the hospital under s. 90 of the National Health Service Act 1977 for capital expenditure on the provision of pay-bed accommodation,[2] or the income of such endowments for maintenance and for better food, a wider choice of food and other amenities, for paying patients and this presumably without such expenditure being taken into account by the Secretary of State in determining pay-bed charges for the class of hospital under s. 65 (3) of the National Health Service Act 1977.[3]

If, however, it were held that, despite payments in respect of provision of pay-bed accommodation and of maintenance of patients therein having been met from endowments, the Secretary of State had

---

[1] The precise expression poor and infirm does not occur in the Statute, i.e. the Statute of Charitable Uses 1601. The expression there used is poor and impotent.

[2] This subject to the difficulty discussed below, viz., that the Secretary of State no longer sets aside pay-bed accommodation, only determining to what extent accommodation shall be made available for paying patients. (1977 Act s. 65 (1), formerly 1968 Act, s. 1 (1).)

[3] For the text of s. 65 (3) see pp. 575–576.

to take such expenditure into account when determining charges for pay-bed accommodation under s. 1 (3) of the 1968 Act, that would consitute an injustice to paying patients in other hospitals classified for determination of charges together with the hospital where the expenditure from endowment funds had taken place, since it would seem to result the cost of additional amenities at one hospital being averaged out so as, in effect, to be paid for by being spread over paying patients in the whole class of hospitals.[1]

The substitution of the provisions of s. 1 of the 1968 Act[2] for those of s. 5 of the 1946 Act relating to the provision of accommodation and services for paying patients, created another difficulty in respect of re Adams type trusts expressly for provision of pay-beds because, whilst under s. 5 of the 1946 Act, and subject to the provisions of that section, the Minister could 'set aside . . . special accommodation' for paying patients in any hospital, under s. 65 of the 1977 Act the Secretary of State does no more than determine the extent to which accommodation in a hospital may be occupied by paying patients at any time; he does not determine which beds. Could it therefore now be said that at any moment in time there existed in any hospital identifiable beds, endowed as pay-beds, particularly as the change in procedure made by s. 1 of the 1968 Act was intended to facilitate the treatment of private patients in whatever beds in whatever part of the hospital best suited their needs? It could certainly have been set of, say, beds in the pay-bed block of a London teaching hospital set aside under s. 5 of the 1946 Act, because — under s. 5 — a bed so set aside could be used for any other than a paying patient only if he urgently needed the accommodation on medical grounds. Under s. 65 of the 1977 Act there is no such restriction on the use of any bed for any patient, whether a paying patient or not. Presumably, therefore, if at any time a hospital had under treatment the maximum number of paying in-patients authorised by the Secretary of State, but one or more of those patients in beds otherwise than those normally reserved for paying patients, it would be the duty of the hospital in accordance with the spirit and intention of the Act and the determination of the Secretary of State, to use the spare pay-patient beds for non-paying patients, and this not necessarily on grounds of urgent medical need. Thus, strict identification of pay-beds for endowment purposes may become extremely difficult. It would seem, therefore, that the substitution of the provisions of s. 1 of the 1968 Act for those of s. 5 of the 1946 Act has given rise to a situation which might constitute something of an obstacle to the establishment of re Adams type endowments in the future. The implementation of the provisions as to common waiting lists in the Health Services Act 1976 will add to the difficulties.[3]

---

[1] As to extra charges for additional personal amenities provided on request, reference should be made to H.M. (69) 25, para.18.
[2] Now s. 65 of the 1977 Act.   [3] See, below p. 105.

13. Whether Nationalisation affects Conditional Gifts: Discretion of Trustees to decide whether Controlled by State

In *Royal College of Surgeons of England* v. *National Provincial Bank Ltd. and Others*[1] a testatrix who died in 1943 had given her residuary estate to trustees to form an 'endowment fund', the income of which was to be used *inter alia* to support the Bland-Sutton Institute of Pathology carried on in connection with the Middlesex Hospital the gift being subject to a proviso that, should the Middlesex Hospital become nationalised or by any means pass into public ownership, the endowment should be transferred to the Royal College of Surgeons. The Bland-Sutton Institute of Pathology before July 5th, 1948, had been part of the medical school of the Middlesex Hospital, the school being carried on as an integral part of the hospital.

The House of Lords decided that although the medical school was not nationalised, being transferred to an independent governing body established in association with the University of London in accordance with s. 15 of the Act of 1946, the hospital had been nationalised within the meaning of the will and that, as the Royal College of Surgeons was a charity, the gift did not fail as a perpetuity.

A Scottish case, *Dundee General Hospital Board of Management* v. *Walker and Another*[2] which reached the House of Lords turned on the question of the limits of the discretion given to the trustees of the will. The gift of £10,000 to the hospital was to be payable 'only if my trustees shall in their sole and absolute discretion be satisfied that at my death the said infirmary has not been taken over wholly or partly or otherwise placed under the control of the State or of a local authority'. The testator died in April 1947 and the hospital was one which was within the National Health Service (Scotland) Act 1947, and so transferred to the Secretary of State on July 5th, 1948, under substantially similar conditions to those for transfer of English hospitals to the Minister of Health on the same day under the 1946 Act. And in the Scottish Act of 1947,[3] as in the English Act of 1946,[4] there was a provision for nullifying any dealing with property after March 21st, 1946, with the intent of defeating the purpose of the Act. Having regard to that provision the trustees decided that the circumstances in which the legacy was not to be paid had arisen. The House of Lords decided that the decision of the trustees could not be questioned as the testator had made them sole judges. They were entitled to take the provisions of s. 9 (8) of the Act of 1947 into account.

Re Buzzacott (deceased). Munday and Another v. *King's College Hospital and Others.*[5] A testator made a will on September 27th, 1948,

[1] [1952] A. C. 631; [1952] 1 T. L. R. 978; [1952] 1 All E. R. 984.
[2] [1952] 1 All E. R. 896. [3] S. 9 (8). [4] S. 9 (7). [5] [1952] 2 All E. R. 1011.

and died on July 23rd, 1949. By his will he left one equal fourth part of his residuary trust fund in trust to divide equally among four institutions including the Royal Eye Hospital and the Royal Cancer Hospital 'provided that if any of the funds of the above-mentioned institutions shall have come under government control at the date of my death then the share payable to such institutions shall not be paid to them . . .'. Each of the two hospitals was designated part of a teaching hospital under the 1946 Act. Held: That on the true construction of the Act a teaching hospital was under the overriding control of the Minister of Health and that they exercised their functions on his behalf. Consequently, the hospitals were, within the meaning of the will, under government control and the gifts to them did not take effect.

In the course of his judgment, Wynn-Parry, J., speaking of the duties of the board of governors of a teaching hospital in relation to transferred endowments said:

'They (*i.e., the transferred endowments*) are, however, even in the case of boards of governors, freed from the trusts which prior to their transfer to such boards of governors affected them, and the boards of governors are placed under the duty, through the use of the word "trust" to give effect to the purposes of the Act, bearing in mind any special trusts or conditions under which the endowment funds were previously held, the giving effect to which would not be inconsistent with the main purposes of the Act. But where there would be any such inconsistency the policy of the Act is to prevail over the wishes of those who established the endowment fund.'

In re *Lowry's Will Trusts; Barclays Bank Ltd.* v. *United Newcastle-upon-Tyne Hospitals Board of Governors and Others*[1] Cross, J., decided that, whilst a voluntary hospital taken over by the Minister of Health under s. 6 of the National Health Service Act 1946 was still a charity, it had ceased to be independent and so could not share in a contingent residual bequest, the continued independence of the hospital at the time of vesting being a condition precedent of the bequest. The facts of the case were as follows.

The testator, who died in 1944 had given his sister and her son successive life interests in a trust fund, known as Mrs. Dalgleish's fund. On the son's death the trust fund was to go to his issue in equal shares and, failing issue, to thirteen named charities in equal shares, the contingent gift to the named charities being subject to the proviso 'if at the time of the failure if the trusts aforesaid any of the said charities shall have ceased to exist as an independent charity Mrs. Dalgleish's fund shall be divided in equal shares among such of the said charities as shall then be in existence'. The son died unmarried and without issue in 1963.

On a motion to determine the effect of the proviso, Cross, J., found that the testator drew no distinction between charities 'in existence' and

[1] [1967] 1 Ch. 638.

'charities in existence as independent charities' and so held that the words 'as independent charities' had to be read in at the end of the proviso. He found too that by 'independent' the testator meant 'self-governing' and that hospitals taken over by the Minister under s. 6 of the National Health Service Act 1946 were no longer self-governing. Accordingly the gift failed.

14. Effect of Amalgamation under the Health Service Acts on Gifts

Re Hutchinson's Will Trusts. Gibbons v. *Nottingham Area No. 1 Hospital Management Committee*[1] was a case in which the facts were quite exceptional. A testator made his will in 1946, making a bequest to a particular voluntary hospital. The hospital in 1947 (*i.e.*, before the transfer to the Minister) was, with the approval of the Minister but without a scheme sanctioned by the Charity Commissioners, amalgamated with another hospital and the work of the first hospital thereafter carried out at the other. The amalgamated hospital passed to the Minister on July 5th, 1948. The testator died in 1952 without altering his will. Held: That the bequest was good as it was the work, and not the particular institution where it was carried on at the date of the will, that it was intended to benefit. The property was therefore declared not undisposed of but the judge (Upjohn, J.) did not declare that the defendant committee were entitled as, in order to allow them to give a valid receipt, a scheme might have to be prepared and approved by the Court or by the Charity Commissioners. This reservation would not have been necessary but for the amalgamation *before* July 5th, 1948.

Gifts for charitable purposes are not subject to the rule against perpetuities. In effect, this means that a gift may be made to a charity in terms that the capital is kept intact without limit of time. Also, there is no obstacle to prevent a gift being given so as to pass from one charity to another on, say, the happening of an event, such as the amalgamation or nationalisation of the first charity at any time. And, provided the donor, by settlement or will, has expressed a general charitable intention, his intention will be carried out, even though he has not named the charity he wishes to benefit in that event. But the rule against perpetuities is not relaxed otherwise than in favour of charities; nor is uncertainty cured, except in favour of charities. And it has been decided[2] that benevolent objects are not necessarily charitable in the legal sense. This led to a peculiar result in *re Bawdon's Settlement. Besant and Others* v. *Board of Governors of London Hospital and Others*.[3] In that case a testator, before July 5th, 1948, left annual income between charities mentioned (including voluntary hospitals

---

[1] [1953] Ch. 387.
[2] *Chichester Diocesan Fund and Board of Finance* v. *Simpson and Others* [1944] A. C. 341, and *re Peel's Settlement* [1921] 2 Ch. 218.
[3] [1953] 2 All E. R. 1235; [1954] 1 W. L. R. 33

subsequently transferred to the Minister), in shares and proportions indicated with a proviso that if any had become amalgamated in any other charities or institutions the trustees might in their discretion pay or apply the share of that charity to or for such other objects or purposes of charity *or benevolence* or amelioration of human suffering . . . as they should in their opinion consider to be in accordance with the original desire and intention of the testator. In the case of those transferred hospitals which had become part of a teaching hospital group under a board of governors it was held that by the provisions of the National Health Service (Designation of Teaching Hospitals (No. 2)) Order 1948,[1] all the institutions under a single board of governors had become a single teaching hospital and so amalgamated. It was further held that the provisions of s. 60 of the National Health Service Act 1946, did not operate so as to override the provisions contained in the trust instrument for diversion of the funds on amalgamation. However, in the event, the hospitals concerned, the London Hospital and the Royal Cancer Hospital, did not lose their share of the income under the will because the clause providing for diversion on amalgamation was held to be void on the authority of, *inter alia, Chichester Diocesan Fund and Board of Finance* v. *Simpson and Others,*[2] and in re *Peel's Settlements,*[3] since the trustees could have applied the whole of the gift over for benevolent, as distinct from charitable, objects, which would have offended against the rule against perpetuities. Consequently the shares were payable to the bodies then carrying on medical teaching work at those transferred hospitals.

Because of the different provisions for grouping non-teaching hospitals under hospital management committees, it was held that Poplar Hospital, which was included in the No. 8 Bow Group, was not amalgamated with the other hospitals in the group and therefore the diversionary clause in the will would not in any event have been operative. Consequently, the income in both cases continued to be received by the hospitals concerned subject to the provisions of s. 60 of the National Health Service Act 1946.

15. Breaches of Trust by Health Authorities

It would appear that there would be no liability as charitable trustees on individual members of Health Authorities within the National Health Service — Regional and Area Health Authorities, Special Trustees and Boards of Governors — in respect of technical breaches of trust (*e.g.,* unauthorised investment in good faith) as distinct from fraudulent breach of trust, since the corporate body is the trustee and not the individuals constituting its membership, members being expressly protected in

[1] S.I. 1948 No. 979.   [2] [1944] A.C. 341.   [3] [1921] 2 Ch. 218.

respect of *bona fide* acts, etc., in the course of their duties by s. 265 of the Public Health Act 1875, as extended by s. 125 of the National Health Service Act 1977.[1] Since there is no power of surcharge on members of Health Authorities, the proviso to s. 265 of the Act of 1875 does not apply to them.

16. Borrowing Powers of Health Authorities as Charity Trustees

Whilst there is nothing in the National Health Service Act to hinder Health Authorities from borrowing against the security of property held by way of permanent endowment[2] on charitable trusts, they — like trustees of other charities, not being exempt or excepted charities[3] — are subject to the provisions of s. 29 of the Charities Act 1960,[4] which section prohibits the mortgaging or charging of permanent endowments[3] without an order of the court or of the Charity Commissioners or the disposal of land without such order.

E. VOLUNTARY HOSPITALS AND NURSING HOMES — ENDOWMENTS OF BEDS FOR PRIVATE PATIENTS

1. General

The provision of pay-beds by voluntary hospitals has been common practice for many years now, having been facilitated by the passing of the Voluntary Hospitals (Paying Patients) Act 1936[5] which, subject to safeguards, allowed trusts of hospitals established for the sick poor to be amended to include the provision of pay-bed accommodation. The decision in *re Adams, decd.*,[6] applies no less to such hospitals than to hospitals within the National Health Service.

The question therefore arises whether that part of the judgment which allows the income of an endowment to be used for current maintenance and, in particular, for the specific purposes referred to by Dankwerts, L.J., allows or requires the hospital to pass on the advantage of the use of the endowment income in the form of reduction of charges to, or increase in amenities of, all paying patients, indifferently without regard to means. In the absence of any direct authority on the point and despite that being a not unreasonable deduction from the judgment in the above case, it is perhaps wise to hesitate to adopt a point of view so much at variance with common practice and with the spirit of the Voluntary Hospitals (Paying Patients) Act 1936, which ordinarily obliges the Charity Commissioners, when approving a scheme for

---

[1] Formerly s. 72 of the 1946 Act as amended.
[2] See p. 64 and ss. 45 (3) and 46 of the Charities Act 1960 for definition of *permanent endowment*.
[3] For definition of *exempt charity* see s. 45 (1).
[4] For the text of s. 29 see pp. 58–59.   [5] See p. 108 *et seq.*   [6] see p. 94 *et seq.*

provision of pay-beds in a voluntary hospital, to see that patients unable
to pay full cost, though able to pay something, should be given priority
in certain beds.[1] Moreover, to charge less than full cost to anyone to
whom it would be no real financial hardship to pay the full cost would
in most cases be contrary to the trusts of the institution. And it may be
suggested that even were there no express obligation to take the means
of the patient into account before making any abatement in the charge,
not to do so would be a less than prudent management of the charity.
To take that standpoint is not to deprive the well-to-do of the benefits
of the hospital which, as necessary to them in the present state of
medical knowledge are as necessary to them as they are to the poor.
They, like all other patients, will have the benefit of the expensive
apparatus and other special facilities of the hospital as well as medical
care and attention, none of which they could perhaps obtain elsewhere,
but they will ordinarily pay full cost. In short, their need is for treatment, not for relief from the cost of providing it; others able to pay
something may be in such financial circumstances that an abatement
of the charge for a pay-bed is, in their case, justified.

2. Endowment of Beds for Private Patients in Nursing Homes

Latterly the Charity Commissioners have been willing to recognise
as a charity a nursing home taking mostly, if not exclusively, paying
patients, most of whom will be expected to pay full cost of maintenance,
subject to the Commissioners being satisfied that its objects — as set
out in its trust deed or memorandum and articles — are exclusively
charitable. In law such a nursing home recognised as a charity would be
indistinguishable from a voluntary hospital and *re Adams, decd.*
would similarly apply. It is, however, interesting to note by way of
example that in the case of one substantial charity incorporated in
1957[2] to provide and finance non-profit nursing homes, the main objects
include the following — 'To prevent, relieve and cure sickness and ill-
health of every kind (including physical injuries) and to promote
health by . . . providing facilities gratuitously or otherwise *according to
their means* for patients resident (and, if thought fit, non-resident) in
nursing homes, hospital pay-beds and similar institutions . . .' Other
objects include building, taking over and managing nursing homes.
In the case of a charitable nursing home with such main objects, it
would seemingly be a breach of trust to make reduced charges to all
patients indifferently without any regard to means, despite its having
an endowment of the Finchley Memorial Hospital type as approved in
re Adams, decd.

[1] S. 3.   [2] Nuffield Nursing Homes Trust (a company limited by guarantee).

CHAPTER 6

PROVISION OF PAY BEDS

A. HOSPITALS UNDER THE NATIONAL HEALTH SERVICE ACTS

S.6 of the National Health Service Act 1977[1] authorises, under certain conditions, provision of hospital accommodation in single rooms or small wards on part payment by or for the patient of the cost of providing it, charges for such accommodation being determined by the Secretary of State for Social Services in accordance with the provisions of the section s. 4 of the Health Services and Public Health Act 1968. Beds so made available are referred to in hospital parlance as 'amenity beds', this to distinguish them from beds for private patients who pay charges, designed to cover the full cost of accommodation and treatment. Ss. 65 to 66[2] of the 1977 Act authorise provision of accommodation and services for private patients on payment of charges determined by the Secretary of State, being charges designed to average out to cover full cost of provision of such accommodation and services.

1. 'Amenity Beds'

Accommodation available on part payment may be provided under s. 63 of the National Health Service Act 1977 reads:

63.—(1) The Secretary of State may authorise the accommodation described in this section to be made available, to such extent as he may determine, for patients who give an undertaking (or for whom one is given) to pay such charges for part of the cost as the Secretary of State may determine, and he may recover those charges.

The accommodation mentioned above is —

(a) in single rooms or small wards which is not for the time being needed by any patient on medical grounds;

(b) at any health service hospital or group of hospitals, or a hospital in which patients are treated under arrangements made by virtue of section 23 above, or at the health service hospitals in a particular area or a hospital in which patients are so treated.

(2) The Secretary of State may allow such deductions as he thinks fit from the amount of a charge due by virtue of an undertaking given under this section to be paid for accommodation in respect of any period during which the accommodation is temporarily vacated by the person for whom it is made available.

[1] Formerly s. 4 of the 1946 Act and see also s. 4 of the 1968 Act.
[2] Formerly ss. 1–3 of the 1968 Act.

F

2. Accommodation for and Treatment of Private In-patients

S. 65 of the National Health Service Act 1977 makes provision for the accommodation for and treatment of private in-patients. Section 65 (1) reads as follows:

65.—(1) Subject to section 71 below, if the Secretary of State is satisfied, in the case of a health service hospital or group of such hospitals or of the health service hospitals in a particular area, that it is reasonable to do so —

(*a*) he may, subject to this section, authorise accommodation and services at the hospital or hospitals in question to be made available to such extent as he may determine; and

(*b*) that accommodation and those services shall be available for resident patients who give an undertaking (or for whom one is given) to pay such charges as he may determine in accordance with the following provisions of this section, and the Secretary of State may recover those charges.

The main difference between the provisions of s. 65 (1) of the Act of 1977 and the roughly corresponding provisions of s. 5 of the Act of 1946, was that under the earlier Act, what the Secretary of State was authorised to do was to 'set aside . . . special accommodation' for private patients whilst under s. 65 of the 1977 Act he may authorise that not more than so many beds in a particular hospital be available for private patients without necessarily setting specific accommodation aside for the purpose.

By the Health Services Act 1976[1] the number of beds authorised for private patients controlled by each Area Authority and preserved Boards had to be reduced by an initial specified number[2] within six months of the coming into force of the Act, *i.e.* 22nd May 1977 (*the initial period*). In carrying out this task each authority was to have regard to the extent to which the treatment of resident private patients was carried out at the hospital before then and the extent to which alternative accommodation and facilities for private practice were (on 31st December 1973) reasonably available (whether privately or at N.H.S. hospitals) in the area served by each hospital.[3]

The Act also set up a Health Services Board.[4] The Board is bound to submit proposals and the Secretary of State to give effect to them for the progressive revocation of any remaining authorisations under s. 65 (1) and s. 66 (1) of the 1977 Act.[5] A timetable is laid down but departures from it are allowed.[6] Representations may be made to the Board.[7]

In formulating its proposals the Board is to have regard to the principles set out in s. 70. They are:

---

[1] Those sections of the Act which have not been consolidated are set out in Appendix B on pages 659–676.
[2] Sch. 2.   [3] S. 3.
[4] S. 1 and 1st Sch. The Board is expressed *not* to be a servant or agent of the Crown.
[5] Ss. 68 and 69 of the 1977 Act.   [6] S. 68 (2).   [7] S. 68 (3).

(*a*) that accommodation or services at any particular N.H.S. hospital should remain authorised only while there is a reasonable demand for accommodation and facilities for private practice in the area served by the hospital;

(*b*) that the authorisation of any accommodation for private use should be revoked only if sufficient accommodation and facilities for private practice is otherwise reasonably available (whether privately or at N.H.S. hospitals) to meet the reasonable demand in the area served by the hospital in question;

(*c*) the continued authorisation of any accommodation for private use should depend on there having been or being taken all reasonable steps to provide, otherwise than at N.H.S. hospitals, sufficient reasonable accommodation for private practice in the area served by the hospital in question;

(*d*) that the failure to take such reasonable steps would itself be grounds for the Board, after giving due warning to persons likely to be affected thereby, to propose the revocation of the authorisations at the hospital in question.

No new authorisations under ss. 65 and 66 are to be allowed.[1]

By s. 76, within the initial period (*i.e.* six months after the coming into force of the Act), the Board must have made recommendations as to what arrangements for affording persons admission as resident private patients are in the opinion of the Board best suited for securing that all persons admitted to N.H.S. hospitals as resident patients are, so far as practicable, admitted on the basis of medical priority alone whether they come as private patients or not. In this way it is hoped to establish what the sub-heading to the section calls *a common waiting list*.

The separation of the public and private sectors of medicine gives added importance to what are now ss. 58 and 61 of the 1977[2] Act. Under these sections the Secretary of State is empowered to allow anybody to make use of any services, the provision of which is involved in the provision of hospital and medical services (s. 58) and to sell, give away or otherwise dispose of goods the production or manufacture by him is involved in the provision of hospital and specialist services (s. 61). By s. 62 of the 1977 Act, the power under s. 61 is exercisable only so long as it does not interfere with his duties under the Acts and it does not operate to the disadvantage of persons seeking admission at N.H.S. hospitals otherwise than as private patients.

By s. 59 of the 1977 Act, in effect the powers in s. 58 of the 1977 Act are: (*a*) not to be exercised at all unless the Secretary of State is satisfied that the accommodation or services are required for the purposes of investigation, diagnosis or treatment which is of a specialised nature (or involves the use of specialised equipment or skills) and is either not privately available in Great Britain or if it is not reasonably accessible to the patient or it is in the interests of the national health services for it to be carried out on that occasion at that N.H.S. hospital; (*b*) nor can

[1] S. 71 (1).   [2] Formerly ss. 31 and 32 of the 1968 Act.

they be exercised unless such services or accommodation are, so far as is practicable, provided on the basis of medical priority alone and even then they must not be provided so as to allow any particular accommodation or facilities at a N.H.S. hospital to be reserved or set aside for regular or repeated use in connection with the treatment of persons as private patients; (c) in the exercise of these powers the Secretary of State must fix charges which involve no increase in the expenditure on the health service (including the capital account) and where the services are provided by a whole-time consultant they may not be less than would be charged by a private consultant. By s. 60 (4), if the Secretary of State so authorises, any fees received in respect of the services of a wholetime consultant shall be retained either by the Area Authority for the purpose of research and development or by the direction of the Secretary of State by the medical school (or university) concerned.

S. 65 (2) provides that the Secretary of State may allow accommodation and services authorised under s. 65 (1) to be made available in connection with the treatment, in pursuance with arrangements made by a medical practitioner or dental practitioner serving, whether in an honorary or a paid capacity, on the staff of a hospital vested in the Secretary of State of private patients of that practitioner as resident patients. Section 5 of the Act of 1946 expressly envisaged a medical practitioner on the staff of a hospital being able to treat his private patients in that hospital *or in any other hospital* with accommodation available. S. 65 (2) of the Act of 1977 could apparently be interpreted in the same sense though in fact, accommodation for private patients at any hospital is usually the close preserve of the consultants on the staff of that hospital and the extent of the availability of private beds to individual consultants usually determined locally — either formally or informally.

It is to be noted that s. 5 (2) of the Act of 1946 having ceased to have effect and the Act of 1977 containing no corresponding provision, the Secretary of State no longer has power by regulations to fix maximum charges by medical and dental practitioners treating their patients in hospital, whether as in-patients or as out-patients.

Section 65 (3) and (4) of the 1977 Act concern the power of the Secretary of State to determine charges for different classes of hospitals and for different types of authorised accommodation. Under s. 65 (5) he may allow a deduction from the charge so determined if the patient is being treated privately under s. 65 (2) and also if the patient temporarily vacates his accommodation.[1] S. 60 (2) of the 1977 Act makes similar

---

[1] The charges determined cover only accommodation and services normally provided at the hospital for private patients. Where a patient asks for additional personal amenities, such as special food or additional nursing services not required on medical grounds, he must pay for them separately, even though the hospital authority may, as a matter of convenience, arrange for them to be supplied. (H.M. (69) 25, para. 18.) Manifestly, a hospital is not obliged to accede to any such request.

provision as regards non-authorised accommodation used privately under s. 58 of the 1977 Act.

Although under s. 65 of the 1977 Act it is no longer neceassry that accommodation for private patients should be specifically set aside, the substance of the proviso to s. 5 (1) of the 1946 Act, giving priority in the use of pay-bed accommodation to non-paying patients on grounds of urgent medical need, is preserved in s. 65 (6) of the 1977 Act, reading as follows:

65.—(6) Nothing in this section shall prevent accommodation from being made available for a patient other than one mentioned in sub-section (1) above if the use thereof is needed more urgently for him on medical grounds than for a patient so mentioned and no other suitable accommodation is available.

Thus, a hospital authority, on urgent medical grounds, may admit a patient other than a private patient to accommodation ordinarily kept for private patients and may do so even though it reduces below the authorised number, the number of private patients who can be accepted anywhere in the hospital, or in a particular department. S. 65 (6) also covers the movement of a private patient already in hospital to some other, possibly less attractive accommodation, or even his discharge if medically reasonable, to make way for a non-paying patient in urgent medical need. These provisions were strengthened by the Health Services Act 1976.

3. Accommodation and Treatment for Private Out-patients

Under s. 66 of the National Health Service Act 1977, the Secretary of State, if he is satisfied that it is reasonable to do so, may authorise out-patient accommodation and services in a hospital to be made available in connection with the treatment of private patients by any medical or dental practitioner serving, whether in an honorary or a paid capacity, on the staff of any such hospital, this subject to the patient, or someone on his behalf, having undertaken to pay such charges as the Minister may determine. No such accommodation and no services are to be made available to private patients to the prejudice of persons availing themselves of services at a hospital otherwise than as private patients.[1]

The separation of the public and private sectors intended by the Health Service Act and applied as noted above as regards in-patients is also applied by the Act to out-patients and to N.H.S. services and facilities generally. In particular the Health Services Board is to apply the principles in s. 70 and the powers in ss. 58 and 61 of the 1977 Act are similarly circumscribed as regards out-patients. Further, by s. 72 general practitioners *etc.* wishing to use any N.H.S. facilities for their

[1] S. 66 (3).

private patients must apply to the Secretary of State. On receiving such an application he shall consider whether anything for which permission is sought would to a significant extent operate to the disadvantage of persons seeking or afforded access otherwise than as private patients to any services provided under the National Health Services Act, and shall grant the permission applied for unless in his opinion anything for which permission is sought would be to a significant extent so operated.[1] There were transitional provisions as regards permissions that were extant when the Act came into force.

B. VOLUNTARY HOSPITALS

1. General

Voluntary hospitals established in recent years are likely to have sufficiently wide powers to permit the use of land, buildings and funds of the charity for provision for pay-bed patients, *i.e.*, patients paying the full cost of maintenance and nursing in hospital including attendance by the resident medical and surgical staff of the hospital.[2] Such patients are also usually required to make a private arrangement for attendance by a physician or surgeon of consultant standing and to pay him his fees. Some older voluntary hospitals, however, were limited by their constitution to the treatment of sick poor so that the treatment of persons able to pay full cost was *ultra vires*. But as was stated in a memorandum attached to the Bill which subsequently became the Voluntary Hospitals (Paying Patients) Act 1936, there are 'patients who, in the event of serious illness or operation, cannot afford the cost of private treatment, but are able and willing to pay for treatment in a hospital at charges proportionate to their means. There are also now many modern methods of diagnosis and treatment which cannot be provided without the aid of the specialised equipment and staff of a hospital except at great expense, if at all'. The Voluntary Hospitals (Paying Patients) Act 1936, was therefore passed to empower voluntary hospitals in pursuance of an order of the Charity Commissioners to provide accommodation and treatment for paying patients.

For the purposes of the Act *voluntary hospital* is defined as an institution (not being an institution which is carried on for profit or which is maintained wholly or mainly at the expense of the rates *or*

---

[1] It will be noted that the Secretary of State himself is responsible for this discretion: it is not like other separations of the public and private sectors given to the non-accountable Health Services Board. It does, however, seem likely, although the directions have not at the time of writing yet been given, that the power will be given to either the Regional or the Area Health Authorities.

[2] It is also understood that some nursing homes, wholly for paying patients have in recent years been established as charities. Apparently the main purpose of such nursing homes is to provide accommodation for patients 'insured' against cost of hospital treatment by subscription to one of the organisations which have generally become known as provident schemes.

which is vested in the Minister of Health[1]) which provides medical or surgical treatment for in-patients. Under the Act such a hospital, if it has not already power to provide pay-beds, may apply to the Charity Commissioners for an order allowing it to do so and such order may be made notwithstanding the trusts express or implied upon which the property and funds of the hospital are held, and notwithstanding any prohibition or restriction imposed by or any local Act relating expressly to the hospital. Any such order made must specify the period for which it is to be operative; how many pay-beds may be maintained, and whether in a new or an old building on land in possession of the hospital. The order must also lay down a scale of charges for accommodation and maintenance (including such medical and surgical attendance and treatment as is given by the resident staff of the hospital).[2] Except when the Charity Commissioners are satisfied that it would be inappropriate in the circumstances to do so, they must include in the scale of charges specified in an order charges fixed with a view to meeting the needs of patients who, though able to make some payment, are unable to pay charges sufficient to meet the full expense to the hospital of their accommodation and maintenance (including such medical and surgical attendance and treatment as is given by the resident staff of the hospital) and must make it a condition of the order that in the use of a specified number of the beds, the maintenance of which is authorised, priority shall be given to such patients. The order may allow the difference between the full expense to the hospital of such patients and the sum authorised to be charged to them to be defrayed out of the general funds of the hospital.[3]

The Act does not allow any order to be made authorising any use of property or funds which apart from the order would involve a breach of trust except:

(*a*) in the case of land unless they are satisfied that if the order were not made the land would not come into use for the purposes for which the trusts were created or the prohibition or restriction was imposed until after the expiration of a substantial period from the date of application.

(*b*) in the case of building either (i) that the use of the buildings or part thereof for the purposes for which the trusts were created or the prohibition or restriction was imposed is impracticable, or likely soon so to become, because the committee of management have not at their disposal, and will be unable to obtain sufficient funds to enable the buildings or that part thereof to be, or to continue to be, so used, or (ii) that the use of the buildings or part thereof for the purposes afore-

---

[1] The words in italics were added by the National Health Service Act 1946. Now, the Secretary of State for Social Services.
[2] S. 2.   [3] S. 3.

said is impracticable, or is likely soon so to become because of a shortage of demand for accommodation on the part of the persons for whose benefit the trusts were created or the prohibition or restriction was imposed; or, (iii) that the committee of management have, or are likely soon to have, at their disposal premises which could be put to the use to which the application related without breach of any trust upon which those premises are held or contravention of any such prohibition or restriction as aforesaid and that the buildings or part thereof will be used by way of exchange for those premises. In any case such authorisation to use land or buildings must not be given if it would diminish or restrict the accommodation for persons who were intended to benefit by the original trust as at the date of the order and which the hospital would have been able to maintain had the order not been made.[1]

The powers of the Charity Commissioners under the above Act are in addition to any other powers exercisable by them.[2] Consequently, it would in principle be possible for the Charity Commissioners, when the original trusts of a voluntary hospital were no longer capable of being carried out or otherwise within the limits of s. 13 of the Charities Act, 1960,[3] to permit the provision of pay beds as part of a scheme of administration *cy-près* independently of that Act, but it would seem unlikely that circumstances could arise which the Charity Commissioners would feel justified them in authorising provision of pay-beds without regard to the conditions laid down in the Act.

2. Part-paying Patients

If the part payment is contractual then its validity must stand or fall on the same considerations as full payment. If it is in the nature of a genuinely voluntary gift by a poor patient who, not being able to afford full cost, makes a contribution of his own free will, then there would seem to be no irregularity even though the hospital is not, by its constitution, allowed to accept payment. This of course does not apply where the promise of the gift is extracted under threat that some service or facility will not be rendered or afforded.

Part III of the Health Services Act 1976 introduces new controls on the building *etc.* of voluntary hospitals. It distinguishes what it calls controlled works from certifiable works.[4] *Controlled works* are works of construction or extension (or adaption) of, or conversion into, *controlled premises*. These are defined in s. 12 (2) as:

premises at which there are or are to be facilities for the provision of all or any of the following services, namely —

---

[1] S. 4 (c).   [2] S. 6 (2).   [3] See pp. 67–68.
[4] Both are liable to inspection under the Health Services Board (Inspectors) Regs. S.I. 1977 No. 673.

(a) the carrying out of surgical procedures under general anaesthesia;
(b) obstetrics;
(c) radiotherapy;
(d) renal dialysis;
(e) radiology or diagnostic pathology,

being premises which, if situated or to be situated in Greater London, provide or will provide one hundred or more beds for the reception of patients or, if situated or to be situated elsewhere, provide or will provide seventy-five or more beds for the reception of patients.

Certifiable works are works of construction or extension (or adaption) of, or conversion into, a hospital premises[1] which are not works for which authorisation is required.

The procedure for certification is that the applicant has to merely satisfy the Health Services Board that the works intended to be carried out do not require authorisation (by the Board)[2]. However, so far as controlled works are concerned, s. 13 provides:

(2) On receiving an application for an authorisation the Board shall consider whether, having regard to the matters mentioned in subsection (3) below, the execution of the works in question —
(a) would to a significant extent interfere with the performance by the Secretary of State of any duty imposed on him by the National Health Service Acts to provide accommodation or services of any kind; or
(b) would to a significant extent operate to the disadvantage of persons seeking or afforded admission or access to any accommodation or services provided by the Secretary of State under those Acts (whether as resident or non-resident patients) otherwise than as private patients,

and shall grant the authorisation unless, having regard to those matters, it is satisfied that the execution of the works would do either or both of the things mentioned in paragraphs (a) and (b) above.
(3) The matters referred to in subsection (2) above are, in relation to the works in question —
(a) how much accommodation or additional accommodation the works would provide;
(b) what facilities or additional facilities the works would enable to be provided;
(c) what staffing requirements or additional staffing requirements the works would give rise to.
(4) An authorisation may contain such terms as the Board thinks appropriate, including in particular, without prejudice to the generality of the preceding provisions of this subsection, terms as to the duration of the authorisation and the place at which or area within which the works may be executed; and the Board may, with the consent of the person to whom an authorisation was issued, alter any of its terms at any time.

The importance of obtaining the appropriate certificate or authorisation is that any application for planning permission under the Town and

[1] Defined in s. 14 (7) and the Health Services Board (Hospital Premises). Regs S.I. 1977 No. 643.
[2] Further procedural matters are dealt with in the Health Services Board (Authorisation and Notification) Regs. S.I. 1977 No. 644.

Country Planning Acts is deemed to have no effect unless accompanied by copies of such documentation. There are transitional provisions as regards planning applications made before the commencement of this part of the Act.[1]

The Act and regulations to be made later set out the procedure for making applications for authorisations or certificates, for the Board either by itself to hear the applicant and other parties and for appeals on points of law to the courts. There is not space in this book to set out these matters in detail. It should however also be noted that contravention of s. 12 of the Health Services Act (executing unauthorised controlled works) has been added to the list of grounds in the Nursing Homes Act 1975 under which registration of a nursing home or mental nursing home may be cancelled.[2]

[1] On 2nd January 1977.   [2] S. 19. See Chapter 25.

CHAPTER 7

HOSPITAL CHARGES

A. VALIDITY OF CHARGES LEVIED

THE subject of charges for treatment of persons injured in motor accidents and falling within the provisions of the Road Traffic Act 1972, is most conveniently dealt with in a separate section. Consequently it is proposed to consider first the question of charges in respect of treatment of other types of case in public authority hospitals and in voluntary hospitals respectively.

1. For other than Road Accident Cases within Road Traffic Act

(a) Hospitals administered under the National Health Service Act

Except as explained below, and subject to what is said on p. 119 *et seq.* about claims under the Road Traffic Act 1972, all hospital and specialist services under the National Health Service Act, 1977, are to be provided free of charge.

(i) *Recovery of expenses of maintenance in-patient engaged in remunerative employment during the day.* S. 64 of the Act of 1977,[1] provides for recovery of expenses of maintenance in hospital from in-patients engaged in remunerative employment during the day. No regulations are necessary and the Secretary of State has full discretion to charge what is reasonable.

(ii) *Persons not ordinarily resident in Great Britain.* By s. 121[2] of the National Health Service Act 1977, the Secretary of State may make regulations providing for the making and recovery in such manner as may be prescribed, of such charges in respect of such services provided under the Act as may be prescribed, being services provided in respect of persons not ordinarily resident in Great Britain as may be prescribed, and such regulations may provide that the charges are only to be made in such cases as may be determined in accordance with regulations. At the time of writing[3] no such regulations have been made.

(iii) *Accommodation available on part payment.* The making available of hospital accommodation on part payment is authorised within the limits laid down in s. 63 of the National Health Service Act 1977, as

---

[1] Formerly s. 28 of the 1949 Act. [2] Formerly s. 17 of the 1949 Act.
[3] September 1977.

amended.[1] The powers under the section are delegated to the Regional Health Authority.[2]

The Secretary of State in a circular to hospital authorities has laid down common form of agreement for signature by patients wishing to have s. 63 accommodation. The same circular states what explanations should be made to them.[3]

(iv) *Accommodation for private patients.* The provision of hospital accommodation for private patients paying charges designed broadly to cover full cost or on whose behalf such charges are paid is authorised within the limits laid down in ss. 65 and 66 of the National Health Service Act 1977.[4]

The powers of the Secretary of State under the Act are delegated in the case of sections 65 (1) and 66 to the Regional Health Authority and in the case of sections 65 (2), (5) and (1) and 66 (so far as he has made no determination and so far as the changes are in respect of a non-resident patient) to the Area Authority.[5]

(v) *Charges for optical and dental appliances, repairs; etc.* Under the National Health Service Act 1977 s. 78 and paragraph 2 of Schedule 12 and regulations made or preserved under the Act, charges may be made in respect of supply — including replacement — of dentures, including bridges, and of supply of glasses, other than children's glasses despite the terms of s. 1 of the Act.

By paragraph 2(5) of Schedule 12 no charge may be made for the supply of lenses for any glasses supplied under the National Health Service Act 1977 if the person for whom the glasses are supplied was at the relevant time[6] of the age of ten or more and either under sixteen years of age or receiving full-time school education; and the frames of the glasses are of any description specified in the Statement of Fees and Charges. Exempt from charges also are patients resident in hospital at the time the appliance is supplied.

Under paragraphs 2 (4) and 3 (4) of the Schedule, no charge is to be made in respect of the supply of (*a*) a dental appliance or (*b*) for relining a denture or the addition of teeth, bands or wires to a denture if at the relevant time[6] the person for whom the appliance has been supplied or the work done was under sixteen years of age or receiving full-time school education, or was an expectant mother or had borne a child within the previous twelve months. Nor is any charge payable for any dental services (other than those in (*b*) above) for patient under 21. Nor also is any charge payable under s. 1 of the 1951 Act in respect of supply

[1] See p. 103.
[2] N.H.S. Functions (Directions to Authorities) Regs. S.I. 1974 No. 24. Regs. 3 (1) (*c*) and 5 (2).
[3] R.H.B. (53) 111.   [4] See pp. 103–104.
[5] N.H.S. Functions (Directions to Authorities) Regs. S.I. 1974 No. 24, Regs. 3 (2) (*a*), (*b*) and (*c*) and 5 (1) and (2).
[6] See para. 2 (7) of the Scedule as to *relevant time*.

(including replacement) of a dental appliance as part of the hospital and specialist services to a person who has undergone operative procedure affecting the mandible, the maxilla or the soft tissues of the mouth as part of treatment for invasive tumours.[1]

Any charges under sections 78 and 79 may be varied by the Secretary of State by regulation.[2] The Minister may also make an order under s. 78 (2) of the National Health Service Act 1977, remitting charges for dentures supplied by a teaching hospital if satisfied that it is in the interests of dental training or education to do so. Moreover, no charges are payable for dental *treatment* at any hospital under the Act although, by s. 79 and paragraph 3 of Schedule 12 of the National Health Service Act 1977, charges are made for such treatment (with certain exceptions) if provided elsewhere by a dentist under Part II of the Act.

(vi) *Charges for drugs, medicines and appliances.* The Act allows regulations to be made for the making of such charges as may be prescribed in respect of the supply (including repair and replacement) of drugs, medicines and appliances. No such charge may be made in respect of (*a*) drugs, medicines or appliances supplied to resident patients; (*b*) drugs supplied for treatment of venereal disease; (*c*) appliances (including contraceptive appliances[3]) supplied to a person under 16 years of age or who is undergoing full-time instruction in a school within the meaning of the Education Act 1944, or, the Education (Scotland) Act 1946;[4] or (*d*) the replacement or repair of any appliance in consequence of a defect in the appliance as supplied. Regulations may also provide for the remission or repayment of any charge payable thereunder in such other cases as may be prescribed.[5] Further, the Secretary of State, in regulations providing for the making of charges in respect of drugs, medicines and appliances, may also make provision for the granting of certificates of exemption to persons who would otherwise be liable to charges, the granting of such certificates being subject to the payment of such sums as may be prescribed in the regulations.[6]

Sections 80-82 give further powers to make regulations to charge for the provision of facilities and appliances. S. 80 covers, in effect, facilities for expectant mothers and young children and for prevention of illness and care and after-care of persons who are or who have suffered from illness. S. 81 deals with the supply of any appliance (or its replacement or repair) which is, at the request of the person supplied, of a more

---

[1] N.H.S. (Charges for Appliances) Regulations S.I. 1974 No. 284, Reg. 9.
[2] National Health Service Act 1977 Sch. 12 paras. 2 (2) and 3 (2).
[2] Supplied under s. 77 (1) and s. 5 (1) (*b*).
[4] National Health Service Act 1977 s. 77. For authorised charges and exemptions, *see* N.H.S. (Charges for Drugs and Appliances) Regulations S.I. 1974 No. 285 and the Amendment Regs. S.I. 1974 No. 627.
[5] Reference should also be made to the provisions of paras. 2 (4) and 3 (4) of Sch. 12 as to children, pregnant women and women within a year after childbirth, as to which see previous page.
[6] S. 77 (2). See also Reg. 6 of the regulations.

expensive type than the prescribed type, S. 82 deals with the replacement or repair of appliances generally. Charges may be recovered if it is determined in the prescribed manner that the replacement or repair is necessitated by an act or omission of the person supplied or (if the act or omission occurred when he was under 16 years of age) of the person supplied or of the person having charge of him when the act or omission occurred.

The current regulations are the N.H.S. (Charges for Appliances) Regulations 1974[1] and the N.H.S. (Remission of Charges) Regulations 1974.[2]

In the previous edition of this book, Dr. Speller argued that the extra charges in what is now s. 81 were those over and above the least cost prescribed by regulation for the type, if any, provided for a particular type of case. However, I take the view that the reference to 'the request of the person supplied' indicates that clinical freedom is not affected and that increased costs are only incurred at the choice of the patient.

(vii) *Charges for wigs and fabric supports supplied by hospitals.* The N.H.S. (Charges) Regulations 1971[3] provides for any out-patient who receives as part of his treatment a wig or fabric support to pay the prescribed charges.

(viii) *Exemptions and refunds.* As a part of the general law of social security, it should be noted that the N.H.S. (Remission of Charges) Regulations 1974[2] provide important exceptions to the principles outlined. Further, if the money is paid by mistake it can be reclaimed. Included but by no means comprising the class of person thus entitled not to pay charges are persons a member of whose family is in receipt of supplementary benefit or family income supplement.

(b) Voluntary hospitals

(i) *Extent of power to charge.* A voluntary hospital can enforce payment of charges for maintenance and treatment of a patient only if the hospital has power to make a charge and a contractual obligation to pay has been expressly or implicitly assumed by the patient or by some other person.

The first point to consider, therefore, is whether the hospital has any power to charge for maintenance or treatment and the answer to this question depends on its objects and constitution. It must not be assumed that because a charity for relief of the sick poor takes in a. patient who could not properly be so described it therefore has a legal right to make a charge in the particular case. Even in the case of a charity, 'for the

---

[1] S.I. 1974 No. 284 as amended by the Amendment Regs. S.I. 1974 No. 609.
[2] S.I. 1974 No. 1377 as extended by S.I. 1977 No. 434. See also S.I. 1971 No. 340 as amended by S.I. 1977 No. 279.
[3] S.I. 1971 No. 340 in Reg. 5 (1) and Sch. 2.

relief of the sick' a power to charge is not implicit, though there is clearly no objection to a patient making a voluntary payment of the full cost of his treatment; nor in the case of a hospital for the relief of the sick poor can there be any legal objection to a voluntary contribution according to means by a person who is a proper object of the charity. This is presumably the position which arises when patients are invited, but not required, to make a payment according to means.

Assuming that a particular hospital has power to make a charge for maintenance and treatment of patients, the next question to ask is whether an enforceable contract has, in fact, been made. Ordinarily, except in the case of accident or other emergency admission, a hospital having power to charge, whether in respect of all admissions or in respect only of admissions to the pay-bed ward or block, can have a routine admission procedure under which the patient, or, in appropriate cases, the husband, parent or other relation or maybe a friend or other interested party, signs a form requesting that the patient be admitted and undertaking in consideration thereof to pay for his maintenance and for services, (e.g., X-ray investigation) on a fixed scale. A request and promise made by word of mouth and not evidenced by writing would be valid in law but there might well be difficulty in proving the promise, especially a promise by a third party, even a husband or parent.

If it is desired to hold both patient and third party liable then the ordinary procedure is for the patient to undertake primary responsibility for payment, the third party acting as guarantor. It must be appreciated that unless a guarantee is by deed, it needs consideration to support it and to avoid any argument as to whether the guarantor did receive any consideration, it should be stated in the form that the guarantee is given 'in consideration of the hospital receiving or retaining the patient at the request of the guarantor'. Even if there is consideration to support it, a guarantee, to be enforceable, must be in writing.[1]

Should nothing have been said about payment at the time of the patient's admission to a voluntary hospital, it is fairly certain that, even though the hospital had the power to charge, it could not do so since there is no well established custom in this country of exacting payment in voluntary hospitals and so no presumption would arise that the patient was accepting services for which a reasonable person would as a matter of course expect to pay. This brings us to the difficult problem of the emergency admission or the accident case.

(ii) *Non-Road Traffic Act accidents and other emergency cases.* An emergency admission from home is ordinarily arranged by the patient's doctor in consultation with the patient, or if the patient is not capable

---

[1] Statute of Frauds 1677, s. 4.

of deciding, with the nearest available relative. Then, if it is arranged that the patient be admitted to a pay-bed there would appear to be some evidence that either he or someone expressly or impliedly authorised by him had made a binding contract on his behalf. Alternatively it could be that there was evidence that a relative authorising the arrangement was acting as principal and accepting personal liability, though such a presumption could hardly ever arise in the case of a doctor who acted simply as a go-between. The only reasonably satisfactory solution, from the point of view of the hospital, is to get the signature of an appropriate relative to a contract on behalf of the patient coupled with an undertaking to be personally liable.

Nowadays, it is seldom that a patient injured in an accident, or taken seriously ill in a public place, would be taken to a voluntary hospital. Presumably, if he were, the old custom would still be followed, *viz.*, of admitting the patient in the first instance to the appropriate general ward for emergency treatment. When that has been done and it has been subsequently ascertained that the patient or responsible relative (*e.g.*, father of a minor or husband) was in a position to pay the maintenance charges in a pay-bed and also the fees of the surgeon or physician in attendance, it has not been unusual, as a condition of continued treatment in a voluntary hospital with pay-beds, to require that the patient be removed to such a bed.

That attitude is entirely proper when the general wards are expressly provided for the sick poor or for persons of more limited means than the patient in question. But, a patient having once been admitted, the hospital should be cautious lest by hasty and ill-advised action it lays itself open to attack and to possible legal action for withdrawing its aid half-way. In the opinion of Dr. Speller, if an accident patient or a patient admitted as an analogous emergency case, does not consent to be removed to a pay-bed, it would probably be better to accept the position rather than risk a legal action or charges, even unfounded, against the reputation of the hospital. The only difficulty in following this advice, apart from the comparatively minor one of some loss of revenue is that the member of the senior medical or surgical staff attending the patient may, perhaps, not be able, under the constitution of the hospital and the terms of his contract, to charge for his services to the patient whilst in a general ward. It is the possibility of abuse of the sometimes, but now less frequently, honorary services of professional staff in the general wards which is one of the main difficulties presented by such cases, but, on balance, it is likely to be as much in the interests of the staff as of the hospital to avoid occasion for dispute on such a question.

2. Road Traffic Act Cases

Statutory authority to enforce payment in respect of treatment of persons injured in road accidents in which a motor vehicle[1] is involved is conferred on medical practitioners and hospitals[2] in respect of emergency treatment, and on hospitals as regards other treatment, by the Road Traffic Act 1972, as explained in the following paragraphs.

(a) *Emergency treatment.* S. 155 of the 1972 Act provides for payment of a fee of £1.25 in respect of *emergency medical or surgical treatment or examination* (referred to in the section as emergency treatment) of any person suffering bodily injury (including fatal injury) caused by or arising out of the use of a motor vehicle on the road, the fee being claimable from the user of the vehicle involved, irrespective of negligence. The fee is payable to the first registered medical practitioner examining or treating the patient and, if no medical examination or treatment had been given when the patient reached hospital then the fee is claimable by the hospital in addition to any payment due from any insurance company in respect of further treatment under (b) below.

A claim on behalf of a hospital in respect of emergency treatment must be made by an executive officer of the Area (or special) Health Authority responsible for its administration and may be made by word of mouth at the time of the incident or subsequently in writing signed by the officer on behalf of the authority, stating the name and address of the hospital, the circumstances in which the treatment was effected and that it was first effected in the hospital. The demand has to be delivered to the user of the vehicle in person or sent to him by prepaid registered letter, or a letter sent by the recorded delivery service,[3] to reach him within seven days of the accident.[4] A chief officer of the police is bound, if so requested by a person who alleges that he is entitled to claim under s. 155 of the 1972 Act to furnish all the information at his disposal as to the identity of the vehicle and of the user.

As to who is the user the better opinion seems to be that when the vehicle is being driven by an employee for his employer, even though the employer is not present, the employer may be regarded as the user, but if a man lends his car to another, then that other is the user.

When more than one vehicle is involved it is proper to claim against that which actually struck the injured person or the car in which he was travelling when the accident occurred. In case of doubt it may be desirable to claim against both or all of the vehicles concerned, though acceptance of double or multiple payment of fee would not be permissible.

[1] In this chapter the expression *motor vehicle* includes *motor cycles* as well as three, four and other multiple-wheel mechanically propelled vehicles.

[2] *Hospital* for the purposes of the Road Traffic Act 1972, means an institution not, being an institution carried on for profit, which provides medical or surgical treatment for in-patients (s. 158).

[3] S. 156 (2).

[4] The Act is not complied with if the claim is sent to the insurers of the vehicle under the Road Traffic Acts instead of to the user, even though in practice payment is usually made by the insurer. The position is different as regards further hospital treatment, as to which see p. 120.

(*b*) *Further hospital treatment.* S. 154 of the Road Traffic Act 1972 makes important provisions for the recovery of costs by hospitals for treatment given to victims of road accidents where a payment has been made with or without an admission of liability by the insurer or the owner to the victim.

The essential points to note are that:

(i) An insurer is liable to make such payment to a hospital only when he has made a payment (whether or not with an admission of liability) under or in consequence of a Road Traffic Act policy[1] in respect of the death or bodily injury of some person arising out of the use of a motor vehicle; or

A motor vehicle owner acting as his own insurer under the Act by security or deposit becomes similarly liable if he makes any payment in respect of death or bodily injury as aforesaid;

(ii) The insurer (or the owner) must have knowledge that the person injured had received hospital treatment.[2] Hence, the owner's insurance company or, under (i), the owner of the vehicle, should be promptly given particulars of patients treated as a result of the accident and notified of the hospital's conditional claim.

(iii) No claim arises under this head in respect of treatment of injuries caused by an accident in which an uninsured vehicle is involved (not being one the owner of which is exempted from taking out a Road Traffic Act policy as aforesaid), but if an insured vehicle is also involved and the insurer of that vehicle makes a payment in respect of death or bodily injury the hospital can maintain its claim against the insurer. It follows that no claim arises by reason of payments made in respect of injuries caused by a vehicle owned by the Crown (*e.g.*, Government Departments) nor by vehicles owned by local and certain other public authorities exempted from insurance by s. 35 of the Act which also applies to tramcars and trolley buses the use of which is authorised by special Act of Parliament. Nor can the hospital claim under the section against the owner or driver of a car which was not insured because the insurance had lapsed, because the car was stolen or being driven by an unauthorised person or for any other reason. See further (*c*) below.

(iv) The charge for out-patient treatment is 'reasonable expenses actually incurred'. Strictly, this involves accurate costing but insurers and other interested bodies and hospital authorities have largely agreed scales of charges.

(v) The provisions of the Road Traffic Act 1972, apply to public

---

[1] A payment is made under a Road Traffic Act policy even though it is in respect of injury to a person against liability for injury to whom the driver is not obliged to be insured if, in fact the policy covers injury to such person. *Barnet Group HMC* v. *Eagle Star Insurance Co. Ltd.* [1960] 1 Q.B. 107.

[2] *Barnet Group HMC* v. *Eagle Star Insurance Co. Ltd.*, above.

authority and voluntary hospitals alike, being hospitals not conducted for profit.[1]

(vi) It is understood that the Minister has authorised hospital authorities exceptionally to agree to waive their claim under the Road Traffic Act, 1972, against an insurer who makes an *ex gratia* payment in respect of personal injury. There must, however, be special circumstances to justify that course. Ordinarily public hospital authorities enforce their legal rights.[2]

(*c*) *Persons injured by uninsured cars.* Insurers transacting compulsory motor vehicle insurance business in Great Britain, under an agreement entered into with the Minister of Transport[3] have established the Motor Insurers' Bureau (M.I.B.) which, subject to the conditions of the agreement, undertakes to satisfy any unsatisfied judgment in respect of liability for any risk compulsorily insurable under the Road Traffic Act, 1972, whether or not the defendant had been insured. M.I.B. may also make an *ex gratia* payment in the case of an unidentified driver who has caused injury or death or a driver who for some reason cannot be sued. But where M.I.B. makes a payment in a case in which the defendant was not insured, the payment not being made under a Road Traffic Act policy, nothing is payable by the M.I.B. under s. 154 of the Road Traffic Act 1972, to a hospital which has given treatment to the injured person.

3. Charges for Treatment of Road Accident Cases apart from Road Traffic Act 1972

If a hospital, not being a hospital within the National Hospital Service, has power to charge and a person injured in a road accident is not regarded as a proper object of charity, there is no obligation on the hospital to receive such person as a patient without charge and to rely on the provisions of s. 154 of the 1972 Act. The hospital may well choose to look to the patient himself for payment of full charges, leaving him to any remedy he might have in law against the owner or user of the vehicle. If it were established that the accident had been due to the fault of the driver of the car (not being the injured person) the full cost of hospital treatment, if reasonable, would be a proper item in the claim for damages. Before the transfer of most voluntary hospitals to the Minister in 1948, when injured persons were very often treated in voluntary hospitals, it is understood that those voluntary hospitals having power to charge patients would frequently enter into an agreement for payment for treatment even in the case of a patient to whom payment out of his own resources would be a hardship, the agreement being so framed that the cost of treatment would be a first charge on

---

[1] See s. 158.　　　　　[2] As to enforcement of claims see p. 122.
[3] The agreement 'Motor Insurers Bureau (Compensation of Victims of Uninsured Driver)' is published by Her Majesty's Stationery Office.

any damages recovered but failing recovery of damages would be waived. In that way voluntary hospitals often received more than they would have done under s. 36 of the Road Traffic Act 1930.[1] Their professional staff also sometimes benefited by such arrangement. To-day the treatment of road accident cases in a voluntary hospital, otherwise than under contractual arrangements with a Regional Health Authority, is but a remote possibility. Presumably, in such circumstances such a hospital could make an agreement of the kind mentioned, provided it was allowed by its constitution to charge patients in the accommodation where the accident patient was being treated.

A hospital administered under the provisions of the National Health Act has no power to refuse to receive a patient into a general ward on the ground that he could afford to pay for treatment and to require that accommodation be taken in the pay-bed block.

B. PROCEEDINGS FOR RECOVERY OF CHARGES AND FEES

1. Hospitals and Institutions

(a) *Hospitals administered under the National Health Service Act*

Charges properly made to part-paying patients under s. 63 or to private patients under ss. 65 and 66 of the National Health Service Act 1977 as well as charges properly made for appliances or for repair of appliances, may be recovered by the Secretary of State. As to method of recovery, s. 121 of the 1977 Act[2] provides that all charges recoverable under the Act by the Secretary of State, or any body constituted under the Acts, may, without prejudice to any other method of recovery, be recovered summarily as a civil debt. Hence, proceedings in a court of summary jurisdiction are an alternative to ordinary civil proceedings in the County Court or the High Court as the case might be.[3] The Secretary of State has made regulations which delegate the recovery of charges to the Area Health Authority.[4]

(b) *Voluntary hospitals*

Liability to pay for a patient's treatment in a voluntary hospital (or in a nursing home) being contractual, the hospital's only remedy, if the patient or other person liable under the contract neglects or refuses to pay, is by ordinary civil proceedings.[5]

In the case of a patient in a pay-bed who has contracted to pay the physician or surgeon for his attendance, or where the circumstances of

---

[1] Corresponding with s. 134 of the 1972 Act.   [2] Formerly s. 71 of the 1946 Act.
[3] Magistrates Court Act 1952, s. 50.
[4] N.H.S. Functions (Directions to Authorities) Regs. S.I. 1974 No. 24, Regs. 3 (1) (d) and 5 (1).
[5] The limits on the power of a voluntary hospital to charge for treatment are discussed at pp. 108–112.

the attendance of the physician or surgeon on the patient are such as to imply an undertaking by the patient to pay him and although the hospital may have laid down maximum charges, it is probably preferable that it should not undertake to render an account on behalf of the consultant, since this could easily blur the limits of the responsibility of the consultant and of the hospital for the patient's treatment. In any event, if both the hospital and the consultant remained unpaid, the hospital could not properly include in its own claim any amount which might be due to the consultant.

2. Medical Practitioners and Dentists

If a medical practitioner or dentist has made a lawful contract with a hospital patient for his treatment as a private patient and the patient does not meet his obligations to pay the agreed fee, the amount owing is an ordinary civil debt.[1] The health authority has no responsibility in the matter.

[1] But a Fellow of the Royal College of Physicians is prohibited by by-law from suing for professional fees.

CHAPTER 8

HOSPITAL RATES AND TAXES AND DUTIES

A. RATES

HOSPITALS administered under the National Health Service Acts 1946–73, being property in occupation of the Crown, are not subject to rates, but contributions in lieu of rates are made on an agreed basis. Real property forming part of a charitable trust under s. 21 of the 1973 Act is not exempt from rates except so far as it can be brought within the provisions of s. 40 (1) of the General Rate Act 1967. This provides that, subject to the provisions of the section, the rate payable in respect of any hereditaments occupied by, or by trustees for, a charity and wholly or mainly used for charitable purposes (*e.g.* for a hospital which is a charity) are not to exceed fifty per cent of what would otherwise have been payable. Thus, whilst the rating authority must give fifty per cent relief, it may at its discretion give relief in excess of that or even to exempt such hereditament altogether.

By s. 40 (5) of the General Rate Act 1967 a rating authority also has power to reduce or remit payment of rates chargeable in respect of any other hereditament which is occupied for the purposes of one or more institutions or other organisations which are not established or conducted for profit and whose main objects are charitable or are otherwise philanthropic or religious or concerned with education, social welfare, science, literature or the fine arts. But in cases falling under s. 40 (5) any relief given is purely discretionary.

In determining the ratable value of property, no account is to be taken of any structure supplied in effect for the benefit of a handicapped or sick or disabled person.[1] This applies even if rates are payable in respect of the premises.

B. INCOME AND CORPORATION TAXES

1. Liability for Tax

As Crown property, hospitals owned by the Secretary of State for Social Services and administered by health authorities under the National Health Service Act, are not liable to income and corporation tax, nor is there any question of such authorities making taxable profits. But the following sections may concern them so far as they administer charitable trusts.

[1] General Rate Act 1967, s. 45.

The law relating to income and corporation tax is such that any full exposition of it here is impracticable, particularly in relation to profit-making activities carried on by a charitable hospital. Therefore, all that it is proposed to do is to outline the general nature of the exemptions in favour of charitable hospitals and other charities and the apparent limits to such concessions, leaving the reader who needs more to refer to specialist works.

The general effect of the Income and Corporation Taxes Act 1970, s. 360, is to relieve hospitals and other charities of liability to tax under the Act within the following definitions and with the modifications and exceptions indicated.

2. Bodies to which Concessions apply

First it must be observed that the general exemption just referred to applies only to a body or fund established under a definite and irrevocable trust for charitable purposes and charitable purposes only[1] but that relief may also be granted if any non-charitable purposes of the body are purely ancillary to the charitable purposes.[2] Further the various kinds of income exempted from tax under the section are exempt only so far as they are applied for charitable purposes only.[3]

(a) Land and Buildings in Occupation of Charity

The rents and profits of any lands and in effect buildings vested in a hospital or other charity trustees are exempt from tax.

(b) Dividends, Interest, etc.

Such income may be received without deduction of tax when (i) the capital securities are in the name of the official custodian of charities or (ii) the interest is on a stock in the public funds in the name of trustees of funds for charitable purposes, as certified by the Charity Commissioners when the Bank of England may pay without deduction of tax. In all other cases, interest, dividends, etc., being paid subject to deduction of income tax at the standard rate, the hospital or other charity may obtain repayment in full. The like position arises as regards claims to repayment of tax on annual subscriptions received under seven-year covenants by donors.

(c) Profits of Trade or Business

The profits of any trade or business carried on by any charity are exempt from tax when such profits are applied solely to the purposes of

---

[1] *Ex parte Ranks's Trustees*, 38 T. L. R. 603.

[2] *Institution of Civil Engineers* v. *Commissioners of Inland Revenue*, 16 T. L. R. 158. See also *Royal College of Surgeons* v. *National Provincial Bank and Others* [1952] A. C. 631; [1952] 1 T. L. R. 978; [1952] 1 All E. R. 984.

[3] *I.R.C.* v. *Educational Grants Association* [1967] Ch. 993.

the charity *and* either (i) the trade is exercised in the conduct of the main and primary purpose of the charity, *or* (ii) the work in connection with the trade is mainly carried on by the beneficiaries of the charity. There could be little doubt that a pay bed block established under the terms of the Voluntary Hospitals (Paying Patients) Act 1936, would be regarded as falling under (i) and also any pay bed block on the same lines but for the establishment of which the powers of the Act had not been invoked, since the provision of accommodation for paying patients by a charity is itself charitable[1] provided that it is within the terms of the trust of the particular charity to help such patients.

In *Coman* v. *Rotunda Hospital*[2] it was decided by the House of Lords that a hospital which regularly let out rooms for entertainments whilst retaining control of the premises could not claim the exemption since neither of the above conditions was fulfilled, but in *R.* v. *Special Commissioners, ex parte Shaftesbury Homes*[3] it was held that where a trade of any kind is carried on by separate trustees who hand over the yearly balance of profits to a 'body of persons or trust established for charitable purposes only' that body is entitled to repayment of tax. Hence in the case of any trade in which a hospital is interested liability to or exemption from tax may, failing compliance with conditions (i) or (ii) above depend on the particular organisational arrangements made.

There appears no authority for a hospital owned by the Secretary of State carrying on a trade or business otherwise than as purely incidental to its main purpose, *e.g.*, farming or market gardening as occupational therapy for psychiatric patients. Also, if a health authority carries on some activity, properly ancillary to the treatment of patients, it would seem properly within its powers to supply the needs of other authorities within the national health service and, for accounting purposes, making a charge therefor. It would not then be liable to tax.

(d) Intermediate Income on Share of Residue of Estate of Deceased Person

If a hospital or other charity is entitled to the whole or any share of the estate of a deceased person, it can recover tax paid by the executors on the income of the residue or proportionate share of the residue from the date of death until the date of distribution. This is now provided by s. 427 of the Income and Corporation Taxes Act 1970, under which intermediate income of the estate of a deceased testator is generally deemed the income of the residuary legatees for income tax purposes.

---

[1] In *re Adams* ([1968] Ch. 80; [1967] 3 All E.R. 285). In this case the Court of Appeal upheld a bequest for 'endowment' of private beds at a hospital even though no additional private beds were needed. See above.

[2] [1921] 1 A. C. 1.

[3] [1923] 1 K. B. 393. See further Konstam's Income Tax, 12th Edition (1952).

C. CAPITAL GAINS TAX

As to exemption of charities from capital gains tax reference should be made to s. 360 (2) of the Income and Corporation Taxes Act 1970, and s. 35 of the Finance Act 1965.[1]

D. CAPITAL TRANSFER TAX

In 1974, death duties were abolished and replaced by CTT. Prior to that date a person could make an *inter vivos* gift with no liability to tax. Now, generally such transfers are taxable under the provisions of the Finance Act 1975, ss. 19–52. However by Schedule 6, paragraph 10, a transfer to a charity is not taxable if (*a*) it is made *inter vivos,* or (*b*) if made within one year of the death of the donor/transferor it does not exceed £100,000[2] *and* in either case the property is given for charitable purposes only.

E. SPIRIT DUTY

By s. 112 of the Customs and Excise Act 1952, a person (which expression includes a hospital) who proves to the satisfaction of the Commissioners of Customs and Excise that he has used spirits on which duty has been paid solely for scientific purposes, or in the manufacture or preparation of an article used for medical purposes, may obtain a refund of the difference between the current rate of duty and that payable immediately before April 23, 1918.

Also, the Department of Health and Social Security is in a position to make further discretionary grants to hospitals in respect of duties paid on spirits for medicinal uses. It must be appreciated, however, that neither partial refund of duty nor grant is available in respect of spirits used for drinking, even by patients on doctors' orders.

F. VALUE ADDED TAX

VAT is a tax on the supply of all goods and services in the United Kingdom. It was introduced by the Finance Act 1972. It has a comprehensive coverage; therefore everything is taxable unless it is exempt. Since the tax is so structured that the ultimate burden falls on the consumer, *exemption* of a supply confers no advantages save that of not keeping records. A business making exempt supplies stands, for the purposes of the tax, as the ultimate consumer and so pays the tax

[1] This position is, broadly, preserved by the Finance Act 1974 which (in ss. 38–44) imposes a tax on development gains from land generally.
[2] If it exceeds this figure only the balance is chargeable.

(without recovery) for the taxable goods and services it itself buys. If a transaction is *zero-rated*, the ultimate consumer pays no tax but the supplier can claim relief from the tax he himself has paid (the input tax), by re-payment if necessary. Schedule 4 of the 1972 Act sets out the transactions which are zero-rated; and Schedule 5 those which are exempt. In both cases the Treasury has power by order to vary the lists.[1]

The lists are too extensive to be set out here and for these lists and a full account of the operation of tax, those who need it are referred to other works.[2] It will be noted that amongst other things Schedule 4, Group 14[3] zero-rates drugs, medicines and appliances supplied by a person registered in the register of pharmaceutical chemists or the prescription of a doctor or a dentist and the supply of certain equipment for the chronic sick or the disabled and it includes renal haemodialysis units, oxygen concentrators, artificial respirators and similar apparatus. Schedule 5, Group 7, exempts the supply of service and in connection with it the supply of goods by a person registered or enrolled as a doctor or dentist etc., a member of a profession supplementary to medicine, a nurse, or a midwife. The supply of services by a registered pharmacist are also exempt. Finally, the Group exempts 'The provision of care or medical or surgical treatment and in connection with it, the supply of any goods, in any hospital or other institution'.

It has been held *per curiam* by the Value Added Tax Tribunal that where the supply of a surgical belt was by an employee of the manufacturer at a hospital and in the presence of the hospital's appliance officer, that the supply was exempt since it took place 'in a hospital'.[4]

In *Crothall and Co. Ltd.* v. *The Commissioners of Customs and Excise*,[5] the appellants supplied ancillary hospital services under contract at some 45 hospitals, and other institutions, no two contracts being the same. They provided 'Domestic Services, Housekeeping Services, Home Warden Services and Ancillary Services'. It was the appellants argument that all the Services they provided were for the welfare and protection of patients and that therefore they amounted to 'the provision of care' within the meaning of Schedule 5, Group 7, Item 4, and were accordingly exempt. The Tribunal held otherwise taking the view that the exemption was limited to 'services supplied for patients necessarily involving in their performance some personal contact with the patients'.

Among the other many decisions of the Tribunal one which might be of particular interest to some hospital staff is *Archer* v. *The Com-*

---

[1] The VAT (Consolidation) Order S.I. 1974 No. 1146 consolidates the amended schedules up to 1st August 1974.
[2] Reference may also usefully be made to circular H.M. (73) 12 which gives guidance on registration and other matter relating to VAT.
[3] For which now see consolidation above.
[4] *Payton* v. *The Commissioners for Customs and Excise* [1974] 1 V.A.T.T.R. 140.
[5] [1973] 1 V.A.T.T.R. 20.

missioners (*No. 2*).[1] Here it was held that the provision for payment by a university of a car park for a member of its staff was exempt as being 'incidental to the provision of education by a university'.[2] It would seem that this decision may be applicable to (and so exempt) charges made by teaching hospitals as part of a university or possibly any made by an Area Health Authority (Teaching) for car parks. Other health authorities do not get this benefit.

A new Group 16 has been added to the Schedule 4 exempting the supply by charities. The text of this Group is now to be found in the VAT (Donated Medical Equipment) Order 1974.[3] Under this Group the supply by a charity established principally for the relief of distress[4] of goods which have been donated for sale and the supply for donation to a designated hospital or research institution, of medical or scientific equipment solely in medical research, diagnosis or treatment where it is purchased by a charity or from voluntary contributions are exempt.

---

[1] [1975] V.A.T.T.R. 1.   [2] See Sch. 5, Group 6.   [3] S.I. 1974, No. 1331.
[4] Relief of distress includes 'the making of provision for the cure or mitigation or prevention of or for the care of persons suffering from or subject to, any disease or infirmity or disability affecting human beings (including the care of women before, during and after child birth)'.

CHAPTER 9

VISITORS WHO REFUSE TO LEAVE

A PERSON entering or remaining on premises, *e.g.*, a hospital or nursing home, without the consent, express or implied, of the occupier or his representative becomes a trespasser,[1] and if he refuses to leave when ordered to do so can be forcibly removed provided no more force is used than the occasion requires. If a trespasser resists such removal he commits an assault and a person lawfully moving him, if attacked, is justified in reasonable self-defence.

It is essential to endeavour to persuade a trespasser to leave quietly. If he refuses he should be clearly and unambiguously ordered to go — if possible, in the presence of at least one witness; then and then only should force be used to eject him. The good offices of a policeman are often useful on such occasions for a show of resistance by the trespasser in the presence of a police officer to the use of reasonable force to remove him, would constitute a breach of the peace in respect of which the police officer would have power of arrest.

The problem of dealing with trespassers on hospital premises is usually practical rather than legal, though it is not always easy to determine whether a person has become a trespasser, and still less to decide whether to treat him as such. It may, therefore, be worth considering one or two examples. First, there is the in-patient who declines to leave on the completion of his treatment. Legally he becomes a trespasser if he refuses to leave when discharged. Yet if by reason of some incapacity, such as blindness, which may be an incapacity unconnected with the illness for which he was treated in hospital, he is not fully able to take care of himself the hospital may feel itself in a practical difficulty if he declines to accept accommodation offered by the local welfare authority because this kind of case is not within s. 47 of the National Assistance Act 1948. Consequently the patient cannot be compulsorily removed to a welfare institution under that section and it is not unknown for such a patient to be unco-operative, because, not only may hospital accommodation be more attractive than that provided in a welfare institution but it has the additional advantage of being provided free whilst accommodation in a welfare institution is subject to payment according to means. In such circumstances, the hospital authority has the difficult task of exercising its legal right of getting rid of the trespasser — as it must in justice to sick people waiting for

---

[1] See Chapter 15 below for a discussion of the duties owed to trespassers.

treatment — without appearing callous. This, however, is not the place to discuss that essentially practical, administrative problem.

Persons who make themselves a nuisance in a ward, whether by their conduct or by their effect on the patient can be required to leave and may, if necessary, be removed. Otherwise unexceptionable visitors may also be excluded from the ward either because, on medical grounds, no visitors or only certain visitors are being allowed, or because a patient does not want to see the visitor. The fact that a visitor excluded at the request of a patient is a near relative — or even husband or wife — of that patient, does not make any less justifiable such exclusion, the patient's wishes being a sufficient justification for exclusion of any person in all but the most exceptional circumstances.

But what if the patient is under the age of 16 and a parent were insistent on access? Refusal might well result in the parent having custody and control claiming to exercise the right to remove the child. If so, although authority is lacking, it would seem most unlikely that any court would uphold his right to do so if removal would be certain to cause the child's death, by depriving him of necessary treatment, or if removal would seriously imperil the child's life or health or subject him to immediate avoidable pain and suffering. It was Dr. Speller's view that accordingly even the parent of a young child could be refused access to the child if that were regarded as medically necessary. He based this view on substantially the same reasoning as adopted[1] for disregarding parental objection to an operation etc. However, I take the view that the parent of a young child should as a matter of practice and possibly as a matter of law only be excluded on medical grounds. This means that so long as the parent remains unobtrusive he may have a right to remain with his child. It is only where he actually interferes with the doctor's higher duty of saving life etc. that he may be excluded. Even if this is right it is unclear how far it imposes a duty on health authorities to provide facilities for parents to remain with their children.[2]

Visitors, so far as allowed, enter the wards, to use the common law term, as licensees, and the ward sister, having full responsibility for her ward may, on behalf of the health authority, withdraw the licence at any time nor, strictly, is she obliged to give a reason for her decision. When, for example, a patient has visitors in excess of such number as may be authorised, the sister can, in her absolute discretion, require such of the visitors to leave as she thinks fit, not necessarily the last — or the first — to come. A person so requested to leave, who does not do so, becomes a trespasser and, if thought desirable, reasonable force may then be used to remove him.

[1] See below, Ch. 13, p. 196 *et seq.*
[2] See H.C. (76) 5 which in any event requires A.H.A.s to provide facilities.

The caller, whether a patient or a patient's relative, who becomes troublesome, as by refusing to leave on the termination of an interview or consultation, should be ordered to leave and, on his persisting in his refusal to do so, may be treated as a trespasser, reasonable force to remove him then being justifiable.

CHAPTER 10

SEARCH AND ARREST OF SUSPECTED PERSONS

FROM time to time thefts occur in most hospitals and similar institutions and a patient or member of staff may be suspected. Sometimes, too, conclusive proof is very hard to come by, especially in respect of a regular course of petty theft, as for example, of comparatively small quantities of foodstuffs. The question then arises as to whether there is any right of search either of the individual or, in the case of a resident, of his or her quarters. Also, there is the question of what justifies the making of a formal charge against a suspected person and of the circumstances in which anyone who is not a policeman may have the right of arrest in respect of theft or of other offences, such as arson or obtaining property by deception.

A. POWERS OF SEARCH

Leaving aside the right of the police to search an arrested person or, under particular statutes, such as the Misuse of Drugs Act 1971, to detain and search a person suspected of a particular offence, it can be said that no-one has the right to search either a person or his quarters except with his consent or on the authority of a search warrant. This statement of general principles will be further analysed and explained in succeeding paragraphs.

1. Search of the Person

Any wrongful act infringing a person's right to his personal liberty, *i.e.* freedom from restraint, generally falls under the head of *false imprisonment* which expression covers any infliction of bodily restraint which is not expressly or impliedly authorised by the law[1] or, put another way, the act of arresting or imprisoning any person without lawful justification or otherwise preventing him without lawful justification from exercising his right of leaving the place in which he is. Similarly any act infringing the right of liberty of the person by direct

---

[1] In the case of a mentally disordered patient liable to detention it may be said that insofar as those in charge of him may do whatever is necessary for his wellbeing or for the safety of others, a search without his consent, *e.g.* for a knife or for drugs would clearly be justified. But it is at least open to some doubt whether, if the patient were volitional, a search for some other purpose (*e.g.* for money or valuables which had been stolen) without his consent would be lawful. The position in the case of an informal patient suffering from mental disorder is more obscure. It is questionable whether, if volitional, he should be searched — even for drugs or weapons — against his will.

application of force, or even threat of force, amounts to battery if force is used and to assault if it is effectively threatened.

From this it follows that to detain a person for search, when he has not consented to remain for the purpose or his consent not having been freely given, generally lays those concerned open to actions both for false imprisonment and for assault and battery. If in the course of an unlawful search stolen property were found on the person searched so as to justify his forthwith being handed over to the police and charged, that would still not technically free those responsible from their liability in respect of the original wrong of false imprisonment and of assault and battery. In such a case however it can be said with some confidence that there would then be little risk of any action by the wrongdoer, or of such action resulting in the award of substantial damages, provided the charge based on the wrongful search had been substantiated. If, however, an illegal search did not lead to the discovery of any stolen property, or if, stolen property having been found, the person searched had been able to give good account of his possession of it, whether at once or to the satisfaction of the criminal court hearing any charge preferred against him, then he would be likely to obtain substantial damages in any action he might bring.

The only effective line of defence to search without lawful authority being consent, it sometimes happens that an employing authority makes the right of search a condition of employment, but even this gives the employer no right of forcible search should an employee, in the event, refuse to be searched. The right of the employer would then be no more than to treat the refusal as a breach of contract.[1]

And what of consent at the time of the search? This to be an effective defence must be genuine consent, real acquiescence in the search with full opportunity to refuse. In particular it is no consent if a person, although he objects, submits to what he conceives to be authority or force. If he feels that he will be searched whether he likes it or not he does not consent by passively submitting to it. On the other hand, in refutation of a suggestion of theft, a person may demand to be searched and unless he withdraws that invitation and passively submits that is clearly 'leave and licence'.

2. Search of Quarters

For search of residential accommodation occupied by a member of the staff of a hospital to be lawful, the consent of the occupant is necessary. In practice the issue may be confused (but not altered in law) by the fact that the right of entry to staff quarters by senior officers may be at least impliedly reserved, for the purpose of supervision, par-

[1] See Annual Report of M.D.U. for 1972 at p. 50 and see further below, Ch. 22 on Labour Law.

ticularly for seeing that the domestic staff are carrying out their duties and that the quarters are being kept clean and used in a proper manner. But such a general right of entry and inspection cannot be expanded into a right of search. Any prying into the personal belongings of a member of the staff, feeling amongst folds of clothing and in pockets and inspecting contents of bags and handbags, is far beyond any such right of general inspection, and, if to be justified at all, must be justified as what it is, namely, a search. Whether in any instance there had been consent sufficient to justify such search would be a matter of fact, relevant factors being substantially the same as in respect of consent to a search of the person. If there has been no effective consent, the search will be actionable as trespass to goods. 'The wrong of trespass includes any unpermitted contact with or impact upon another's chattel . . . Probably the courts will hold that direct and deliberate interference is trespass even if no damage [to the goods] ensues.'[1]

3. Search of Staff Lockers

What has been said about the search of staff quarters applies equally to search of staff lockers intended to be used exclusively for personal belongings. The existence of a master key in the hands of a senior officer makes no difference. Nor, without the consent of the member of the staff who has been given the use of the locker, is any search by a police officer lawful, unless authorised by a search warrant or, exceptionally, by the terms of some statute.[2]

4. Search of Patients' Lockers etc.

What has been said in this section of the chapter about searching staff quarters would no less apply to the deliberate searching of a patient's possessions, though this is less likely to be at issue. Certainly the *bona fide* tidying up of a patient's locker would not constitute the wrong we are here discussing.[3]

B. ARREST

Apart from arrest to stop a threatened breach of the peace or to bring

---

[1] Clerk and Lindsell, *Torts* 14th Edn. (1975). See also: Salmond, *Torts* 16th Ed., p. 93; Street, *Torts* 5th Ed., p. 31; Winfield, *Torts* 9th Ed., p. 412.

[2] Search of lockers without warrant has been known to occur when the chief administrative officer of a hospital has called in the police to investigate suspected theft and has provided them with the master key of staff lockers.

[3] Those treating a patient in hospital may sometimes have the strong suspicion that he has a supply of and is using dangerous drugs. Such suspicion does not in law justify any member of the hospital staff searching possible hiding places such as wallets, purses and handbags. The hospital may, however, be in a position to exercise some control over what a patient may keep with him in the ward and could possibly find a reason for having a suspect container removed from the ward for safe custody. Also, as ordinarily a hospital has power to exclude visitors, it could on occasion consider use of that power to exclude visitors who might be possible sources of supply of drugs, giving no more than a conventional reason to anyone excluded. As to giving information to the police, see p. 137.

to an end an existing breach of the peace and one or two other similarly anomalous cases, the right of summary arrest is strictly limited, being in respect only of *arrestable offences*[1] and of attempts to commit such offences.

Any person may arrest without warrant anyone who is, or whom he, with reasonable cause, suspects to be, in the act of committing an arrestable offence.[2] Also, where an arrestable offence has been committed, any person may arrest without warrant anyone who is, or whom he, with reasonable cause, suspects to be guilty of the offence.[2] A policeman has additional powers of arrest, for where he, with reasonable cause, suspects that an arrestable offence has been committed, he may arrest without warrant anyone whom he, with reasonable cause, suspects to be guilty of the offence.[3] He may also arrest without warrant any person who is, or whom he, with reasonable cause, suspects to be, about to commit an arrestable offence.[4] Moreover, for the purpose of making an arrest in any of the circumstances set out above, a policeman — but no-one else — may enter (if need be by force) and search any place where that person is or where the policeman, with reasonable cause, suspects him to be.[5]

It may also here be said that if a private person makes a charge against another to a policeman, so that that other is arrested, the arrest is usually regarded as being the responsibility of the private person so that, if it should afterwards appear that the circumstances were not such as to justify arrest by a private person, the person making the charge may be held liable in an action for false imprisonment. A further risk in the event of irresponsible and unjustifiable prosecution is an action for wrongful arrest and malicious prosecution.[6]

If a hospital officer detained someone for theft it now seems, on the basis of *Tims* v. *John Lewis & Co. Ltd.*,[7] that the arrest would not be invalidated, nor the detention support an action for false imprisonment,

---

[1] An arrestable offence is any offence for which the sentence is fixed by law (*e.g.* murder) or for which a person, not previously convicted, may under or by virtue of any enactment be sentenced to imprisonment for a term of five years. (Criminal Law Act 1967, s. 2 (1).) It is manifestly impossible to give a comprehensive list of such offences but some arrestable offences subject of the Theft Act 1968 which may concern hospitals are theft (which now includes, *inter alia*, embezzlement and conversion); robbery; burglary, which the 1968 Act defines much more widely; abstracting electricity; obtaining property by deception; obtaining pecuniary advantage by deception; false accounting; suppression of documents for the purpose of gain for oneself or another; blackmail; handling stolen goods, knowing or believing them to have been stolen. Taking a motor vehicle or other conveyance, except a bicycle, without the owner's consent or other lawful authority is also ordinarily an arrestable offence, although the maximum sentence is under five years; (s. 12 of 1968 Act). Also, any person may arrest without warrant, anyone who is, or whom he, with reasonable cause, suspects to have with him, away from his abode any article for use in the course of or in connection with any burglary, theft or cheat. (S. 25 (4) of the 1968 Act.)
[2] Criminal Law Act 1967 S. 2 (2) (3).   [3] *Ibid.*, s. 2 (4).
[4] *Ibid.*, s. 2 (5).   [5] *Ibid.*, s. 2 (6).
[6] An action for malicious prosecution lies when a person is prosecuted on a criminal charge, maliciously and without reasonable and probable cause.
[7] [1952] A. C. 676.

merely because the person arrested had been detained a reasonable time for reference to be made to a senior officer in accordance with hospital rules, for him to decide whether a charge should be made. It must be observed, however, that in the *Tims* case there was justification for a charge being made although, in the event, the accused person was acquitted. Consequently the *Tims* case will not help if the arrest was unjustified *ab initio*. But the prompt release of the arrested person without his being charged might go in mitigation of damages in an action for wrongful arrest and false imprisonment.

C. LIABILITY FOR WRONGFUL SEARCH AND ARREST

Should a member of the staff or a patient be searched in circumstances giving rise to an action for assault or for false imprisonment; or should quarters or possessions be searched so as to result in an action for trespass to goods; or should a person be charged so as to give rise to an action for false imprisonment or, perhaps, malicious prosecution — who may be made defendants?

Certainly the individual officer concerned could be made a defendant as well as any other members of the staff who might have assisted him and 'superior orders' does not exonerate from such liability. But the aggrieved person would, if possible, usually prefer to sue the Area Health Authority either alone or jointly with the officer or officers concerned, since any judgment in his favour would then be more likely to be effective than if solely against individuals who might prove insolvent. And in most cases it is probably safe to say that the authority could be made liable, the test being whether the officer concerned acted in the course of his employment.[1]

The practical conclusion to be drawn from this outline of the law as to arrest is that only in absolutely clear-cut cases of manifest and serious wrongdoing should a private person, such as a hospital officer, take the responsibility of arresting or formally charging another person with an arrestable offence such as theft. Otherwise, unless the situation is one of extreme urgency, he should seek advice and instructions.

Another possibility is to place the facts before the police without formally making a charge, leaving the police to decide whether the circumstances are such as to justify an arrest.[2]

---

[1] For a full discussion of the principle that an employer is jointly and severally liable for any tort committed by his employee while acting in the course of his employment and as to the limits of its application, see Clerk and Lindsell, *Torts* 14th Ed. (1975) at 221 *et seq.*

[2] The police cannot require a person who takes that course to make a charge or to undertake responsibility for prosecution. On the other hand, it seems that the informant cannot oblige the police to prosecute. (See *Blackburn* v. *Commissioner of Metropolitan Police* [1968] 2 Q. B. 118; [1968] 1 All E. R. 763.) If, however, the informant, having made an accurate statement to the police, the police advise him to make a charge, that would appear to be a strong defence to an action for malicious prosecution, should the charge fail. See *Malz* v. *Rosen* [1966] 1 W. L. R. 1004.

For completeness it may be added that in discussing these topics the writer has left aside all questions concerning naval and military establishments, Royal dockyards, prisons and similar establishments for which there may be special statutory provisions outside the scope of this book.

CHAPTER 11

THE HOSPITAL CHAPEL AND CHAPLAINS

A. THE CHAPEL

IN one case only, Saint Bartholomew's Hospital, London, a parish church — St. Bartholomew-the-Less, the whole parish being within the bounds of the hospital — serves as the hospital chapel and the incumbent, in effect, as the Anglican chaplain of the hospital. One of the results of St. Bartholomew-the-Less being a parish church is that banns of marriage can be called there and marriages there solemnised by the incumbent or, with his authority, by any other ordained clergyman of the established church.

Ordinarily, the hospital chapel will either be consecrated or dedicated as such. In neither case does it come under the jurisdiction of the minister of the parish in which it is situated. Even so, an important distinction has to be drawn between a legally consecrated chapel and one which has simply been dedicated. A consecrated chapel is one which has been formally set aside for religious purposes in accordance with canon law and the rites and ceremonies of the established Church of England and it is unlawful to use a consecrated chapel for any secular purpose. Nor may it be used for Roman Catholic or Free Church services without the authority of the bishop of the diocese.

The holding of a service of dedication, whether conducted by the bishop of the diocese or by some other minister of the established church, and whether by him alone or in conjunction with ministers of other Christian churches, does not bring the chapel under the jurisdiction of the bishop of the diocese, nor prevent its use for secular purposes at any time.[1] However, if a hospital authority had accepted the gift of a building for use as a chapel, and that building had only been dedicated, there might still arise the question whether, having regard to the terms of the gift, the hospital authority or the Secretary of State could thereafter, without breach of trust, allow the building to be used for secular purposes, either at all or exclusively; or could allow it to be demolished at any time.[2] The same problem could arise in respect of a building which had been given to the hospital authority for the purpose of religious observances according to the Jewish faith.

[1] But a sense of what is seemly might limit the secular purposes for which it was used so long as still used for religious services.

[2] If, say, demolition in connection with a rebuilding scheme were necessary, it would be expected that the charity commissioners would give their consent subject to satisfactory provision for replacement being made in the scheme.

B. HOSPITAL CHAPLAINS

So far as N.H.S. hospitals are concerned, the appointment of hospital chaplains is in the hands of the Area Health Authority or committee responsible for the administration of the hospital or group of hospitals to which the appointment is being made, the appointing authority being bound by nationally negotiated scales of pay and conditions of service.[1]

The method of appointment of chaplains to other types of hospital or residential home depends on the constitution and rules of the hospital or institution. Now, because there are some differences in law, we must consider separately the position of Church of England chaplains and others.

1. Church of England Chaplains

(a) *Appointment*

The immediately relevant law regarding the appointment and official position of a Church of England chaplain is now to be found in the Extra-Parochial Ministry Measure 1967 of the Church Assembly (now the General Synod of the Church of England).[2] Section 2 of the Measure, in effect, requires the chaplain to have been licensed to the chaplaincy by the bishop of the diocese and provides that, being duly licensed, he performs his ministry independently of the minister of the parish in which the hospital is situated: his licence does not, however, extend to the solemnisation of marriage. The relevant subsections of s. 2 read as follows:

2. (1) The Bishop of the diocese in which any university, Ministry at college, school, hospital or public or charitable institution is situated, whether or not it possesses a chapel, may license a clergyman of the Church of England to perform such offices and services as may be specified in the licence on any premises forming part of or belonging to the institution in question, including residential premises managed by the institution and occupied by the members or staff of the institution;
Provided that no such licence shall extend to the solemnization of marriage.
(2) The performance of offices and services in accordance with any such licence shall not require the consent or be subject to the control of the Minister of the parish in which they are performed. . . .
(4) A licence granted under this section may be revoked at any time by the Bishop of the diocese.

Since a Church of England chaplain needs the licence of the bishop of the diocese, it follows that he could and, presumably, should have his appointment terminated if, at any time, it becomes known to the hospital authority that his licence has been withdrawn.[1]

---

[1] Further as to dismissal see '2. Other chaplains', p. 141 and references there given.
[2] See also circulars H.M. (63) 80; H.M. (63) 81; H.M. (68) 18; and H.M. (72) 78.

(b) Alms collected at Church of England Services

S. 2 (3) of the Extra-Parochial Ministry Measure 1967 provides that alms collected in the course of or in connection with the performance of such offices and services as under s. 2 (1) a hospital or other chaplain is authorised to perform, shall be disposed of in such a manner as the Minister performing the office or service, subject to the direction of the Bishop of the diocese, may determine.

2. Other Christian Chaplains

(a) Appointment

The Extra-Parochial Ministry Measure 1967 has no application to the appointment of chaplains other than a clergyman of the Church of England. There is thus no recognition in law that, say, a Roman Catholic chaplain may need the licence of his bishop — a licence which might be withdrawn; nor that a chaplain — other than a Church of England chaplain — being placed under some kind of ecclesiastical censure, might properly be regarded as unfitted for the task, by those to whom he had been appointed to minister. Probably in such circumstances, the hospital would have the right of dismissal, always provided that the chaplain had either not had recourse to, or had exhausted, any rights of appeal he might have had within his own religious organisation. If, however, the position were not sufficiently clear to justify summary dismissal, or it appeared that during possibly protracted proceedings in the domestic tribunal of the particular church, the ministry to patients and staff might suffer, the better plan would appear to be to terminate the services of the chaplain with notice or with salary in lieu of notice.[1]

(b) Alms collected at Offices and Services

There is no statutory provision as to the disposal of alms collected at or in connection with offices and services, save in respect of offices and services of the Church of England but obviously the sensible and seemly thing would be for a hospital authority to assume without question that a similar rule applies, if only as a matter of custom.

3. Non-Christian Chaplains

The position of a Jewish or other non-Christian chaplain attached to a hospital or group of hospitals is substantially the same as that of a Christian chaplain who is not a minister of the established church.

[1] For a discussion of the position which may arise on dismissal of a person occupying hospital accommodation see p. 419; also as to free meals as part of a person's remuneration pp. 417–418. As to suspension see pp. 414–415.

CHAPTER 12

MEDICINES, POISONS, CONTROLLED DRUGS AND RADIO-ACTIVE SUBSTANCES

THE purpose of this chapter is to draw attention to, and in outline only, those aspects of the law relating to medicines,[1] poisons,[2] controlled drugs[3] and radio-active substances which are likely to concern hospitals and nursing home proprietors and members of their staffs which are not dealt with elsewhere in this book. Those who need more detailed information must look in other places.

A. MEDICINES

Although at the time of going to press none of the orders which would bring those provisions of the Medicines Act 1968 which touch hospitals and similar institutions have been made, it seems they will be fairly soon. That being so, it is here assumed that the relevant provisions of the Act will be in force and the previous law is accordingly omitted. I would like to express my gratitude to certain of the staff of the D.H.S.S. for giving me a sight of the orders in draft.

1. Introductory

The Medicines Act 1968 provides a broad legislative framework for the making of orders and regulations by the appropriate Ministers[4] for controlling the manufacture, importation, exportation, sale and supply, including supply on prescription, of what, in the Act, are referred to as *medicinal products*. When the Act is fully operational, it will govern all those products used as medicines; the Poisons Act 1972 will deal with substances without a medicinal use. In other words medicines will be removed from the Poisons List. As regards any poisons still in medical use (i.e. substances not manufactured etc. wholly or mainly for medical purposes) this purpose will be exempt from the restrictions in the Poisons Act. The effect therefore of the new legislation is to change the basis of control from *substances* to *medicinal products*.

The 1968 Act also makes new provision respecting the registration and inspection of retail pharmacies, at the same time conferring on

---

[1] Under the Medicines Act 1968.
[2] Under the Pharmacy and Poisons Act 1933 and the Poisons Act 1972.
[3] Under the Misuse of Drugs Act 1971.
[4] Section 1. The appropriate Minister for England and Wales, in respect of medicinal products for treatment of human beings, is the Secretary of State for Social Services.

registered pharmacies the exclusive right of retail sale and supply of medicinal products except those on the General Sales List contained in an order made by the appropriate Minister[1] and, except as otherwise provided in the Act in respect of supply by doctors, hospitals *etc*. Among other things for which the Act makes provision is the possible assignment to the Crown of the copyright in the British Pharmacopoeia and also the possibility of reference for official purposes to other similar publications.[2]

Some sections of the Act come into force only on an appointed day.[3] as do various consequential repeals. Other sections become operative in practice only on the making of those orders and regulations which alone can give meaning and effect to their provisions.

2. Definitions

The parts of the Act relevant to our present purpose are those concerning supply *etc.*, of medicinal products and only so far as relates to such products for treatment of human beings and use in clinical trials on human beings. Consequently, references in the Act to medicinal products for animals and to the position of veterinary surgeons and veterinary practitioners are here generally ignored, though it may be noted that the expression *practitioner* when used in the Act includes them as well as medical practitioners and dentists. *Doctor* means a fully registered person within the meaning of the Medical Act 1956 and *hospital* includes a clinic, nursing home or similar institution. These and other expressions used in the Act are defined in s. 132 (1). Also particularly to be noted are the following:

(a) Medicinal product[4]

130.—(1) Subject to the following provisions of this section, in this Act 'medicinal product' means any substance or article (not being an instrument, apparatus or appliance) which is manufactured, sold, supplied, imported or exported for use wholly or mainly in either or both of the following ways, that is to say—

  (*a*) use by being administered[5] to one or more human beings or animals for a medicinal purpose:

  (*b*) use, in circumstances to which this paragraph applies, as an ingredient in the preparation of a substance or article which is to be administered to one or more human beings or animals for a medicinal purpose.

  (2) In this Act 'a medicinal purpose' means any one or more of the following purposes, that is to say—

  (*a*) treating or preventing disease;

  (*b*) diagnosing disease or ascertaining the existence, degree or extent of a physiological condition;

  (*c*) contraception;

  (*d*) inducing anaesthesia;

[1] Ss. 51 to 54.   [2] Part VII of the Act.   [3] Under s. 16 (1) 17 or s. 136.
[4] See also ss. 104 and 105.   [5] S. 130 (9).

(*e*) otherwise preventing or interfering with the normal operation of a physiological function, whether permanently or temporarily, and whether by way of terminating, reducing or postponing, or increasing or accelerating, the operation of that function or in any other way.

(3) In paragraph (*b*) of subsection (1) of this section the reference to use in circumstances to which that paragraph applies is a reference to any one or more of the following, that is to say—

(*a*) use in a pharmacy or in a hospital;

(*b*) use by a practitioner;

(*c*) use in the course of a business which consists of or includes the retail sale, or the supply in circumstances corresponding to retail sale, of herbal remedies.

(4) Notwithstanding anything in subsection (1) of this section, in this Act 'medicinal product' does not include any substance or article which is manufactured for use wholly or mainly by being administered to one or more human beings or animals, where it is to be administered to them—

(*a*) in the course of the business of the person who has manufactured it (in this subsection referred to as 'the manufacturer'), or on behalf of the manufacturer in the course of the business of a laboratory or research establishment carried on by another person, and

(*b*) solely by way of a test for ascertaining what effects it has when so administered, and

(*c*) in circumstances where the manufacturer has no knowledge of any evidence that those effects are likely to be beneficial to those human beings, or beneficial to, or otherwise advantageous in relation to, those animals, as the case may be,

and which (having been so manufactured) is not sold, supplied or exported for use wholly or mainly in any way not fulfilling all the conditions specified in paragraphs (*a*) to (*c*) of this subsection.

(5) In this Act 'medicinal product' shall also be taken not to include—

(*a*) substances used in dental surgery for filling dental cavities;

(*b*) bandages and other surgical dressings, except medicated dressings where the medication has a curative function which is not limited to sterilising the dressing:

(*c*) substances and articles of such other descriptions or classes as may be specified by an order made by the Ministers, the Health Ministers or the Agriculture Ministers for the purposes of this subsection. . . .

(*b*) *Administer*

(5) In this Act 'administer' means administer to a human being or an animal, whether orally, by injection or by introduction into the body in any other way, or by external application, whether by direct contact with the body or not; and any reference in this Act to administering a substance or article is a reference to administering it either in its existing state or after it has been dissolved or dispersed in, or diluted or mixed with, some other substance used as a vehicle.

(*c*) *Wholesale dealing; retail sale; supplying in circumstances corresponding to retail sale*

These expressions, as concerning medicinal products and substances and articles made subject of the Act by order under ss. 104 and 105 are defined in s. 131 (1) to (4) as follows:

131.—(1) In this Act any reference to selling anything by way of wholesale dealing is a reference to selling it to a person as being a person who buys it for one or more of the purposes specified in subsection (2) of this section, except that it does not include any such sale by the person who manufactured it.

(2) The purposes referred to in the preceding subsection, in relation to a person to whom anything is sold, are the purposes of—

(a) selling or supplying it, or

(b) administering it or causing it to be administered to one or more beings, in the course of a business carried on by that person.

(3) In this Act any reference to selling by retail, or to retail sale, is a reference to selling a substance or article to a person as being a person who buys it otherwise than for a purpose specified in subsection (2) of this section.

(4) In this Act any reference to supplying anything in circumstances corresponding to retail sale is a reference to supplying it, otherwise than by way of sale, to a person as being a person who receives it for a purpose other than that of—

(a) selling or supplying it, or

(b) administering it or causing it to be administered to one or more human beings.

in the course of a business carried on by that person.

3. Application of the 1968 Act to Hospitals, Nursing Homes etc.

Since, as used in the Act, the expression *business* includes a professional practice and includes any activity carried on by a body of persons, whether corporate or unincorporate,[1] the provisions of the Act, so far as they relate to sale and supply of medicinal products (and of substances and articles within ss. 104 and 105), apply to hospitals, clinics, nursing homes and similar institutions generally, subject to any specific exemptions in or under the Act. However, the Act does not bind the Crown, and it does not apply to institutions, such as N.H.S. hospitals, which are a service of the Crown. Hence, what is properly done in the course of their duties by persons working in such institutions is not subject to the provisions of the Act,[2] though it is understood that, by administrative action, the Secretary of State will secure that N.H.S. hospitals apply safeguards equivalent to those required by the Act.

4. Licences and Certificates

Part II of the Act is largely concerned with control of manufacture, importation, exportation, sale and supply of medicinal products,[3] apart from retail dealings by pharmacists at registered pharmacies and retail

---

[1] S. 132 (1).

[2] The purpose of the reference in s. 131 (5) to provision of services by the Secretaries of State is simply to enable a manufacturer or wholesaler to sell medicinal products to one of the Health Departments on N.H.S. central contract without turning himself into a retailer. The effect of s. 131 (4) is to cover, as though they were retail sales on prescription, the dispensing at a registered pharmacy of N.H.S. prescriptions, the supply of medicines on such prescriptions not being a sale, even though, unless exempt, the patient is required to pay a charge.

[3] And of substances within ss. 104 and 105.

sales by other persons of medicinal products on a general sales list.[1] The control is by way of a system of licensing, the basic principles being set out in ss. 6, 7 and 8. Unlicensed dealing with any medicinal products, unless exempted by the Act itself or by the appropriate Minister acting within his powers under the Act, is illegal.

By regulations under s. 61, licence holders and wholesalers may be prohibited from supplying medicinal products otherwise than to persons within a class specified in regulations; whilst under s. 62 regulations may be made prohibiting the supply *etc.*, where it is necessary in the interests of safety, of medicinal products of any description.

Part III of the Act makes further provision as to dealings with medicinal products. Amongst other things it enables regulations to be made to distinguish those medicines which may be sold by a retail chemist[2] and those which are to be available only on prescription.[3] The matter is discussed further below.

5. Exemptions

Apart from certain transitional provisions, the following exemptions from the licencing system are expressly provided for in the sections of the Act quoted or referred to below:

(a) Doctors and dentists

9.—(1) The restrictions imposed by sections 7 and 8 of this Act do not apply to anything done by a doctor or dentist which—
  (a) relates to a medicinal product specially prepared, or specially imported by him or to his order, for administration to a particular patient of his, and consists of manufacturing or assembling, or procuring the manufacture or assembly of, the product, or of selling or supplying, or procuring the sale or supply of, the product to that patient or to a person under whose care that patient is, or
  (b) relates to a medicinal product specially prepared at the request of another doctor or dentist, or specially imported by him or to his order at the request of another doctor or dentist, for administration to a particular patient of that other doctor or dentist, and consists of manufacturing or assembling, or procuring the manufacture or assembly of, the product, or of selling or supplying, or procuring the sale or supply of, the product to that other doctor or dentist or to that patient or to a person under whose care that patient is.

The Medicines (Prescription Only) Order will provide first for those medicinal products which are to be available only on prescription and secondly for the manner in which prescriptions may be issued. It also will make provision for certain ancillary matters such as emergency supply. Section 58 says that these provisions do not apply where a doctor supplies a patient of his.

---

[1] S. 51.   [2] See the Medicines (General Sale List) Order.
[3] See the Medicines (Prescription Only) Order.

(b) *Pharmacists, including hospital and health centre pharmacists*

10.—(1) Subject to the next following subsection,[1] the restrictions imposed by sections 7 and 8 of this Act do not apply to anything which is done in a registered pharmacy, a hospital[2] or a health centre[2] and is done there by or under the supervision of a pharmacist and consists of—

(a) preparing or dispensing a medicinal product in accordance with a prescription given by a practitioner, or

(b) assembling a medicinal product;

and those restrictions do not apply to anything done by or under the supervision of a pharmacist which consists of procuring the preparation or dispensing of a medicinal product in accordance with a prescription given by a practitioner, or of procuring the assembly of a medicinal product.

Also, by s. 10 (4), and subject to s. 10 (2) as to animal vaccines *etc.*, the restrictions imposed by sections 7 and 8 do not apply to anything which is done in a hospital[2] or a health centre[2] by or under supervision of a pharmacist and which consists of preparing a stock of medicinal products with a view to dispensing them as mentioned in subsection (1) (a) of that section.

(c) *Nurses and midwives*

The restrictions imposed by s. 8 of the Act do not apply to the assembly[3] of any medicinal product by a person in the course of that person's profession as a nurse registered under the Nurses Act 1957[4] or as a state certified midwife or as an exempted midwife.[5]

Further by the Medicines (Prescription Only) Order,[6] such midwives are also to be exempt from the provisions of s. 58 (2) (b) so that, in effect, they may administer such medicines as are necessary in the course of their professional duties. The particular medicines are to be specified in the order.

(d) *Exemption in respect of herbal remedies*

The manufacture, supply *etc.*, of herbal remedies, as defined in s. 132 (1) is exempt from the licensing provisions of ss. 7 and 8.[7] Retail sale of herbal remedies, otherwise than by a pharmacist is also permitted under, and subject to the provisions of, s. 56.[8]

(e) *Exemption of imports*

13.—(1) The restriction imposed by section 7 (3) of this Act does not apply to the importation of a medicinal product by any person for administration to himself or to any person or persons who are members of his household, and does not apply to the importation of a medicinal product where it is specially

---

[1] Sub-section (2) refers only to vaccines for administration to animals.
[2] See s. 132 (1) for definition.   [3] See s. 132 (1) for definition.
[4] *i.e.* on any 'part' of the register.
[5] S. 11. For definition of *exempted midwife* see s. 11 (2) (a).
[6] Art. 11 (2) Sch. 3 Part III.   [7] S. 12.
[8] See Medicines (Retail Sale or Supply of Herbal Remedies) Order.

imported by or to the order of a doctor or dentist for administration to a particular patient of his.

(2) Without prejudice to the preceding subsection, the restriction imposed by section 7 (3) of this Act shall not apply to the importation of a medicinal product in such circumstances as may be specified in an order made by the Ministers for the purposes of this section.

(3) Any exemption conferred by an order under this section may be conferred either in relation to medicinal products generally or in relation to a class of medicinal products specified in the order, and (in either case) may be so conferred subject to such conditions or limitations as may be so specified.

(f) Other exemptions

The appropriate Ministers,[1] by order under s. 15, may provide that ss. 7 and 8 shall have effect subject to such other exceptions and to such conditions and limitations as may be specified in the order.

6. Clinical Trials

Section 31 provides:

(1) In this Act 'clinical trial' means an investigation or series of investigations consisting of the administration of one or more medicinal products of a particular description—
  (a) by, or under the direction of, a doctor or dentist to one or more patients of his, or
  (b) by, or under the direction of, two or more doctors or dentists, each product being administered by, or under the direction of, one or other of those doctors or dentists to one or more patients of his,
where (in any such case) there is evidence that medicinal products of that description have effects which may be beneficial to the patient or patients in question and the administration of the product or products is for the purpose of ascertaining whether, or to what extent, the product has, or the products have, those or any other effects, whether beneficial or harmful.

(2) Subject to the following provisions of this Act, no person shall, in the course of a business carried on by him,—
  (a) sell or supply any medicinal product for the purposes of a clinical trial, or
  (b) procure the sale or supply of any medicinal product for the purposes of a clinical trial, or
  (c) procure the manufacture or assembly of any medicinal product for sale or supply for the purposes of a clinical trial,
unless one or other of the conditions specified in the next following subsection is fulfilled.

(3) Those conditions, in relation to a person doing any of the things specified in the preceding subsection, are—
  (a) that he is the holder of a product licence which authorises the clinical trial in question, or does it to the order of the holder of such a licence, and (in either case) he does it in accordance with that licence;
  (b) that a certificate for the purposes of this section (in this Act referred to as a 'clinical trial certificate') has been issued certifying that, subject to the provisions of the certificate, the licensing authority have consented

[1] See s. 1.

to the clinical trial in question and that certificate is for the time being in force and the trial is to be carried out in accordance with that certificate.

(4) Subject to the following provisions of this Act, no person shall import any medicinal product for the purposes of a clinical trial unless either—

    (*a*) he is the holder of a product licence which authorises that clinical trial or imports the product to the order of the holder of such a licence, and (in either case) he imports it in accordance with that licence, or

    (*b*) a clinical trial certificate has been issued certifying as mentioned in subsection (3) (*b*) of this section and that certificate is for the time being in force and the trial is to be carried out in accordance with that certificate.

(5) Subject to the next following subsection, the restrictions imposed by the preceding provisions of this section do not apply to a doctor or dentist in respect of his selling or supplying, or procuring the sale or supply of, a medicinal product, or procuring the manufacture or assembly of a medicinal product specially prepared to his order, or specially importing a medicinal product, where (in any such case) he is, or acts at the request of, the doctor or dentist by whom, or under whose direction, the product is to be administered.

(6) The exemptions conferred by the last preceding subsection do not apply in a case where the clinical trial in question is to be carried out under arrangements made by, or at the request of, a third party (that is to say, a person who is not the doctor or dentist, or one of the doctors or dentists, by whom, or under whose direction, one or more medicinal products are to be administered in that trial).

(7) The restrictions imposed by subsection (2) of this section do not apply to anything which is done in a registered pharmacy, a hospital or a health centre and is done there by or under the supervision of a pharmacist in accordance with a prescription given by a doctor or dentist: and those restrictions do not apply to anything done by or under the supervision of a pharmacist which consists of procuring the preparation or dispensing of a medicinal product in accordance with a prescription given by a doctor or dentist, or of procuring the assembly of a medicinal product.

(8) The restrictions imposed by subsection (2) of this section also do not apply to anything done in relation to a medicinal product where—

    (*a*) it is done by the person who, in the course of a business carried on by him, has manufactured or assembled the product, where he has manufactured or assembled it to the order of a doctor or dentist who has stated that it is required for administration to a patient of his or is required, at the request of another doctor or dentist, for administration to a patient of that other doctor or dentist, or

    (*b*) it is done by the person who, in the course of a business carried on by him, has manufactured or assembled the product to the order of a pharmacist in accordance with a prescription given by a practitioner, or

    (*c*) it consists of selling the product by way of wholesale dealing where it has been manufactured or assembled in the circumstances specified in paragraph (*a*) or paragraph (*b*) of this subsection.

(9) For the purposes of this section a product licence shall be taken to be a licence which authorises a particular clinical trial if—

    (*a*) the trial is to be a trial of medicinal products of a description to which the licence relates, and

    (*b*) the uses of medicinal products of that description which are referred to in the licence are such as to include their use for the purposes of that trial.

(10) A clinical trial certificate may certify as mentioned in subsection 3 (*b*) of this section without specifying the doctor or dentist (or, if there is to be more than one, any of the doctors or dentists) by whom, or under whose direction, any medicinal product is to be administered, or the patient or patients to whom any medicinal product is to be administered.

Ancillary matters are dealt with in s. 35, and applications for clinical trial certificates in s. 36. For duration, renewal and revocation, see ss. 38 and 39.

7. Retail Sale and Supply of Medicinal Products

(*a*) *Generally*

Subject to exemptions by or under the Act, medicinal products may only be sold, or exposed for sale, retail or supplied in circumstances corresponding to retail sale,[1] at a registered pharmacy and in accordance with ss. 52 and 53. Exemptions already mentioned are of medicinal products on a general sale list[2] and herbal remedies.[3] By s. 55 supply by doctors and dentists and from a hospital[4] or health centre is exempt from the restrictions imposed by ss. 52 and 53. The section also gives more limited exemption in respect of medicinal products sold or supplied by nurses and midwives in the course of professional practice. The section reads:

55.—(1) The restrictions imposed by sections 52 and 53 of this Act do not apply to the sale, offer for sale, or supply of a medicinal product—
  (*a*) by a doctor or dentist to a patient of his or to a person under whose care such a patient is, or
  (*b*) in the course of the business of a hospital or health centre, where the product is sold, offered for sale or supplied for the purpose of being administered (whether in the hospital or health centre or elsewhere) in accordance with the directions of a doctor or dentist.
(2) Those restrictions also do not apply—
  (*a*) to the sale or supply of a medicinal product of a description, or falling within a class, specified in an order made by the Health Ministers for the purposes of this paragraph,[5] where the product is sold or supplied by a registered nurse in the course of her professional practice, or
  (*b*) to the sale or supply of a medicinal product of a description, or falling within a class, specified in an order[5] made by the Health Ministers for the purposes of this paragraph, where the product either is sold or supplied by a certified midwife (or, in relation to England and Wales, by a certified midwife or exempted midwife) in the course of her professional practice or is delivered or administered by such a midwife on being supplied in pursuance of arrangements made by *the Secretary*

---

[1] For definition of 'supplying in circumstances corresponding to retail sale', see s. 131 (4), covering the dispensing of N.H.S. prescriptions, which are not, strictly, sales.
[2] S. 51.
[3] S. 56 as amended by the Transfer of Functions (Wales) Order 1969.
[4] *Hospital* includes nursing home, clinic or similar institution. (S. 132 (1).)
[5] See the Medicines (Exemption from Pharmacy Sale) Order.

of State or the Ministry of Health and Social Security[1] in Northern Ireland.....

(4) Expressions to which a meaning is assigned by subsection (2) of section 11 of this Act have the same meanings in this section as in that section.

(b) Medicinal products on prescription only

Under s. 58 (1) and (2) the appropriate Ministers may by order specify descriptions or classes of medical products which may only be sold retail, or supplied in circumstances corresponding to a retail sale, in accordance with a prescription given by a doctor or, if the order so states, a dentist, but this does not prevent the sale or supply of a medicinal product to a patient of his by a doctor or dentist.[2] No sale or supply of a medicinal product on prescription will be within the provisions of s. 58 unless such conditions or limitations as may have been specified in any order made under s. 58 (1) are fulfilled. Also, any order may be subject to such exemptions as are specified therein.[3] The provisions of s. 59 apply to orders in respect of new medicinal products as therein defined.

(c) Restricted sale, supply and administration of medicinal products, the supply and administration of which requires specialised knowledge

60.—(1) Subject to the following provisions of this section, regulations made by the appropriate Ministers may provide that no person shall sell by retail, or supply in circumstances corresponding to retail sale, a medicinal product of a description specified in the regulations, or falling within a class so specified, unless —

(a) he is a practitioner holding a certificate issued for the purposes of this section by the appropriate Ministers in respect of medicinal products of that description or falling within that class, or a person acting in accordance with the directions of such a practitioner, and the product is so sold or supplied for the purpose of being administered in accordance with the directions of that practitioner, or

(b) he is a person lawfully conducting a retail pharmacy business and the product is so sold or supplied in accordance with a prescription given by such a practitioner.[4]

(2) Any regulations made under this section may provide that no person shall administer (otherwise than to himself) a medicinal product of a description specified in the regulations, or falling within a class so specified, unless he is such a practitioner as is mentioned in subsection (1) (a) of this section or a person acting in accordance with the directions of such a practitioner.

(3) The powers conferred by the preceding subsections shall not be exercisable in respect of medicinal products of a particular description, or falling within a particular class, except where it appears to the appropriate Ministers that the sale by retail, or supply in circumstances corresponding to retail sale, or the administration, of such products requires specialised

[1] Words in italics inserted by N.H.S. Reorganisation Act 1973.
[2] S. 58 (3). See the Medicines (Prescription Only) Order.
[3] S. 58 (5).
[4] The expression *practitioner* used in s. 60, as also in a number of other places in the Act, besides doctors and dentists also includes, as regards treatment of animals, veterinary surgeons and veterinary practitioners.

knowledge on the part of the practitioner by whom or under whose directions they are sold, supplied or administered.

(4) Any regulations made under this section in respect of a particular description or class of medicinal products may specify the qualifications and experience which an applicant for a certificate in respect of that description or class of medicinal products must have, and may provide for the appointment of a committee to advise the appropriate Ministers, in such cases as may be prescribed by or determined in accordance with the regulations, with respect to the grant, renewal, suspension and revocation of such certificates.

Retail sale or supply of medicinal products subject of regulations under s. 60 of the Act is also subject to such conditions as may be prescribed in the regulations.[1] Regulations made will also contain provision as to the granting, renewal, suspension and revocation of certificates.[2] The coming into force of the section will enable the Radioactive Substances Act 1948, ss. 2 and 3 to be repealed.[3]

(d) Further powers to regulate dealings with medicinal products

Under section 66 the appropriate Ministers[4] are given extensive powers, by regulation, to prescribe the conditions under which medicinal products are prepared, dispensed, sold and supplied, ranging from the manner in which, or persons under whose supervision, medicinal products may be prepared or dispensed to the construction of the premises in which these things are done, sanitation and disposal of refuse.

8. Containers, Packages and Identification of Medicinal Products

Regulations may be made of the Act as to containers and packages of medicinal products and as to the colours, shapes and markings of medicinal products and their containers and packaging. The Medicines (Labelling) Regulations 1976[5] impose requirements relating to the labelling of containers and packages of medicinal products. The Medicine (Child Safety) Regulations[6] (as amended) make provision for all aspirin and paracetamol preparations (whether for children or adults) to be used in retail sales[7] to be assembled in child resistant containers.

At the time of writing other regulations have not been published. They will replace, for medicinal products, rules 20–26 of the 1972 Poisons Rules.

9. Supply and Storage of Poisons within Institutions

Power to regulate these matters is contained in s. 66 of the medicines Act. Pending the making of such regulations and the coming into force of the Poisons Act 1972, the Poisons Rules 1972 are still in force.[8]

---

[1] S. 60 (6).   [2] S. 60 (5).
[3] For this reason those sections are not discussed in this edition. See further, pp. 170 below.
[4] S. 1 (1).   [5] S.I. 1976 No. 1726.   [6] SI. 1975 No. 2000 as amended by S.I. 1976 No. 1643.
[7] Or in circumstances corresponding to retail sales. See above p. 150 note 1.
[8] See also the note on page 155 at the beginning of section B of this chapter 'Poisons'.

For the purposes of rules 31 and 33 dealing with the supply and storage of poisons within hospitals and similar institutions, '*institution*' means any hospital, infirmary, health centre, dispensary, clinic, nursing home, or other institution at which human ailments are treated.[1] For the purposes of r. 33 the definition also includes any family planning clinic as defined in r. 32, which rule deals with the supply of contraceptives from such clinics. In this part of the chapter the expression 'institution' is therefore used with that meaning, public, charitable and other institutions being distinguished as necessary. The following rules are additional to the requirements of the Misuse of Drugs Act 1971 and of the regulations made thereunder, which will be dealt with later in the chapter.[2]

(a) Institution with a special dispensing or pharmaceutical department

The Poisons Rules in rule 31 provide:

(1) In any institution in which medicines are dispensed in a dispensing or pharmaceutical department in charge of a person appointed for that purpose, no medicine containing a poison shall be issued from that department for use in the wards, operation theatres or other sections of the institution, except in accordance with the requirements contained in the following provisions of this Rule.

(2) The medicines must not be issued except upon a written order signed by a duly qualified practitioner, registered dentist, or by a sister or nurse[3] in charge of a ward, theatre or other section of the institution: Provided that in a case of emergency a medicine containing a poison may be issued notwithstanding that no such written order is produced, on an undertaking by the person ordering the medicine to furnish such a written order within the twenty-four hours next following.

(3) The container of the medicine must be labelled:

    (a) with words describing its contents; and

    (b) in the case of a substance included in Schedule 1 to these Rules with a distinguishing mark or other indication, indicating that the poison is to be stored in a cupboard reserved solely for the storage of poisons and other dangerous substances.

All poisons other than those issued for use within the institution in accordance with r. 31 must be stored within the dispensing or pharmaceutical department.[4]

(b) Institutions not having a dispensing or pharmaceutical department

All poisons other than those issued for use within the institution must be stored:[5]

    (i) in charge of a person appointed for the purpose by the governing

[1] See r. 31 (4) and r. 33 (5).   [2] See pp. 158–170.
[3] *Sister or nurse* is a somewhat wider expression than *matron or acting matron* used in Reg. 8 of the Misuse of Drugs Regulations S.I. 1973 No. 797. For a discussion of the meanings of the expressions in both regulations, see p. 161 *et seq.*
[4] R. 33 (1).   [5] R. 33 (2).

body or person in control of the institution (*e.g.*, the matron of a cottage hospital or a nursing home);

(ii) otherwise than on an open shelf, unless the container of the poison is distinguishable by touch from containers of substances other than poisons kept on the same premises; and

(iii) in the case of substances included in Schedule 1 to the Rules, either in a cupboard or drawer or on a shelf reserved solely for the storage of poisons.

(*c*) *Storage of poisons in wards etc.*

In every institution[1] whether or not having a dispensing or pharmaceutical department, every substance included in Schedule 1 kept in a ward shall be stored in a cupboard reserved solely for the storage of poisons and other dangerous substances.[2]

(*d*) *Inspection of all places in which poisons are kept in an institution*[3]

All places in which poisons are kept in an institution shall be inspected at intervals of not more than three months by a pharmacist or other person appointed for the purpose by the governing body or person in control of the institution.[3]

(*e*) *Other matter relating to supply and storage*

Other provisions of the Rules which apply no less to hospitals, infirmaries, nursing homes, *etc.*, than to commercial establishments are as follows:

It is not lawful to sell whether by wholesale or retail or to supply any poison except in a container impervious to the poison and sufficiently stout to prevent leakage from the container arising from the ordinary risks of handling and transport[4] nor to store any Schedule 1 poison unless the container is sufficiently strong to withstand the ordinary risks of handling.[5]

It is not lawful to consign any poison for transport unless it is sufficiently stoutly packed to avoid leakage arising from the ordinary risks of handling and transport.[6]

It is not lawful to consign for transport by carrier any poison included in Schedule 8 to the Rules unless the outside of the package containing the article is labelled conspicuously with the name or description of the poison as set forth in the schedule and a notice indicating that it is to be kept separate from food and from empty containers in which food has been contained. Nor may any person knowingly transport any such poison either on his own behalf or for another person, in any vehicle

---

[1] Rs. 31 (4) and 33 (5).
[2] R. 33 (3). Oddly, this provision does not apply to such places as out-patient departments.
[3] R. 33 (4).   [4] R. 26 (1).   [5] R. 27 (1).   [6] R. 28.

in which food is being transported, unless the food is being carried in a part of the vehicle effectively separated from that containing the poison, or is otherwise adequately protected from the risk of contamination. This rule does not apply to medicines.[1]

10. Enforcement

Exemption of hospitals, clinics, nursing homes and similar institutions from enforcement provisions of s. 108 (2) to (8) of the Medicines Act 1968.

By s. 108 (1) overall responsibility of enforcing or securing the enforcement of the Act is placed on the appropriate Ministers,[2] the broad effect of s. 102 (2) to (8)[3] being to provide that certain powers of enforcement in various respects may be shared by them with the Pharmaceutical Society of Great Britain, food and drugs authorities, county councils, London borough councils and the Common Council of the City of London. It is however provided by s. 108 (9) that notwithstanding anything in subsections (2) to (8) of the section, no duty or power conferred or imposed by or under any of those subsections shall be performed or be exercisable in relation to, *inter alia*, any hospital, which expression includes any clinic, nursing home or similar institution.[3] That does not, however, free hospitals from such obligations as they may have under the provisions of the Act, nor prevent the Secretary of State from taking any other steps that may be open to him to satisfy himself that hospitals are observing the Act.

B. POISONS

When Part III of the Medicines Act comes into force, the Poisons Act 1972 will be automatically activated. The 1972 Act is itself a consolidating measure which repeals and re-enacts much of the previous law including the Pharmacy and Poisons Act 1933. Unfortunately, there could be a source of even further confusion. The 1972 Poisons Rules[4] were also a consolidating measure. These however have been made under the 1933 Act and they came into force in 1973.

The 1933 Act was concerned with *poisons* but the 1972 Act deals only with *non-medicinal poisons*. What follows is based on the 1972 Act (with appropriate references to the Act of 1933) and on the 1972 Rules. It is hoped that this arrangement will both sufficiently state the law as it stands at the time of writing and anticipate such changes as are to be made on the commencement of Part III of the 1968 Act.

[1] R. 29   [2] S. 1 (1).
[3] As amended by the Local Government Act 1972 Sch. 30.
[4] S.I. 1972 No. 1939. The Poisons Rules generally deal with such matters as the sale, labelling, storage, transport and use of poisons. They have since been amended by the Poisons (Amendment) Rules S.I. 1974 No. 81, S.I. 1975 No. 1073 and S.I. 1976 No. 978 and the Local Authorities etc. (Miscellaneous Provision) (No. 2) Order S.I. 1974 No. 595.

1. Generally

Since the Poisons Act 1972 does not bind the Crown, it does not apply to National Health Service Hospitals,[1] though its provisions are applied administratively.

There are very detailed rules relating to the sale and purchase of poisons made under the legislation which may be summarized as follows.

Substances in Part I of the Poisons List[2] may be sold retail only by a person lawfully conducting a retail pharmacy whilst substances on Part II may also be sold by a person entered on the local authority's list for the purpose.

Various strict rules as regards sales, including regulations as to labelling *etc.*, also have to be complied with by the seller. Also, if the poison is in Schedule 1 to the Poisons Rules 1972, the buyer must be known to the seller or vouched for in writing by a householder.[3] The buyer of a poison in Schedule 1 must also sign the supplier's book, stating the reason for his purchase. But except as provided by Poisons Rules, these provisions which in effect restrict the sale of poisons to members of the public to retail pharmacists do not apply *inter alia* to the sale of an article to a doctor[4] or dentist for the purpose of his profession, nor to the sale of an article for use in or in connection with any hospital, infirmary, health centre, dispensary or clinic. In such a case, unless the poison is listed in Schedule 2, 3 or 4 of the Misuse of Drugs Regulations 1973,[5] there is no need to state the purpose for which the sale is required. Further when a retail sale of a poison in Part I of the Poisons List is made to such a person, a specific written order may take the place of a signed entry in the pharmacist's 'poison book'. In an emergency, the poison may be supplied on an undertaking that the written order (or the signing of the book) will be given within 24 hours.[6]

Substances included in Schedule 3 to the Poisons Rules 1972 are excluded from the provisions of the Act and of the Rules to the extent therein specified.[7] Machine-spread plasters, surgical dressings and certain corn paints, together with certain poisons for destruction of rats and mice, are excluded by r. 11.

Strychnine and certain other substances such as monofluoroacetic acid and salts of thallium may not ordinarily be sold to the public

---

[1] Nor did the Pharmacy and Poisons Act 1933.

[2] S.I. 1972 No. 1938 as amended.

[3] Pharmacy and Poisons Act 1933, s. 18 (2) (Poisons Act 1972, s. 3 (2)). Poisons Rules r. 36 and Sch. 11. It will be noted that this applies to those poisons set out in Sch. 1 of the Poisons Rules and not those in the Poisons List.

[4] *Doctor* as used in the 1972 Act means 'a fully registered person within the meaning of the Medical Act 1956'.

[5] S.I. 1973 No. 797, see p. 167 *et seq.* This exception is included in the Poisons Rules by the Amendment Rules S.I. 1974 No. 81.

[6] See the proviso to Poisons Rules r. 8 (3).   [7] R. 12.

except as the ingredient of a medicine, and other substances named in Rule 18 may be sold only in accordance with that rule[1] and Sched. 13.[1] Substances in Schedule 4 to the Rules may be sold to the general public only on a prescription from a medical practitioner, dentist or veterinary surgeon in accordance with the provisions of r. 13.

2. Hospitals and Health Centres etc.

Where the wholesale or retail seller of a poison is reasonably satisfied that the poison is required for the purpose of medical, dental or veterinary treatment, and the buyer is a hospital, infirmary, health centre, dispensary or clinic the purchaser is not required to state his trade, business or profession nor the seller to be satisfied with respect thereto, nor in the case of a poison, not being a poison to which the Misuse of Drugs Act 1971 applies, to require the purchaser to state the purpose for which the poison is required.[2]

The general rules governing retail sales do not apply as regards any medicine for the treatment of human ailments dispensed from a hospital, infirmary, health centre or dispensary maintained by any public authority, or out of public funds, or by a charity.[3] In such cases, the medicine must only be supplied on and in accordance with a prescription of, a duly qualified medical practitioner for the purposes of medical treatment, or a registered dentist for the purposes of dental treatment. In a case where a substance in schedule 1 of the Poisons Rules 1972 is supplied, a record must be kept on the premises in such a way that at any time during a period of two years after the date on which the substance was supplied, the following particulars can readily be traced: (a) the name and quantity of the poison supplied; and (b) the date on which it was supplied; and (c) the name and address of the person to whom it was supplied; and (d) the name of the person who supplied the poison or gave the prescription upon which it was supplied. But these records need not be kept as regards National Health prescriptions. The container of the medicine must be labelled:

(a) With a designation and address sufficient to identify the hospital, infirmary, health centre or dispensary from which it was supplied.[4]

(b) Except in the case of a medicine made up ready for treatment, with the word 'Poison'.

In addition to the foregoing requirements of r. 30, in the case of an embrocation, liniment, lotion, liquid antiseptic, or other liquid medicine for external application, the container must be labelled with the name

---

[1] As amended by S.I. 1974 No. 81.

[2] R. 8 (4).   [3] R. 30.

[4] The actual name of the hospital need not be included nor perhaps its principal address, but only a designation and address sufficient to identify the institution. Sometimes, as in the case of a V.D. clinic or hospital the full name and address of the institution might embarrass the patient and the rules were framed with such cases in mind.

of the article (*e.g.*, *Liniment*, and not the names of the ingredients) and also with the words 'For external use only'.[1]

3. Supply of Oral Contraceptives from a Family Planning Clinic

Rule 32[2] regulates the supply of oral contraceptives. Briefly the Poisons Rules do not apply if the contraceptive is supplied on a doctor's prescription and the container in which they are supplied indicates the name of the family planning clinic or registered pharmacy from which they came. 'Family planning clinic' here means a health centre, dispensary or clinic which is maintained by any public authority or by a charity or by an institution approved for the purpose of para. 4 of s. 20 of the Act or by an order made thereunder and at which contraceptive substances are supplied.

4. Nursing Homes

If a trust by which a nursing home is controlled is registered as a charity as it is understood, some are, it seems that the nursing home, although it may charge the patients received full cost of accommodation and board, as well as for all services provided, is maintained by a charity and so comes within the above rules.

Nursing homes, clinics, *etc.*, which are not charitable institutions are not within the exempting provisions of r. 30 and so cannot supply poisons, not being authorised sellers nor exempt institutions. It seems, however, that r. 30 applies only to medicines supplied to out-patients since the expression used in that rule is 'any medicine for the treatment of human ailments dispensed *from* a hospital . . .'[3]

C. CONTROLLED DRUGS

1. Introductory

The Misuse of Drugs Act 1971 has taken the place of the Dangerous Drugs Acts 1965 and 1967 as well as of Drugs (Prevention of Misuse) Act 1964, all of which have been repealed. Regulations made under the repealed Acts were revoked or ceased to have effect and have been replaced by regulations made under the 1971 Act.

The range of substances to which the provisions of the Misuse of Drugs Act 1971 apply is much wider than of those to which the Acts of 1965 and 1967 applied. Substances within the 1971 Act are known as 'controlled drugs'[4] and are as specified in Parts I, II and III of Schedule

---

[1] R. 24 (1) (*b*). This rule is applicable to the supply of out-patients r. 30 (4).
[2] As amended.
[3] This interpretation is supported by the italic heading to the rule '*Supply of medicines to out-patients* . . .' and by italic heading to r. 31 '*Supply of medicines for use in institutions*'.
[4] S. 2.

2[1] of the Act, being known respectively as Class A, Class B and Class C drugs.[2] The interpretation of expressions used in Parts I, II and III of the schedule is in Part IV. Broadly, the effect of the Act is to make unlawful the manufacture, supply or possession of any controlled drug except so far as is expressly permitted by any provision of the Act itself or of any regulation made under it.

The provisions relating to the production, possession and supply of controlled drugs for medical use in hospitals, nursing homes and similar institutions and for supply to out-patients, either directly or on prescription, are set out in the Misuse of Drugs Regulations 1973.[3] Rules as to safe custody of controlled drugs are in the Misuse of Drugs (Safe Custody) Regulations 1973[4] and those relating to supply of controlled drugs to addicts and as to notification of addicts are in the Misuse of Drugs (Notification of and Supply to Addicts) Regulations 1973.[5]

The Misuse of Drugs Act 1971 does not bind the Crown, neither do regulations made thereunder apply to servants or agents of the Crown unless expressly made so applicable.[6]

2. Misuse of Drugs Regulations 1973

(a) Generally

Leaving aside altogether exceptional cases and classes of persons mentioned in the Misuse of Drugs Regulations 1973, it can be said that for all practical purposes a member of the public can be in lawful possession of a controlled drug only if, being a drug within Schedule 1 of the regulations, he has obtained it from a retail pharmacist or from a doctor or dentist or, being a drug within Schedule 2 or Schedule 3, if it has been supplied by a practitioner or by a pharmacist on the prescription of a practitioner,[7] for administration for medical, dental or veterinary purposes in accordance with the practitioner's directions. But even possession of a drug supplied or prescribed by a practitioner is illegal if the practitioner had been misled into doing so by any concealment or false statement.[8] Any person may administer to another any drug in Schedule 1 of the regulations; a doctor or dentist may also administer any drug specified in Schedule 2 or 3 and any person may do so in accordance with the directions of a doctor or dentist.[9]

---

[1] As modified by the Misuse of Drugs Act 1971 (Modification) Orders S.I. 1973 No. 771 and S.I. 1977 No. 1243.

[2] This classification relates to maximum punishments for offences against the Act, see Sch. 4. What is important for our present purpose is not that classification but the classification of drugs into three different categories, *viz.* Sch. 1, 2 and 3 drugs in the Misuse of Drugs Reg. 1973.

[3] S.I. 1973, No. 797.

[4] S.I. 1973, No. 798 as amended by S.I. 1974, No. 1449.

[5] S.I. 1973, No. 799.

[6] S 22 (c).

[7] S. 37.   [8] Reg. 10.   [9] Reg. 7.

(b) *Production, possession and supply of controlled drugs — Hospitals, nursing homes and research laboratories*

Subject to what is said above concerning the circumstances in which an ordinary member of the public may be in possession of controlled drugs or may have such drugs supplied or administered to him, the position in respect of the supply of controlled drugs to or by a hospital or nursing home or research laboratory and possession of such drugs by such institution or, more accurately, by any person therein who is a member of an authorised group (*e.g.* the pharmacist or, in a hospital where there is no pharmacist, the matron) is as follows.

(i) *Practitioners and pharmacists.* A practitioner or pharmacist acting in his capacity as such may manufacture or compound any drug specified in Schedules 1 or 2[1] or Schedule 3.[2] Likewise a practitioner or pharmacist may, when acting in his capacity as such, have in his possession and supply or offer to supply any such drug to any person who may lawfully have that drug in his possession.[3]

(ii) *Matron or acting matron in a hospital or nursing home not having a pharmacist responsible for the dispensing and supply of medicines.* In a hospital or nursing home which is wholly or mainly maintained by a public authority out of public funds or by a charity or by voluntary subscriptions, not having a pharmacist responsible for the dispensing and supply of medicines, the matron or acting matron,[4] when acting in her capacity as such, may possess, supply or offer to supply any drug specified in Schedule 1, 2 or 3 to any person who may lawfully have that drug in his possession. She cannot, however, herself sign an order or requisition for Schedule 2 or 3 drugs.[5] If a hospital or nursing home is not within the above definition which in the great majority of cases must mean that it is an institution conducted for profit, the authority given to matron to possess and supply controlled drugs if there is no pharmacist, is restricted to Schedule 3 drugs.[6] If in any hospital or nursing home there is a pharmacist responsible for the dispensing and supply of medicines, the matron or acting matron as such has no authority to obtain, possess or supply any drug within Schedule 1, 2 or 3 even if she obtains them from the pharmacist.

(iii) *Sister or acting sister in charge of a ward, theatre or other department of a hospital or nursing home.* The sister or acting sister in charge of a ward, theatre or other department of a hospital or nursing home is authorised to possess Schedule 1, 2 or 3 drugs supplied to her by a person responsible for the dispensing and supply of medicines at that hospital or nursing home, but only for administration in accordance

---

[1] Reg. 8 (1).   [2] Reg. 9.   [3] Regs. 8 (2), 9 (2) and 10.
[4] *Matron or acting matron* and *sister or acting sister* includes any male nurse occupying a similar position, Reg. 2 (1).
[5] Regs. 8, 9, 10 and 14 (5).   [6] *Cf.* Reg. 8 (2) (*d*) and 9 (2) (*d*).

with the directions of a doctor or dentist to a patient in the ward, theatre or department.[1] It follows also from what has been said that if in the hospital or nursing home where the sister or acting sister works the drugs are in charge of matron and, because it is not a public or charitable hospital, matron cannot hold Schedule 1 or 2 drugs, neither can a sister, except, in the case of a sister, in the form of medicine supplied or prescribed by a practitioner for an individual patient. She could, however, hold a ward or departmental stock of a Schedule 1 or 2 drug were she in a private hospital or nursing home where the hospital stock of drugs was in charge of a pharmacist.

(iv) *Midwives*. A midwife, so far as it is necessary to the practice of her profession as such, may have in her possession and administer pethedine, but she can lawfully obtain supplies only on a midwife's supply order signed by the appropriate medical officer[2] to whom she must surrender any stocks no longer required by her.[3] This method of obtaining supplies would not be relevant if she were on the staff oᶜ a public or charitable hospital as defined in Reg. 8 but if she worked on the staff of a private nursing home where matron had charge of the drug stock, it would give her a source of supply of pethidine, which is a Schedule 2 drug.

(v) *Person in charge of a laboratory in which is conducted scientific education or research.* The following mentioned provisions for the availability of controlled drugs for use in educational and research laboratories are sufficient to provide for the needs, *inter alia*, of medical schools and also of research laboratories in hospitals.

Controlled drugs within Schedule 2 of the regulations may be possessed and supplied by any person in charge of a laboratory the recognised activities of which consist in, or include, the conduct of scientific education or research and which is attached to a university, university college, or a hospital wholly or mainly maintained by a public authority out of public funds or by a charity or by voluntary subscriptions, or to any other institution approved for the purpose by the Secretary of State.[4] The class of laboratory where Schedule 3 drugs may similarly be made available is much more widely drawn, including any laboratory the recognised activities of which consist in, or include, the conduct of scientific education or research.[5] In both cases it will be noted that the distribution of drugs by the person in charge of the laboratory is restricted, since he may lawfully supply drugs only in that capacity which means, in effect, only to persons carrying out research in the laboratory of which he is in charge.

There is also provision in the regulations for the Secretary of State to grant licences for the cultivation of plants of the genus *cannabis* and

---

[1] Reg. 8 (2) (*e*) and proviso, Reg. 9 (2) (*e*) and proviso and Reg. 10.
[2] *Appropriate medical officer* is defined in Reg. 11 (3) as amended by the Amendment Regs. S.I. 1974, No. 402.
[3] Reg. 11 (1).   [4] Regs. 8 and 10.   [5] Regs. 9 and 10.

for the smoking of cannabis or cannabis resin for the purposes of research.[1]

(c) Documentation and record keeping

(i) *Requisitions.* The requirements as to requisitions[2] for controlled drugs specified in Schedules 2 and 3 are contained in Reg. 14. So far as hospitals and nursing homes are concerned those requirements apply, to the extent indicated below, not only to supply to the institution, but also to requisition and supply within it. Thus, the regulation applies, *inter alia*, to supply to a practitioner, a hospital pharmacist, a matron (or acting matron) of a hospital or nursing home where there is no pharmacist, and to a person in charge of a laboratory the recognised activities of which consist in, or include, the conduct of scientific education or research. Also, somewhat modified, the same provisions apply to requisitions by a sister of acting sister.[3] Expressly excluded from the provisions of Reg. 14 is supply on prescription or by way of administration.

The following is a summary of the relevant provisions of Reg. 14: Every requisition for a Schedule 2 or Schedule 3 controlled drug must be in writing and signed by the recipient, whose name, address and profession or occupation must be stated, as well as the purpose for which the drug is required and the total quantity to be supplied.[4] Nor may the supplier[5] supply the controlled drug until he has actually obtained such a requisition[6] and is reasonably satisfied that the signature is that of the person purporting to have signed the requisition and that that person is engaged in the profession or occupation specified in the requisition.

(ii) *Controlled drugs procured by a practitioner in urgent need without requisition.* To the requirement that a controlled drug within Schedule 2 or 3 of the regulations can be supplied only if a signed requisition has been received there is a limited exception in favour of a practitioner in urgent need of such a drug, the proviso to Reg. 14 (2) and Reg. 14 (3), reading as follows:

Provided that where the recipient is a practitioner and he represents that he urgently requires a controlled drug for the purpose of his profession, the supplier may, if he is reasonably satisfied that the recipient so requires the

---

[1] Regs. 12 and 13.

[2] *Requisitions* as here used includes orders and purchases.   [3] Reg. 14 (6).

[4] Reg. 14 (2) (5) (*a*). The position in respect of requisitions of controlled drugs for use in private hospitals or nursing homes seems somewhat obscure but the effect of the regulation appears to be that as only a doctor or dentist 'employed or engaged in that hospital or nursing home' could sign a requisition, one who was only in contract with and attending an individual patient could not; but he could sign prescriptions for, or supply, medicines and medicaments needed by his patient.

[5] *Supplier* includes a pharmacist, or a matron or acting matron supplying on requisition within a hospital or nursing home as well as a retail pharmacist or wholesale supplier.

[6] Reg. 14 (2) (*a*), but see below as to supply to practitioner of drug urgently needed.

drug and is, by reason of some emergency, unable before delivery to furnish to the supplier a requisition in writing duly signed, deliver the drug to the recipient on an undertaking by the recipient to furnish such a requisition within the twenty-four hours next following.

(3) A person who has given such an undertaking as aforesaid shall deliver to the person by whom the controlled drug was supplied a signed requisition in accordance with the undertaking.

(iii) *Requisitions by sister or acting sister.* The special requirements relating to requisitions by a sister or acting sister[1] in charge of a ward, theatre or other department of a hospital are set out in Reg. 14 (6) which provides:

(6) Where the person responsible for the dispensing and supply of medicines at any hospital or nursing home supplies a controlled drug to the sister or acting sister for the time being in charge of any ward, theatre or other department in that hospital or nursing home (hereafter in this paragraph referred to as 'the recipient') he shall —
   (*a*) obtain a requisition in writing, signed by the recipient, which specifies the total quantity of the drug to be supplied; and
   (*b*) mark the requisition in such manner as to show that it has been complied with,
and any requisition obtained for the purposes of this paragraph shall be retained in the dispensary at which the drug was supplied and a copy of the requisition or a note of it shall be retained or kept by the recipient.

(iv) *Delivery to a messenger of Schedule 2 or 3 drugs requisitioned under Reg. 14.* Even though a signed requisition has been obtained by the supplier — which expression here includes a pharmacist or matron or acting matron of a hospital or nursing home issuing drugs to members of the medical staff or to sisters or acting sisters in charge of wards, theatres or other departments of the institution — he may not supply the drug to a messenger, *e.g.* to a nurse other than a requisitioning sister herself, save in accordance with the provisions of Reg. 14 (1) reading as follows:

(1) Where a person (hereafter in this paragraph referred to as 'the supplier'), not being a practitioner, supplies a controlled drug otherwise than on a prescription, the supplier shall not deliver the drug to a person who —
   (*a*) purports to be sent by or on behalf of the person to whom it is supplied (hereafter in this paragraph referred to as 'the recipient'); and
   (*b*) is not authorised by any provision of these Regulations other than the provisions of Regulation 6 (*f*) to have that drug in his possession,
unless that person produces to the supplier a statement in writing signed by the recipient to the effect that he is empowered by the recipient to receive that drug on behalf of the recipient, and the supplier is reasonably satisfied that the document is a genuine document.

(v) *Supply of controlled drugs on prescription.* The form of prescription for controlled drugs or medicines containing them and the pro-

---

[1] *Appropriate medical officer* is defined in Reg. 11 (3) as amended by the Amendment Regs. S.I. 1974, No. 402.

visions as to supply on prescription are the subject of Regs. 15 and 16, set out below.

15.—(1) Subject to the provisions of this Regulation, a person shall not issue a prescription containing a controlled drug other than a drug specified in Schedule 1 unless the prescription complies with the following requirements, that is to say, it shall —

(*a*) be in ink or otherwise so as to be indelible and be signed by the person issuing it with his usual signature and dated by him;

(*b*) in so far as it specifies the information required by sub-paragraphs (*e*) and (*f*) below to be specified, be written by the person issuing it in his own handwriting;

(*c*) except in the case of a health prescription, specify the address of the person issuing it;

(*d*) have written thereon, if issued by a dentist, the words 'for dental treatment only' and, if issued by a veterinary surgeon or a veterinary practitioner, the words 'for animal treatment only';

(*e*) specify the name and address of the person for whose treatment it is issued or, if it is issued by a veterinary surgeon or veterinary practitioner, of the person to whom the controlled drug prescribed is to be delivered;

(*f*) specify the dose to be taken and —

    (i) in the case of a prescription containing a controlled drug which is a preparation, the form and, where appropriate, the strength of the preparation, and either the total quantity (in both words and figures) of the preparation or the number (in both words and figures) of dosage units, as appropriate, to be supplied;

    (ii) in any other case, the total quantity (in both words and figures) of the controlled drug to be supplied;

(*g*) in the case of a prescription for a total quantity intended to be dispensed by instalments, contain a direction specifying the amount of the instalments of the total amount which may be dispensed and the intervals to be observed when dispensing.

(2) Paragraph 1 (*b*) shall not have effect in relation to a prescription issued by a person approved (whether personally or as a member of a class) for the purposes of this paragraph by the Secretary of State.

(3) In the case of a prescription issued for the treatment of a patient in a hospital or nursing home, it shall be a sufficient compliance with paragraph (1) (*e*) if the prescription is written on the patient's bed card or case sheet.

It must be appreciated that para. (3) of the regulation only makes an entry on an in-patient's bed card or case sheet sufficient compliance with para. (1) (*e*). The entry must in all other respects comply with the relevant requirements of the rest of para. (1), notably those of sub-para. (*a*). It must be written in ink, or otherwise so as to be indelible, and be signed *with his usual signature* by the medical practitioner making the entry on the bed card and be dated by him.

Regulation 16 provides:

(1) A person shall not supply a controlled drug other than a drug specified in Schedule 1 on a prescription —

(*a*) unless the prescription complies with the provisions of Regulation 15;

(*b*) unless the address specified in the prescription as the address of the person issuing it is an address within the United Kingdom;

(*c*) unless he either is acquainted with the signature of the person by whom it purports to be issued and has no reason to suppose that it is not genuine, or has taken reasonably sufficient steps to satisfy himself that it is genuine;

(*d*) before the date specified in the prescription;

(*e*) subject to paragraph (3), later than thirteen weeks after the date specified in the prescription.

(2) Subject to paragraph (3), a person dispensing a prescription containing a controlled drug other than a drug specified in Schedule 1 shall, at the time of dispensing it, mark thereon the date on which it is dispensed and, unless it is a health prescription, shall retain it on the premises on which it was dispensed.

(3) In the case of a prescription containing a controlled drug other than a drug specified in Schedule 1, which contains a direction that specified instalments of the total amount may be dispensed at stated intervals, the person dispensing it shall not supply the drug otherwise than in accordance with that direction and —

(*a*) paragraph (1) shall have effect as if for the requirement contained in sub-paragraph (*e*) thereof there were substituted a requirement that the occasion on which the first instalment is dispensed shall not be later than thirteen weeks after the date specified in the prescription;

(*b*) paragraph (2) shall have effect as if for the words 'at the time of dispensing it' there were substituted the words 'on each occasion on which an instalment is dispensed'.

Certain test prescriptions issued under a scheme for testing the quantity and quality of drugs supplied are exempted from the provisions of Regs. 15 and 16.[1]

(vi) *Marking of bottles and other containers.* Regulation 18 provides:

(1) Subject to paragraph (2), no person shall supply a controlled drug otherwise than in a bottle, package or other container which is plainly marked —

(*a*) in the case of a controlled drug other than a preparation, with the amount of the drug contained therein;

(*b*) in the case of a controlled drug which is a preparation —

(i) made up into tablets, capsules or other dosage units, with the amount of each component (being a controlled drug) of the preparation in each dosage unit and the number of dosage units in the bottle, package or other container;

(ii) not made up as aforesaid, with the total amount of the preparation in the bottle, package or other container and the percentage of each of its components which is a controlled drug.

(2) Nothing in this Regulation shall have effect in relation to the drugs specified in Schedule 1 or poppy-straw or in relation to the supply of a controlled drug by or on the prescription of a practitioner.

The provisions of Reg. 18 must be complied with not only in respect of the central supply of drugs in charge of a pharmacist or matron or acting matron but also in respect of ward, theatre and departmental stock in charge of a sister or acting sister, except so far as a controlled

[1] Reg. 17.

drug may be contained in a medicine supplied on prescription for administration to a particular patient.

(vii) *Keeping and preservation of registers.* The provisions of Reg. 19 and Schedule 5 and of Reg. 20 as to the keeping of registers of Schedule 2 drugs received and supplied apply to a pharmacist or matron or acting matron in charge of the central drug stock of a hospital or nursing home but not to a sister or acting sister in charge of a ward, theatre or other department. Reg. 21 (3) requires that a midwife authorised by Reg. 11 (1) to have pethidine in her possession shall:

(a) on each occasion on which she obtains a supply of pethidine, enter in a book kept by her and used solely for the purposes of this paragraph the date, the name and address of the person from whom the drug was obtained, the amount obtained and the form in which it was obtained; and

(b) on administering pethidine to a patient, enter in the said book as soon as practicable the name and address of the patient, the amount administered and the form in which it was administered.

All registers and books kept in pursuance of Reg. 19 or Reg. 21 (3) must be preserved for a period of two years from the date on which the last entry was made and every requisition, order or prescription (other than a health prescription[1]) on which a Schedule 2 or 3 drug is supplied in pursuance of the regulations must be preserved for a period of two years from the date on which the last delivery under it was made.[2]

(d) Destruction of controlled drugs

Destruction of controlled drugs must be in accordance with Reg. 24 which reads:

(1) No person who is required by any provision of, or by any term or condition of a licence having effect under, these Regulations to keep records with respect to a drug specified in Schedule 2 or 4 shall destroy such a drug or cause such a drug to be destroyed except in the presence of and in accordance with any directions given by a person authorised (whether personally or as a member of a class) for the purposes of this paragraph by the Secretary of State (hereafter in this Regulation referred to as an 'authorised person').

(2) An authorised person may, for the purpose of analysis, take a sample of a drug specified in Schedule 2 or 4 which is to be destroyed.

(3) Where a drug specified in Schedule 2 or 4 is destroyed in pursuance of paragraph (1) by or at the instance of a person who is required by any provision of, or by any term or condition of a licence having effect under, these Regulations to keep a record in respect of the obtaining or supply of that drug, that record shall include particulars of the date of destruction and the quantity destroyed and shall be signed by the authorised person in whose presence the drug is destroyed.

---

[1] In effect a prescription issued by a doctor or dentist under the National Health Service Act or on a form issued by a local authority for use in connection with the health services of the authority, but more precisely defined in Reg. 2 (1).

[2] Reg. 22.

(e) Crown immunity

Under s. 22 of the Act, and The Misuse of Drugs Regulations 1973, the Regulations do not bind the Crown, its servants or agents, since Reg. 2 (4) provides that nothing in the regulations 'shall be construed as derogating from any power or immunity of the Crown, its servants or agents'.

3. The Misuse of Drugs (Safe Custody) Regulations 1973

(a) Obligation on certain hospitals, nursing homes and similar institutions to keep controlled drugs in conditions of security

In the Misuse of Drugs (Safe Custody) Regulations 1973, the first two regulations are, as customary, formal and interpretative. Regulation 3 applies to any premises occupied by a retail dealer for the purposes of his business;[1] to any nursing home or mental nursing home.[2] In effect Regulation 3 requires that on all such premises all controlled drugs, other than those specifically excluded,[3] shall, as far as circumstances permit, be kept in a locked safe, cabinet or room which is so constructed and maintained as to prevent unauthorised access to the drugs[4] and which complies with the specifications laid down in Schedule 2 of the Regulations.[5] It is not, however, necessary to keep in such a locked safe, cabinet or room any controlled drug which is for the time being under the direct supervision of the person in charge of a hospital or nursing home within the regulation, or of any member of the staff designated by him for the purpose.[6]

The relevant parts of Regulation 3 read as follows:

(2) Subject to paragraph (4) of this Regulation, the occupier and every person concerned in the management of any premises to which this Regulation applies shall ensure that all controlled drugs (other than those specified in Schedule 1 to these Regulations) on the premises are, so far as circumstances permit, kept in a locked safe, cabinet or room which is so constructed and maintained as to prevent unauthorised access to the drugs.

(3) Subject to Regulation 4 of these Regulations, the relevant requirements of Schedule 2 to these Regulations shall be complied with in relation to every safe, cabinet or room in which controlled drugs are kept in pursuance of paragraph (2) of this Regulation.

(4) It shall not be necessary to comply with the requirements of paragraph

---

[1] Reg. 3 (1) (a).

[2] Reg. 3 (1) (b) (d); sub-paragraphs (c) (d) make the Regulations applicable to similar institutions in Scotland. The Regulations still refer to the old legislation which has been consolidated in the Nursing Homes Act 1975. However by s. 22 of that Act, the Interpretation Act 1889 is applied so that the references to the old legislation are now to be taken as references to the new statute.

[3] Reg. 3 (2) and Schedule 1.   [4] Reg. 3 (2).

[5] Reg. 3 (3). The Schedule is not here reproduced.

[6] To ascertain whether the person in charge of the premises or any member of the staff so designated by him is authorised to be in possession of such controlled drugs, reference must be made to Reg. 10 of the Misuse of Drugs Regulations 1973.

H

(2) of this Regulation in respect of any controlled drug which is for the time being under the direct personal supervision of —

> (a) in the case of any premises falling within paragraph (1) (a) of this Regulation, a pharmacist in respect of whom no direction under section 12 (2) of the Act is for the time being in force; or
> (b) in the case of premises falling within paragraph (1) (b) to (e) of this Regulation, the person in charge of the premises or any member of his staff designated by him for the purpose.

The definitions of *nursing home* and of *mental nursing home* for the purposes of the Acts named in Reg. 3 are sufficiently wide to comprehend not only nursing homes conducted for profit, including so-called private hospitals, but also voluntary and co-operative hospitals and clinics. Excluded only are National Health Service hospitals and other public authority hospitals.

(b) *Obligation on person in possession of controlled drug to keep it in locked receptacle when not stored in a locked safe, cabinet or room*

Regulation 5, which imposes the obligation of keeping controlled drugs in a locked receptacle when not in a locked safe, cabinet or room, reads:

(1) Where any controlled drug (other than a drug specified in Schedule 1 to these Regulations) is kept otherwise than in a locked safe, cabinet or room which is so constructed and maintained as to prevent unauthorised access to the drug, any person to whom this Regulation applies having possession of the drug shall ensure that, so far as circumstances permit, it is kept in a locked receptacle which can be opened only by him or by a person authorised by him.

(2) Paragraph (1) of this Regulation applies to any person other than —

> (a) a person to whom the drug has been supplied by or on the prescription of a practitioner for his own treatment or that of another person or an animal; or
> (b) a person engaged in the business of a carrier when acting in the course of that business; or
> (c) a person engaged in the business of the Post Office when acting in the course of that business.

Regulations made under the Misuse of Drugs Act 1971 do not bind the Crown, neither do they apply to servants or agents of the Crown unless explicitly so stated,[1] Reg. 5 has not been made so applicable. Hence, it does not apply to persons working in any hospital directly administered by a government department, because persons working in such a hospital are either servants or agents of the Crown.[2] The regulation equally does not apply to a pharmacist or any other person on the staff of a statutory hospital authority established under the provisions of the National Health Service Act 1977, such a person being either a

---

[1] See Misuse of Drugs Act 1971, s. 22 (c).
[2] For example, persons working in a special hospital managed and administered by the Secretary of State, s. 4 of the National Health Service Act 1977.

servant or an agent of the Crown, although employed by the corporate health authority with which he is in contract.

Nowhere in the Misuse of Drugs (Safe Custody) Regulations 1973 is there any interpretation of the word *receptacle* as used in Reg. 5, but it seems reasonable that the word should be given its most ample meaning so as to include as a *locked receptacle* not only such things as a locked bag, as carried by a general practitioner, but also a 'locked safe, cabinet or room'. Most people would certainly regard a safe, or even a cabinet, as a receptacle, though it has to be admitted that to extend the meaning to include a room is hardly common usage. Even so, unless the meaning of 'receptacle' is so extended, the pharmacist, or matron if she is in charge of controlled drugs, or any sister in charge of controlled drugs in a N.H.S. hospital, would be placed in an impossible position. Take the case of the pharmacist: the only practicable thing for him to do is to keep his store of controlled drugs under lock and key in such safe, cabinet or room as his authority may have provided for the purpose, whether or not that safe, cabinet or room is so constructed and maintained as to prevent unauthorised access. Indeed, since Reg. 3 does not apply to N.H.S. hospital authorities, they neither are nor will be compellable to provide accommodation so constructed and maintained.[1] So, if *receptacle* were narrowly interpreted as excluding a safe, cabinet or room, a N.H.S. hospital pharmacist could be held liable or to be held to have committed an offence if he used the storage accommodation provided. If the wider interpretation were accepted that would not be so. Similar considerations apply in the case of a matron having charge of the stock of controlled drugs and of a sister having charge of ward, theatre or departmental stocks in such a hospital.

The acceptance of the wider interpretation of *receptacle* does not weaken the security arrangements required in hospitals, nursing homes and similar institutions subject to Reg. 3.

The words 'or by a person authorised by him' at the end of Reg. 5 (1) also call for comment. It must be appreciated that the inclusion of those words does not enlarge the categories of persons who may have access to controlled drugs, such categories being as laid down in the Misuse of Drugs Regulations 1973.[2]

(c) Exempted drugs

Controlled drugs to which the provisions of the regulations do not apply and which need not, therefore, be kept in a locked safe, cabinet

---

[1] The Secretary of State may give advice or directions to N.H.S. Health Authorities concerning provision of properly secure storage accommodation for controlled drugs but failure of an authority to follow any such advice or obey any such direction would not be an offence.

[2] See above, pp. 160–162.

or room or, so far as permitted, in a locked receptacle are set out in Schedule 1 of the Misuse of Drugs (Safe Custody) Regulations 1973.

Another way of putting the position is to say that all controlled drugs in Schedules 2 and 3 of the Misuse of Drugs Regulations 1973 excepting only those listed in paragraph 2, are within the Misuse of Drugs (Safe Custody) Regulations 1973.

D. RADIOACTIVE SUBSTANCES[1]

There are two Acts dealing with radioactive substances which may concern hospitals. They are the Radioactive Substances Act 1948, which makes provision with respect to radioactive substances and certain apparatus producing radiation; and the Radioactive Substances Act 1960, which regulates the keeping and use of radioactive material and the disposal and accumulation of radioactive waste.

1. Radioactive Substances Act 1948

(a) *Generally*

The Radioactive Substances Act 1948, which provides machinery for a strict control of the manufacture, supply and use of radioactive substances[2] and of certain apparatus producing radiation, does not bind the Crown and so does not apply to hospitals owned by the Secretary of State and administered by hospital authorities constituted under the provisions of the National Health Service Act 1977.

The two sections of the Act most likely to concern other hospitals are s. 3[3] which relates to the control of the sale and supply of substances containing radioactive chemical elements intended to be taken internally by, injected into or applied to a human being and s. 4[3] concerning the use of irradiating apparatus for therapeutic purposes. Both those sections are repealed by s. 135 (2) of the Medicines Act 1968, which comes into operation on the making of an appointed day order under s. 136 (3) of that Act. The order will be made on the relevant provisions of the 1968 Act becoming operative. Other provisions of the Act which will still be operative and which may concern hospitals are discussed below.

[1] See also the Radiological Protection Act 1970 as amended by the National Radiological Protection Board (Existing Functions) Order S.I. 1974 No. 1230.

[2] S. 12 provides:
'substance' means any natural or artificial substance, whether in solid or liquid form or in the form of a gas or vapour, and also includes any manufactured article or article which has been subjected to any artificial treatment or process'.
'radioactive substance' means any substance which consists of or contains any radio-active chemical element, whether natural or artificial.

[3] The provisions of ss. 3 and 4 are dealt with in the fourth edition of this book at pp. 341 to 345, but must be read subject to the Act 2 (2) and Sched. 1 of the Transfer of Functions (Wales) Order 1969.

(b) Safety regulations for occupations involving radioactive substances and irradiating apparatus

S. 5 provides:

(1) The appropriate Minister[1] may, as respects any class or description of premises or places specified in the regulations, being premises or places in which radioactive substances[2] are manufactured, produced, treated, stored or used or irradiating apparatus is used, make such provision by regulations as appears to the Minister to be necessary —

  (a) to prevent injury being caused by ionising radiations to the health of persons employed at those premises or places or other persons; or

  (b) to secure that any radioactive waste products resulting from such manufacture, production, treatment, storage or use as aforesaid are disposed of safely;

and the regulations may, in particular and without prejudice to the generality of this subsection, provide for imposing requirements as to the erection or structural alteration of buildings or the carrying out of works.

(2) The appropriate Minister may, as respects the transport of any radioactive substances, make such regulations as appear to him to be necessary to prevent injury being caused by such transport to the health of persons engaged therein and other persons.

(3) Regulations made under this section may provide for imposing requirements, prohibitions and restrictions on employers, employed persons and other persons.

(4) Any person who contravenes or fails to comply with any regulation made under this section or any requirement, prohibition or restriction imposed under any such regulation shall be guilty of an offence.

Before making any regulations under this section, the appropriate Minister shall consult with the National Radiological Protection Board.[3]

(5) In this section the expression 'the appropriate Minister' means such Minister, or such Ministers acting jointly, as may be designated by Order in Council, and different Ministers may be designated, for the purposes of subsection (1) of this section, for different classes or descriptions of premises of places and, for the purposes of subsection (2) of this section, for different forms of transport or for the transport of different classes or descriptions of substances.

(6) This section shall be without prejudice to the provisions of the Factories Act 1937, as amended by any subsequent enactment.

S. 7 provides:

The Secretary of State has not so far made any regulations under s. 5 to prevent injury being caused by ionising radiations to the health of persons employed in hospitals and other persons. He has, however, issued a code of practice for the protection of persons exposed to ionising radiations.[4] Doubtless, this code, so far as hospitals are concerned, will be regarded as good practice and failure to observe its provisions may give strength to a claim for common law damage in respect of any injury suffered.

[1] See ss. (6).   [2] See s. 12.
[3] Established under the Radiological Protection Act 1970.
[4] Circulars H.M. (59) 48, (60) 99, (66) 70.

(c) *Power of entry and inspection*

(1) Any person authorised by the appropriate Minister to act under this section shall, on producing, if so required, a duly authenticated document showing his authority, have a right to enter at all reasonable hours any premises (other than premises wholly or mainly used for residential purposes) or any vehicle, vessel or aircraft, for the purpose of ascertaining whether there has been committed, or is being committed, in or in connection with the premises, vehicle, vessel, or aircraft an offence under any provision of this Act except section two.

Presumably a hospital must be regarded as an entity and not as a mere collection of different departments. Hence it would seem that it might be that it is wholly or mainly used for residential purposes so as to be exempt from entry without warrant under this subsection. On the other hand it could be argued that the main use of a hospital is for the treatment of patients and not as their place of residence, this even though they be in-patients. If that argument were accepted, a hospital would not be exempt from entry under the subsection. On balance the present writer holds the view[1] that they must be regarded as used wholly or mainly for residential purposes so that, failing permission to enter, a justice's warrant must be obtained in accordance with s. 7 (2),[2] which subsection may also be availed of without prior request when an application or request for admission would defeat the object of entry. However, such right of entry under the Act as there might be would apply only to voluntary and private hospitals and nursing homes and not to hospitals acquired by the Secretary of State for Social Services under the provisions of the National Health Service Act 1977, which,

---

[1] It was also Dr Speller's view.

[2] (2) If it is shown to the satisfaction of a justice of the peace on sworn information in writing by a person authorised as aforesaid —

    (a) that the exercise of the right conferred by the preceding subsection has been refused or, in the case of premises wholly or mainly used for residential purposes, that a request for admission has been refused, or that the case is one of urgency or that an application or request for admission would defeat the object of the entry; and

    (b) that there are reasonable grounds for suspecting that an offence under any provision of this Act (except section two) has been or is being committed in or in connection with the premises, vehicle, vessel or aircraft in question;

the justice may by warrant under his hand authorise that person and any other person named in the warrant and any constable to enter and search any premises, vehicle, vessel or aircraft, if need be by force.

(3) Every warrant granted under this section shall continue in force until the purpose for which it was granted has been satisfied.

(4) If any person wilfully obstructs any person exercising powers under this section, he shall be guilty of an offence.

(5) If any person discloses any information obtained by means of the exercise of powers under this section, being information with regard to any manufacturing process or trade secret, he shall, unless such disclosure was made in accordance with the directions of the appropriate Minister or for the purpose of proceedings for an offence under this Act or any report of those proceedings, be guilty of an offence.

(6) In this section the expression 'the appropriate Minister' means, in relation to the exercise of powers for enforcing any section of this Act, the appropriate Minister within the meaning of that section.

being Crown property, administered by health authorities on his behalf are not within the ambit of the Act.[1]

(d) Offences and penalties

Penalties for offences under the sections already dealt with are covered by s. 8 (1)–(3). Continuing offences are dealt with in s. 8 (4), responsibility of officers for acts and omissions of corporate bodies in s. 8 (5) and power to order forfeiture of substances and apparatus in s. 8 (6).

8.—(4) If the act or omission constituting an offence under any provision of this Act in respect of which a person is convicted is continued after conviction, he shall be guilty of a further offence and may, on summary conviction, be punished accordingly.

(5) Where an offence under any provision of this Act has been committed by a body corporate, every person who at the time of the commission of the offence was a director, general manager, secretary or other similar officer of the body corporate, or was purporting to act in any such capacity, shall be deemed to be guilty of that offence unless he proves that the offence was committed without his consent or connivance and that he exercised all such diligence to prevent the commission of the offence as he ought to have exercised having regard to the nature of his functions in that capacity and to all the circumstances.

(6) The court by which any person is convicted of an offence under any provision of this Act in respect of any substances or apparatus may order that the substances or apparatus shall be forfeited to the Crown.

2. The Radioactive Substances Act 1960

(a) Generally and application to N.H.S. hospitals

The Radioactive Substances Act 1960, regulates the keeping and use of radioactive material and makes provision as to the disposal and accumulation of radioactive waste.[2] The Act applies to hospitals and others using such material for therapeutic purposes. The Minister of Housing and Local Government is the responsible Minister under the Act.[3]

The special position of hospitals within the National Health Service under the Act is set out in s. 14 (1) reading:[4]

14.—(1) In relation to any hospital in Great Britain which is a hospital with respect to the management and control whereof any functions are exercised by an *Area Health Authority* or Board of Management,
   (a) the *Area Health Authority* or Board of Management shall, notwithstanding that their functions are exercised (directly or indirectly) on

---

[1] The Secretary of State may by administrative action impose standards on N.H.S. hospitals and, if necessary, use his power of direction to do so. He may similarly confer powers of inspection on his officers.
[2] Defined in s. 18 (4).
[3] Now the Secretary of State for the Environment.
[4] As amended by the 1973 Reorganisation Act. Words in italics added by that Act.

behalf of the Minister of Health or of the Secretary of State, be treated for the purposes of sections six and seven of this Act (but not for the purposes of section one thereof) as persons by whom the premises of the hospital are used for the purposes of an undertaking carried on by them, and

(*b*) no other person shall, for the purposes of any provisions of this Act, be treated as a person by whom the premises of the hospital are so used;

and the provisions of this Act (other than section one thereof) shall have effect in relation to any such premises accordingly.

But although hospitals covered by the provisions of s. 14 (1) are exempted from the statutory obligation under s. 1 in respect of any premises where radioactive material[1] is kept, or used the Government have accepted that similar control should be applied to such hospitals administratively and the Secretary of State has given instructions accordingly.[2] But there being no offence under the Act if the instructions of the Secretary of State are disregarded, they can be enforced only by administrative measures.

Apart from the special case of National Health Service hospitals covered by s. 14 (1), the provisions of the Act have no effect with respect to any premises which are in the occupation of a government department or, being premises in which there is an interest belonging to Her Majesty in right of the Crown and forming part of the Crown Estate, are occupied in right of that interest.[3]

Premises occupied by or for the purpose of a visiting force under the Visiting Forces Act 1952 (*e.g.*, for a hospital) are in the same position under s. 14 (2) (3) of the Act as if in the occupation of the government department by arrangement with whom the premises are so occupied.

(*b*) *Registration of users of radioactive material*

It is provided by s. 1 (1) as follows:

1.—(1) As from the appointed day no person shall, on any premises which are used for the purposes of an undertaking carried on by him, keep or use, or cause or permit to be kept or used, radioactive material of any description, knowing or having reasonable grounds for believing it to be radioactive material, unless either —

(*a*) he is registered under this section in respect of those premises and in respect of the keeping and use thereon of radioactive material of that description, or

(*b*) he is exempted from registration under this section in respect of those premises and in respect of the keeping and use thereon of radioactive material of that description, or

---

[1] Defined in s. 18 (1), (2), (3) and the 3rd Sch. Note also the power to amend the definition by order.

[2] Ministry circular H.M. (63) 14. This circular sets out the position of N.H.S. hospitals and covers a memorandum explanatory of the Act.

[3] S. 14 (2). The provisions as to removal of waste, use of mobile apparatus, *etc.*, and the position of Crown servants and agents in respect thereof will be noted in the appropriate place.

(c) the radioactive material in question consists of mobile radioactive apparatus in respect of which a person is registered under section three of this Act or is exempted from registration under that section.

Application for registration has to be made to the Secretary of State for the Environment in accordance with the provisions of s. 1 (2) and of any regulations made under the Act. The Minister has power to refuse registration[1] and any registration may be subject to such limitations or conditions as the Minister thinks fit.[2] On registering a person in respect of any premises under s. 1, the Minister is to furnish him with a certificate and (unless, for reasons of national security, it is in the Minister's opinion necessary that knowledge of the registration should be restricted) he is also to send a copy of the certificate to each local authority in whose area the premises are situated. A registration may be cancelled or varied at any time.[3]

National Health Service hospitals are exempt from registration by virtue of s. 14 (1). So would be any other hospital 'with respect to the management and control of which any functions are exercised by an Area Health Authority'. *Hospital* is not defined for the purposes of the Act of 1960, but the wording of s. 14 (1) leads to the irresistible conclusion that that word has the same meaning as in the National Health Service Act 1977.

Special hospitals under the National Health Service Act 1977 s. 4,[4] as well as Service and prison hospitals and any other hospitals directly controlled by a government department, are exempt from registration under s. 14 (2) and hospitals in occupation of visiting forces under s. 14 (5).

(c) Registration of mobile radioactive apparatus

Section 3 relates to the registration of mobile radioactive apparatus[5] for testing, measuring or otherwise investigating any of the characteristics of substances or articles situated elsewhere than on the premises occupied by the person providing the services or the lending or letting on hire of mobile radioactive apparatus for the purpose. A registration may be cancelled or varied at any time.[6] The section does not refer to mobile radioactive apparatus for therapeutic or diagnostic purposes.

If, however, an Area Health Authority or the Board of Governors of a teaching hospital, did own mobile apparatus within s. 3, seemingly it would be required to register unless exempted by order of the Minister under s. 4 (2).

(d) Accumulation and disposal of radioactive waste

The power to grant any authorisation necessary in respect of the disposal (s. 6) or the accumulation (s. 7) of radioactive waste by hospital

---

[0] S. 1 (3).   [2] S. 1 (4) (5) which should be referred to if greater detail is desired.
[3] S. 5.   [4] See p. 2.   [5] Defined in s. 18 (5).   [6] S. 5.

authorities and similar bodies is vested in the Secretary of State for the Environment.[1] Should a public or local authority take any special precautions in respect of radioactive waste disposed of in accordance with an authorisation granted under s. 6 of the Act and those precautions are taken in compliance with the conditions subject to which the authorisation was granted, the public or local authority has power to make such charges, in respect of the taking of those precautions, as may be agreed between that authority and the person to whom the authorisation was granted, or as, in default of such agreement, may be determined by the Minister, and to recover the charges so agreed or determined from that person.[2]

Where an authorisation granted under s. 6 requires or permits radioactive waste to be removed to a place provided by a local authority as a place for the deposit of refuse, it is the duty of that local authority to accept any radioactive waste removed to that place in accordance with the authorisation, and, if the authorisation contains any provision as to the manner in which the radioactive waste is to be dealt with after its removal to that place, to deal with it in the manner indicated in the authorisation.[3]

Sections 6–9 as to accumulation and disposal of radioactive waste apply to Area Health Authorities and to Boards of Governors, as well as to voluntary hospitals and to nursing homes. They do not, however, apply to special hospitals under s. 40 of the N.H.S. Re-organisation Act 1973 or to Service or prison hospitals or to visiting forces hospitals. Where, in the case of premises in occupation of the Crown, etc., to which ss. 6 and 7 do not apply,

(a) arrangements are made whereby radioactive waste is not to be disposed of from those premises except with the approval of the Minister, and

(b) in pursuance of those arrangements the Minister proposes to approve, or approves, the removal of radioactive waste from those premises to a place provided by a local authority as a place for the deposit of refuse.

the provisions of subsections (3) to (5) of s. 9 of the Act apply as if the proposal to approve the removal of the waste were an application for an authorisation under s. 6 of the Act to remove it, or (as the case may be) the approval were such an authorisation.[4]

By s. 10, the Minister is empowered to provide additional facilities for disposal of radioactive waste and to charge therefor.

---

[1] S. 8 (3). See Radioactive Substances (Hospital Waste) Exemption S.I. Order 1963 No. 1833.
[2] S. 9 (4).   [3] S. 9 (5).
[4] S. 9 (3) relates to consultation with the local authority before authorisation is granted and s. 9 (4) (5) as to special precautions and recovery of charges therefore by the local authority providing for disposal.

(e) Procedure in connection with registrations and authorisations

It is provided in s. 11 (1) that before the Minister refuses or attaches limitations or conditions to a registration or authorisation or varies a registration or authorisation otherwise than by revoking a limitation or condition subject to which it has effect, the Minister must afford the person directly concerned, and may afford to such local authorities or other persons as he may consider appropriate, an opportunity to appear before, and to be heard by, a person appointed for the purpose by the Minister. 'The person directly concerned' means the person applying for the registration or to whom the registration relates or the person applying for the authorisation or to whom the authorisation has been granted.[1]

(f) Rights of entry and inspection

Section 12 (2) and (3) provides that any person appointed by the Minister as an inspector under s. 12 (1) or any person authorised in that behalf by the Minister (referred to as an 'inspector') may at any reasonable time enter and inspect any premises in respect of which any person is licensed under s. 1 or exempted under s. 2 (1) and (2) and also any premises in respect of which an authorisation has been granted under s. 6 (1) or s. 7. The inspector is also given necessary power to have equipment with him, to take samples, obtain information and inspect documents.

Where an inspector has reasonable grounds for believing that radioactive material has been or is being kept or used on any premises not registered or exempt, or that radioactive waste has been or is being disposed of or accumulated on or from premises without any necessary authorisation, he may enter and inspect those premises—

(a) with consent given by or on behalf of the occupier of the premises; or

(b) under a warrant under the provisions of the Second Schedule; or

(c) where entry is required in a case of emergency, there being reasonable cause to believe that circumstances exist which are likely to endanger life or health, and that immediate entry to the premises is necessary to verify the existence of those circumstances or to ascertain their cause or to effect a remedy.[2]

(g) Offences

Offences under the Act are set out in s. 13 and the penalties are increased by the Control of Pollution Act 1974.

---

[1] S. 11 (4).
[2] S. 12 (4), (6) and (9).

3. Atomic Energy Act 1946 — Uranium Parts

'Uranium parts' are now supplied on hire to hospitals. Uranium is a prescribed substance under the Atomic Energy Act 1946, s. 18 (1). The pieces must be kept in a safe place and a certificate showing where they are held must be given to the Department of Atomic Energy at the end of every quarter. The full definition of prescribed substances under s. 18 (1) is uranium, thorium, plutonium, neptunium or any of their respective compounds or any other substance prescribed, being a substance which in the opinion of the Minister[1] is or may be used for the production or use of atomic energy or research into matter connected therewith.

[1] *i.e.*, originally the Minister of Supply, now the Secretary of State for Education and Science (S.I. 1964 No. 490).

CHAPTER 13

CONSENT TO TREATMENT AND KINDRED MATTERS

1. Introductory

IN this chapter will be discussed the extent of the duty of a medical practitioner not to undertake any medical or surgical procedure without the consent of the patient or of some other person in his stead. Also will be discussed such closely related matters as the extent of the obligation of the medical practitioner to afford the patient or other person some explanation about the nature and effect of the procedure proposed and of any risk involved when seeking to obtain any necessary consent. It will be observed that a signature on a 'consent form' is powerful evidence of consent; however, it is only evidence of it. Consent forms are therefore discussed here. Even at this stage however it is important to note that the legal question is whether the consent was full, free and voluntary[1] and not whether a form was signed. Cases which reach the courts and to which one looks for authority usually concern operative procedures, reference is generally made here to the duty of a surgeon in this or that set of circumstances. But the same principles apply no less to things done by any other medical practitioner, e.g., a physician undertaking an investigation or treatment involving significant risk to the patient.[2]

2. Patients of Full Age and Understanding

(a) General principles

An operation, or any other surgical or medical procedure, or even a medical examination, carried out without the consent, express or implied, of the person concerned will usually amount to actionable trespass to the person, for it is a direct, unauthorised interference with the patient's body for which the surgeon or other responsible medical practitioner and those helping him may be held personally liable.[3]

---

[1] Compare *Burnett* v. *British Waterways Board* [1973] 1 W.L.R. 700; [1973] 2 All E.R. 631.

[2] It will be noted that in general the law is only concerned with those methods of treatment or investigation that involve a physical touching of the person. It follows that, generally, no action lies for a psychiatric examination carried out without consent. However in *Re R.* (*P.M.*) [1968] 1 W.L.R. 385; [1968] 1 All E.R. 691, such an examination was carried out on an infant ward of court without the consent of either the Court or the Official Solicitor. The Court condemned this practice. See also *Re D.* (*A Minor*) (*wardship: sterilisation*), [1976] Fam. 185; [1976] 1 All E.R. 326.

[3] As to the vicarious liability of hospital authorities, nursing home proprietors, *etc.*, see p. 262.

But in *Fowler* v. *Lanning*[1] Diplock, J., laid down the general principle that an action for trespass to the person does not lie if the injury to the plaintiff has been caused unintentionally and without negligence on the defendant's part. Does this help if the surgeon honestly believes that the patient's consent to an operation has been obtained, *e.g.*, if he is so informed by another member of the hospital staff? And does it help if, through carelessness on the part of, say, the houseman or nurses, the wrong patient is brought into the theatre and the surgeon is thereby led to perform an unauthorised operation?

The answer appears to be 'No' in both instances. In the first instance, *i.e.*, absence of consent, it may be argued that the surgeon was entitled to rely on other members of the hospital staff to obtain consent and may reasonably have accepted the assurance of, say, the theatre sister or the house officer that consent had been obtained, and therefore, in operating in reliance on such assurance, he had not been negligent.[2] But, unfortunately for the surgeon, to bring himself within the protection of *Fowler* v. *Lanning*,[3] he must not only have acted without negligence but must also have acted unintentionally. In fact, he has performed the operation on the patient intentionally. It would seem however, that if sued personally the surgeon could join as third parties the other member or members of the hospital staff who, by their negligence, had misled him and could also bring in the hospital authority, either as being vicariously liable for the negligence of those other members of the staff, or as answerable for a negligent system of working. What indemnity, if any, the surgeon might thereby obtain would depend on the Court's assessment of the extent to which his own negligence might have been a contributory factor.

In the second instance, *i.e.*, an operation performed on the wrong patient, the trespass to the person is again intentional and therefore the defence that he had acted without negligence would not be open to the surgeon. And in this case the surgeon's position may be weaker since the Court might take the line that he ought to have known his own patient and what he intended to do for him.

Obvious exceptions to the rule that a patient's own consent to an operation or analogous procedure must be obtained are children up to the age of 16[4] and persons suffering from mental disorder if that disorder be of such a nature and degree as to render them incapable of giving a valid consent. In the case of the former it is the parent or guardian who ordinarily gives the necessary consent whilst in the case

[1] [1959] 1 Q.B. 426.
[2] He might however be under a duty to ensure that there was a duly signed consent form in the patient's notes. See, *e.g.*, Annual Report of M.D.U. 1974 at pp. 48–9. As to consent forms, see below, p. 187 *et seq.*
[3] [1959] 1 Q.B. 426.
[4] Not necessarily in the wider sense of minors or legal infants. See further, p. 193 *et seq.*

of the latter it is possibly the responsible medical officer if the patient is liable to detention in hospital or, otherwise, the patient's guardian if one has been appointed. Not infrequently the consent of the patient's nearest relative is relied on. Those, as well as certain other apparent exceptions, such as an operation on an unconscious accident patient will be considered more fully later in this chapter. It is sometimes said that the consent of the husband is necessary in the case of a proposed operation on his wife if the operation may or will result in sterility. This too will be considered.

If a person presents himself for treatment as a patient at a hospital his co-operation is ordinarily sufficiently obvious to make clear his consent to ordinary external physical examination. Also, the nature of his trouble when he voluntarily attends, *e.g.*, a severe cut, manifestly needing stitches, a broken arm requiring setting, or an eye with a piece of metal in it, may sufficiently indicate his desire for and assent to the necessary treatment. But we now reach a point at which it is exceedingly difficult to draw a line and to say whether the patient's consent may reasonably be inferred or not. What if the broken arm does not set properly and needs resetting to make a satisfactory job of it, or if the patient's trouble is internal and for purposes of diagnosis the surgeon wishes an internal examination with the aid of instruments? Prudence would dictate that even if the patient's formal consent had not already been obtained it should not be neglected at this stage. It would however not seem necessary, even in respect of in-patients, in every case to obtain the patient's consent in writing, though it is highly advisable to do so for surgical treatment and also for internal examination under anaesthetic, aortography and other procedures in respect of which there is more than a minimum degree of risk and also where the proposed treatment is truly elective.[1] Illustrative of the kind of case in which written consent might be dispensed with is that of a pregnant woman who had been having ante-natal care before entering hospital for what was expected to be a normal delivery. But if it were known at the time of the woman's admission, or became known before the onset of labour, that surgical intervention, *e.g.* Caesarian section, would be necessary, then it would be desirable to obtain consent in writing.[2]

It is attractive to some that the patient's signature to a form of consent, couched in the most general terms, should be obtained when he first

[1] The kind of case in which the patient might have the choice, say, between having an operation entailing considerable risk which, if successful, would result in a complete cure, or of not having the operation and going on living subject to a disability and all its consequences.

[2] Whether consent in writing might usefully be sought after the onset of labour would depend on whether the patient was in a condition meaningfully to consent and this without distress. If she were under any degree of sedation when she signed the form its value would be significantly diminished. In such circumstances, being in the nature of an unforeseen emergency, whether a form is signed or not matters little, provided that what is best is done for the patient.

attends hospital, this so that nothing for which consent is requisite should unwittingly be done without it. Such procedure is strongly to be deprecated since, in all but the most obvious conditions of ill-health, no one has any idea what operative or other procedure is involved until the patient has been examined and, maybe, until he has been under observation for some time. Moreover it may well be found that alternative courses of treatment are possible, treatments of such different nature and such different possible consequences that the choice whether to undergo a particular operation is truly elective. Then there is a real choice to be made by the patient and in such circumstances it is more than a little doubtful how effective would be a general consent given by a patient on entering hospital and in complete ignorance of what was proposed to be done and of any possibility of choice. It is therefore preferable that, in all cases, the patient's consent should be sought only when the surgeon has decided to advise a particular operation and that such explanation as is thought necessary or desirable be given to the patient by the responsible surgeon or other senior member of the surgical team.

(b) The nature of the required explanation

What explanation is necessary? In most instances, where there is no question of a truly elective operation, the patient is likely to be well content with a quite simple, rather sketchy, non-technical explanation which concentrates attention more on the object sought to be attained by the proposed operation than on its precise nature. Above all, the average patient wants reassurance. But is there any obligation on the surgeon in any circumstances to warn the patient of particular risks? In answering that question we must distinguish the following cases: (i) the statement made in answer to a question asked by the patient; and (ii) the volunteered statement, whether or not there is a truly elective element in the decision the patient has to make.

(i) *Replies to patients' questions.* If a patient asks a question about the risk involved in the operation or procedure (*e.g.*, aortography) or about the possible consequences (*e.g.* the effect on the voice of thyroidec- tomy), may the question be answered untruthfully or evasively, or just avoided by a contrived turn of conversation? Or must the surgeon answer frankly? On the basis of *Smith* v. *Auckland Hospital Board*[1] a decision of strong persuasive authority in the New Zealand Court of Appeal, and taking into full account the summing up of Denning, L.J., in *Hatcher* v. *Black and Others*,[2] the answer would seem to be that the surgeon — or other medical practitioner — should ordinarily answer accurately. He is not, however under a duty to volunteer information beyond that positively asked for by the patient, it being for the patient

----

[1] [1965] N.Z. 191.   [2] [1954] *The Times*, 2nd July.

to ask supplementary questions if the answer to his original question, being a truthful answer, has not told him all he wanted to know. Also, the surgeon is not at risk by refraining from answering provided it should have been clear to the patient that he was deliberately not answering. It may be otherwise if — as in *Smith's case*[1] — he answers so evasively as to mislead the patient. And even if *Smith's case* were followed, it would seem that there might be the exceptional case in which an untruthful or evasive answer would be justified, but the onus would then be on the defendant to satisfy the court that the circumstances were exceptional and the untruth or evasion in the patient's own interest. This exception is however of questionable validity for, in maintaining it, one is, in fact, asserting the validity of consent to an operation obtained by deceit. Finally it has to be said that even if a patient's consent to a procedure or operation were given after the surgeon had made an untrue or evasive statement about the risk involved,[2] the patient would not succeed in an action for damages unless the court were satisfied that he would have been likely to refuse consent had a truthful answer been given.

The facts of *Smith* v. *Auckland Hospital Board* were as follows. The plaintiff suffered from an aortic aneurism and a surgeon in one of the defendant Board's hospitals sought his consent to a preliminary exploratory procedure, aortography, before deciding on the next step. Aortography involved passing a catheter through the femoral artery to the aorta to inject an opaque fluid to outline the aorta for photography. In answer to a question by the patient whether there was any risk, the surgeon W. gave an answer which was so evasive as to mislead the plaintiff into the belief that there was no risk, although W. was aware that there was a slight risk of the mishap which unfortunately did occur, a gangrenous condition of the right leg consequent upon the formation of a clot which necessitated the amputation of the leg below the knee. The evasive answer was given for no other reason than to reassure the patient.

The plaintiff brought an action claiming damages alleging that W., employed by the Board had been negligent in answering his question whether there was any danger in aortography and that the answer had misled him into giving his consent. The plaintiff failed in his action in the lower court,[3] Woodham, J., setting aside a finding by the jury that the Board by its servants or agents had been negligent so as to involve him in the loss of his leg by failing to inform him adequately of the risks of conducting a femoral aortogram upon it — this on grounds that there

---

[1] [1965] N.Z. 191.
[2] Presumably the position would be the same if the untruthful statement had been made after the consent had been given and, in consequence of it, the patient refrained from withdrawing his consent.
[3] [1964] N.Z. 241.

was no evidence on which the jury could find any breach of duty and, alternatively, that, even if there had been such evidence, the answer given by the surgeon could not reasonably be found causative of the damage suffered by the plaintiff. Both these conclusions were attacked in the Court of Appeal where the Court allowed the plaintiff's appeal and, applying *Hedley, Byrne & Co. Ltd.* v. *Heller & Partners Ltd.*,[1] held that the particular relationship of doctor and patient is sufficient to impose upon a doctor a duty to use due care in answering a question put to him by the patient where the patient, to the knowledge of the doctor, intends to place reliance on that answer in making a decision as to a treatment or procedure to which he is asked to consent. If in answering such a question the doctor fails to use due care and, as a result of submitting to the treatment or procedure the patient suffers injuries, the doctor will be liable to the patient in tort if the evidence shows that it is probable that if a proper answer had been given the patient would have refused to undergo the treatment or procedure either immediately or after further questions.

In the course of his judgment, Sir Harold Barrowclough, C.J., said:

'I do not think that it will be disputed, and I cannot imagine Mr Windsor disputing that he had not answered truthfully in this case. Of course I do not mean that he acted mendaciously. He meant only to be reassuring and he avoided a real answer, and one can understand his reasons for that. But what he said was so reassuring as to be capable of the construction that there was no risk. That would not have been the truth: at least it fell short of the truth.'[2]

But to establish liability on the principle of *Hedley Byrne's case*, the plaintiff had not only to establish that the surgeon had not answered him frankly but also that his injury resulted therefrom. The verdict of the jury in the lower court that that was so was not disturbed though Sir Harold Barrowclough said:

'Had I been trying the action myself and without a jury I might have come to the conclusion that this was not proved — even on balance of probabilities — that had he received a proper answer to his inquiry about the risks involved, the appellant would have declined to submit himself to the aortogram procedure.'[3]

Other members of the court expressed themselves to similar effect. It would seem then that if *Smith's case*[4] is followed in the English courts a plaintiff making a similar claim will not succeed unless the court is satisfied that, as an ordinary, reasonable man, he would — in all the circumstances — have refused the operation or procedure if he had been answered frankly.

---

[1] [1964] A.C. 465.   [2] [1965] N.Z. 191, 198.
[3] This passage from the judgment of Barrowclough, C.J., is in line with the guidance given to the jury by McNair, J., in *Bolam's* case ([1957] 1 W.L.R. 582; [1957] 2 All E.R. 118). See below pp. 185–186.
[4] [1964] A.C. 465.

(ii) *Statements volunteered to the patient.* Although the guidance of decided cases is lacking it seems generally accepted today that if a patient's consent to an operation or other procedure is to be relied on he must have been given — even without his having asked — such reasonable explanation of the nature and effect of what is proposed to be done as is appropriate and practicable in the circumstances, taking into account such things as the patient's level of understanding and his physical condition.

But should the information be volunteered about any risk involved? The line generally taken by members of the medical profession of not volunteering information about a slight but inevitable risk involved in undergoing a necessary operation or procedure, *i.e.*, an operation or procedure which affords the only reasonable chance of saving the patient's life or of curing the condition from which he is suffering, is no more than common sense, since any interference with the human body must entail some risk of danger to life or at least ill effects, however remote that risk may be. To warn a patient of such minimal risk without the patient himself raising the question could not but be unsettling to even the most level-headed patient, for such a patient would inevitably assume that the risk was much greater than it really was and that by being referred to as a slight risk it was being played down. And this view gains support in the summing up of McNair, J., in *Bolam* v. *Friern H.M.C.*[1]

The plaintiff had agreed to undergo electro-convulsive therapy (ECT) and, in the course of that treatment sustained serious injury, bi-lateral stove-in fractures of the acetabula. In his action against the hospital management committee he alleged negligent treatment[2] and also that he should have been warned of the risk involved in the operation to which his consent had been sought and obtained.

On the question of whether a warning should have been given, McNair, J., told the jury that they should consider two questions, 'First, does good medical practice require that a warning should be given to a patient before he is submitted to E.C.T. treatment; and, secondly, if a warning had been given what difference would it have made'? Having summed up the evidence, including the opinions of expert witnesses on both sides, he continued:

'Having considered the evidence on this point you have to make up your minds whether it has been proved to your satisfaction that when the defendants adopted the practice they did (namely, the practice of saying very little and waiting for questions from the patient), they were falling below a proper standard of competent professional opinion on this question of whether or not it is right to warn. Members of the jury, though it is a matter entirely for you,

[1] [1957] 1 W.L.R. 582; [1957] 2 All E.R. 118. Followed in *Chin Keow* v. *Government of Malaysia* [1967] 1 W.L.R. 813 (P.C.).
[2] This aspect of the case is further discussed on pp. 233–234.

you may well think that when dealing with a mentally sick man and having a strong belief that his only hope of cure is E.C.T. treatment, a doctor cannot be criticised if he does not stress the dangers which he believes to be minimal involved in that treatment.'

On the second question, viz., whether a warning, if given, would have had any effect, he suggested that unless the plaintiff had satisfied the jury that he would not have taken treatment if he had been warned, there was really nothing in that point.

If then we leave aside the case of the operation or procedure in respect of which any sensible person, as a potential patient, would feel that there was a truly elective element[1] and restrict ourselves to the operation which is the only course reasonably practicable if anything is to be done for a patient whose condition is grave, it would seem that what was said by McNair, J., in his summing up in *Bolam's case*,[2] gives reasonable guidance.[3] It will be observed, however, that in this case McNair, J., carefully left on one side what the position might have been, had the patient asked questions. Hence, there is no conflict between *Bolam's case*[7] and the later decision of the New Zealand Court of Appeal in *Smith* v. *Auckland Hospital Board*[4] which concerned only the surgeon's duty to answer questions frankly. Nor does the summing up of McNair, J., in *Bolam's case*[5] give blanket cover to the surgeon even where no questions are asked, for he was addressing himself properly only to the case in hand where the surgeon himself reasonably believed not only that the operation was the patient's only hope of cure but also that the risk was minimal — a belief which, though not universal among practitioners in his speciality, was shared at the date of the injury, by his clinical chief and also by others of similar standing in his field. Hence are left open both the case where the risk is more than slight and also what explanation is called for in the case of the truly elective operation.

If the risk involved in a proposed operation is more than slight and the patient's life is not in immediate danger[6] if he does not undergo it, though possibly if he does not do so his expectation of life may be shortened or he may have to live the rest of his days under some serious disability, it would seem only proper that such operation should be regarded as an elective one[7] and that the patient should be told as

---

[1] For meaning of *elective element* see footnote 1 on p. 181.

[2] [1957] 1 W.L.R. 582; [1957] 2 All E.R. 118.

[3] One is, however, left to speculate on whether the lead given in the summing up in this case would have been quite so strong, had the patient's disability been not mental but physical, bearing in mind that his life was not apparently in danger.

[4] [1965] N.Z. 191.   [5] [1957] 1 W.L.R. 582; [1957] 2 All E.R. 118.

[6] 'Immediate danger' probably means not only death within days but also inevitable death within a matter of months if the operation be not done, *e.g.*, from carcinoma.

[7] A further example of the elective operation is the operation as an alternative to medical treatment, as by a course of injections. This is illustrated by the facts of *Hatcher* v. *Black* ([1954], *The Times*, July 2). The plaintiff had suffered from goitre and could apparently have

simply as may be what the position is and invited to make his own choice, though one would see no reason why, if he were then content to place himself in the surgeon's hands, the surgeon should not then guide the patient in his choice. But where there is an immediate danger to life if the operation be not done, it would be in keeping with medical practice and common sense not usually to emphasise or, perhaps, even mention the risk. But here another question, probably ethical rather than legal, comes to mind, *i.e.*, the desirability on occasion of saying sufficient to a patient who may be near death to give him opportunity of putting his affairs in order.

(c) Forms of consent

(i) *Generally.* This part of the chapter touches on some major considerations of practical importance in relation to the use of forms of consent — the content of the forms currently recommended and the advice given by the Department of Health and Social Security and by the medical defence societies concerning the use of those forms is the subject of closer examination in Appendix E.

It is advisable that the consent form be kept with the case papers, and that the duty should be laid on a particular person of seeing that a consent form has been completed in respect of any patient in the ward upon whom it is proposed to operate or to undertake any other procedure for which it is the practice to obtain consent in writing. Exceptions, such as accident cases, must arise. Such exceptions should always be brought to the notice of the operating surgeon as a matter of course and, if there is any grave doubt as to the advisability of proceeding, referred to the most senior administrative officer available. Failure to observe these elementary precautions might involve the surgeon and all who collaborated with him, as well as the area health authority or the hospital, in a civil action for assault, an action in which, if there were any unfortunate sequel to the operation, heavy damages might be awarded.

At the time of writing it seems that different advice is being given to their members by the Medical Defence Union and the Medical Protection Society on the extent to which it is desirable to use specially

been treated with drugs, but that would have been over a long period. She was, however, apparently encouraged to undergo the alternative operative procedure, partial thyroidectomy. During the operation her larangeal nerve was damaged, this affecting her voice. She claimed against the surgeon, alleging negligence, and against her physician for allegedly having advised her that there was no risk whatever. The action, a jury case, failed. The summing up of Denning, L.J., has been quoted as authority for the view that a surgeon is justified in telling a patient, untruthfully, that there is no risk, should he regard it as in the patient's interest to do so. However, the passage relied on is, at best, only persuasive authority as it was *obiter*, the surgeon not having been sued on that ground, though the allegation was made. The line taken in *Smith* v. *Auckland Hospital Board*, (see p. 182), *viz.*, that only in an exceptional case would an untruthful or evasive answer be justified, the onus being on the defendant to satisfy the court that the circumstances were exceptional, is to be preferred.

designed consent forms in particular circumstances, *e.g.*, for gynae-cological operations; or when a patient or the parent of a child-patient, whilst consenting to an operation, refuses consent to a blood trans-fusion; or when a child suffering from severe burns of congenital abnormality may need several operations, sometimes at short notice. And these are matters on which the Department has failed to give any real guidance, being content to say in the communication to hospital authorities in which it advises the use of a standard form for the generality of operations that 'there is no objection to the use of special consent forms for particular purposes . . . either adapted from the standard form or specially designed for the purpose, as advised by the appropriate medical defence society.[1]

(ii) *Single consent for more than one operation.* Does a single consent cover more than one operation during a period in which the patient was being treated continuously as an in-patient? As an example may be cited sub-total gastrectomy performed on December 8th, 1976, laparo-tomy on December 29th, 1976, and laparotomy–enterostomy on January 12th, 1977.

On the face of it, if gastrectomy was named in the form, being the standard form recommended by the Department, that operation would be authorised to be done and also 'such further or alternative operative measures as might be found to be necessary during the course of the above-mentioned operation'. But the wording used in the form is ambiguous. It could mean either any such further or alternative measures as might be found to be necessary *and also carried out* at the time of the original operation or such further or alternative measures then found to be necessary *but carried out subsequently.* What it cannot mean is any further operative treatment known or believed to be necessary but not so found during the course of the operation.

How the courts would interpret the formula in any particular case cannot be forecast with confidence and so it would be preferable when-ever a further operation is to be performed at any time after the patient has fully recovered his faculties after undergoing the first, that he should be invited to sign a fresh form. If, however, it is known at the outset that two or more related operations will be necessary, it is suggested that the form used originally might be amended appropriately. If an operation, in its very nature, involves two separate surgical procedures, the second after a lapse of maybe weeks or even months after the first, the original form of consent might suffice, at all events if the position had been explained to the patient. Nevertheless, the patient is free at any time after the performance of the first part of the operation and before the carrying out of the second to withdraw his consent. If he does so, it is important that the risk he is running should be clearly

---

[1] For text of Departmental advice and commentary thereon, see Appendix E.

explained to him and, if possible, his acknowledgment in writing of the explanation be obtained.[1,2]

(iii) *Removal of male organs and fashioning of artificial vagina*. The removal of a patient's male organs and the fashioning of an artificial vagina, for therapeutic reasons, *i.e.* for the sake of his mental health and done with the consent of the patient is not illegal but the patient does not thereby become a female and any marriage he contracts as such will be a nullity.[3]

(iv) *Hypnotism*. The Hypnotism Act 1952, which regulates the use of hypnotism for the purpose of entertainment, places no restriction on its use for medical and scientific purposes, s. 5 provides as follows:

Nothing in this Act shall prevent the exhibition, demonstration or performance of hypnotism (otherwise than at or in connection with an entertainment) for scientific or research purposes or for the treatment of physical or mental disease.

Consequently it is lawful — with the patient's consent[4] — to use hypnotism for producing anaesthesia or otherwise for the purpose of treatment. Whether or not it is lawful to use hypnotism for any such purpose without the patient's consent remains an open question.[5]

(v) *Breath tests and specimens of blood and urine under the Road*

---

[1] A somewhat more difficult situation from the hospital's point of view would arise if, say, valuable radium needles had been implanted and the patient would not submit to the procedure necessary for withdrawal. It would not be lawful to compel the patient to submit but it is suggested that, provided the patient had understood the nature of the implantation when he accepted it, he could be sued for damages if he refused to allow the hospital to recover the needles.

[2] As to consent to a series of operations on a child suffering from severe burns, congenital abnormality, *etc.*, see pp. 199–200.

[3] If the patient were married at the time he sought surgical intervention, it is questionable whether the operation should be undertaken without the consent of his wife (see *Bravery* v. *Bravery* [1954] 1 W.L.R. 116) even though for the sake of his mental health unless evidence of a psychiatrist were available that the effect on the patient's mental health of his not having it would be grave. *Corbett* v. *Corbett* ([1971] P. 83) was the first case in which an English court has been called on to pronounce on the sex of a male who has undergone such an operation. Ormrod, J., himself medically qualified, having referred to the various possible factors taken into account in determining sex in doubtful cases and which should be taken into account in deciding whether a 'sex-change' operation should be undertaken, reached the common sense conclusion that a person who has male primary sex organs is in law a male and does not become a female by having them removed and an artificial vagina substituted. The report is also interesting because a form of consent for such a 'sex-change' operation is there referred to. It reads as follows —

'I . . . of . . . do consent to undergo the removal of the male genital organs and the fashioning of an artificial vagina as explained to me by . . . (name of surgeon).

'I understand it will not alter my male sex and that it is being done to prevent deterioration of my mental health.'

Those wishing to pursue the matter even further than is done in the judgment are referred to Sir Roger Ormrod's paper 'Medico–Legal Aspects of Sex Determination', Medico–Legal J., Vol. 40, p. 78.

[4] It would seem advisable as always when consent is required to obtain it in writing.

[5] The general question of when consent to an operation or other procedure is unnecessary or when the consent of some person other than the patient is required or suffices is discussed elsewhere in this chapter. The position would be the same in respect of use of hypnotism if, ordinarily, the patient's consent is necessary.

Traffic Act 1972. Under the Road Traffic Act 1972 ss. 7 and 8[1] a constable in uniform may require a driver in hospital[2] after a road accident to take a breath test and to provide a specimen of blood or urine. The law is summarised in a departmental circular.[3]

It will be noted that the doctor in immediate charge[4] of the case (even an out-patient case[5]) must be told of the procedure and its consequences[6] and must consent to the tests being carried out.[7] There is no objection to him giving consent to both tests at once[8] and indeed he can sign a *pro forma* supplied by the police for this purpose.[9]

If the patient is discharged from the hospital the 'hospital' procedure does not apply and the police must resort to their practices.[10] This applies even if the motorist absconds from the hospital before being asked to provide the specimens.[11] It also applies where although the patient is still in the hospital, the treatment has been given and he is leaving.[12]

If the doctor objects to the test on the ground that the procedure proposed would be prejudicial to the proper care or treatment of the patient it is not to be carried out. Also, tests may not be made on a patient, nor any specimen taken from him without his consent, nor may they be made on or taken from an unconscious patient. If the constable honestly and reasonably believes that the patient/driver can hear and understand even if the patient cannot do this he can be convicted.[13] Consent is a matter entirely between the patient and the constable. Hospital staff are not required to take part in taking specimens nor is hospital equipment to be used in the tests. A patient in hospital is not liable to arrest without warrant under the 1972 Act, nor can he be required to go elsewhere to give specimens of breath, blood or urine.

(d) *Accident cases and other emergency patients*

Sometimes it is possible in these cases to obtain the usual consent before operating, but sometimes the patient is either unconscious or so affected by his physical condition as to be in no state of mind either to

---

[1] Previously the Road Safety Act 1967 ss. 2 and 3.

[2] *Hospital* here means an institution which provides medical or surgical treatment for in-patients or out-patients. It does not include an ambulance, *Hollingsworth* v. *Howard* [1974] R.T.R. 58.

[3] H.M. (67) 64. For the text, see pp. 761–763.

[4] This would include, *e.g.*, a houseman treating a patient in 'casualty' or on admission to a ward at night, even though — in hospital parlance — it would probably not be 'his' patient but rather the patient of the consultant under whom he worked.

[5] *MacNeill* v. *England* [1972] Crim. L.R. 255.   [6] *Burke* v. *Jobson* [1972] R.T.R. 59.

[7] This applies where a police officer makes a request for a breath test before the patient reaches the hospital but the request is not complied with until after he gets there *R.* v. *Crowley* [1977] R.T.R. 153.

[8] *Rutledge* v. *Oliver* [1974] R.T.R. 394.   [9] *Taylor* v. *Armand* [1975] R.T.R. 225.

[10] *R.* v. *Porter, The Times,* 6th December 1972.

[11] *Cunliffe* v. *Bleasdale* [1973] R.T.R. 90, but if he absconds deliberately he may be guilty of obstructing the police in the execution of their duties.

[12] *A.–G's. Reference (No. 1 of 1976), The Times* 29th March 1977.

[13] *R.* v. *Nicholls* [1972] 1 W.L.R. 502; [1972] 2 All E.R. 186.

consent or to object. Then, if the operation is urgently necessary in order to save the patient's life or even to reduce grave pain or for his ultimate well-being (*e.g.*, to save a limb), it is ordinarily carried out with the consent of the husband or wife or of the nearest relative immediately available. But if even that consent is unobtainable there is no alternative but to operate. If what is done is reasonable in the circumstances, no action against the surgeon or the hospital could be sustained.

But what should be done if, as occasionally happens, the spouse or nearest relative refuses to sign a form of consent? Such refusal may well be accompanied by what purports to be a positive prohibition on the proposed procedure being carried out, *e.g.* a therapeutic abortion; or the purported prohibition may be more limited but none the less fundamental, *e.g.*, of the administration of a blood transfusion. Such purported prohibitions are most frequently on religious grounds and may or may not include an assertion that it is the patient's view which is being expressed. A husband, for example, may say something to the effect, 'My wife is a Catholic and would not, therefore, consent to a therapeutic abortion.' Or he might say, 'I am a Catholic and I therefore cannot consent to my wife having a therapeutic abortion.'[1] There might be similar alternative possibilities in a refusal by husband, wife or near relative to the administration of a blood transfusion to the patient on the grounds of adherence to the sect known as Jehovah's Witnesses.

There are no legal grounds on which any relative has the right to refuse to allow a patient to receive necessary medical treatment. Therefore, if on refusing consent, the spouse or near relative of the patient does not purport to be expressing the patient's own wishes, there seems to be no alternative but to disregard the purported prohibition. But, if the spouse or near relative purports to be conveying what he believes to be the patient's own wishes, a more difficult situation arises, for when an operation is done in an emergency without consent, the hospital and its staff act on the higher ground of duty to save the patient.[2] Is that duty displaced by the information that the patient, because he is a Jehovah's Witness, would refuse consent to a blood transfusion? The answer is probably not, since there is no certainty that if the patient were told, 'Either you have this procedure carried out or you will be in danger of almost certain death,' he would refuse his consent to the advised procedure. Therefore, if a blood transfusion or other procedure is necessary in order to attempt to save life, or similarly, to prevent serious disablement or suffering, it should as a rule still be carried out despite objection by a spouse or relative, even if, in objecting, that

---

[1] Further as to married persons, see p. 202 *et seq.*

[2] See *per* Chisholm, C.J., in *Marshall* v. *Curry* 3 D.L.R. 260; 60 Can. C.C. (Nova Scotia Supreme Court); and see also '*The Right of the Mental Patient to his Psychosis*' [1976], M.L.R., p. 17, 34, J. Jacob. In previous editions Dr Speller argued for a similar result on the basis of an 'agency of necessity'. It may be a distinction without a difference.

spouse or relative purports to be expressing what he believes would be the patient's wishes.[1]

3. Minors[2]

A person now reaches full age on attaining 18.[3] In looking at minors we must distinguish minors who have attained the age of 16 from those who have not, because, by s. 8 of the Family Law Reform Act 1969, a minor who has attained the age of 16 can, to the same extent as a person of full age in like circumstances, give consent to surgical, medical and dental treatment.

(a) Minors who have attained the age of 16

Any doubt whether a person who had attained the age of 16 and who needed surgical, medical or dental treatment may himself give consent thereto has been finally removed by s. 8 (1) (2) of the Family Law Reform Act 1969 which reads as follows:

8.—(1) The consent of a minor who has attained the age of sixteen years to any surgical, medical or dental treatment which, in the absence of consent, would constitute a trespass to his person, shall be as effective as it would be if he were of full age; and where a minor has by virtue of this section given an effective consent to any treatment it shall not be necessary to obtain any consent for it from his parent or guardian.

(2) In this section 'surgical, medical or dental treatment' includes any procedure undertaken for the purposes of diagnosis, and this section applies to any procedure (including, in particular, the administration of an anaesthetic) which is ancillary to any treatment as it applies to that treatment.

[1] There are reasonable grounds for the view that if a patient who has consented to an operation, whilst expressly refusing consent to a blood transfusion, were nonetheless given such transfusion because, during the course of the operation to which he has consented, it became apparent that the only reasonable hope of saving his life was to give it, no civil liability for trespass to the person would be incurred by any of those concerned. An argument in support of that view is based on the fact that the decision whether or not the giving of such transfusion was vitally necessary could have been made only at a time when the patient was no longer in a fit state to be consulted and that, could he have made the decision at that time, he would not necessarily have opted as he did when he signed the limited form of consent specifically excluding blood transfusion. In such an emergency situation it seems reasonable that the surgeon, acting either under the higher ground of duty or as an agent of necessity, should do what ought to be done in the best interests of the patient. The position seems analogous to that of the rescuer of the would-be suicide by drowning who, by physical force, if necessary, overcomes any resistance and brings the drowning person safely to shore. However even if that approach be wrong, it may be suggested that, were the patient afterwards to sue for damages for trespass to the person, this solely because he had been given the transfusion and without any allegation of ill-consequences, or of any ill-consequences not outweighed by the harm which would have resulted had the transfusion not been given, he would be unlikely to obtain more than nominal damages — maybe no more than the contemptuous halfpenny. The M.D.U. have made it clear that they will stand by any member whichever course he adopts (Annual Report 1974, p. 85).
[2] It is provided in s. 12 of the Act that a person who is not of full age may be described as a minor instead of as an infant and, in the Act, 'minor' means such a person.
[3] Family Law Reform Act 1969 s. 1. By s. 9 a person attains a particular age expressed in years at the commencement of the relevant anniversary of his birth (i.e., on his birthday). This changes the old common law rule and is, of course, subject to any other provision in any written document (including a statute) that has to be construed.

Among other things authorised to be done with the patient's own consent as being necessary surgical, medical or dental treatment is any necessary medical or surgical attention to a pregnant unmarried girl who has reached the age of 16, whether or not such help is in respect of a normal delivery.[1] What the section apparently does not cover is consent by the minor to the use of his body for purposes of experimentation or research. As to the use of patients and others, including minors, whether patients or volunteers, and on the general question of consent to any such use, see section 10 of this chapter, at page 218.

The possibility of parental consent[2] as an alternative to consent by the minor himself is preserved by s. 8 (3) of the Act reading as follows:

8.—(3) Nothing in this section shall be construed as making ineffective any consent which would have been effective if this section had not been enacted.

It must, however, be added that another interpretation of sub-section (3) is that it does no more than to preserve the right of a minor under 16 years of age, if capable of understanding what he is doing, himself to give consent to operative or other treatment. Read literally s. 8 (3) is apt to cover both cases so, applying it to the one, does not imply the exclusion of the other. But whatever view of its meaning may prevail, what is beyond all doubt is that no parent of a minor who has reached the age of 16 can veto any treatment, whether necessary or only desirable, which the minor is willing to accept.

(b) Minors who have not attained the age of 16

So far as a child who has not attained the age of 16 is concerned there has been no alteration of the common law rule that he is ordinarily in the custody and control of a parent[3] and that any interference with his body, as by medical or surgical treatment, without the consent of his parent and without lawful excuse[4] may lay anyone concerned open

---

[1] The question whether, in such a case or in any other, it is permissible without the consent of the patient to communicate with the parents of a patient between the ages of 16 and 18 is discussed in Chapter 20, at pp. 360–361.

[2] If treatment to which a minor had himself refused consent were such that his co-operation or his willing submission thereto, were necessary to its success, parental consent would be practically useless. But there are other circumstances in which such consent would afford cover for a procedure to which the minor had refused his consent or to which he was unable to give it, e.g. the administration of a blood transfusion during an operation or a therapeutic abortion to save the life of a young girl or, indeed, any other operation necessary o attempt save life or prevent permanent disability. There could also be circumstances, e.g. an elective operation, not being a matter of extreme urgency, when the surgeon — acting for himself and for the hospital authority — might think it desirable that the minor should have the advice of a parent or guardian in reaching a decision and so might indicate to the minor that — assuming the parent or guardian were available — his consent was required. But the absence of such consent would not be a defence in an action by a minor who had suffered harm because necessary treatment which he was willing to undergo had been withheld. In any case in which parental consent might be appropriate, either mother or father could ordinarily give that consent without the other. See pp. 194–195.

[3] See below (pp. 194–195) as to effect of s. 1 of the Guardianship Act 1973 which gives the mother equal rights with the father in matters concerning the child's welfare.

[4] In the present context, emergency treatment without parental consent is the best illustration of a lawful excuse. See further pp. 190–191.

to an action for trespass to the person of the child. Also, as is stated above, s. 8 (3) of the Family Law Reform Act 1969 may be interpreted as preserving the right of a child under 16 years of age who understands the nature and effects (both legal and medical) of his consent himself to give it to any treatment,[1] including operative treatment.

If by 'treatment' is meant treatment immediately necessary for relieving present pain and suffering; for preventing or alleviating pain and suffering foreseen as an immediate consequence of the child's condition; for averting or minimising any permanent disability; for reducing the prospect of a shortened life; for saving life, or attempting to do any of those things it can be accepted that if the child has sufficient understanding of what he is doing, his consent is sufficient. But if the child objected to having such treatment and it were practicable to give it without his active co-operation, a medical or dental practitioner, whether in hospital or elsewhere, could none the less lawfully undertake that treatment on the basis of the higher duty owed by a practitioner to his patient. But treatment which, though necessary, was not immediately necessary or which, although desirable,[2] was not necessary, should ordinarily be undertaken only with parental consent.[3] If however the child understands, it would appear unwise to impose treatment against a specific refusal. Thus if a girl under the age of 16 becomes pregnant and she refuses an abortion it would appear that her parents cannot compel her to have it; at least so long as she understands the consequences not only of the abortion which she is refusing but also of bearing the child.

In all ordinary cases,[4] since the coming into force of s. 1 of the Guardianship Act 1973, either the father or the mother of a child may — without the other — give a valid consent to treatment, this being a matter concerning the child's welfare.[5] Nor apparently need the hospital

---

[1] In previous editions Dr Speller has argued that the child's right to give consent to treatment is confined to 'necessary treatment'. Whether this is right or not undoubtedly the more important question is the extent of the consequences of the proposed treatment and the child's appreciation of them. Thus a comparatively young child can consent to the administration of a sticking plaster over a grazed knee; the more complex the medical procedures so the greater degree of understanding is required.

[2] An example of treatment which may not always be necessary but may nevertheless be desirable is cosmetic surgery.

[3] Except where the context otherwise requires *parental consent* includes the consent of a lawful guardian or custodian and *parent* includes *guardian* or *custodian*.

[4] Exceptional cases referred to in s. 1 of the Guardianship Act 1973 include the child who is in the custody and control of one or other parent by agreement (s.1 (2)) and the illegitimate child (s. 1 (7)) who is in the custody and control of its mother. We are not here immediately concerned with children in the lawful or actual custody of any person or authority under a court order. In that case that person or an officer on behalf of the authority will have the responsibility of consenting or withholding consent to treatment.

[5] The relevant provisions of the Guardianship Act 1973 are as follows —

S. 1—(1) In relation to the custody or upbringing of a minor, . . . a mother shall have the same rights and authority as the law allows to a father, and the rights and authority of mother and father shall be equal and be exercisable by either without the other. . . .

(3) Where a minor's father and mother disagree on any question affecting his welfare,

or practitioner even inquire whether the other parent, whether father or mother, knows what is proposed to be done, though one can envisage circumstances in which — unless the treatment were urgently necessary — it would be sensible to make sure that both parents were in the picture, this from a social rather than a legal point of view. This could be so in the case of an elective operation not immediately necessary, being one of which a successful outcome was by no means certain, even leaving aside unforeseen accidents. The position which might arise if the father and mother were known to disagree on a particular course or action, one consenting, the other objecting, is discussed later.

The Guardianship Act does not seemingly affect regulations made under the Health Service Acts 1946 to 1973 under which, assuming the child is to be treated as a N.H.S. patient, a child's mother is responsible for choosing its family doctor. It does, however, raise the question whether, if for good reason, the father disagreed with the mother's choice, the court might, on application by him, order the mother to choose a different doctor. Whatever might be the answer to that question, it seems plain from s. 1 (1) (3) of the 1973 Act that, once a child is on a doctor's N.H.S. list, both parents have equal rights in the matter of accepting or refusing advice as to treatment. These rights may be exercised by either parent without the other.

The surviving parent, whether father or mother, is the child's natural guardian, but the deceased parent may have appointed a testamentary guardian to act with the survivor.[1] The possibility of awkward legal problems arising in these cases is sufficiently remote to be ignored, and, in all ordinary circumstances, a medical practitioner would be safe in acting on the authority of the surviving mother or father alone as he would have been under s. 1 of the Guardianship Act 1973 during the lifetime of both parents. What is not so clear is his right to act on the sole authority of the testamentary guardian whilst there is a surviving parent except so far as the guardian may, in the absence of the surviving

either of them may apply to the court for its direction, and . . . the court may make such order regarding the matters in difference as it may think proper.
The provisions of s. 1 (3) for settling differences between parents on questions concerning the child's welfare, although only 'custody and upbringing' are mentioned in s. 1 (1), lead to the reasonable and inevitable conclusion that questions relating to a child's welfare are within the compass of 'upbringing' in s. 1 (1). So, as any question relating to provision of medical or dental treatment clearly concerns a child's welfare, it follows that in the matter of giving or withholding consent to treatment the rights and authority of a child's mother and father are equal and are exercisable by one without the other. This is now confirmed by the Children Act 1975 s. 85 (3). But see text and footnote 1 as to exceptional cases.

[1] Guardianship of Minors Act 1971. Generally as to guardianship, including guardians appointed by the court, see Bromley's Family Law, 4th edition, Professor Bromley, at p. 331, refers to the dictum of Lord Hardwicke in *Mendes* v. *Mendes* ([1784] 1 Ves. Sen. 89, 91) that the right of custody of a daughter ceases if she marries under the age of 21 [presumably now 18]; and, referring to *R.* v. *Wilmington* ([1822] 5 B. & Ald. 525, 526) and to *Lough* v. *Ward* ([1945] 2 All E.R. 338, 348), suggests that that is equally true of a son. In respect of consents to operations the question of the effect of marriage of the minor is now relevant only where, under s. 8 (3) of the Family Law Reform Act 1969, it is desired to administer treatment relying on the consent of a parent or lawful guardian or custodian.

parent, be acting as in actual custody. But, taking into account the duty of parents, guardians and custodians alike to provide a child with necessaries, a hospital or practitioner should never withhold treatment which is immediately necessary because of doubts about the validity of any consent obtained.

A stepparent has no parental rights in respect of a stepchild,[1] so, as between a stepfather and his wife — the child's surviving natural parent, it is her consent which is necessary. Hence, if the child's mother consents any objection by its stepfather should be disregarded except so far as any reason given for that objection might merit consideration on medical grounds. But, failing evidence to the contrary, it can usually be reasonably assumed that a stepfather giving consent to treatment of his stepchild is doing so on behalf of his wife, just as it might be assumed that, if the wife took her stepchild to hospital, any consent she might give would be as agent of the child's father who had entrusted his child to her care. Moreover, if a man or woman is *de facto* in charge of a stepchild either in the absence of the child's natural parent whom he/ she had married, or after that parent's death, his consent would ordinarily be acceptable as that of a person *in loco parentis*.

(c) Child under 16 years of age: refusal of parental consent

There are circumstances in which, if there is to be any hope whatever of saving the life of a child, the necessary treatment must be given without delay. A clear example is that of a new-born baby whose only hope of survival — because of rhesus factor incompatibility — is that his blood should be wholly and speedily replaced by blood transfusion. From time to time, parents — mostly adherents of particular religious sects — refuse consent to that procedure being undertaken. In such circumstances there is no time for a care and protection order to be obtained by the local children authority[2] so that an authorised officer of the authority can give consent in place of the parents. Consequently, either the blood transfusion has to be given despite parental objection or, although the child is in the care of the hospital staff who have available means whereby its life might be saved, it must be left to die. The choice is the same whatever may be the age of any child urgently needing a blood transfusion; and so also whatever else may be the proposed treatment to which parents have refused consent if, in fact, the medical practitioner[3] treating the child in hospital believes on good grounds

---

[1] In *re N (Minors) (Parental Rights)* [1974] Fam. 40; [1974] 1 All E.R. 126 [1973] 3 W.L.R. 866, unless, of course a custodianship order under s. 33 of the Children Act 1975 is in force.
[2] Children and Young Persons Act 1969 s. 28.
[3] Ordinarily a child in hospital will be under the care of the consultant surgeon or physician into one of whose beds he has been admitted and under whose general or specific guidance treatment may be given by other members of his team. Nevertheless, if, say, an emergency admission has to be dealt with without reference to him, then the immediate responsibility will be on the practitioner who has to deal with the situation, *e.g.* a registrar

that, failing that treatment, the child could not survive. The position would be the same if the practitioner, on good grounds, believed that without the recommended treatment the child's chance of survival would be significantly less.

Assuming, in a case within the above general description, that the child is in hospital under the care of a medical practitioner,[1] is that practitioner justified in doing what is necessary to attempt save the child's life, despite parental objection? It seems beyond doubt that he is justified, since in doing all he can to try save the child's life the medical practitioner is doing no more than it is the duty of the parents to have had done. That being so, it is inconceivable that an action against the hospital or against any member of its staff for trespass to the person of the child, solely on the ground that parental consent had not been obtained, could succeed.[2] A parent's duty to provide necessary medical aid for his child and his liability to prosecution for manslaughter if he wilfully fails to do so and the child dies in consequence, upon which the above statement is based, are brought out in *R.* v. *Senior*.[3] He might also be convicted of manslaughter if the failure to provide medical aid had been reckless, though not deliberate as in *R.* v. *Senior*.[4]

In *R.* v. *Senior*, the father of a child suffering from pneumonia, being a member of a sect known as the Peculiar People, omitted — on religious grounds — to supply the child with medical aid or medicine although he was aware of the danger to the child's life. The child died and, medical evidence having been given that the child's life would have been prolonged and might have been saved if a doctor had been allowed to treat it, the father was convicted of manslaughter. On appeal it was held that the defendant had been rightly convicted. But in *R.* v. *Spencer and Spencer*[5] on somewhat similar facts in an unreported case tried at the Nottingham Assizes in 1958 the defendants were acquitted. In this case the defendants belonged to the Jehovah's Witnesses and, on religious grounds, had refused to allow their newborn child to be given the blood transfusion which offered the only hope of saving its life. Under cross-examination the family doctor, who had attended the patient and had been called by the prosecution, admitted that, although he had told the father that the child should go into hospital for a

---

or — especially at night — a house officer. Also, if the consultant instructed a registrar to perform an operation to which parents had objected, it is then the registrar who, as well as the hospital authority, might be sued if the parents thought that they had a case. Medical practitioner must also here be understood to include dental practitioner.

[1] See footnote 3 on p. 196.

[2] The position of a medical practitioner who feels obliged to disregard objection by one parent, say, the child's father, is immensely strengthened if he has obtained the consent of the other parent. This is because of s. 1 (1) and (3) of the Guardianship Act 1973, there being no time for the parents to resolve their differences by an application to the court under s. 1 (3).

[3] [1899] 1 Q.B. 283. See also the Childrens and Young Persons Act 1969.

[4] *R.* v. *Lowe* [1973] Q.B. 702; [1973] 1 All E.R. 805.   [5] *The Times*, March 1, 1958.

transfusion, he might not have warned the parents that failure to give a transfusion would result in the child's death. At that point in the trial the prosecution offered no further evidence and, on the direction of Paull, J., the defendants were acquitted. But in discharging them the judge said, 'If after all you have learned in this court anything like this happens again, the position may be quite different. Just remember that.'

So far the conclusion has been reached only that a medical practitioner treating a child in hospital is justified in doing all that he can to attempt — notwithstanding parental objection — to save the life of a child, and this even though the objection may be on religious grounds. But there are strong grounds for going further and suggesting that not only may the medical practitioner do all he can to save the child's life, but that it is his duty to do so and that, if he failed in that duty and the child died in consequence, he might be charged with manslaughter. Whatever may be the right of the parents to custody and control of the child, coupled with responsibility for its welfare, it is the responsible medical practitioner in hospital who, at the time of the child's extreme need, has immediate care of the child, with the nursing staff looking after his needs in accordance with the doctor's orders. In such case, if the medical practitioner withheld treatment he believed to be necessary and the child died, it is hardly likely that, if he were charged with manslaughter, the parents' refusal of consent would constitute a defence, the parents themselves being under a duty to provide for the child that medical aid which had been withheld. Indeed, if such defence were available the life of the child in hospital would be less protected by the criminal law than that of a child at home since neither medical practitioner nor parent would be answerable, for a parent would surely never be convicted of manslaughter for refusing to sign a form, especially as it is manifest that, in case of need, parental objection can be ignored.[1]

So far we have been considering only operations and other medical procedures done, despite parental objection, in order to attempt to save the life of the child. But what of a child in hospital whose life is not in immediate danger but who, unless appropriate treatment is given without undue delay, will suffer, or be very likely to suffer, some permanent disability or degree of ill-health, and have a shorter expectation of life, parental consent to such treatment having been refused? What, too, of the case where failure to carry out promptly the necessary treatment would subject the child to a period of otherwise avoidable pain and suffering, though without foreseeable long-term consequences?

[1] The position of a general practitioner advising treatment which, in his opinion, is necessary for saving the child's life is different from that of the medical practitioner on the staff of a hospital where the child is an in-patient, since it is not within the power of the general practitioner to give the necessary treatment in face of parental objection, or to have the child removed to hospital for that purpose. The position of the general practitioner in such circumstances is more fully discussed in Dr Speller's *Law of Doctor and Patient* (Lewis, 1973), at p. 35.

To find an answer to those questions, as in cases in which the child's life is in immediate jeopardy, it is relevant to consider the legal responsibility of the parents. *Oakey* v. *Jackson*[1] is authority for the view that the unreasonable refusal by a parent to the carrying out on a child of an operation which ought to be done may constitute wilful neglect, whilst *R.* v. *Hayles*[2] supports the view that a parent not providing a child with necessary medical aid may be convicted of ill-treatment under s. 1 (1) of the Children and Young Persons Act 1933. Nor did *Hayles's* case concern neglect to obtain medical help which put the child's life in immediate danger, the position being that a conviction for neglect or ill-treatment may be obtained whenever a parent fails to provide medical aid for the child when a reasonable parent, similarly circumstanced, would have done so and the child suffers in any way in consequence. But except in extreme cases parental failure or wrong-headedness seldom results in prosecution. More likely, the local children authority would obtain a care and protection order and then have done — or have authorised to be done — whatever was necessary for the child's welfare, say, the provision of spectacles or of a hearing aid, or the carrying out of a tonsillectomy.

However, in the case of a child in hospital needing immediate treatment for present pain and suffering or to avert permanent disability or prospect of a shorter life, the obtaining of a care and protection order may be just as impracticable as where the operation is to save life. In this case, too, it can be argued that if the necessary treatment is given despite parental objection, the parents will have no cause of action either against the hospital or against those members of its staff who actually gave that treatment, for they will have done no more for the child than the parents were under a legal duty to have done. It could be otherwise if, in any action alleging trespass to the person of the child, the parents' case was supported by medical experts who satisfied the court that a significant body — though not necessarily a majority — of medical practitioners qualified to express an opinion would not have considered the disputed treatment necessary. Even so, it is not to be expected that the court would readily find against a medical practitioner who, in a case in which prompt action was required, had taken a course approved by a substantial body of professional opinion, this notwithstanding that some other practitioners might have done otherwise.[3]

But the risk of challenge on medical grounds discussed above is a remote one, especially if the member of the hospital staff who believes it urgently necessary to treat a child in a manner not approved by the parents obtains a second opinion before doing so and that second, concurring, opinion is recorded in the patient's case notes.

[1] [1914] 1 K.B. 216. [2] [1969] 1 Q.B. 364; 53 Cr. App. R. 36 (C.A.).
[3] *Bolam* v. *Friern H.M.C.* [1957] 1 W.L.R. 587. See pp. 233–234.

I

(*d*) *Child under* 16 *years of age: operation or other treatment not immediately necessary*

If a desirable, or even necessary, operation or other treatment can be deferred without immediate ill-consequence to the child, it should not be performed or given against the wishes of the parents. If, however, it is considered necessary in the child's interest, the position should be brought to the attention of the appropriate medical officer of the area health authority or of the appropriate officer of the local social services authority for the area in which the child lives, leaving it for that officer to consider what steps it might be desirable for his authority to take for the child's welfare, *e.g.*, the obtaining of a care and protection order. However, if the parents refuse the recommended treatment, the child, if in hospital, may properly be discharged, unless to do so would plainly and seriously be detrimental to his health.

It is convenient here to mention *Re D.* (*A Minor*) (*wardship: sterilisation*).[1] In this case a girl of twelve was suffering from Sotos Syndrome, a form of mental handicap which might have led her to give birth to an abnormal child. Both the mother and consultant paediatrician considered sterilisation to be desirable. This view was challenged by an educational psychologist on the staff of the local social services authority. She applied to make the girl a ward of court with a view to preventing the operation. Heilbron, J. held that since the right of a woman to reproduce is a basic human right and since the girl was likely to be able to appreciate the nature of the operation when she was eighteen, she should be a ward of court. She also held that a decision to carry out a sterilisation operation on a minor for non-therapeutic purposes was not solely within a doctor's clinical judgment. She also suggested that there is no regular machinery for reviewing proposed operations where the parents and the doctors are agreed.

(*e*) *Child in charge of someone other than a parent*

If a child who is not yet sixteen years of age is living with or at the time he needs treatment is in the care of an adult other than a parent, and parental consent is not obtainable or is not obtainable in time, the consent of such other person should, if practicable, be obtained. When a child has been committed to the custody and control of a local authority, the person to give any requisite consent is the proper officer of that authority. There seems no doubt that a guardian has power to consent and only very little doubt that a person with legal custody[2] also has such power. It is less clear that a person with mere actual custody[3] has the power since he apparently only has the duties of the

---

[1] [1976] Fam. 185; [1976] 1 All E.R. 326.
[2] Defined in s. 86 of the 1975 Children Act.   [3] Defined in s. 87 of the 1975 Children Act.

legal custodian without the rights. Nevertheless such a consent would be useful evidence of the desirability of the treatment.

(f) Forms of consent

For the Form of Consent to treatment at the present time recommended by the Department of Health and Social Security for use in the case of children under 16 years of age, reference should be made to Appendix E.[1] For use in the case of a child suffering from a condition, such as severe burns or congenital abnormality, in respect of which more than one operation may be necessary and a second or subsequent operation have to be performed at short notice, an appropriately modified form is recommended by the Medical Defence Union.[2]

(g) Blood test on child for purpose of matrimonial proceedings in which paternity of child questioned

The circumstances in which the court should permit a blood test on a young child for the purpose of matrimonial proceedings in which the paternity of the child is in question were summarized and explained by Lord Reid in S. v. McC. and M. as follows:[3]

'The court ought to permit a blood test of a young child to be taken unless satisfied that it would be against the child's interest. I say a young child because as soon as a child is able to understand these matters it would generally be unwise to subject it to this operation against its will. The court must protect the child, but it is not really protecting the child to ban a blood test on some vague conjecture that it may turn out to be to its disadvantage; it may equally well turn out to be for its advantage or at least do it no harm.'

That the court may permit a blood test on a child does not place a doctor under any obligation to undertake the procedure, whether he be, say, a doctor on whose N.H.S. list the child is, or one working on the staff of a hospital where the child is an in-patient. Moreover, even if so requested by both 'parents' a doctor would be unwise to undertake a blood group test on a young child without a court order if he knew or had reason to suspect that matrimonial proceedings had been or were likely to be commenced. If he did, he could, almost unwittingly, find himself in contempt of court. There is, however, nothing to prevent a doctor at any time doing a blood test on a child for therapeutic reasons, whatever the state of relations might be at that time between the parties to the marriage of which the child was the ostensible offspring. But in that case, the blood group of the child should not be communicated to either of the 'parents' for use in matrimonial proceedings between them. Leaving aside matrimonial proceedings, there may be very good grounds for parents being made aware of the child's blood group.

What of performing a blood test on an older child? It having been

[1] See p. 765.   [2] See p. 766.   [3] [1972] A.C. 24, 45; [1970] 3 All E.R. 107.

so clearly stated by Lord Reid in *S.* v. *McC. and M.*[1] that it would generally be unwise to subject the child to such an operation against its will and, by inference, that the court would not very readily compel the child to submit to it against its will, it would plainly be wrong for a medical practitioner, even at the request of both parents, to make blood tests on the child against his will, otherwise than for therapeutic purposes. Nor should he do so, other than for therapeutic purposes, if the child appears to be acquiescing under parental pressure. Nor should an older child, though perfectly willing be subjected to a blood test in relation to matrimonial proceedings or possible proceedings, at the request of either or even both parents, since his interests should be under the protection of the court.[2]

4. Married Persons

As to refusal of consent by a spouse or relative in case of emergency, the patient being unable to make a decision for himself, reference should be made to p. 191. In this part of the chapter are dealt with only those problems specially concerning married persons as such.

(a) *Married women — operative treatment on medical grounds*

A married woman[3] has the right to decide for herself whether or not to undergo operative or other treatment which may be advised on medical grounds. This applies no less to gynaecological operations,[4] including therapeutic abortion,[5] than to any other medical or surgical procedure.

It follows that what is necessary for preserving a woman's life or health need not, and should not, be withheld because her husband refuses his consent. The fear that he might have an independent claim for damages against the surgeon or the hospital because an operation on his wife, performed on competent medical advice, seems entirely without foundation. Certainly there is no English case which upholds the husband's veto. It is, however, most important that the woman should herself understand both the effect of the operation and equally the consequences of not having it, so that she may not afterwards be able to allege that her consent was given under a misapprehension

---

[1] [1972] A.C. 24, 45; [1970] All E.R. 107.

[2] It must be remembered that if a medical practitioner does undertake a blood test on a child, he may be called to give evidence about it in any subsequent matrimonial proceedings. Also, had he been a party to making a blood test, in circumstances when it ought not to have been done without an order of the court, he might be open to criticism and, had he acted knowingly, possibly to contempt proceedings.

[3] What follows also applies to treatment on husbands. The particular gender is adopted in the text merely to confront the ancient out-moded conception that somehow wives are a chattel of their husbands.

[4] See p. 203.

[5] Therapeutic abortion may now be carried out only in accordance with the provisions of the Abortion Act 1967, as to which see p. 210. The Act does not alter the position as regards consent of the patient.

induced by the surgeon. This is particularly important to bear in mind because some patients may have religious scruples.

The gravest complication that one can imagine is in the case of a young married woman who has not had sexual intercourse with her husband up to the time when an operation resulting in sexual incapacity is performed. Such incapacity might possibly afford grounds for a decree of nullity. This would not seem to impose any legal responsibility on the surgeon, but in view of its grave effect on the woman's position should not be overlooked. On this account, an informal explanation to the husband *with the patient's consent*, may be useful.

The position may be summed up in the statement that if a suitably qualified registered medical practitioner exercising a reasonable degree of care and skill advises a married woman to have an operation on medical grounds, the woman's own consent to that operation is all that is necessary even though it is a gynaecological operation which may result in sterility or hinder sexual intercourse. If, however, such advice were given negligently, the operation being unnecessary, then the husband, as well as the wife, might well have a cause of action. Nor, seemingly, would the position be any different had the husband's consent been obtained, were it shown that the advice that the operation was necessary or desirable had been given negligently. But although in respect of some gynaecological operations it may be desirable to seek the husband's understanding co-operation whenever, with the consent of the patient, the position can be explained to him, a surgeon in charge of a patient who refused to operate solely because the husband's consent was not forthcoming might be in a difficult predicament professionally if the woman died as a result. Further, he might be liable in damages if he had failed for such reason to give the appropriate treatment and she had either died or suffered ill-health, disability or pain in consequence.[1]

(b) Married persons — operations on generative organs

It was said *obiter* in *Bravery* v. *Bravery*[2] that an operation for sterilisation should not be performed on the one spouse — in that case the husband — without the consent of the other. Not only is that opinion not binding but it must be appreciated that in the case quoted the operation was not medically necessary. It would seem, however, that any operation or procedure on either spouse without medical need (*e.g.*, on eugenic or social grounds) without the consent of the other spouse, being an operation or procedure which took away the capacity for procreation or child-bearing, or even suspended such capacity, might, but by no means certainly, lay the medical practitioner open to

---

[1] See also p. 189 as to consent to an operation for the removal of male organs and the fashioning of an artificial vagina, this for the sake of the patient's mental health.
[2] [1954] 1 W.L.R. 1169.

action by an aggrieved spouse. Plainly therefore where the operation is medically necessary *Bravery* is of little guidance. Where it is not medically necessary but is *e.g.* desirable on social grounds, it is suggested that attitudes have changed so much in the last twenty years that the *obiter dicta* there can be ignored. Consent from the other spouse may be required for a surgical operation (even a minor one) which either permanently or possibly permanently takes away the capacity for child-bearing or procreation. It is most dubious if it is required for any other medical procedures, *e.g.*, the prescription of an oral contraceptive or the fitting of an intra-uterine contraceptive device. It is plain however that in the case of any reversible process, *e.g.*, a husband cannot by withdrawing his 'consent' compel a doctor to restore the fertility.[1]

5. Mentally Disordered Patients

The Mental Health Act 1959 offers no guidance on who should give consent to an operation on a mentally disordered patient detained in hospital under the provisions of that Act, but it appears to be a common assumption[2] that — if the patient is unfit to give consent — the area Health Authority, acting through an appropriate officer, is the proper person to give or withhold consent to any operation on the patient, since it is the Authority which is authorised to detain the patient and, therefore, has custody of him. And it is suggested that for operative or other treatment for the patient's mental disorder the appropriate officer to act for the Authority would be the 'responsible medical officer', *i.e.*, the medical practitioner in charge of the treatment of the patient, though it may be more appropriate that the consent should be given on behalf of the Authority by an administrative officer if the proposed operation is for some physical condition.

There are, however, some grounds for suggesting that the proper person to give consent to an operation would be the patient's nearest relative, since, subject to the provisions of the Act and except in the case of patients subject to a hospital order as a result of criminal proceedings, or transferred from prison, *etc.*, that relative ordinarily has the right to discharge the patient.[3] But the fact that the nearest relative has to give seventy-two hours notice of discharge; that his power is not absolute; and that he might, if circumstances justified, be defeated by a barring report by the responsible medical officer under s. 48; or be

---

[1] See Annual Report of the M.D.U. 1971 at p. 67 where a husband was in prison and wanted an I.V.C.D. removed from his wife. The advice given that to do this without the consent of the wife would be an assault is undoubtedly right.

[2] The propositions set out in this section of the chapter differ from those I have offered in my article 'The Right of the Mental Patient to his Psychosis' [1976] M.L.R., p. 15. There I argued that a mental patient was no different in law from any other patient and that apart from the doctor's higher duties of care for his patients, particularly in an urgent situation, there was no power to impose treatment. Dr Speller's view is left in the text because it is not at this stage possible to say it is wrong.

[3] Ss. 47 (2); 48.

deprived of his powers by the county court under s. 52, modifies his position. Common sense suggests, however, that if the nearest relative is reasonably co-operative it is desirable to obtain his consent to any operation on the patient, the operation not being a matter of urgency to save the patient's life or to prevent pain and suffering.

But what of the case of the patient whom it is necessary to detain — possibly for the safety of others, as in the case of some patients suffering from *psychopathic disorders*[1] — and yet who, apart from his particular mental twist, is of full understanding and is capable of making a decision for himself? In such cases, if the responsible medical officer is satisfied that the patient is volitional and of a sufficient understanding, the patient himself could give consent. This might be the case not only with many psychopaths but also with some patients suffering from mental illness and even — though more doubtfully — with some *sub-normal*[1] patients.[2] However, the question appears largely academic for if an operation performed on such a patient with his consent were one which, in the patient's interests, ought to have been performed, Dr Speller could see no possibility of an action for trespass to the person, subsequently brought against the hospital authority or against any member of its staff on the ground that the patient had not been mentally capable of exercising the necessary judgment when he purported to give consent, being successful.[3]

A more difficult situation arises if a patient liable to detention in hospital is advised to have an operation for a physical condition and refuses to do so, even though the operation is regarded as necessary to save his life. If the patient's understanding and judgment were very seriously impaired by his mental disorder there would presumably be grounds for carrying out the operation without his consent, were it reasonably practicable to do so. But if the patient were volitional, although suffering from some mental disorder justifying his detention, one would hesitate to say that he ought to be deprived of the choice he would have had, had he not been so detained.

Patients informally admitted to hospital for treatment for mental disorder also raise problems, since not all 'informal' patients are volitional, for even a *severely sub-normal* patient[4] who is virtually without understanding, and possibly no better than a common law idiot,[5] may be admitted informally unless he objects. Consequently, the class of 'informal' patients will cover all types of mentally disordered patient from those with slight mental illness and fully volitional to what

[1] For definition see s. 4.
[2] For a discussion of forms recommended and advice given by the Medical Defence Union in the 1971 edition of 'Consent to Treatment', including forms and advice relating to mentally disordered patients, see Appendix E, page 765.
[3] The present editor whilst tending to agree, does so with less emphasis.   [4] S. 4.
[5] 'An idiot is a person who from birth has had no mind' (*R.* v *F.* (1910), 74 J.P. 384, quoted in footnote in Halsbury's Laws of England, 3rd Edition, vol. 10, p. 749).

would formerly have been called idiots. All that can be done is to obtain the patient's consent in the case of patients who are in any degree volitional and of sufficient understanding and, for the rest, do whatever is considered for the good of the patient so long as he does not object. It may be in some cases that the necessary procedure should be gone through to make an uncooperative patient liable to detention, so that someone else may have the right to give consent for him. But even Dr Speller was not happy with that solution if the patient were volitional. Nor is it necessarily a practicable solution in all cases, since the patient's cooperation or at least his acquiescence may be vital to the success of the treatment.

If a patient is not liable to detention in hospital but is under guardianship under the Mental Health Act 1959, it is the patient's guardian who should give consent to any operation, he having all such powers in relation to the patient as would be exercisable by him in relation to the patient if he were the father of the patient and the patient were under the age of fourteen years.[1] Should the guardian not act in the best interests of the patient, as by refusing to consent to an operation which ought to be performed, it is possible that he might be removed under s. 52 (3) of the Act. But the necessary procedure in the county court might take too long to be effective and, in those circumstances, if an urgent operation were carried out without consent, the hospital and its staff would incur no liability.[2] If a mentally disordered patient under guardianship needed hospital treatment for his mental disorder, it is likely that he would be transferred to hospital under the provisions of s. 41 (2) of the Mental Health Act 1959, this bringing the guardianship to an end.[3] Then, the position as regards consent to treatment would be as for any other patient liable to detention.

If a mentally disordered person, not being under guardianship, nor liable to detention in hospital as a mentally disordered person, is sent to hospital for treatment for a physical illness, his consent to any operation — for what it is worth — should be obtained. In so far as the patient may be unable to give a valid consent and needs the proposed treatment, the hospital and its staff, doing what is reasonably necessary, may be regarded as acting as agents of necessity. This, in the last analysis, may well be the position in respect of all others — except those under guardianship — who cannot themselves give a valid consent.

6. Artificial Insemination

There have by now undoubtedly been a fair number of cases of artificial insemination, although, understandably, little is heard of

[1] S. 34.   [2] Cf. p. 196 *et seq.*, 'Minors'.
[3] But he could thereafter, by transfer, again be placed under guardianship under the provisions of the Act.

them.[1] Although authority is lacking it is obvious that artificial insemination from a donor other than the woman's husband may have serious legal implications for the woman concerned, for the donor of semen, for any doctor assisting and, above all, for the possible offspring, and for relatives whose material expectations might be prejudiced by the arrival of an apparently legitimate but, in fact, illegitimate child.[2]

This book is not concerned with the moral aspects of the practice of artificial insemination, but only to examine the legal implications. Dr Speller considered the undertaking of such procedure on any 'patient' by members of the staff on hospital premises is most inadvisable except in the case of a married woman when the donor is her own husband,[3] the adoption of the procedure then being simply to overcome some physical disability in either man or woman not amounting to sterility. The objection to the hospital being a consenting party in other cases is that whenever the husband is not the donor the child must, in the present state of the law, be illegitimate and, furthermore, there is as yet no clear guidance as to whether the procedure amounts to fornication or adultery, as the case may be, nor — if it does — what might be the legal liability of the hospital authority or any other party assisting in the transaction. No hospital authority should knowingly be a party to a practice of such doubtful validity and possibly grave legal consequences.

The case of the husband as donor to his own wife as mentioned above is quite straightforward. Difficulties arise only when the donor is not the woman's husband, the woman being either single or married to someone other than the donor. The responsibility of the doctor may also vary according as to whether he actually undertakes responsibility for finding a donor who remains anonymous to the donee, or whether he merely acts as an intermediary for donation by a man known to the woman.

It is but an elementary precaution that no doctor should be a party to arranging for artificial insemination of a married woman from a third party without the consent of her husband. Authority is completely lacking as to whether the husband would have good grounds for divorce and equally as to whether the doctor concerned might be cited in the proceedings, but the practice of artificial insemination seems such an obvious infringement of marital rights that it is difficult to imagine that the courts would not aid the husband. Moreover, guidance appears to be equally lacking as to whether the doctor acting as agent would be guilty of serious professional misconduct.

If the husband consents and the circumstances are such that it would

---

[1] See *Status of the A.I.D. Child* D. J. Cusine [1977] S.L.T. 161 and *The Legal Status of the A.I.D. Child in Australia* M. Mayo (1977) 50 A.L.J. 562.
[2] But see now footnote 2 on p. 208.
[3] When the husband is donor the procedure is usually referred to as 'A.I.H.': when the donor is a third party, 'A.I.D.'.

seem reasonable for a doctor to help with artificial insemination of the wife from a donor (*e.g.*, where the wife cannot have a child by her husband), one would not expect that the doctor would run any risk of disciplinary proceedings by the General Medical Council for giving his aid. It is, however, important that before he acts he should see that both the husband and wife understand what is involved. They should be told plainly that in law any child born as a result of the procedure of artificial insemination with a third-party donor will be illegitimate and that it should be registered as such. But they may also be told of the possibilities of legal adoption of the child so born to the wife and encouraged to consult their solicitor before proceeding with the project. If the husband — with full knowledge of the facts — gives his consent, the doctor's responsibility is at an end.

It has, however, sometimes been suggested that the procedure might be secret and the husband and wife, without any guidance from doctor or solicitor, left to register the child as their own when born. The danger of this, apart from the fact that such false registration would be an offence, lies in the possibility of wrongful disturbance of rights of succession to titles of honour or to any right to property, whether on intestacy, or under a will or settlement.[1] No assurance that the husband and wife can give, even in the utmost good faith, can afford a complete guarantee that connivance in false registration would not deprive someone else of his rights.

A further, yet unresolved, legal problem arises if the donor is married. Does the fact that he, by being a donor, becomes the father of the child of a woman other than his wife give his wife good grounds for divorce? The question is merely academic if the donor and his wife have no knowledge of the donee or even as to whether the semen given has been used at all, but it may be a very practical one if the circumstances are such that the donor's name is known in relation to a particular donee so that he can be said to be the father of her child.

Marriage within the prohibited degrees, or even incest, might also occur in the next generation as a result of insemination of a woman from an unknown donor or from a donor whose identity was not disclosed to the resultant child, if any.[2]

It may here be suggested that a medical practitioner who assists with an artificial insemination from a donor should keep a careful record of the occasion or occasions and of the identity of the donor or donors as his evidence might be of vital importance, maybe after a long interval of time.

[1] The position may have been made more rather than less complicated by the liberalising provisions of Part II of the Family Law Reform Act 1969 (ss. 14 to 19) which, for purposes of inheritance, has — for the most part — put an illegitimate child on the same footing as a legitimate child of his parents, whether or not they marry or could marry.

[2] This statement is made on the assumption that, in law, the donor would be regarded as the child's father

7. Illegal Operations

No examination of the subject of consents to operations would be complete without some reference to operations which are in themselves illegal, this whether or not the consent of the patient or of someone on his behalf has been obtained. There are also fields in which operative or other treatment is subject to statutory limitations and conditions, and this again even though consent may have been obtained, *viz.*, medical termination of pregnancy and treatment of drug addiction. Here, however, we shall be considering illegal operations, only reserving the other two matters for succeeding sections of the chapter.

(a) *Abortion outside the provisions of the Abortion Act* 1967

Abortion or attempted abortion, except so far as permitted by the Abortion Act 1967, remains an offence under ss. 58 and 59 of the Offences against the Person Act 1861 and, in the case of viable foetus, under the Infant Life (Preservation) Act 1929, it being expressly provided in s. 5 (2) of the Act of 1967 that, for the purposes of the law relating to abortion,[1] anything done with intent to procure the miscarriage of a woman is unlawfully done unless authorised by s. 1 of the Act. It has been held that the penalties imposed by a court in respect of an abortion, illegal even under the 1967 Act, should be greater than those imposed before it.[2]

(b) *Other operations without medical need*

Any operation done without medical need, which necessarily resulted in serious injury to the person on whom it was performed, or had more than a minimal probability of doing so, could lay the person who performed it open to the risk of prosecution, the consent of the person injured ordinarily being no defence in such circumstances. Leaving aside medical termination of pregnancy, the only procedures likely to be carried out by a registered medical practitioner, is sterilisation of a patient of either sex otherwise than on medical grounds, the sterilisation being undertaken at the request of the person sterilised and cosmetic surgery.

(c) *Tattooing of minors*

It is now lawful to tattoo a person under the age of 18 only if the tattoo is performed for medical reasons by a duly qualified medical practitioner or by a person working under his directions.[3]

[1] *the law relating to abortion* here means ss. 58 and 59 of the Offences against the Person Act 1861 and any rule of law relating to the procurement of abortion (Abortion Act 1967, s 6)
[2] *R.* v. *Scrimaglia and Young* (1971) 55 Cr. App. R. 280.
[3] Tattooing of Minors Act 1969, s. 1.

8. Medical Termination of Pregnancy

(a) Abortion Act 1967

A pregnancy may only be lawfully terminated, and only by a registered medical practitioner, in accordance with the provisions of the Abortion Act 1967. The provisions of the Act are as follows.[1]

Medical Termination of Pregnancy

1.—(1) Subject to the provisions of this section, a person shall not be guilty of an offence under the law relating to abortion[2] when a pregnancy is terminated by a registered medical practitioner if two registered medical practitioners are of the opinion, formed in good faith[3] —

(a) that the continuance of the pregnancy would involve risk to the life of the pregnant woman, or of injury to the physical or mental health of the pregnant woman or any existing children of her family, greater than if the pregnancy were terminated; or

(b) that there is a substantial risk that if the child were born it would suffer from such physical or mental abnormalities as to be seriously handicapped.

(2) In determining whether the continuance of a pregnancy would involve such risk of injury to health is mentioned in paragraph (a) of subsection (1) of this section, account may be taken of the pregnant woman's actual or reasonably foreseeable environment.

(3) Except as provided by subsection (4) of this section, any treatment for the termination of pregnancy must be carried out in a hospital vested in the Minister of Health or the Secretary of State[4] under the National Health Service Acts, or in a place for the time being approved for the purposes of this section[5] by the said Minister or the Secretary of State.

Termination of Pregnancy in Emergency

1.—(4) Subsection (3) of this section, and so much of subsection (1) as relates to the opinion of two registered medical practitioners, shall not apply to the termination of a pregnancy by a registered medical practitioner in a case where he is of the opinion, formed in good faith, that the termination is immediately necessary to save the life or to prevent grave permanent injury to the physical or mental health of the pregnant woman.

---

[1] It is to be noted that since, by s. 7 of the Act, the provisions of the Infant Life (Preservation) Act 1929 are preserved, the extended grounds on which abortion is permitted under s. 1 (1) do not apply in the case of a viable foetus, *i.e.* a foetus capable of being born alive. In such case, the foetus may be destroyed only if it is necessary to do so to preserve the life of the pregnant woman and for no other purpose. For the purposes of the 1929 Act a foetus is *prima facie* viable after the twenty-eighth week of pregnancy.

[2] For the meaning of *law relating to abortion*. By s. 6 this means 'ss. 58 and 59 of the Offences against the Person Act 1861, and any rule relating to the procurement of abortion'.

[3] Although evidence of professional practices and medical probabilities is relevant, the question as to whether a doctor has acted in good faith is for the jury to decide on the totality of the evidence. *R.* v. *Smith* [1973] 1 W.L.R. 1510.

[4] 'Secretary of State' here means the Secretary of State for Scotland in respect of termination of pregnancy in Scotland. The duties of the Minister of Health are now performed by the Secretary of State for Social Services and, for Wales and Monmouthshire by the Secretary of State for Wales.

[5] *E.g.* Service hospitals and some nursing homes. Lists of approved places are supplied to local Social Services authorities and Area Health Authorities.

Notification

2.—(1) The Minister of Health in respect of England and Wales,[1] and the Secretary of State in respect of Scotland, shall by statutory instrument make regulations[2] to provide —

(*a*) for requiring any such opinion as is referred to in section 1 of this Act to be certified by the practitioners or practitioner concerned in such form and at such time as may be prescribed by the regulations, and for requiring the preservation and disposal of certificates made for the purposes of the regulations;

(*b*) for requiring any registered medical practitioner who terminates a pregnancy to give notice of the termination and such other information relating to the termination as may be so prescribed;

(*c*) for prohibiting the disclosure, except to such persons or for such purposes as may be so prescribed, of notices given or information furnished pursuant to the regulations.

(2) The information furnished in pursuance of regulations made by virtue of paragraph (*b*) of subsection (1) of this section shall be notified solely to the Chief Medical Officer of the *Department of Health and Social Security, or of the Welsh Office or of the Scottish Home and Health Department*[3] respectively.

(3) Any person who wilfully contravenes or wilfully fails to comply with the requirements of regulations under subsection (1) of this section shall be liable on summary conviction to a fine not exceeding one hundred pounds.

Application of Act to Visiting Forces, etc.

3.—(1) In relation to the termination of a pregnancy in a case where the following conditions are satisfied, that is to say —

(*a*) the treatment for termination of the pregnancy was carried out in a hospital controlled by the proper authorities of a body to which this section applies; and

(*b*) the pregnant woman had at the time of the treatment a relevant association with that body; and

(*c*) the treatment was carried out by a registered medical practitioner or a person who at the time of the treatment was a member of that body appointed as a medical practitioner for that body by the proper authorities of that body,

this Act shall have effect as if any reference in section 1 to a registered medical practitioner and to a hospital vested in a Minister under the National Health Service Acts included respectively a reference to such a person as is mentioned in paragraph (*c*) of this subsection and to a hospital controlled as aforesaid, and as if section 2 were omitted.

(2) The bodies to which this section applies are any force which is a visiting force within the meaning of any of the provisions of Part I of the Visiting Forces Act 1952 and any headquarters within the meaning of the Schedule to the International Headquarters and Defence Organisations Act 1964; and for the purposes of this section —

(*a*) a woman shall be treated as having a relevant association at any time with a body to which this section applies if at that time —

(i) in the case of such a force as aforesaid, she had a relevant association within the meaning of the said Part I with the force; and

[1] *See* note 4 on p. 210.
[2] The text of the Abortion Regulations 1968 S.I. No. 390 are set out on pp. 213–214.
[3] Words in italics substituted by the Transfer of Functions (Wales) Order 1969.

        (ii) in the case of such a headquarters as aforesaid, she was a member of the headquarters or a dependant within the meaning of the Schedule aforesaid of such a member; and

  (b) any reference to a member of a body to which this section applies shall be construed —

        (i) in the case of such a force as aforesaid, as a reference to a member of or of a civilian component of that force within the meaning of the said Part I; and

        (ii) in the case of such a headquarters as aforesaid, as a reference to a member of that headquarters within the meaning of the Schedule aforesaid.

Conscientious Objection to Participation in Treatment

4.—(1) Subject to subsection (2) of this section, no person shall be under any duty, whether by contract or by any statutory or other legal requirement, to participate in any treatment authorised by this Act to which he has a conscientious objection:

Provided that in any legal proceedings the burden of proof of conscientious objection shall rest on the person claiming to rely on it.

(2) Nothing in subsection (1) of this section shall affect any duty to participate in treatment which is necessary to save the life or to prevent grave permanent injury to the physical or mental health of a pregnant woman.

It will be appreciated that s. 4 applies to anyone else, *e.g.*, a nurse or a theatre attendant, who may have a conscientious objection to participation in a termination of pregnancy, no less than to a medical practitioner.

Section 4 continues:

(3) In any proceedings before a court in Scotland, a statement on oath by any person to the effect that he has a conscientious objection to participating in any treatment authorised by this Act shall be sufficient evidence for the purpose of discharging the burden of proof imposed upon him by subsection (1) of this section.

Supplementary Provisions

5.—(1) Nothing in this Act shall affect the provisions of the Infant Life (Preservation) Act 1929 (protecting the life of the viable foetus).

This has the effect of imposing the '28 week rule' — *i.e.* an abortion may only be carried out within the first 28 weeks of a pregnancy. The Act provides that it is an offence to destroy the life of a child capable of being born alive and that after the twenty-eighth week of the pregnancy it shall *prima facie* be presumed that the child was capable of being born. The Act does not apply where the foetus was destroyed in good faith for the purpose only of preserving the life of the mother.

Section 5 continues:

(2) For the purposes of the law relating to abortion, anything done with intent to procure the miscarriage of a woman is unlawfully done unless authorised by section 1 of this Act.

(b) Abortion Regulations 1968

The *Abortion Regulations 1968* provide as follows:

Certificate of Opinion

3.—(1) Any opinion to which section 1 of the Act refers shall be certified in the appropriate form set out in Schedule 1 to these regulations.[1]

(2) Any certificate of an opinion referred to in section 1 (1) of the Act shall be given before the commencement of the treatment for the termination of the pregnancy to which it relates.

(3) Any certificate of an opinion referred to in section 1 (4) of the Act shall be given before the commencement of the treatment for the termination of the pregnancy to which it relates or, if that is not reasonably practicable, not later than 24 hours after such termination.

(4) Any such certificate as is referred to in paragraphs (2) and (3) of this regulation shall be preserved by the practitioner who terminated the pregnancy to which it relates for a period of three years beginning with the date of such termination and may then be destroyed.

Notice of Termination of Pregnancy and Information Relating Thereto

4.—(1) Any practitioner who terminates a pregnancy shall within 7 days of the termination give to the Chief Medical Officer of the Ministry of Health[2] notice thereof and the other information relating to the termination in the form set out in Schedule 2[3] to these regulations.

(2) Any such notice and information shall be sent in a sealed envelope to the Chief Medical Officer, Ministry of Health, Alexander Fleming House, Elephant and Castle, London, S.E.1.

Restriction on Disclosure of Information

5. A notice given or any information furnished to the Chief Medical Officer in pursuance of these regulations shall not be disclosed except that disclosure may be made —

(a) for the purposes of carrying out their duties,
    (i) to an officer of the Ministry of Health[2] authorised by the Chief Medical Officer of that Ministry, or
    (ii) to the Registrar General or a member of his staff authorised by him; or
(b) for the purposes of carrying out his duties in relation to offences against the Act or the law relating to abortion, to the Director of Public Prosecutions or a member of his staff authorised by him; or
(c) for the purposes of investigating whether an offence has been committed against the Act or the law relating to abortion, to a police officer not below the rank of superintendent or a person authorised by him; or
(d) for the purposes of criminal proceedings which have begun; or
(e) for the purposes of bona fide scientific research; or
(f) to the practitioner who terminated the pregnancy; or
(g) to a practitioner, with the consent in writing of the woman whose pregnancy was terminated.

[1] Schedules not here reproduced.
[2] Now Department of Health and Social Security or, for Wales and Monmouthshire the Welsh Office (see Abortion (Amendment) Regulations S.I. 1969 No. 636.)
[3] See footnote 1.

(c) Assisting suspected illegal abortion

A medical practitioner (e.g., an anaesthetist or a houseman) who, in hospital, cooperated with another practitioner who was performing an unlawful abortion or other illegal operation, would ordinarily also be guilty of an offence unless he satisfied the court that he had had no knowledge of the illegality, the circumstances being such that the suspicions of a reasonable man in his position would not have been aroused. But if the circumstances were such that his suspicions ought to have been aroused, he would not escape liability if it appeared that he had deliberately shut his eyes to what was going on. The position of a nurse or midwife assisting in an illegal operation is substantially the same as that of a medical practitioner. So also is the position of non-medical staff although probably the burden on them of showing they acted reasonably is probably easier.

Should a nurse or midwife assisting become suspicious of the legality of an abortion only after the operation has been started, it may be suggested that she is entitled to continue to assist in order to safeguard the life of the patient. But the choice could be a grave one since, by continuing to help, she would inevitably be open to *some* suspicion of being an accomplice. A nurse so involved should be careful not to make to any third party any statement about the practitioner which she cannot fully substantiate since it might easily be defamatory. But, of course she would be allowed to make a statement to the police or to her superiors, e.g., a matron or supervising midwife or member of her Health Authority, to both seek advice and guidance and provide some evidence to rebutt any suspicion. Such a statement would, if made in good faith, be privileged under the general law of defamation.

A nurse or midwife should in no circumstances procure a miscarriage nor even assist in procuring a miscarriage, except when acting as an assistant to a registered medical practitioner in circumstances apparently within the provisions of the Abortion Act 1967 and having no reason to doubt the legality of the practitioner's intentions. Moreover, neither a medical practitioner nor a nurse or midwife should tell a woman desiring to have an abortion what drug or appliance she might use; still less procure for her any such drug or appliance. To do so would, at best, involve risk of erasure from the register or loss of certificate and, at worst, a criminal charge. The only proper course for a nurse or midwife consulted by a woman desiring an abortion is to refer her to a doctor for advice.

9. Drug Addicts

(a) Generally

In this section of the chapter will be noted the provisions of the Misuse of Drugs Act 1971 and of the Misuse of Drugs (Notification of

and Supply to Addicts) Regulations 1973[1] made thereunder concerning the obligation of doctors[2] to give to the Chief Medical Officer of the Home Office particulars of any drug addicts they attend and as restricting the authority to treat certain addicts to doctors[2] licensed for the purpose by the Home Secretary. The remaining provisions of the Act, which are designed to tighten up control of drugs of addiction and of other dangerous drugs are dealt with, so far as relevant, in Chapter 12. There is power to make regulations and under s. 22 (c) to make them applicable to agents of the Crown.
them applicable to agents of the Crown.

The relevant part of s.10 of the Act reads as follows:

10.—(1) Subject to the provisions of this Act, the Secretary of State may by regulations make such provisions as appears to him necessary or expedient for preventing the misuse of controlled drugs.

(2) Without prejudice to the generality of subsection (1) above, regulations under this section may in particular make provision —

(*h*) for requiring any doctor who attends a person who he considers, or has reasonable grounds to suspect, is addicted (within the meaning of the regulations) to controlled drugs of any description to furnish to the prescribed authority such particulars with respect to that person as may be prescribed.

(*i*) for prohibiting any doctor from administering, supplying and authorising the administration and supply to persons so addicted, and from prescribing for such persons, such controlled drugs as may be prescribed, except under and in accordance with the terms of a licence issued by the Secretary of State in pursuance of the regulations.

The word *addicted* not being defined in the Act it must be read in context as bearing the meaning ordinarily given to it when used by the medical profession. For the purposes of the Misuse of Drugs (Notification of and Supply to Addicts) Regulations 1973 its application has been more precisely limited in Reg. 2 (2) reading as follows:

2.—(2) For the purposes of these Regulations, a person shall be regarded as being addicted to a drug if, and only if, he has as a result of repeated administration become so dependent upon the drug that he has an overpowering desire for the administration of it to be continued.

By Reg. 2 (1) the expression *drug* in the Regulations means a controlled drug specified in the Schedule thereto, *viz.*, cocaine, dextromoramide, diamorphine, dipipanone, hydrocodone, hydromorphone,

---

[1] S.I. 1973 No. 799.

[2] The expression *doctor*, not *medical practitioner*, is used in the Act and Regulations, being defined in s. 37 (1) of the Act as meaning 'a fully registered person within the meaning of the Medical Acts 1956 to 1969. Hence, a *medical practitioner* who is not such a fully registered person, has no authority under the Act or regulations in respect of controlled drugs in so far as it depends on his being a *doctor* within the meaning of the Act. Even where, as in Reg. 9 of the Misuse of Drugs Regulations 1973, the expression used is *practitioner*, that is no help since by s. 37 (1) of the Act, *practitioner* means 'a doctor, dentist, veterinary practitioner . . .', *i.e.* in the case of a doctor, a doctor as defined in the Act.

levorphanol, methadone, morphine, opium, oxycodone, pethidine, phenazocine, piritramide. Also, any stereoisomeric form of any of the foregoing substances, not being dextrorphan.

(b) *Notification of addicts*

Reg. 3 of the 1973 Regulations provides as follows:

3.—(1) Subject to paragraph (2) of this Regulation, any doctor who attends a person who he considers, or has reasonable grounds to suspect, is addicted to any drug[1] shall, within seven days of the attendance, furnish in writing to the Chief Medical Officer at the Home Office such of the following particulars with respect to that person as are known to the doctor, that is to say, the name, address, sex, date of birth and national health service number of that person, the date of the attendance and the name of the drug or drugs concerned.

(2) It shall not be necessary for a doctor who attends a person to comply with the provisions of paragraph (1) of this Regulation in respect of that person if —

(a) the doctor is of the opinion, formed in good faith, that the continued administration of the drug or drugs concerned is required for the purpose of treating organic disease[2] or injury; or

(b) the particulars which, apart from this paragraph, would have been required under those provisions to be furnished have, during the period of twelve months ending with the date of the attendance, been furnished in compliance with those provisions —

  (i) by the doctor; or
  (ii) if the doctor is a partner in or employed by a firm of general practitioners, by a doctor who is a partner in or employed by that firm; or
  (iii) if the attendance is on behalf of another doctor, whether for payment or otherwise, by that doctor; or
  (iv) if the attendance is at a hospital,[3] by a doctor on the staff of that hospital.

A doctor on the staff of a hospital attends a person each time he sees him as a patient, whether as an in-patient or as an out-patient and so, should he consider a patient he attends on any particular occasion to be a drug addict or has reasonable grounds for suspicion that he is, the practitioner must within seven days notify the Home Office unless he or some other member of the medical staff of the hospital has notified the Home Office within the previous twelve months ending with the date of attendance and unless the drug of addiction is being medically administered or prescribed by way of treatment of organic

---

[1] See p. 215 above and Reg. 2 (2) and Sch. to Regs. for meaning of *drug*.

[2] The expression *treating organic disease or injury* is wider in scope than *relieving pain due to organic disease or injury*, that used in the Dangerous Drugs (Notification of Addicts) Regulations 1968, S.I. No. 136, replaced by the 1973 Regulations. Nor does the expression *treating organic disease or injury* exclude treatment of mental disorder, provided that that disorder be attributable to organic disease or injury, the brain being an organ.

[3] The expression *hospital*, (a) in respect of England and Wales, now has the same meaning as in the National Health Service Acts and includes a nursing home and mental nursing home within the meaning of the Nursing Homes Act 1975 and a special hospital within the meaning of the 1977 Act; (b) and as respects Scotland, see Reg. 2 (1).

disease or injury. If, howevêr, the doctor has no reasonable grounds for suspicion at the time he attends him as an out-patient that a person is a drug addict but is given grounds thereafter he is under no obligation to notify the Home Office until he next attends the patient.[1] Even in hospital, the obligation of notification of drug addiction is still laid personally on the medical practitioner who attends the patient, and this whether he be a physician or a surgeon and whether a house officer or a consultant or in any of the grades between those two extremes in the hospital hierarchy, always provided he be a doctor as defined in the Misuse of Drugs Act 1971, *i.e.*, 'a fully registered person within the meaning of the Medical Acts 1956 to 1969'. Consequently, a junior doctor who on any occasion sees a patient and considers or has reasonable grounds for suspicion that he is an addict, is not relieved of his personal responsibility for notifying the Home Office by reporting his opinion or grounds for suspicion to his senior.[2]

No standard form of notification having been prescribed, any notification to the Home Office may be given either by letter or in such other form as the doctor sending it thinks fit. It is, however, understood that in N.H.S. hospitals a standard form is generally in use.[3]

(c) Supply to addicts

The rules generally relating to the supply of controlled drugs by doctors[4] to patients, or by pharmacists on prescription, are to be found in the Misuse of Drugs Regulations 1973,[4] the administration and supply of the more dangerous drugs of addiction (cocaine and diamorphine and their salts and preparations containing them) by way of treatment of addiction being also subject to the provisions of Reg. 4 of the Misuse of Drugs (Notification of and Supply to Addicts) Regulations 1973, reading as follows:

4.—(1) Subject to paragraph (2) of this Regulation, a doctor shall not administer or supply to a person who he considers, or has reasonable grounds to suspect, is addicted to any drug,[5] or authorise the administration or supply to such a person of, any substance specified in paragraph (3) below, or prescribe for such a person any such substance, except —
(*a*) for the purpose of treating organic disease or injury; or

---

[1] This view was expressed by the Department of Health and Social Service in a circular to Hospital Authorities (H.M. (68) 6, para. 6) relating to the corresponding regulation under the now repealed Dangerous Drugs Acts. The circular added: 'In practice the practitioner would no doubt forward the notification as soon as he formed the opinion that the patient was addicted without waiting for a subsequent attendance.'

[2] In para. 9 of the circular referred to in footnote 6 the position was put thus, 'Each medical practitioner who considers or has reasonable grounds to suspect that a patient he is attending is addicted within the terms of the regulations comes under a liability to notify'. The following gloss is then added: 'Hospital medical staff below consultant rank would however normally inform the consultant responsible for the patient's treatment before notifying particulars of that patient.'

[3] See Circular H.M. (68) 6, para. 7.   [4] See pp. 159–167.

[5] *I.e.* any controlled drug specified in the schedule to the Regulations (Reg. 2 (1)). For list, see pp. 215–216.

(*b*) under and in accordance with the terms of a licence issued by the Secretary of State in pursuance of these Regulations.

(2) Paragraph (1) of this Regulation shall not apply to the administration or supply by a doctor of a substance specified in paragraph (3) below if the administration or supply is authorised by another doctor under and in accordance with the terms of a licence issued to him in pursuance of these Regulations.

(3) The substances referred to in paragraphs (1) and (2) above are —

(*a*) cocaine, its salts and any preparation or other product containing cocaine or its salts other than a preparation falling within paragraph 2 of Schedule 1 to the Misuse of Drugs Regulations 1973(**a**);

(*b*) diamorphine, its salts and any preparation or other product containing diamorphine or its salts.

(*d*) *Application of the Misuse of Drugs (Notification of and Supply to Addicts) Regulations 1973 to the Crown*

Regulation 5 provides as follows:

5. These Regulations and, in relation only to the requirements of these Regulations, sections 13 (1) and (3), 14, 16, 19 and 25 of and Schedule 4 to the Misuse of Drugs Act 1971 (which relate to their enforcement) shall apply to servants and agents of the Crown.

Hence, the regulations are binding on doctors and other staff of Service and prison hospitals and also of special hospitals under s. 4 of the National Health Service Act 1977 and on doctors otherwise acting as servants or agents of the Crown. They apply to the staff of hospitals, clinics, *etc.*, administered by health authorities on behalf of the Secretary of State under the provisions of the 1977 Act.

10. Use of Patients for Clinical Teaching or as Controls or otherwise for Research or as Donors of Organs

(*a*) Use of patients for clinical teaching

We are here concerned with the legal implications of the use of patients in connection with clinical teaching, in particular to examine when, and in what circumstances, such use of a patient might constitute a tort. To that end we have to consider the use of patients in connection with the clinical teaching of medical and dental students, as when a student takes a patient's history or makes a physical examination; or when a clinical teacher demonstrates on a patient, whether to a single student or to a group of students, large or small, whether in the ward, in the operating theatre or elsewhere and whether by closed circuit television or video-tape or by the use of still photographs. It covers also the similar use of patients in postgraduate courses for medical practitioners, including, *inter alia*, refresher courses for general practitioners. Equally to be included is the essentially similar use of patients in connection with the clinical teaching of student and pupil nurses, pupil midwives and of those training for other paramedical professions, as well as in post-qualification courses for members of such professions. But for our present purpose the actual treatment of a patient by a medical student or by a medical practitioner being trained in a particular speciality, or by a student nurse, a pupil midwife or other paramedical student, is not to be regarded as the use of a patient for clinical teaching.[1] Equally excluded is the use of a patient for purposes of research, as for example, by using him as a control or — otherwise than primarily in his own interest — subjecting him to a method of treatment still in its experimental stage.[2]

Whether if use were made of a patient in connection with clinical teaching without his consent that would constitute a tort depends on what was actually done. If it were something, such as medical examination by a student, which involved interference with the patient's body otherwise than in the ordinary course of treatment, done without consent it would be actionable as trespass to the person. So, too, would the use of a patient for demonstration purposes if it involved touching him in any way.[3] Hence it is important that no patient should be used in connection with clinical teaching without his consent, this as a safeguard not only against the possibility of a claim for trespass to the person but also against a claim on any other ground, being a claim which could not have been made had consent been obtained.[4]

But although, if a patient is to be used for clinical teaching, it should be only with his consent,[5] that consent is sufficiently manifested by the patient's having not in any way indicated his unwillingness to be so used, always provided that, being aware that it was intended that he

[1] In so far as it is customary to use student grades, most notably student and pupil nurses, in the treatment of patients and for medical students to carry out procedures on them, e.g., when serving as dressers, their proper dealings with the patient by way of treatment are fairly covered if any necessary consent to treatment has been obtained. Such consent, whilst safeguarding the student from an action for trespass to the person would not protect him from a claim based on negligence. As to that and the vicarious liability of the Health (or Hospital) Authority, as well as the possibility of liability of the practitioner in charge of the treatment of the patient for negligent delegation, see Chapter 14.

[2] As to use of patients for research, etc., see pp. 219–220.

[3] If something for which the patient's consent was necessary were done without that consent but no harm resulted therefrom, the probability of an action for trespass to the person being brought is very remote and, were such action brought, the likelihood of more than nominal — or even contemptuous — damages being awarded no less remote unless what had been done had been done wilfully in the face of the patient's objection. But if some harm had been done, then the patient could claim substantial compensatory damages without proving negligence. Had what was done been done with the patient's consent, he could succeed in an action for damages only if he could establish negligence.

[4] For example, it is arguable that the communication of information about a patient to a group of medical students in the course of a demonstration could be a breach of professional confidence and for this the patient *might* have a remedy in damages had he sustained any material loss or loss of reputation as a consequence thereof. If what had been done had been done with the patient's consent, such remote risk would have been avoided.

[5] Consent in the case of children and other persons under a disability is discussed separately, see p. 192 *et seq.*

was to be so used and also aware of matters relevant to a decision, (*e.g.*, whether his refusal would prejudice his treatment) he had had reasonable opportunity to object. Useful guidance for making the position abundantly clear to patients in N.H.S. hospitals is given in a departmental circular 'Teaching on Patients'.[1] When they first attend hospital, it is to be made known to patients, out-patients and in-patients alike, that they may refuse to be used for teaching, this without prejudicing their treatment. Moreover, there should be a personal explanation by the clinical teacher to the patient when the patient is to be used for demonstration purposes, explicit mention being made of demonstrations by closed-circuit television or by use of video-tape or still photographs.[2] Moreover, there is the following admonition:

The Secretary of State would deprecate any attempt to overpersuade an unwilling patient to participate in teaching and the provision of necessary treatment available at a hospital should, of course, never be prejudiced by the patient's attitude in this respect.[3]

On the presence of students when emergency procedures are being carried out, the patient being unconscious or otherwise unable to give consent, the departmental advice is as follows:

... while it may be impossible to seek the consent of a patient or his next of kin to the presence of students at emergency procedures this should be done whenever possible and when it is not possible the teacher should remember that the students are present without the patient's consent, and should keep their numbers to a minimum.[4]

The apparent inference of the reference to the next of kin, *viz.*, that, if available, the next of kin could give effective consent on behalf of a patient is unwarranted. The reason is that, the presence of students not being for the good of the patient, there would be no ground for anyone to give consent on his behalf. It could, of course, be otherwise if the patient's acceptance for necessary treatment had been made conditional on consent being given to the presence of students.[5] However, the matter is relatively unimportant for the presence of students at emergency procedures would not, in itself, appear to infringe any of the patient's rights save possibly that of medical, confidentiality, and that — if actionable at all[6] – would be so only on proof of special damage.

But what of the use of child patients or of the mentally disordered

---

[1] H.M. (73) 8. The Secretary of State has expressed broad agreement with paragraphs 287 to 293 of the Report of the Royal Commission on Medical Education 1965–68 (Cmd 3569), set out as an appendix to the circular.
[2] H.M. (73) 8, paragraph 4.　　　　　　[3] H.M. (73) 8, paragraph 7.
[4] H.M. (73) 8, paragraph 5.
[5] This is not so in N.H.S. hospitals. See paragraphs 3 and 7 of H.M. (73) 8.
[6] That breach of medical confidentiality is actionable is not yet beyond the slightest possible doubt, though a medical practitioner, not sufficiently restrained by professional ethic, who acted on the assumption that it was not, would be exceedingly rash. See further, Chapter 20.

in clinical teaching, and this whether or not the patient is conscious? On this matter, the departmental advice is as follows:

> Consent for child patients to participate in teaching should be secured from their parents[1] and for mentally handicapped patients[2] from parent[1] or next of kin as appropriate.[3]

Presumably, 'parents' here includes 'guardians' and 'custodians' and might also include persons in actual control. In the case of a mentally handicapped patient under statutory guardianship as such,[4] who might be admitted to hospital otherwise than for treatment of his mental disorder, e.g., admitted for treatment of a physical injury or acute physical illness, the consent of the statutory guardian would be appropriate.

Although any such consent to the use of a child or mentally handicapped patient for use in connection with clinical teaching within the limits discussed in the departmental circular[5] would ordinarily suffice in ordinary circumstances, it would not be effective to authorise the use of the patient for purposes of research, as by using him as a control or subjecting him to experimentation.

(b) *Use of patients as controls and otherwise for research or as donors of organs*

Although patients may reasonably be expected to understand that in a teaching hospital — or, indeed, today possibly in any other hospital — they will, incidentally to their treatment, serve as material for the teaching of medical students. This is ordinarily brought to their notice by an explanatory leaflet, and even in a non-teaching hospital they will possibly serve an analogous purpose, e.g., as examples for general practitioner refresher courses, and that medical students, student nurses, student physiotherapists, etc., may, under proper supervision and subject to suitable safeguards take a part in their treatment. However they cannot be held, by merely attending hospital, to have agreed to submit to any procedures or the administration of any drugs not directed towards the treatment of their disease. Also, having regard

---

[1] There seems no reason for *parents* in the plural in the first place and *parent* in the singular in the other. Presumably it is meant that, whether in the case of a child patient or of one who is mentally handicapped, the consent of either parent would be regarded as sufficient unless it were known that the other parent objected.

[2] The expression *mentally handicapped patient* used in the circular does not correspond with the name of any of the forms of mental disorder named in s. 4 of the Mental Health Act 1959. The implication of the use of the expression seems to be that it refers only to those mentally disordered patients who, whatever their form of mental disorder, are thereby rendered incapable of reaching a rational decision on the matter. Since, according to the nature and extent of his disorder, every mentally disordered person is more or less mentally handicapped, the only other rational interpretation would be to equate *mentally handicapped* with *mentally disordered*. If that were the intention, there would be no good reason for using the expression at all.

[3] H.M. (73) 8, para. 6.

[4] Under the Mental Health Act 1959, see Chapter 28.   [5] See H.M. (73) 8.

to the provisions of the Health Service Acts, it would appear that if a hospital which had in any way committed itself to the treatment of a patient, *e.g.*, by having had him on a waiting list and then calling him in when a bed was available or, in the case of any other patient, having admitted him to a bed or commenced his treatment as an outpatient, afterwards — because the patient was unwilling to be used for teaching — refused to give or continue any treatment necessary, it would be liable for any ill consequences suffered by the patient unless satisfactory alternative arrangements had been made for his treatment at another hospital. This could apparently be done since there is no statutory right to treatment at any particular hospital.[1] Moreover, it is suggested that no experimental treatment of the disease involving risk to the patient is permissible when a well-tried treatment involving less risk to the patient or with greater degree of probability of a successful outcome is available. The only obvious cases justifying experimental treatment are when the patient's condition is not serious (*e.g.*, the common cold) or when it is virtually hopeless and the proposed experiment is the only apparent hope of either saving his life or restoring or partially restoring his health. Even so, the position should be explained to the patient or, if he is not in a fit condition to understand, to the appropriate relative and consent obtained. But even if the patient were not in a condition to give or withhold consent, the consent of a relative on his behalf to any experimental procedure involving unnecessary pain, suffering or discomfort to the patient would be valueless.

But if experimental treatment which, at the time of its use had not gained any acceptance among members of the relevant sector of the profession caused injury to the patient, the practitioner would lay himself open to a claim for damages based on negligence, this unless the patient had been made aware of the experimental nature of the treatment and of the risk involved.[2] This is illustrated by the facts in a very old case, *Slater* v. *Baker and Stapleton*,[3] in which damages were awarded against an eminent surgeon and an apothecary for negligently causing injury, the award being upheld on appeal. The surgeon, Baker, had been called in by the apothecary, Stapleton, to set Slater's broken leg. But things did not go well and then the surgeon tried out a new instrument, apparently to straighten the leg. The leg broke again at the point

---

[1] It has, however, to be added that refusal to treat or continue treatment in these circumstances, even if coupled with reference to another hospital, would be contrary to official policy, the Secretary of State for Social Services having stated clearly that the minority of patients who refuse to be taught on should not, on that account, be denied treatment at a teaching hospital. (See Parliamentary reply of the then Secretary of State (Mr Crossman) on 14th April, 1969 (Hansard Col. 785–787) confirming the assurances given by his predecessor.)

[2] See also pp. 226–227 as to criminal liability for negligence and *R.* v. *Long* (1830, 1831) 4 C P.. & 398, 423.

[3] (1767) 95 E.R. 860. See now *Haluska* v. *University of Saskatchewan* (1963) 53 D.L.R. (2d) 436 (Sask. C.A.).

of the original fracture and this led in Slater's successful claim against both practitioners[1] for 'unskilfully disuniting the callous of the leg after it had set'. In the judgment in appeal proceedings by the defendants when the judgment in favour of the plaintiff was upheld, it was said:

'For anything that appears to the Court this was the first experiment made with this new instrument and, if it was, it was a rash action and he who acts rashly, acts ignorantly: and although the defendants in general may be as skilful in their respective professions as any two gentlemen in England, yet the Court cannot help saying, that in this particular case they acted ignorantly and unskilfully, contrary to the known rules and usages of surgery. . . ."

It is to be doubted whether today the courts would use quite that language but it is certain that they would still hold a practitioner liable for experimental treatment which caused injury, unless it could in some way be justified as, for example, by showing that it had been the only chance of saving the patient's life or limb.

If it is desired to use a patient of full age and understanding as a control or otherwise for research, involving procedures or administration of drugs not directed primarily to the treatment of his disease, or, maybe, deprivation of some substance normally included in his diet, his express consent, freely given, should be obtained. Moreover, he should be told quite clearly what is involved in terms of discomfort, pain and risk, if his consent is to be relied on.[2] Even so, it is suggested that such consent would not avail in all cases for it is, to say the least, questionable whether anyone can lawfully consent to any surgical procedure or the administration of any drug or to any deprivation involving danger to life or limb. Reasonable use of volunteers, there being no recklessness is not, however, likely to involve conflict with the law.

It may be appropriate here to say a word about the use of an organ, *e.g.*, a kidney, from a living person with his consent to try to save the life of another person. Could such procedure result in either a criminal charge or in civil proceedings if the donor died or suffered serious injury?

Authority is lacking on both these points. But it is suggested that provided that the operation is not one which must inevitably result in the death or serious impairment of the health of the donor and that the surgeon has reasonable grounds for believing that in the ordinary course

[1] It seems unlikely that if today a general practitioner called in a surgeon to his patient and remained in attendance whilst the surgeon dealt with a fracture or other condition needing skilled surgical attention, the general practitioner as well as the surgeon would be held liable for the negligence of the latter. From the report, the evidence against the apothecary in *Slater's* case seemed but slight.

[2] For a very useful survey of the legal requirements for consent, see Professor B. M. Dickens, *Information for Consent in Human Experimentation*, University of Toronto Law Journal 1975 p. 381. The obligation to disclose risks known to the researcher probably increases in proportion to the lack of benefit likely to be gained by the 'patient'. Note also *Halushka* v. *University of Saskatchewan* (1965) 53 D.L.R. (2d) 436 (Sask. C.A.) which appears to be the only modern case in a common law jurisdiction which deals with consent in an entirely experimental setting.

of things the donor will not be subjected to grave risk of death or serious impairment of health, there would be no risk of a prosecution if, without criminal negligence, the donor, unfortunately, suffered harm. Even if a donor, with full knowledge, had consented to, or even requested, a procedure which must result in his death or serious disability even to save the life of another, the surgeon who performed the procedure would possibly be liable for manslaughter — if not indeed for murder — if rhe donor died, for causing grevious bodily harm if he lived, though consent, freely given would, even in this case, almost certainly be a bar to civil proceedings.

Apart from circumstances in which death or injury to the donor *must* result from the procedure, it is reasonable to assume that a responsible surgeon will be willing to effect such operations as transfer of a kidney from a donor to a dangerously ill patient only when he is satisfied that the operation does not involve an excessively grave risk to the donor. If he has explained the position to the donor, making it plain that there must be some risk in the procedure, with the added long-term risk — if such there be — of the donor's relying on one kidney only for the future, then it would seem that, provided the procedure is properly carried out and any necessary after-care properly given, there can be no civil liability either for bodily harm to the donor or even for his death. *Volenti non fit injuria.*[1]

The position as regards persons under a disability, notably children and mentally disordered patients, is different. They clearly cannot themselves consent to be controls or subject of research nor can anybody else, such as a parent or guardian, do so on their behalf.[2] Dr R. E. W. Fisher has stated as the ethical rule as regards children as follows: 'No medical procedure involving the slightest risk or accompanied by the slightest physical or mental pain may be inflicted on a child for experimental purposes unless there is a reasonable chance, or at least a hope, that the child may benefit thereby.'[3] This seems to be a fair

---

[1] In a presidential address at the congress of the Royal Society of Health, Lord Cohen of Birkenhead rejected outright, as entirely unethical, the use of live organs or tissue from a dying person to save another's life 'even if permission is sought and given by relatives or guardians' (*J. Roy. Soc. Health*, 1966). Not only would such procedure be 'entirely unethical', but it would also be tortious and, if it could be shown to have hastened the death of the patient, criminal.

[2] Compare *Re Taylor's Application* [1972] 2 All E.R. 873 and see Skegg, *Consent to Medical Procedures on Minors* (1973), 36 M.L.R. 370.

[3] *Lancet*, Nov. 7, 1953, p.993. The draft code of ethics on human experimentation issued by the World Medical Association in 1963 and published in *Brit. Med. J.*, 1963, 1119, is not sufficiently strong on this point to reflect the legal — let alone ethical — responsibility of the medical profession towards children in this country. Readers desirous of following up practical problems in applying legal principles in this field and of weighing different ethical standpoints might refer to Sir Austin Bradford Hill's 'Medical Ethics and Controlled Trials', *Brit. Med. J.*, 1963, 1, 1043. A most balanced statement of both the legal and the ethical limits to experimentation on human beings — well or ill — is that included in the report for 1962/3 of the Medical Research Council, being entitled 'Responsibility for Investigation on Human Subjects'. It must, however, be said that even this statement is

statement also of the position in law as regards persons under a disability generally, provided it is understood that even the hope of the child's benefiting by the experimental procedure is not sufficient justification if some other procedure involving less pain or risk is known to be available and, but for the desire to experiment, would have been used. In short, in the case of a child, treatment is paramount and nothing must be done which cannot be justified as treatment. Maybe, however, the use of young people between 16 and 18 — not being mentally disordered persons — as controls or for research with their own consent, as well as with the consent of their parent or guardian, is not entirely ruled out. But it is suggested that they should be used with the greatest discretion.[1] It may here be recalled that s. 8 (3) of the Family Law Reform Act 1969 refers only to consent to treatment and has no relevance to use minors for research or as controls.

The basis of the opinion expressed that a parent or guardian cannot lawfully consent to or permit the use of a child under 16 years of age or of a mentally disordered person as a control or for purposes of research, assuming it involves any pain, discomfort or risk, is that the authority of the parent or guardian[2] exists only for the protection and well-being of child or of the person under the disability. So he may consent to something involving pain, discomfort or even risk for the good of the child or other such person himself, but not for any other purpose, not even the good of other children or of other sick persons, however many in number.

(c) Clinical trials, etc.

If patients and other volunteers are to be used in clinical trials additionally the provisions of ss. 31 to 39 of the Medicines Act 1968 have to be complied with.[3]

open to some criticism, not least concerning what it says — and does not say — about the use of children for purposes of research. The statement is printed in full in Appendix F.

[1] In the statement by the M.R.C. referred to in note 3 on p. 224, above, it is said '. . . . it may be safely assumed that the courts would not regard a child of 12 years or under . . . as having the capacity to consent to any procedure which may involve him in an injury'. That statement is unexceptionable so far as it goes; but it does not go far enough. Our view is as stated above. Although of no authority in clarifying the legal position and rather glossing over some issues, the report of a committee of the Royal College of Physicians of London on the supervision and ethics of clinical investigations in institutions, circulated to N.H.S. hospitals under cover of Departmental circular H.M. (68) 33, is interesting for the following statement: 'The design and conduct of clinical investigation should be guided by a code of clinical practice and the Code of Ethics of the W.M.A. ("Declaration of Helsinki") is accepted throughout the civilised world. The Medical Research Council has also issued a statement on 'Responsibility in Investigation on Human Subjects'. . . . The Committee accepts that these statements define the ethical situation and considers that all clinical investigators should be familiar with their recommendations.' It must, however, be appreciated that these statements do not necessarily reflect accurately the law of England: in places they seem to fall short of its demands.

[2] The expression 'parent or guardian' does not here include a step-parent, as to whose position in respect of consent to treatment see page 200 and Re N. (Minors) (Parental Rights) [1974] Fam. 40.

[3] See pp. 148–150.

CHAPTER 14

INJURIES TO PATIENTS

A. INTRODUCTORY

IN this chapter, after a brief examination of the circumstances in which the criminal law may be invoked for harm done to a patient, there will be discussed the nature and extent of the civil liability attributable to medical negligence or incompetence. Commonly such liability arises by reason of a wrong diagnosis or of some mistake in the course of treatment. Far too frequently it arises because of a failure to communicate information or instructions, whether to another member of the medical team or to the patient or sometimes to the relative of the patient. Left over for the next chapter is the extent of the liability for the safety of hospital premises. Later chapters deal with loss and damage to the property of patients and staff and other complaints machinery. The question of the quantum of damages is not discussed since it is not related in any way to liability for wrongs done in the course of medical treatment. It suffices here to say that the extent of the damages to be awarded following a finding of liability are determined in medical cases as in other cases in the light of the general law.

Many of the cases dealing with liability involve actions against the former hospital management committees. Such liability is known as vicarious liability. It forms a separate section of this chapter. It should however be noted at the outset that whether the liability be personal or vicarious, the principles are similar and accordingly the cases involving the one are relevant to the other.

B. CRIMINAL LIABILITY FOR INJURY

This is not the place for a detailed exposition of that part of the criminal law concerned with wrongful acts causing either death or injury to the person and of the nice gradation of possible charges, having regard to the nature and circumstances of the injury and the apparent intention of the wrongdoer. Broadly, however, it may be said that any person who *wilfully* does a wrongful act whereby another is killed or injured is liable to prosecution in respect of the death or injury, if it was the necessary consequence of the wrongful act (*e.g.*, assault; wounding). Criminal responsibility also arises in respect of injury caused recklessly (*e.g.*, death or injury caused by reckless driving of a car) though not intended. It may also sometimes arise if someone is killed or injured in or in consequence of the commission of another offence, *e.g.*, illegal abortion or attempted abortion. Neither the prior consent of the victim to the offence, nor his subsequent unwillingness for a criminal charge to be brought against the wrongdoer, is a bar to prosecution. The victim, if available, will usually be a compellable witness, though this is not so in the case of injury due to an illegal abortion or attempted abortion, because the victim, having been a consenting party to the offence, could herself be charged with participation therein and is not compellable to give what would be self-incriminatory evidence in the proceedings against the abortionist. Anyone who knowingly assists in preparations for committing an offence or in carrying it out, although not the principal wrongdoer and getting no benefit from it, will normally be answerable in law. Anyone who assists in concealing a crime, or who actively helps the wrongdoer to escape, may also be punishable.[1]

The above basic principles have been roughly stated because they may, on infrequent occasions, have application to happenings in medical practice, especially in hospitals and nursing homes. By way of example may be taken such obvious and rare instances of criminal liability as that of a medical practitioner who, without lawful excuse such as self-defence and otherwise than by negligence not amounting to criminal negligence, injures a patient, or who actively assists in concealing an offence against a patient (*e.g.*, a crime of violence in a psychiatric hospital). Yet another possibility, if an operation had been performed badly or an overdose of a drug had been administered, or there had been some other serious mistake in treatment as a consequence of which the patient had died, the responsible practitioner at the time of the happening had been so far under the influence of drink or drugs that his judgment had been impaired, the mere fact that the practitioner did not intend the patient's death would not alone suffice to save him from liability for manslaughter.

That the number of prosecutions for manslaughter in respect of recklessness or the plainest negligence in an obviously serious matter relating to the care or treatment of a patient is even lower than might be expected from the occasional reports of such things is to be attributed to the strict standard of proof required to obtain a conviction in the criminal courts, *i.e.* proof beyond all reasonable doubt.[2] But a much

---

[1] Criminal Law Act 1967, s. 4.

[2] *R.* v. *Spiller* (5 C. & P. 333; 336) was a case in which a charge of manslaughter was based on an allegation of failure of a medical practitioner to exercise due care. In that case, Bolland, B., in his summing up said — 'The law . . is this — if any person, whether he be a registered or licensed medical man or not, proposes to deal with the life or health of his Majesty's subjects he is bound to have competent skill to perform the task that he holds himself out to perform, and he is bound to treat his patients with care, attention and assiduity.' Alternatively, as stated in *R.* v. *Long* (1830, 1831 — two separate cases) 4 C. & P. 398, 423; 172 E.R. 756, 767) 'A person acting as a medical man, whether licensed or unlicensed, is not criminally responsible for the death of a patient, occasioned by his treatment

slighter degree of negligence will support a civil action, turning as the verdict does on balance of probabilities. Moreover, ordinarily, the outcome of a successful civil action in which damages have been awarded is much more likely to be to the patient/plaintiff's satisfaction than the defendant's conviction on a criminal charge.

The question of possible criminal liability of those helping a surgeon to perform an operation when he is under the influence of drink or drugs would be likely to arise only if it were obvious before he began that he was unfit to perform it. In that case those assisting, especially those medically qualified, might also lay themselves open to prosecution. If the fact that something was wrong became apparent only after the operation had started, one can only suggest that those assisting should do what they consider is in the best interest of the *patient* at the time. Conceivably that could mean that, if practicable, someone present who was competent to do so should take over.[1]

C. CIVIL LIABILITY FOR INJURY

1. Personal Liability for Negligence

(a) *Personal responsibility of medical practitioners and of others*

Except in rare cases, none of which is relevant to our present subject, no one is liable for any injury to person or property due to an accident not arising from incompetence or carelessness, unless he assumes such a liability by contract. Hence, if a patient is injured or dies as a result of a wrong diagnosis, but one made with proper care and skill,[2] or of an operation or other medical treatment performed with such skill as in all the circumstances, was reasonable, there is no liability on the medical practitioner, nurse or other medical auxiliary concerned.[3] Examples readily come to mind. A patient may die under anaesthetic, all normal precautions having been taken by the surgeon and the anaesthetist. Or a sudden, violent and unexpected movement by a patient who is being catheterised may cause injury to the patient, the nurse having warned him not to move and all due precautions having been taken. Or again,

unless his conduct is characterized either by gross ignorance of his art or gross inattention to his patient's safety.' and 'Where a person undertaking the cure of a disease (whether he has received a medical education or not) is guilty of gross negligence in attending his patient after he has applied a remedy, or a gross rashness in the application of it, and death ensues in consequence of either, he is liable to be convicted of manslaughter.' Further in cases of manslaughter by neglect, a reckless breach of an assumed duty to care for a patient rather than mere inadvertance is required *R. v. Store* [1977] 2 W.L.R. 169.

[1] For advice given by the Department to Hospital Authorities for preventing harm to patients resulting from physical or mental disability of hospital medical and dental staff, including disability due to addiction to drugs or alcohol, reference should be made to Circular H.M. (60) 45 and to circulars and reports there mentioned. This advice does nothing to alter the criminal responsibility of a wrongdoer nor his civil liability nor that of the employing authority for his negligence or incompetence.

[2] *Whiteford v. Hunter* (1950) 94 S. Jo. 758 (H.L.); [1950] W.N. 533.

[3] See Scott, L.J., in *Mahon v. Osborne* [1939] 2 K.B. 14 quoted on p. 230.

a drug for injection is wrongly labelled by the manufacturers and a patient suffers harm in consequence.[1] In this type of case there is no liability on the professional person or on any hospital or other authority or person by whom he may be employed unless, maybe, something ought to have put the user on inquiry, *e.g.*, the appearance or smell of the drug.

But if a medical practitioner or anyone else concerned has been negligent,[2] the negligent person may be liable in damages. Generally, too, it may be observed that if a person is negligent in the course of his duties, it does not follow that any exemption from liability enjoyed by his employer, either by contract or as a condition of a voluntary benefit an injured person, will avail the negligent employee.[3]

It is not within the province of this work to examine closely the limits of the common law duty of care, but it may be said that the courts have been very ready to fix the duty of care on a defendant whenever his negligent act or omission has directly led to the loss or injury suffered by another or when such loss or damage should have been within his contemplation, as in *Donoghue* v. *Stevenson*.[4] A series of cases in which damages have been claimed for shock due to seeing or fearing a road accident due to the negligence of the defendant have now brought the law to a point at which the courts have begun to say that such plaintiffs may be outside the scope of the duty owed by the defendant. This type of case, however, is not here our concern. Generally, therefore, we can say that in any ordinary activity of life the customary degree of care and skill is to be exercised and, if it is not, and anyone is injured in person or property thereby, the wrongdoer may be liable in damages provided the damage suffered is of a kind to be contemplated for failing to exercise the customary skill and care.[5] It may, however, here be observed that the injury or damage reasonably to be foreseen from a negligent act or omission, and for which damages may therefore be awarded, may be less closely circumscribed than it has in the past been thought. In *Chadwick* v. *British Railways Board*,[6] the Board was held liable to a rescuer in a rail disaster who suffered in health as a result of shock, and this even though he had not been in fear for his own safety or that

[1] As to liability of manufacturer see *Donoghue* v. *Stevenson* [1932] A.C. 562.
[2] Incompetence usually imports negligence.
[3] *Genys* v. *Matthews* [1966] 1 W.L.R. 759, referred to on p. 295.
[4] [1932] A.C. 562 and particularly Lord Atkin at p. 580.
[5] The words 'provided . . . care' have been added as a very rough indication of the effect of *Wagon Mound (The)*; *Overseas Tankship (U.K.)* v. *Mort's Dock and Engineering Co.* [1961] A.C. 388; *Wagon Mound (The) (No. 2); Miller Steamship Co. Pty.* v. *Overseas Tankship (U.K.); Miller (R.W.)* v. *Same* [1963] [1967] A.C. 617. For a full discussion of the effect of the *Wagon Mound* decision, the reader must refer to a standard work on torts. But see *Robinson* v. *The Post Office* (1973) 16 K.I.R. 12. The plaintiff suffered a minor injury at work, an anti-tetanus injection was given but he suffered encephatis. The doctor was held to be negligent. However on the facts, the plaintiff would have so suffered without the negligence and therefore the defendants were liable for the whole of the damages. Note also *Stephenson* v. *Waite Tileman* [1973] N.Z.L.R. 152 and *Malcolm* v. *Broadhurst* [1970] 3 All E.R. 508 on specially susceptible plaintiffs.
[6] [1967] 1 W.L.R. 912.

of his children. The basis of the decision was that the risk of injury to a rescuer or his suffering from shock was foreseeable.[1] It is not only the professionally qualified expert to whom such liability applies. Any employee is equally obliged to exercise the skill and care appropriate to his respective calling and, if he fails to do so, and harm results, he may personally be answerable in damages.[2]

A person who undertakes work for which special skill is required if injury to the person or property of another is to be avoided is ordinarily under a duty to that person to exercise the requisite degree of care and skill, even though he undertakes the work gratuitously and for the benefit of that other person. Incompetence or lack of care by his own standards makes the expert liable in damages.[3] However the skill to be demonstrated is at least that which ordinary professional opinion would impose. Accordingly it is no defence to show that an incompetent person (or a person with an incompetent method) behaved normally and according to his own (too low) standards.[4]

The measure of the responsibility of the professional man with special reference to the surgeon was clearly laid down in *Mahon* v. *Osborne*[5] when Scott, L.J., said:

'It is desirable to recall the well-established legal measure of a professional man's duty. If he professes an art he must be reasonably skilled in it. There is no doubt that the defendant surgeon was that. He must also be careful, but the standard of care the law requires is not insurance against accidental slips. It is such a degree of care as a normally skilful member of the profession may reasonably be expected to exercise in the actual circumstances of the case in question. It is not every slip or mistake which imports negligence and, in applying the duty of care to the case of a surgeon, it is peculiarly necessary to have regard to the different kinds of circumstances that may present themselves for urgent attention.'

This principle applies to anyone whose work requires some special skill. It is applicable to the work of a medical practitioner,[6] a nurse or

---

[1] The principle also applies where a doctor is killed or injured when attempting to rescue or treat victims of an accident. In *Baker* v. *T. E. Hopkins* ([1959] 1 W.L.R. 966) a doctor had descended a well to rescue two workmen overcome by fumes and was himself overcome. The defendant company being found liable for the accident to the workmen was also held liable in damages to the doctor's widow.

[2] *Lister* v. *Romford Ice and Cold Storage Co. Ltd.* [1957] A.C. 555; [1957] 1 All E.R. 125. In practice, if such a Health Service employee causes injury by his negligence, he is not likely to be sued personally, either because he is not worth suing, not having the money to satisfy a judgment or, sometimes, because not identified, any action being brought against the Hospital Authority.

[3] *Coggs* v. *Bernard* (1704) 2 Ld. Raym. 909 Salk, 26; *Wilson* v. *Brett* (1843) 11 M. & W 113.

[4] *Cowan* v. *Wilcox* (1973) 44 D.L.R. (3d) 42 (New Brunswick Sup. Ct.). A nurse was held negligent where the doctrine of *res ipsa loquitur* applied and it was not rebutted by proof that the technique used in the particular case was the same as had been used in other cases. See S. 1 (5) of the Congenital Disabilities (Civil Liability) Act 1976 applying the rule in *Roe* v. *Minister of Health* [1954] 2 Q.B. 66.

[5] *Mahon* v. *Osborne* [1939] 2 K.B. 14. In *Urry and Anor.* v. *Bierer and Anor.* (*The Times*, July 15, 1955) the Court of Appeal discussed responsibility of a surgeon for packs left in patient.

[6] *R.* v. *Bateman* (1925) 19 Cr. App. R. 8.

a medical auxiliary such as a radiographer[1] or physiotherapist. If any such person fails to exercise reasonable care and skill and the patient suffers injury, he will be personally liable, nonetheless so because he may be working as a whole-time salaried officer for a hospital authority. The question of the extent of the concurrent liability of the hospital authority and of contribution towards damages is reserved for further discussion.[2]

(b) Extent of medical practitioner's duty to keep up to date

What is a reasonable degree of care and skill is a matter of fact to be determined in accordance with the evidence in the particular case and may vary from time to time as knowledge increases. Thus in *Roe* v. *Ministry of Health and Others; Woolley* v. *Same*[3] which reached the Court of Appeal in 1954, the two plaintiffs had been given a spinal anaesthetic in 1947, the ampoules of which had, unfortunately, become contaminated with phenol. In the result the two patients suffered very serious and permanent incapacity. From the evidence it appeared that the ampoules had been kept in phenol as an antiseptic precaution, it not being then appreciated that there was any danger of the phenol seeping in through microscopic cracks or molecular flaws not visible on ordinary inspection. It was held by the Court of Appeal that in the state of medical knowledge in 1947 neither the anaesthetist nor any other member of the hospital staff had been guilty of negligence.

Somervell, L.J., said in his judgment in *Roe's* case that the attention of the profession was first drawn to the risk in this country only by the publication of Professor Mackintosh's book 'Lumbar Puncture and Spinal Anaesthesia' in 1951. From that it follows that the defence on the facts in *Roe's* case would not now succeed. On the other hand, members of the medical profession are not placed under the impossible duty of reading every technical paper as soon as it appears, still less of agreeing with the suggestions of every contributor to a medical journal. This was illustrated by *Crawford* v. *Board of Governors of Charing Cross Hospital.*[4] In that case the plaintiff had suffered permanent injury — brachial palsy — as a consequence of the position of his arm during the operation, during which blood transfusion to that arm had been necessary. An article had appeared in *The Lancet* some six months before the operation was performed in which the writer had condemned the positioning of the arm which had given rise to Crawford's injury. The anaesthetist agreed that he had seen letters in *The Lancet* commenting on the article but had not, in fact, referred back to it. It was sought on this ground to say that he had been negligent in not knowing that the position should never be adopted. The Court of Appeal rejected

---

[1] *Gold* v. *Essex C.C.* [1942] 2 K.B. 293; 58 T.L.R. 357; [1942] 2 All E.R. 237.
[2] See p. 253 *et seq.*   [3] [1954] 2 Q.B. 66.   [4] *The Times*, Dec. 8, 1953.

K

that contention, the obligation on a medical practitioner in respect of articles in the medical press being succinctly stated by Denning, L.J., who said:

'It would, I think, be putting too high a burden on a medical man to say that he has to read every article appearing in the current medical press; and it would be quite wrong to suggest that a medical man is negligent because he does not at once put into operation the suggestions which some contributor or other might make in a medical journal. The time may come in a particular case when a new recommendation may be so well proved and so well known and so well accepted that it should be adopted. But that was not so in this case.'

As an example of technical writings which medical practitioners in hospital as well as other officers of hospital authorities may disregard only at their peril are advisory circulars, often supported by memoranda prepared by appropriate working parties, issued by the Department of Health and Social Security. As an illustration may be mentioned Departmental circular HM(72)37 on precautions for the avoidance of surgical accidents. In that circular hospital authorities were asked to review the procedures at their hospitals to ensure that the precautions against operations on the wrong patient, side, limb or digit and against swabs, *etc.*, being left in a patient after an operation were as closely as possible in line with those recommended in the joint memoranda of the Medical Defence Union and the Royal College of Nursing as revised in 1969. The circular also required hospital authorities to investigate any such accidents which might occur in their hospitals and to take steps to avoid a recurrence. The results of such investigations were to be reported to the Department which, in turn, would circulate to all hospital authorities any recommendations arising which might be of general interest and application.[1] Other illustrations are circulars on provision of safe cots for babies, on anaesthetic explosions in operating theatres and on control of staphylococcal infections in hospitals.

Whilst such publications do not afford conclusive proof that anyone who, without good reason, falls short of the standard of care suggested in them has been negligent, they would certainly afford some, and possibly strong, evidence of the appropriate standard of care, especially if it were proved that precautions advised were generally taken and there was no substantial reason why they should not have been in the

---

[1] Another Departmental circular which requires untoward incidents to be reported to the Department, and to be reported immediately, so that other hospitals can be advised or warned against possible harm to patients and staff, is H.M. (73) 9 which relates to incidents caused by defects in medicinal products or in other medical supplies and equipment. At page 252 is discussed the possible liability of the Secretary of State if, such a report of an incident having been received by the Department, a second incident — and one which causes harm — occurs and this time at a different hospital and one which has not received any warning from the Department. What is said at page 252 relating to reports under H.M. (73) 9 applies equally to failure of the Department to issue any warning or advice which might be appropriate after receiving a report under any other circular.

particular instance. Such evidence might be against a defendant medical practitioner if the fault were alleged to be his but, as in the matter of provision of safe cots, the responsibility might rest squarely on the Health Authority if, for example, it had refused to authorise expenditure on necessary alterations or replacements. Indeed, in this instance, any liability might be on the authority as occupier of the premises, by virtue of the Occupiers' Liability Act 1957. The limits of such liability are discussed in the next chapter.

It may also be suggested that if through departmental circulars and official reports the desirability of particular precautions being taken for the safety of patients becomes known to and adopted by most of the medical and nursing profession, it is a well-nigh inevitable conclusion that private hospitals and nursing homes and those who work in them will be held liable if they fail to take such precautions and harm results.

It follows that the degree of skill and the standard of care required of a medical practitioner if he is to avoid civil liability is not static but is conditioned by the level of knowledge and skill current among those with whom a defendant practitioner may fairly be compared at the time of the accident. Thus the acts or omissions of a person who holds himself out as an anaesthetist will be judged by current knowledge and skill of ordinarily competent anaesthetists at the time of the act or omission, and similarly in the case of other specialities.[1] But in none of these cases will the standard of skill and competence achieved by the practitioner be judged against that of a giant in his field. But in so far as the leaders in a speciality make known better techniques which can be adopted by others, and so far as those techniques have become accepted by competent practitioners in the speciality, a defendant practising that speciality will invite a finding of negligence if he does not follow that accepted technique, and the harm it was designed to avoid occurs. Thus a practitioner allows his knowledge and techniques to become out of date at his peril.[2]

(c) Duty of practitioner where there is more than one school of thought on the treatment to be given

In *Bolam* v. *Friern Hospital Management Committee*,[3] an action in which the plaintiff failed in a claim for damages for injury in the course of an operation, injuries which he alleged to be due to negligence, and in which he also alleged negligent failure to warn him of the risk of injury, McNair, J., in his summing up to the jury took substantially the same

[1] He will therefore be bound to recognise known, if very rare, phenomena such as ether convulsions *O'Donovan* v. *Cork C.C. and others* [1967] I.R. 173 (Eire).

[2] As an example of the necessity of keeping up to date may be suggested the need to be aware of the possible ill-effects of newer drugs as they come into common use, from penicillin to the contraceptive pill. (See *Chin Keow* v. *Government of Malaysia and Another* [1967] 1 W.L.R. 813, summarized in footnote 2 on page 234.

[3] [1957] 1 W. L. R. 582; [1957] 2 All E. R. 118.

line as the Court of Appeal in *Crawford* v. *Board of Governors of Charing Cross Hospital*,[1] In *Bolam's* case the plaintiff had been given electro-convulsive therapy (ECT) in 1954, by a member of the professional staff who, following his normal practice and that of his clinical chief, a consultant psychiatrist attached to the hospital, gave the treatment 'unmodified', *i.e.*, without the prior administration of a relaxant drug and without applying any form of manual restraint, though certain other precautions were taken. The plaintiff, who had sustained bilateral 'stove-in' fractures of the acetabula, brought an action for damages against the hospital, alleging negligence in the failure to administer a relaxant or the provision of manual control; also in failing to warn him of the risks which he was running when he consented to the treatment, in particular, failing to warn him that it was proposed to carry out the treatment without relaxant drugs being previously administered and without manual control being available. McNair, J., said:

'When you get a situation which involves the use of some special skill or competence . . . the test . . . is the standard of the ordinary skilled man exercising and professing to have that special skill. A man need not possess the highest expert skill; it is well-established law that it is sufficient if he exercises the ordinary skill of an ordinary competent man exercising that particular art. . . .[2] In a Scottish case, *Hunter* v. *Hanley*,[3] Lord President Clyde said:
   ' "In the realm of diagnosis and treatment there is ample scope for genuine difference of opinion and one man clearly is not negligent merely because his conclusion differs from that of other professional men, nor because he has displayed less skill or knowledge than others would have shown. The true test for establishing negligence in diagnosis or treatment on the part of a doctor is whether he has been proved to be guilty of such failure as no doctor of ordinary skill would be guilty of, if acting with ordinary care."
'If that statement of the true test is qualified by the words "in all the circumstances", Mr Fox-Andrews[4] would not seek to say that that expression of opinion does not accord with the English law. It is just a question of expression. I myself would prefer to put it this way, that he is not guilty of negligence if he has acted in accordance with a practice accepted as proper by a responsible body of medical men skilled in that particular art. I do not think there is much difference in sense. It is just a different way of expressing the same

[1] See above p. 231.
[2] [1957] 1 W.L.R. 582, 596; [1957] 2 All E.R. 118. This test of the standard of care required of a professional man if he is to escape liability for negligence was approved by Sir Hugh Wooding, delivering the judgment of the Privy Council in *Chin Keow* v. *Government of Malaysia and Another* ([1967] 1 W.L.R. 813). In *Chin Keow's* case, a young woman had been given an injection of procaine penicillin by a clinic doctor and had died within an hour. The death occurred as a result of a reaction due to the patient's having at some previous time been given an injection of penicillin, such reaction being known to be a remote risk in such circumstances. In an action for damages, Ong, J., had found for the plaintiff, the mother of the deceased on grounds that the doctor had been negligent in failing to enquire whether the patient had ever previously been injected with penicillin before administering the drug. The Privy Council, applying the test approved from the summing up of McNair, J., in *Bolam's* case, and reversing the Malaysian Court of Appeal, restored the judgment of Ong, J.
[3] [1955] S.L.T. 213, 217.   [4] Counsel in the case.

thought. Putting it the other way round, a man is not negligent, if he is acting in accordance with such a practice, merely because there is a body of opinion who would take a contrary view. At the same time, that does not mean that a medical man can obstinately and pig-headedly carry on with some old technique if it had been proved to be contrary to what is really substantially the whole of informed medical opinion. Otherwise you might get men today saying: "I do not believe in anaesthetics. I do not believe in antiseptics. I am going to continue to do my surgery in the way it was done in the eighteenth century." That clearly would be wrong.

'Before I get to the details of the case, it is right to say this, that it is not essential for you to decide which of two practices is the better practice, as long as you accept that what the defendants did was in accordance with a practice accepted by responsible persons; if the result of the evidence is that you are satisfied that his practice is better than the practice spoken of on the other side, then it is really a stronger case. Finally, bear this in mind, that you are now considering whether it was negligent for certain action to be taken in August 1954, not in February 1957; and in one of the well-known cases on this topic it has been said you must not look with 1957 spectacles at what happened in 1954.

'Before I leave this question of liability it is right to refer you to some wise words used recently in the Court of Appeal in *Roe* v. *Minister of Health*,[1] a case not dissimilar to this. That was a case where two men in the prime of life were submitted to an anaesthetic for, in both cases, some trivial condition requiring operative treatment and, as the result of a mishap in the anaesthetic, both men came off the operating table paralysed. After a very long inquiry, the trial judge came to the conclusion that it had not been established that, by the standard of care and knowledge operating at the time, the anaesthetist was negligent. The Court of Appeal took the same view, and Denning, L.J., said:

' "If the anaesthetists had foreseen that the ampoules might get cracked with cracks that could not be detected on inspection they would no doubt have dyed the phenol a deep blue; and this would have exposed the contamination. But I do not think that their failure to foresee this was negligence. It is so easy to be wise after the event and to condemn as negligence that which was only a misadventure. We ought always to be on our guard against it, especially in cases against hospitals and doctors. Medical science has conferred great benefits on mankind, but these benefits are attended by considerable risks. Every surgical operation is attended by risks. We cannot take the benefits without taking the risks. Every advance in technique is also attended by risks. Doctors, like the rest of us, have to learn by experience; and experience often teaches in a hard way. Something goes wrong and shows up a weakness, and then it is put right. That is just what happened here. . . . One final word. These two men have suffered such terrible consequences that there is a natural feeling that they should be compensated. But we should be doing a disservice to the community at large if we were to impose liability on hospitals and doctors for everything that happens to go wrong. Doctors would be led to think more of their own safety than of the good of their patients. Initiative would be stifled and confidence shaken. A proper sense of proportion requires us to have regard to the conditions in which hospitals and doctors have to work. . . . We must insist on due care for the patient at every point, but we must not condemn as negligence that which is only a misadventure." '

[1] [1954] 2 Q.B. 66; [1954] 2 All E.R. 131.

The cases fairly point to the conclusion that whilst a medical practitioner in his dealings with his patient, whether by way of diagnosis, warning or treatment, acts in a manner which would find favour with a substantial proportion, albeit of minority, of his competent colleagues, he is unlikely to be found negligent. By the word 'competent' is here meant competent in the particular branch of medicine or surgery concerned or in general practice, as the case may be.

(d) Failure of communication

Another case which may be mentioned, which reached the House of Lords, was *Chapman* v. *Rix*.[1] The facts of the case were somewhat unusual. Chapman, a butcher, when boning a rump of beef, slashed his abdomen. He was taken to Brentwood District Hospital, a 'cottage hospital'[2] where, there being no resident medical staff, he was dealt with by a local general practitioner, Dr. Rix, who happened to be there. Dr. Rix concluded that, though the deep fascia had been cut, the wound had not penetrated the peritoneum, and ordered that the wound be stitched[3] and dressed. He then sent Chapman home, giving him emphatic instructions to see his own doctor, Dr Mohr, that evening. Chapman told Dr Mohr that the hospital had told him that the wound was 'superficial'. Dr Mohr, not appreciating that the hospital was a cottage hospital and that Dr Rix was not a casualty officer, examined the patient and diagnosed a digestive disorder. The patient died and a *post mortem* revealed that the wound had penetrated the small intestine. In an action by the widow, Barry, J., found that Dr Rix had been negligent in failing to communicate directly by telephone or letter with the man's own doctor after he had dealt with him. The judgment was reversed by the Court of Appeal. The plaintiff's further appeal to the House of Lords, which turned solely on the question whether the failure of the defendant to communicate directly was negligent, was also dismissed.[4]

Dismissing the appeal, Lord Goddard[5] said that it was true that Dr Rix did not communicate directly with Dr Mohr, but he had emphatically warned the patient to call in his own doctor — and he did — and to tell him exactly what had happened and what had taken place at the hospital — and that was done. It was easy to say after the event: 'Well, Dr Rix might have told him more.' But if he had written

[1] *The Times*, Nov. 19, 1959. See also *Crichton* v. *Hastings* (1972) 29 D.L.R. (3d) 692 (Ontario C.A.). The plaintiff had a tendency to phlebitis. The defendant operated and prescribed an anti-coagulent drug which when taken in overdose could cause a haemorrhage He gave no warning because he did not think the plaintiff would be discharged from the hospital whilst taking the drug. This was held to be negligence.

[2] The expression 'cottage hospital' is generally taken to mean a very small hospital without any resident medical staff and which will not necessarily often be visited by consultants.

[3] The report does not say who stitched the wound.　　　　　[4] *The Times*, Dec 21, 1960.

[5] Lord Morton agreed with the speech of Lord Goddard.

or spoken directly to his fellow practitioner, his Lordship doubted whether he would have told him more than that after observation and probing he had formed the opinion there was no penetration. He might have added: 'He needs watching', but that he might well assume Dr Mohr would understand without being told.

Lord Hodson, also concurring with dismissing the appeal, said that it was true that the patient would be expected to pass on to his own doctor the reassuring statement that the wound was, in the opinion of Dr Rix, superficial, but that did not cancel out the main sense of the message, which was an emphatic one. An object of that message must have been to guard, by observation, against what Dr Rix thought an outside chance, that penetration of the peritoneal cavity had occurred.

In his dissenting speech Lord Keith said that Chapman had fallen between two stools and that was due chiefly to the failure of communication. The patient himself was made the medium of communication. The question was, was that communication adequate and, if not, was Dr Rix responsible for the inadequacy, and did his failure amount to negligence? Dr Mohr would have acted differently if he had known of the observed penetration through the deep fascia down to the muscles of the abdomen. A doctor who was expected to look after a patient with an abdominal wound, which had already been diagnosed and treated by another doctor who had decided that the injury did not require operative or observational treatment in a hospital, should be put in possession of information on what had been observed and done by the first doctor. The question had to be dealt with in relation to the risks run by the patient in the absence of proper medical and surgical treatment. The non-communication, in his Lordship's view, amounted to negligence in law.

Lord Denning, also dissenting, said that misleading information was a dangerous thing to throw about. There was no telling where it would finish up. A medical man might sometimes feel justified in giving misleading information to a patient so as not to worry him. But if he did so, he must be very careful to give the true information to his relatives and those about him, and most important of all, to the patient's own doctor who had to treat him. It was the failure of Dr Rix to observe that rule, which his Lordship would regard as elementary, which was his mistake here.

The division of judicial opinion both in the Court of Appeal and in the House of Lords on the somewhat unusual facts of *Chapman* v. *Rix* leave one of the mind that with but a slight variation of the facts, or even, perhaps, in their presentation, the decision might have been different. It could certainly not be deduced from the case that a medical practitioner treating at a hospital, without admitting him as an in-patient, a person who has met with an accident, is never under an

obligation to communicate directly with the patient's own doctor. All
that can be said is that in all the circumstances of *Chapman* v. *Rix* and
at that time, the failure of the defendant medical practitioner to do so
was not negligent. So, if in a later case, it could be shown that since
Chapman v. *Rix* it had become common practice for a medical practitioner treating at a hospital, without admitting him as an in-patient,
the victim of an accident, to communicate directly with the patient's
own doctor, even if the injury appeared superficial, *Chapman* v. *Rix*
would be no obstacle to a finding of negligence. But although *Chapman*
v. *Rix* is a case of little importance, the judgment of Romer, L.J., in
the Court of Appeal, included a significant passage on the criteria for
establishing medical negligence.

Having referred to evidence of eminent medical men in support of
the course Dr Rix had taken, his Lordship said that he knew of no case
in which a medical man had been held guilty of negligence when eminent
members of his own profession had expressed on oath their approval of
what he had done. He adopted the views of Lord Clyde in *Hunter* v.
Hanley[1] when he said that to establish liability by a doctor where
deviation from normal practice was alleged, it must be proved:

> that there was a usual and normal practice; that the defendant had
> not adopted that practice; and that the course the doctor had adopted
> was one which no professional man of ordinary skill would have taken
> if he had been acting with ordinary care.

(e) Failure of communication by hospital staff and negligent treatment by general practitioner

That it could be unsafe to regard *Chapman* v. *Rix* as a sure guide to
the limit of liability for failure of communication may be illustrated by
reference to *Coles* v. *Reading and District Hospital Management Committee and Another*,[2] in which the facts were not very dissimilar, yet
sufficiently differentiated to have justified the trial judge in not
following the House of Lords in *Chapman* v. *Rix*, if indeed, that case
was quoted to him, the short report in *The Times* giving no indication
whether it was or not.

The plaintiff in *Coles's* case was the father of a deceased man and
sued on behalf of the estate for loss of expectation of life and also for
special damages on the ground that his son's death had resulted from
negligent failure of communication by the staff of the hospital where he
had first been seen and from negligent treatment by the general practitioner who had attended him thereafter. The facts of the case were as
follows. At 8.40 a.m. on November 5th, 1959, a man who afterwards
died of tetanus was shovelling coal from a railway truck when a large
lump of coal fell on his hand, causing a crush injury to his left index

[1] [1955] S.L.T. 213.   [2] *The Times*, Jan 31, 1963.

finger. The wound was covered with dust and dirt and its nature was such that the deceased should have been given an anti-tetanus injection at the first reasonable opportunity. Immediately after the accident the deceased received first aid treatment and then went to Wallingford Hospital — a cottage hospital — at about 9.00 a.m. where he was examined by a nurse. After further examination by a sister, the nurse obtained instructions from the duty doctor by telephone,[1] whereupon she cleansed and covered the wound. The deceased was then instructed by the sister that he must proceed immediately to Battle Hospital at Reading for further examination and treatment. A friend who had accompanied him said he would drive him there. But the deceased did not then or at any time attend Battle Hospital. Instead, he went home, where he was seen by the second defendant, M his general practitioner, who told him to call the following day, November 6th. The deceased was seen again by M at his surgery on November 6th and 11th, and at the deceased's home on November 21st and 22nd. The wound became infected and the deceased was admitted to the Park Hospital, Reading, where he died of tetanus on November 25th. The judge found against both defendants on grounds of negligence. He said that it was manifestly clear that tetanus infection had entered through the wound on the occasion of the accident and also that if an appropriate anti-tetanus injection had been given on November 5th or 6th or within a day or two later, the deceased would probably still have been alive at the time of the hearing.

The finding of negligence against the hospital authority was on the ground of failure of proper communication. After some general observations on the duty of 'proper communication' which his Lordship defined as 'that which was reasonably necessary for safeguarding a patient's interests', he said that the responsibility of ensuring that a proper system of communication existed rested on whoever was in charge of a hospital. It should not be left to individual sisters or nurses to decide without any guidance. It was evident that there were many places where there existed difficulties of communication but the witnesses were reluctant to say what was reasonably necessary. . . . Turning to the particular case the judge said that having regard to the evidence as a whole the probabilities were that the deceased was not given to understand either the importance of his going to Battle Hospital or that there was any risk involved in not going. When transferring a patient from one hospital to another there ought to be some communication. Any system which failed to provide for adequate communication of the type in question was wrong, and negligently wrong. None of the potentially appropriate steps relating to anti-tetanus precautions were taken and that resulted from the breakdown in communications. His Lordship

[1] See footnote 1 on p. 240.

came to the conclusion that the hospital authorities were negligent.

The judge also found the general practitioner negligent, because he took the case too lightly. It seemed probable that, having learnt that the deceased had come from the hospital, the doctor assumed that all that was necessary had been done. It was clear that he should have made some inquiries. Had he done so, he would have been put on the right track and the deceased would still have been alive. Even taking the doctor on his own evidence that he had considered anti-tetanus and decided that no precautions were necessary, it was equally clear that he was neglecting elementary precautions.

The judge's criticism of the sister and the nurse having been left responsible for communication invites the further question whether, in the case of an injury of the kind in question, it is a reasonable system of working for the duty doctor to give directions on the telephone without having seen the patient. In effect that appears to be leaving responsibility for diagnosis to the nursing staff. Although, in this particular case, it might have made no difference had the duty doctor seen the patient, it may be suggested that if, on any occasion, a patien, suffered harm through not having been seen by a doctor at a hospitalt even at a cottage hospital, a finding of negligence against the hospital authority would be almost inevitable. It seems probable, too, that a doctor who attempted to deal with a hospital casualty case by telephone might also be made liable unless neither he nor any other practitioner could attend or it was most unlikely that he could have reached the hospital in time to be of any use.[1] That it would have been very inconvenient for a general practitioner on call as a member of the staff of a cottage hospital to deal with accident and emergency cases, or for any other practitioner similarly on call as a member of the staff of a hospital to have attended on a particular occasion, would not, in itself, be sufficient justification for relying entirely on the telephone for diagnosis and for instructions for treatment. Further, it may be suggested that if it is reasonably practicable in a larger hospital to obtain the attendance of a more senior member of the staff, even though at some inconvenience — a case should not be dealt with at night by a junior houseman which, at any other time, would certainly be seen by a specialist. However, a doctor might be able to avoid personal liability for not attending a patient if he could show that on the information available to him it was not necessary. To this extent communication by telephone is allowed.[2]

Coles's case differed from *Chapman* v. *Rix* in that the patient's own general practitioner was sued in *Coles's* case and not in *Chapman* v. *Rix*.

---

[1] The giving of instructions by telephone for the immediate treatment of a patient in an emergency pending the arrival of the doctor on the scene is an altogether different matter, whether such instructions be given to someone looking after the patient at home or to a member of the nursing staff of a hospital where the patient may be.

[2] *Cavan* v. *Wilcox* (1973) 44 D.L.R. (3d) 42 (New Brunswick Sup. Ct.)

Also, the hospital doctor, who advised the nursing staff on the telephone, was not made a party. Besides, there was the question of communication between one hospital and another.

(f) Casualty officer — negligent failure to see and examine patient

In *Barnett* v. *Chelsea and Kensington H.M.C.*,[1] the question of the duty of a hospital with a casualty department and of a medical casualty officer and of nurses working in such a department towards a patient presenting himself there complaining of illness or injury came up for consideration. The patient in this case, having been referred from the hospital casualty department to his own doctor without having been seen by the duty medical casualty officer, died a few hours later of arsenical poisoning. The circumstances were as follows: Three night-watchmen presented themselves at eight o'clock in the morning at the casualty departmant of St. Stephen's Hospital, London, a hospital for which the defendant hospital authority were responsible, complaining that they had been vomiting ever since drinking some tea three hours earlier. The nurse to whom they spoke reported their complaints *by telephone* to the duty medical casualty officer who thereupon instructed her to tell the men to go home and call in their own doctor. That she did. The men left and, some five hours later, one of them died from poisoning by arsenic which had been introduced into the tea. A claim being made by the widow of the deceased that his death had resulted from the defendants' negligence in not diagnosing or treating her husband's condition when he presented himself at the casualty department, Nield, J., held that since the defendants provided and ran the casualty department to which the deceased had presented himself complaining of illness or injury, such a close and direct relationship existed between him and them that they owed him a duty to exercise the skill and care to be expected of a nurse and medical casualty officer acting reasonably, notwithstanding that he had not been treated and received into the hospital wards. He also found that the medical casualty officer was negligent in not seeing, and not examining the deceased, in not admitting him to the wards and in not treating him or causing him to be treated and that, accordingly, the defendants were in breach of their duty to the deceased. Nevertheless, the plaintiff failed in her action because she failed to establish on the balance of probabilities that the negligence of the defendants had caused her husband's death, the judge accepting the view put forward by witnesses for the defence that the poisoned man must have died even had he been promptly admitted to hospital.

Giving judgment Nield, J., was at pains to say that he was not suggesting that a duty casualty officer at a hospital was obliged to see

[1] [1969] 1 Q B 428; [1968] 1 All E.R. 1068.

everyone who presented himself. 'If a receptionist, for example, dis-covers that the visitor is already attending his own doctor and merely wants a second opinion, or if the caller has a small cut which the nurse can perfectly well dress herself, then the casualty officer need not be called.' It must, however, be appreciated that this was *obiter*, since the judge had been able to decide without difficulty that the patient whose death had given rise to the action ought to have been seen. Even so, no one would doubt the first of the two examples given by his Lordship of visitors who need not be seen by a doctor. But the second example is more open to question since for a nurse to decide that the cut is so trifling that a doctor need not be called must involve her to a greater or less degree in diagnosis as well as in making a decision on what treatment is, in fact, necessary. What, for example, of a small wound, in itself trifling, but covered in dirt and dust for which, perhaps, an anti-tetanus injection should be given as well as a dressing applied? Here the treatment would surely be a matter for decision by a medical practitioner and, if an anti-tetanus injection had to be given it should be given by him or under his supervision, having regard to the patient's possible adverse reaction to it. That the Department apparently now accepts that every patient who presents himself at a N.H.S. hospital, at whatever time of the day or night he does so, should be seen by a doctor,[1] would seem to constitute a serious obstacle to a successful defence by a hospital authority in an action based on alleged negligence where a patient had been sent away without being so seen. Furthermore, in most instances, the facts would probably be sufficient to support an action for negligence against any medical practitioner on the staff of the hospital who had been a party to sending the patient away.

(g) *House officer acting reasonably in accordance with instructions of consultant, not negligent even though treatment given was inadequate*

In *Junor* v. *McNicol and Others*,[2] a Scottish case concerning a boy who lost his arm because of inadequate treatment in hospital, it was decided that a house officer is not personally liable on grounds of negligence if the treatment he gives a patient on the instructions of the

---

[1] See paragraph 18 of the memorandum sent to hospitals under cover of Departmental Circular H.M. (68) 11, dated March 25, 1968. The relevant passage reads as follows —
'. . . The hospital out-patient clinics for the treatment of addicts are therefore not planned to operate on a 24-hour basis, nor is it intended to provide facilities for addicts to obtain a prescription for heroin at any time of the day or night. But, *as in the case of all other patients*, it is important that an addict presenting himself at a hospital *at any time* should not be turned away by non-medical staff without being seen by a doctor on duty and, if the doctor considers it necessary, being given emergency treatment. . . .' (The italics are mine, J.J.) There seems here to be the further inescapable inference that, except by way of 'first aid' pending the arrival of a duty doctor, no treatment should be given by a nurse until the patient has been seen by a doctor and that even if the nurse's first aid may, in fact, appear to have met the patient's need, he should not be sent away until a duty doctor has satisfied himself that that is so.
[2] *The Times*, March 25, 1959.

consultant is faulty or inadequate, the house officer not being in charge of the case. Lord Kilmuir, L.C., in his judgment, speaking of the house officer, Dr McNicol, said there was no doubt that a mistake had been made in letting the boy out of hospital, but the question was whether Dr McNicol was negligent. There was no doubt that there was a duty on her to display the care and skill of a prudent qualified house surgeon, it being remembered that such a position was held by a comparative beginner. There was also a duty to carry out the instructions of the consultant . . . unless those instructions were manifestly wrong.

On the conflict of evidence his Lordship found it impossible to disbelieve Dr McNicol. On the probabilities he could not believe that a house surgeon, with her reputation, would have refrained from giving the boy the course of penicillin treatment, had those been her instructions. As to the fact that — of her own motion — she did give *some* penicillin the answer to that was that she felt herself bound to accept the consultant's view and treat this case as a simple fracture, in which case the patient would be discharged after the operation. But because she was unhappy about the wound she decided on the anti-tetanus serum and also penicillin as a prophylactic. It would seem unreasonable, and indeed unreal, to hold her guilty of negligence because she had been careful.[1]

Primarily her duty was to follow instructions. His Lordship did not question the authorities which stated that where instructions were manifestly wrong, duty and common sense combined to say that they must not be followed. But in view of the opinion which the consultant had conveyed in regard to the wound in this case, his Lordship could not say that it was one where Dr McNicol should have disregarded what she believed her instructions to be. On these facts the appellant had failed to show that Dr McNicol was 'in charge' of the case in the sense of being fully answerable for it. The appeal should be dismissed.

(*h*) *Extent of liability of member of medical staff senior to house officer acting on instructions or advice of a consultant*

There seems no reason to doubt that the decision in *Junor* v. *McNicol and Others* also fairly reflects the law of England. Presumably, the same principle applies to all hospital medical and surgical staff below the consultant grade when working on the instructions of a medical practitioner in a higher grade than themselves even though that senior officer is not the consultant ultimately in charge. For example, a house officer, in the absence of the consultant, is expected to accept instructions from a registrar who is working under the general supervision of the consultant on his cases. And it applies also even to the senior registrar who carries out the instructions of his chief. But in this case, his own quali-

[1] *i.e.*, she had gone a little beyond the instructions of her chief in the precautions she took.

fications often being the same as those of his chief, and his experience very much greater than that of a house officer, he, much more readily than a house officer, will presumably be held liable for negligence in carrying out instructions which he ought to have known were wrong.

(*i*) '*Special difficulties*' *as answer to claim in respect of injuries alleged to be due to negligence*

In *Williams* v. *North Liverpool Hospital Management Committee and Others*[1] the Court of Appeal allowed the appeal of the hospital management committee and the medical practitioner concerned, that administration of pentothal into the tissue of the patient's arm, instead of intravenously, to induce anaesthesia, thus causing injury to the arm was negligent. The difficulties the anaesthetist had to contend with were summed up by Hodson, L.J., as follows:

'The patient was exceedingly fat. This made her veins more difficult to find. The existence of fat was itself a handicap to the administration of pentothal because fat was not sensitive to pain, and one of the indications that pentothal had not gone into the vein but had gone into the tissues was the sensation of pain.'

Then, having outlined the course of events, he concluded that there was no basis for a finding of negligence against the doctor and that the appeal should be allowed.

Ormerod, L.J., concurring, said that no one would question the accuracy of the judge's (Elwes, J.) statement of the law:

'There are risks inherent in most forms of medical treatment, and anaesthetics is certainly no exception. All one can ask of a practitioner is that he should keep those risks to the minimum to which reasonable skill and care can reduce them. If he does this, no injury which occurs, however serious, will be actionable.'

(*j*) *Importance of expert evidence in rebutting claim based on alleged negligence in treatment*

The importance of expert evidence in any case involving an allegation of medical negligence causing injury to a patient is also illustrated by *Moore* v. *Lewisham Group Hospital Management Committee*,[2] another case in which the judgment and skill of an anaesthetist came into question. The patient had been anaesthetised by means of spinal anaesthesia (for the purpose of an operation for the removal of her gall bladder) as a result of which she suffered paralysis of the left leg. The plaintiff's case was that, having regard to the risks of spinal anaesthesia the operation should have been performed under one of the

[1] *The Times*, Jan. 17, 1959.　　　　[2] *The Times*, Feb. 5, 1959.

relaxant drugs. The judge, giving judgment for the defendant hospital authority, referred to the very great assistance given to the court by expert evidence of eminent anaesthetists, and said:

'No one suggested that Dr Piney was anything other than a highly competent anaesthetist or that he failed to acquaint himself with up-to-date techniques. . . . On the whole of the evidence it would not be difficult to find that on balance it might have been better for this operation to be performed under one of the relaxant drugs. But it was impossible to hold that Dr Piney's decision was a negligent one: it was one which could have been made by a competent and properly informed anaesthetist exercising a proper degree of skill and care.'

But *Moore's* case may be contrasted with *Smith* v. *Lewisham Group Hospital Management Committee*,[1] tried before Gorman, J., and a jury, in which a claim on grounds of negligence was made in respect of injury to a woman of eighty-six years of age who fell off a hospital trolley whilst left unattended for a few minutes. The judge, in his summing up, having directed the jury on negligence, referred to the expert evidence. A surgeon, Lord Uvedale, had given evidence that in his hospital, not a general hospital, there was one attendant per trolley night and day: he said that in his opinion it was unwise to leave the patient unattended, but — said the judge — he had not said it was improper. Also plaintiff's counsel had admitted in his speech to the jury that if the plaintiff had only been left unattended for thirty seconds, they might find it difficult to say there was negligence.

The jury having returned a verdict for the plaintiff with a rider that someone should have been in attendance at all times on a patient on a trolley or else the trolley should be supplied with guard rails, counsel for the defendant hospital authority moved that judgment be not entered for the plaintiff on the grounds that there was no evidence on which the jury could find for her. He asked that the court should hold as a matter of law, that to say that hospital staff must always, at all times, have an attendant upon a trolley was too high, and that there was no such duty. Gorman, J., said that he was not justified in determining the case purely because of the rider, or to say that that was the only reason why the jury came to their verdict. There was evidence which the jury could accept that the plaintiff had been left for four or five minutes. It was open to the jury to accept Lord Uvedale's evidence, speaking of leaving such a patient for four or five minutes, that 'it was unwise, it was a mistake, and it did cause serious injury'. He had given as his reason, in the first place, that an elderly lady of eighty-five or eighty-six should not be left unattended, and, taking that and other factors into account, he considered that the plaintiff should not have been left.

[1] *The Times*, June 21, 1955.

(k) Failure to protect patient from other risks

This case also raises the question of the duty owed by the hospital to protect a patient whilst he is in its care. The duty includes, in the case of a suicidal patient, such supervision as is reasonably practicable to prevent his making an attempt on his life. This is illustrated by *Selfe* v. *Ilford and District H.M.C.*[1] In that case a 17-year-old youth had been admitted to hospital after taking an overdose of sleeping pills. He was placed in a ground floor ward with a window — left open — at the back of his bed, his bed was grouped at one end of the ward with those of three other suicidal patients. He escaped through the window and climbed some steps to a roof, from which he threw himself, as a result suffering serious injuries. His claim against the hospital authority on, grounds of negligence succeeded. In his judgment, Hinchcliffe, J. adopted what had been laid down in *Thorne* v. *Northern Group H.M.C.*[2] as the duty of the hospital. They had to use reasonable care and skill in looking after the plaintiff. They had to use reasonable care to avoid acts and omissions which they could reasonably foresee would be likely to harm. The degree of care which was reasonable was proportionate to the degree of risk and to the magnitude of the mischief which might be occasioned. It was accepted that reasonable care demanded adequate supervision, which included continuous observation by duty nurses in the ward. There had been a breach of that duty by the hospital. To leave unobserved a youth of 17 with suicidal tendencies and an unlocked window behind his bed was asking for trouble.

There had been three nurses on duty in Selfe's ward and each knew that he was a suicide risk and had to be kept under constant supervision. Besides the charge nurse, there was another nurse who, just before the occurrence giving rise to the action, and without a word to the charge nurse, had gone to the lavatory. The third, a nursing auxiliary, went to the kitchen, neither of those nurses being able to see into the main ward. The charge nurse answered a call for assistance by a patient and went to him. Thus, no one had an eye on Mr Selfe, who was able to get out of bed. The judge thought that the charge nurse had been let down by the other two nurses. The incident should never have been allowed to happen, should not have happened, and would not have happened if three, or even two, nurses had been in the ward keeping Mr Selfe under observation. The case may be contrasted with one in which a subnormal patient ate a lavatory freshener and died of the consequent poisoning. In this case, which was not litigated, the Coroner found that no one was to blame.[3]

---

[1] *The Times*, Nov. 26, 1970.　　　[2] *The Times*, June 5, 1964.
[3] See Annual Report of the M.D.U. for 1971, at p. 46.

(l) Treatment given in an emergency, normal facilities not being available, or by a practitioner or nurse not specially qualified to give it

The cases which have been quoted are illustrative not only of the basis of liability for negligence in medical and nursing treatment which, after all, is but one application of a much wider principle of common law, but also illustrate the protection afforded to medical practitioners and others concerned, by the fairly high onus of proof on the plaintiff, except, that is, in cases where the doctrine of *res ipsa loquitur*[1] applies. *Cassidy* v. *Minister of Health*[2] and *Urry* v. *Bierer*[3] are cases in which the plaintiff relied on that doctrine. Further, it must be appreciated that an emergency may justify a practitioner or a nurse undertaking a procedure for which, strictly, he has not been trained. Thus, a general practitioner or some other medical practitioner acting outside his own speciality or normal sphere of work in an emergency who has done his best will be judged not according to the more exacting standards by which the work of a specialist would be judged but by what, in the circumstances, it is reasonable to expect of a practitioner who is not a specialist. Hence, whilst a general practitioner who undertook a surgical procedure beyond his competence when he could have referred the case to a surgeon, would be liable. He would not, however, be liable, if in an emergency, he did his best which, although inadequate, did not fall short of what could reasonably be expected of a general practitioner.

As a simple example might be suggested the case of a patient who came to harm through failure in aseptic technique. If something had to be done on the spot for victims of a road accident it can be imagined that the risk inevitably and therefore legitimately taken would be greater than it would be if a general practitioner tackled an emergency operation or put in stitches in his own surgery, or even at the patient's home. But even then, with the limited resources available, he could not be judged by the same standards as if he were working in hospital. His major

---

[1] *Res ipsa loquitur* in this context means no more than that where the thing giving rise to an accident (*e.g.* moving bales or barrels about on the top floor of a warehouse, or performing a surgical operation or giving other medical treatment) is shown to be under the management of the defendant or his employees and the accident is such as in the ordinary course of things does not happen if those who have the management use proper care, the injury itself affords reasonable evidence, in the absence of explanation by the defendant, that the accident arose from lack of care. (See Erle, C.J., in *Scott* v. *London and St. Katherine Docks Co.* (1865) 3 H. & C. 596). In *Lloyd* v. *West Midlands Gas Board* ([1971] 1 W.L.R. 749, 755), Megaw, L.J., said 'I doubt whether it is right to describe *res ipsa loquitur* as a "doctrine". I think that it is no more than an exotic, though convenient phrase to describe, what is in essence no more than a common sense approach, not limited by technical rules to the assessment of the effect of evidence in certain circumstances. It means that a plaintiff *prima facie* establishes negligence where: (i) it is not possible for him to prove precisely what was the relevant act or omission which set in train the events leading to the accident; but (ii) on the evidence as it stands at the relevant time it is more likely than not that the effective cause of the accident was some act or omission of the defendant or of someone for whom the defendant is responsible, which act or omission constitutes a failure to take proper care for the plaintiff's safety.' See also *Turner* v. *Mansfield Corporation* (1975) 119 S.J. 629. *The Times*, May 15, 1975.
[2] See p. 253 *et seq.*   [3] See pp. 260–263.

risk is a claim that, without necessity, he had attempted something which he ought to have known was beyond either his capacity or his resources.

It may perhaps be usefully mentioned that there is no case known to the editor of this book in any common law jurisdiction in which a doctor has been successfully sued for injuries inflicted by him on the victim of a road accident.

(m) *Medical practitioners in hospital hierarchy — extent of liability for failure to use requisite degree of skill in treating patient*

(i) *Generally.* In a hospital, between the specialist of consultant[1] rank and the newly qualified house officer come various grades of medical and surgical officer. Medical assistants, assistant dental surgeons and senior registrars are high up the professional ladder, standing in for consultants and carrying out operations and treatment unsupervised. Below them are registrars, practitioners of some experience — or gaining experience — in a particular specialty, who have either obtained, or are preparing for, a higher qualification. Below them again are the various grades of house officer,[2] the most junior in many hospitals being newly qualified medical practitioners, still only conditionally registered.[3] In any action for injury to a patient in which negligence is alleged, all these will be judged according to the skill they hold themselves out as possessing and the circumstances of the case. Thus a medical assistant, an assistant dental surgeon or a senior registrar in any specialty would ordinarily have to accept the full responsibilities of a specialist. A house officer if he had failed to use the skill of a specialist, when such skill was called for, would — like a general practitioner — have to justify his having undertaken something beyond his competence, *e.g.*, by pleading that in an emergency it had been impossible to obtain the help of a better qualified person.

It is apparent that the range of responsibilities that a house officer is qualified to undertake is more limited than that which senior members of the staff can perform. It is the more obvious if the houseman is only conditionally registered and is still engaged in serving the twelve months in approved hospital posts now a prerequisite of full registration. Consequently, the house officer is more likely to err not by negligently doing something he is qualified to do but by failing to seek the aid of a senior member of the staff when he should, and tackling something for which he had neither the skill nor the experience. Unless he has acted in an emergency, there being no more experienced practitioner available in time, he will have no defence if harm results, for by his very

---

[1] See also p. 257 for extract from judgment of Denning, L.J., in *Razzel* v. *Snowball* [1954] 1 W.L.R. 1382, 1386, in which case the position of the consultant was considered.
[2] There are also grades not mentioned, some of which are becoming obsolete.
[3] See p. 373.

actions he has claimed the requisite skill and will be judged as if he had it. Here it may be interpolated that if a house officer, on grounds of emergency, does escape personal liability for harm done to a patient by reason of his lack of special skill, it by no means follows that the hospital will also escape liability. The question of such vicarious liability is discussed later. As to the position of a houseman following the instructions of the consultant, the treatment ordered being inappropriate or inadequate (see *Junor* v. *McNicol* above).

(ii) *Nurses, midwives, members of professions supplementary to medicine etc.* The general principles by which are determined the limits of liability of a medical practitioner for injury to his patient apply equally in the case of nurses,[1] radiographers,[2] physiotherapists and pharmacists and of any other professionally qualified persons. Any such professionally qualified person is liable in damages if the patient suffers harm as a result either of his negligence or of his failing to exhibit that degree of skill which he had held himself out as possessing.

(iii) *Nurses in particular.* It is, however, more difficult to apply those principles if a nurse is concerned, if she has done something inefficiently and thus caused harm to the patient. This is because of the continuous, but sometimes barely perceptible, shifting of the dividing line between those things which are within the exclusive province of the medical profession and those which may properly be delegated to a trained nurse who has been properly instructed and trained in procedures necessary in a particular department. The giving of injections is a case in point; their number is now legion and their effects of varying gravity. Some injections — insulin is a case in point — patients are taught to give themselves; others, such as morphia, are usually administered by a nurse on medical orders; still others, such as spinal anaesthetics, are always administered by a doctor. But there will always remain debatable territory in this and in other procedures and it is beyond the scope of this work and of the editor's competence to discuss such matters.[3]

Somewhat similar problems arise as regards the competence of nurses of greater or less experience and qualifications. These are experienced, fully qualified ward and theatre sisters who, in their respective spheres can properly be assumed to be fully competent. There are staff nurses, also qualified, *i.e.*, on the appropriate part of the Register, but who may either have had experience as wide as the sister under whom they serve or who may only just have become fully fledged. But what of the State enrolled nurse, the requirements for admission to the Roll being significantly lower than those for admission to the Register? There are

---

[1] *Collins* v. *Herts. C.C.* [1947] 1 All E.R. 639.
[2] *Gold* v. *Essex C.C.* [1942] 2 K.B. 293; 58 T.L.R. 357; 2 All E.R. 237.
[3] Note however *Cavan* v. *Wilcox* (1973) 44 D.L.R. (3d) (New Brunswick Sup Ct.) discussed above, p. 240, and *Junor* v. *McNicol and Others, The Times*, March 25, 1959, above pp. 242–243.

no grounds in law for saying that an enrolled nurse may not become a fully responsible staff nurse or be promoted sister of a ward or department if the appointing authority is satisfied that the duties are within her competence. An obvious example might be appointment as sister in a geriatric ward. But even if an enrolled nurse were promoted sister in, say, a major surgical ward for which post her instruction as a pupil nurse might not have fitted her, that would not, in itself, afford proof that anything which went amiss with a procedure which she carried out was due to her incompetence. Also it must be appreciated that she might have learned by experience in such a ward after qualification as an enrolled nurse.

There are also student nurses who may be completely new hands and so of minimal use or who may have completed their training and be as competent as many staff nurses. Then there are pupil nurses and nursing aides and orderlies. It would be idle speculation here to try to decide what each should be allowed to do, either under supervision or unsupervised. Whilst, in law, if a nurse undertook some task beyond her competence and caused harm to a patient, she might be personally liable even though she had been ordered by her superior to do the task, if she knew or ought to have known that the order was wrong, it is fairly certain that if the authority for which she worked were joined in the action the nurse would, in such circumstances, be given full indemnity against it under the provisions of the Law Reform (Married Women and Tortfeasors) Act 1935.

What has been said about nurses is substantially true of radiographers and physiotherapists and student radiographers and student physiotherapists and of any other medical auxiliary such as a pathological laboratory technician who may undertake a procedure in connection with the treatment of a patient.

(iv) *Medical students, student radiographers or physiotherapists, etc.* Except for *Collins* v. *Herts. C.C.*,[1] which had special features, a senior medical student under war conditions having been employed as a house officer, there does not appear to be a case in which a claim has been made alleging negligence of a medical student or, for that matter, of a student radiographer or physiotherapist. But the principles would be substantially the same. The student acts carelessly, or attempts something beyond his competence, at his peril.

(n) *Liability of Secretary of State for harm to a patient or to a member of the staff of a hospital attributable to failure to communicate notice or warning of a danger of which the Department has been made aware by a report from a Health Authority. Position of an authority which fails to make such report*

[1] [1947] 1 All E. R. 639.

Under some departmental circulars, it is required that if a specified type of incident occurs which causes harm to a patient or to a member of the staff, or which might have caused such harm, the hospital authority or one of its officers report the incident to the Department. This is with the express intention of putting the Department into a position to advise or warn authorities managing other of the Secretary of State's hospitals. A question which presents itself, and one which has not yet reached the courts, is whether if harm to a patient or member of the staff in a N.H.S. hospital be caused by an incident of a kind which has already been reported to the Department as having happened in another hospital, the Secretary of State would be liable for negligence had there been failure by the Department to warn or advise the hospital where the second incident occurred. That question is most conveniently considered against the background of a departmental circular issued to hospital authorities in 1973,[1] being a strengthened version of one sent to them in 1967,[2] requiring immediate report to the Department of any incidents arising from defects in medicinal products and other medical supplies and equipment which lead to injury, however slight, and also of incidents where harm was avoided but potential danger suggested. Moreover, suspicion as well as hard facts are to be reported.[3]

The main purpose of the Department in requiring immediate report of any such incident is expressly stated to be 'so that warnings can be issued simultaneously when necessary to all authorities concerned[4] and appropriate action taken under the Medicines Act 1968 where medicinal products are affected.' The great importance the Department attaches to the requirements of the circular being observed is stressed in paragraph 18, which reads:

No arrangements can be effective unless hospital staffs at all levels have in mind that untoward incidents may have a significance going far beyond their own hospitals and that there is a duty in the interests of all patients and staff to see that they are reported even in some cases of suspicion only. Therefore doctors and hospital authorities should do everything within their power to see that all staff, both senior and junior, are conscious of their responsibilities in this respect. It may be that action on these lines is what is needed above all else. Without it, the reporting system will never be fully effective.

So, by clear inference from the terms of the circular, the Department which, by the National Health Service Act 1977 has the duty of providing the hospital service,[5] accepts that it has a duty to advise those authorities which manage the hospitals,[6] of dangers to patients and to staff which are brought to its notice. From this it seems inevitably to follow that the

---

[1] H.M. (73) 9.   [2] H.M. (67) 31, now cancelled.
[3] H.M. (73) 9, para. 6; see also paras. 7 and 8 for amplification.
[4] Not all Hospital Authorities are necessarily concerned. The use of a particularly sophisticated piece of equipment or scarce medicinal product may be restricted to a few hospitals.
[5] S. 2.   [6] S. 7.

negligent failure of the Department to give to authorities concerned any warning or other advice which ought to have been given following report of an incident within the terms of the circular, could form the basis of an action for damages by anyone who suffered harm attributable thereto.

It seems, however, more than a little doubtful whether there would be a good cause of action if the failure in communication had been between the authority managing the hospital where the first incident had occurred and the Department and not between the Department and the authority managing another hospital where subsequently someone suffers harm for want of the warning which ought to have been given. There seem to be no grounds, on which the injured person could claim from the authority where the breakdown in communication occurred, there being no relationship between that person and such authority and the chain of causation being too tenuous. But could the negligence of that authority be attributed to the Department, so as to make the Department answerable in damages to the person harmed in the second incident; this because of its own failure in communication? It is, to say the least, unlikely that, without more, a court would hold that the Department was, or ought to be, burdened with such vicarious liability.

2. Contributory Negligence

In any case in which damages for injury or loss due to negligence are claimed and the party sued satisfies the court that the plaintiff was himself guilty of negligence which contributed to those injuries or losses, *i.e.*, that had he taken due care and acted reasonably he could have avoided or lessened the loss or injury caused by the defendant's negligence the court will reduce the award of damages in proportion to the plaintiff's share of the responsibility. This also applies to actions for damages in respect of negligence leading to death of any person[1].

This book is not the place to discuss the operation of this branch of the law and all that can be usefully said is that when a dispute arises, the defendant's legal advisers would do well to consider whether such a defence may apply. It will, however, be noted that a doctor may be negligent not only in his diagnosis or the treatment he prescribes but also in failing to give adequate information to a patient about the future steps the patient should take.

A somewhat related topic, also not discussed in this book, is the duty on any person who suffers injury or loss at the hand of another, to take reasonable steps to limit the extent of the injury or loss and hence the damages. Whilst a defendant must take a plaintiff as he finds him, he is not bound to take the plaintiff's unreasonableness. Thus

[1] Law Reform (Contributory Negligence) Act 1945.

if a plaintiff was injured in an operation (on *e.g.* a swab was left inside him) he might be under a duty to submit to a further operation to limit the ill-effects of the injury.[1] On the other hand if the further operation were serious or dangerous it might be reasonable for him to refuse. In the former case, the doctor in the first operation would be liable for not the actual injuries suffered but for (*a*) causing the necessity of the second operation and (*b*) the extent of the injuries would probably have been suffered had the second operation been performed. In the second case the doctor would be liable for all the injuries suffered.

3. Vicarious Liability

(*a*) *Application of principle*

The general principle that if a person does anything negligently when he owes a duty of care, and harm results, he is answerable in damages applies no less if the person who is under the duty to take care, has entrusted the actual task to an employee or agent. Such are the grounds of vicarious liability of employers for acts of their employees.[2] The test is whether the employer has undertaken responsibility. If he has, it makes no difference that he can only carry out the undertaking through the intervention of an employee or agent possessed of special skill or qualifications. But as Denning, L.J., pointed out in his judgment in *Cassidy's* case[3] it may be relevant to a decision on vicarious liability to know whether the actual wrongdoer was an employee or an agent, if the wrongdoing was in some collateral matter. Thus, to take one of Denning, L.J.'s, illustrations, if an employer has a lamp which overhangs his front door he is under a duty to use reasonable care to see that it is safe and he cannot escape that duty by employing an independent contractor to do it. He is liable, therefore, if the contractor fails to discover a defect which a reasonably careful man would have discovered and the lamp falls and injures a passer-by, but he is not liable if, whilst doing the job, the independent contractor drops a hammer on someone's head. On the other hand, if the man's own employee had been doing the job and had dropped a hammer his employer would be liable.

If then it were accepted that a hospital undertook to provide treatment for patients, the way would seem clear for a simple statement that the Health Authority was liable for harm resulting to a patient from the negligence or incompetence of any member of the staff, including

---

[1] See *F. Morgan* v. *T. Wallis* [1974] 1 Lloyds Rep. 165 and *Steel* v. *R. George* [1942] A.C. 497.

[2] See cases referred to by Denning, L.J., in *Cassidy* v. *Ministry of Health* [1951] 2 K.B. 343, 363.

[3] *Ibid.*, pp. 364–5.

medical staff,[1] whether employed whole-time or part-time and whether under a contract of service or a contract for services. This was the view expressed by Denning, L.J., in *Cassidy's* case[2] and also in *Roe* v. *Minister of Health, Woolley* v. *Same*,[3] a view with which the present editor respectfully agrees.[4] But the majority of the court both in *Cassidy*[2] and in *Roe*[3] felt unable to make a clean break with the line of cases beginning in 1909 with *Hillyer* v. *St. Bartholomew's Hospital*[5] which was at one time taken as authority for the view that hospital authorities were not liable for the acts of their medical staff, but only for not taking due care in making appointments. In later years *Hillyer's* case had been distinguished most decisively by a majority in *Cassidy's* case, so that the apparent non-liability of a hospital authority was limited to consultants employed under a contract for services, it being held in that case that a hospital authority would be liable for the negligence or incompetence of a whole-time officer employed under a contract of service even though qualified as a specialist and working as a surgeon. Thus the majority judgments in the Court of Appeal in *Cassidy's* case appeared to make liability or non-liability of the hospital authority depend on the nature of its contract with the surgeon or physician concerned, a most unreal distinction, which left the patient's possible recourse against the hospital for negligent injury to be determined by reference to a contract to which he was not a party and of the terms of which he could know nothing. Fortunately the difficulties created by the majority judgments in *Cassidy's* case seem now to have been largely removed by the judgments delivered in the Court of Appeal in *Roe* v. *Minister of Health, Woolley* v. *Same*.[6]

In *Roe's* case two patients in a voluntary hospital, before that hospital had been taken over by the Minister of Health under the Health Service Acts, suffered serious injury by reason of injection with a spinal anaesthetic contaminated with phenol which had seeped through microscopic cracks in the ampoules. The injured men alleged negligence on the part of the anaesthetist and, the hospital having been taken over, they sued the Minister as successor to the liabilities of the former voluntary hospital under s. 6 (2) of the 1946 Act. It was finally decided that the anaesthetist had not been negligent. The trial judge[7] had also held, on the authority of *Gold* v. *Essex C.C.*[8] and of the majority judgments in *Cassidy's* case,[9] that the hospital authority was not liable

---

[1] The hospital or Health Authority would also be vicariously liable for the negligence of a medical student who helped in the treatment of patients or who — as part of his medical education — was allowed to examine them, *etc.* Whether the student received any remuneration for such work as he performed would be wholly immaterial to the question of vicarious liability.

[2] [1951] 2 K.B. 343.
[3] [1954] 2 Q.B. 66; 2 All E.R. 131.
[4] It was also Dr Speller's view.
[5] [1909] 2 K.B. 820.
[6] [1954] 2 Q.B. 66; 2 All E.R. 131.
[7] McNair, J.
[8] [1942] 2 K.B. 293; 58 T.L.R. 357; [1942] 2 All E.R. 237.
[9] [1951] 2 K.B. 343.

for the wrongful acts and omissions of the anaesthetist, whom he assimilated to the consulting physicians and surgeons referred to by Lord Greene in *Gold's* case.[1] On appeal, the trial judge's finding that there had been no negligence was upheld, but his finding that the hospital authority would not in any event have been liable was not approved. This is of special significance having regard to the terms of the anaesthetist's contract, which certainly was not one of employment.

In 1940 the anaesthetist G and another P had been appointed visiting anaesthetists to the hospital being between them under obligation to provide a regular anaesthetic service for the hospital, it being left to them to decide how to divide up the work. The hospital set aside a sum of money out of their funds derived from investments, contributions and donations for division among the whole of the medical and surgical staff, including visiting and consulting surgeons as the participants might decide. Dr G participated in the fund but otherwise received no remuneration from the hospital. He was at all times allowed to continue his private anaesthetic practice. Somervell, L.J., accepting those as the facts and that the trial judge, on the authority of *Gold's*[2] case and of his own and Singleton, L.J.'s, judgments in *Cassidy's* case,[3] had concluded that Dr G was a consultant for whom the hospital was not responsible said:

'The line suggested in that case[4] and in *Cassidy's* case in the judgments of Singleton, L.J., and myself may not be a very satisfactory one but I would have regarded Dr P and Dr G as part of the permanent staff and, therefore, in the same position as the orthopaedic surgeon in *Cassidy's* case. . . . The position of surgeons and others under the National Health Service Act 1946, will have to be decided when it arises. The position of hospitals under the Act may or may not be different from when they were voluntary or municipal hospitals.'

Denning, L.J., consistently with his judgment in the *Cassidy* case said:

'. . . I think that the hospital authorities are responsible for the whole of their staff, not only for the nurses and doctors, but also for the anaesthetists and the surgeons. It does not matter whether they are permanent or temporary, resident or visiting, whole-time or part-time. The hospital authorities are responsible for all of them. The reason is because, even if they are not servants, they are the agents of the hospital to give the treatment. The only exception is the case of consultants or anaesthetists selected and employed by the patient himself.'[5]

The concluding sentence of this extract from the judgment of Denning, L.J., is his reconciliation of his decision in this and in *Cassidy's* case[6] with *Hillyer* v. *St. Bartholomew's Hospital*.[7]

[1] [1942] 2 K.B. 293; 58 T.L.R. 357; [1942] 2 All E.R. 237.
[2] [1942] 2 K.B. 293.   [3] [1951] 2 K.B. 343.
[4] *i.e., Gold's* case.   [5] [1954] 2 W.L.R. at p. 922.
[6] [1951] 2 K.B. 343.   [7] [1909] 2 K.B. 820; 78 L.J. (K.B.) 958.

Morris, L.J., was no less definite. He said, '. . . I have come to the conclusion that Dr G was the servant or the agent of the hospital.' Then applying the test suggested by Lord Greene, M.R., in *Gold's* case[1] he reached the conclusion that the hospital had in this case undertaken the responsibility, *inter alia*, for anaesthetising the patient for the surgical operation. He adopted Lord Green's opinion that in such case the principal cannot escape liability because he has employed another person, whether an employee or agent, to discharge the obligation on his behalf, and that that is equally true whether or not the obligation involved the use of skill. Hence, although the work Dr G was employed to do at the hospital was work of a highly skilled and specialised nature the hospital authority did not avoid the application of the rule of *respondeat superior*. But although Morris, L.J., thus came down in favour of the vicarious liability of the voluntary hospital authority for the work of a visiting anaesthetist he left open the question of liability for visiting surgeons saying:

'If a patient in 1947 entered a voluntary hospital for an operation it might be that if the operation was to be performed by a visiting surgeon the hospital would not undertake, so far as concerned the actual surgery itself, to do more than to make the necessary arrangements to secure the services of a skilled and competent surgeon. The facts and features of each particular case would require investigation.'[2]

It seems that here Morris, L.J., was perhaps paying undue deference to the majority judgments in *Gold's* case[1] and in *Cassidy's* case[3] especially as neither did, in fact, involve directly consideration of the extent of the liability of a hospital authority for a visitng member of the staff. After all, Somervell, L.J., has since himself indicated that the line drawn may not have been a very satisfactory one. Moreover, in *Roe's* case the terms and conditions of appointment of the anaesthetists were indistinguishable from those of the other senior visiting staff — physicians and surgeons. How then could it seriously be suggested that the hospital authority could be made liable for the negligence of the anaesthetist but not for that of the surgeon? The only way out of the dilemma appears to be that taken by Denning, L.J., *i.e.*, to say that the only consultants for which a hospital authority was not liable were those selected and employed by the patient.

That a hospital authority, now Health Authority, under the National Health Service Act being under a duty to provide hospital accommodation and medical and nursing treatment is vicariously liable for the negligence of its staff in the performance of their duties, whether in respect of treatment of patients or otherwise, has never been in doubt, save only in the case of the specialists, whose title in the hierarchy is 'consultant'.[4]

---

[1] [1942] 2 K.B. 293.   [2] [1954] 2 Q.B. 66; [1954] 2 All E.R. 131.
[3] [1951] 2 K.B. 343.   [4] See p. 248 as to grades in the hospital medical hierarchy.

Many consultants are also in private practice and, by the terms of their contract, committed to only a specified number of hospital, clinic or health centre sessions per week. In the early days of the National Health Service, many of them tended to regard themselves as outside experts distinguishable from other hospital medical staff in the nature of their relationship both to the patient and to the hospital authority with whom they were in contract.

That specialists might be in a fundamentally different position from other hospital medical staff received some slight — very slight — support from the wording of s. 3 (1) of the National Health Service Act 1946 which — until repealed and replaced by s. 2 (2) of the National Health Service Reorganisation Act 1973[1] — set out the hospital and specialist services it was the duty of the Secretary of State to provide. They included '(a) hospital accommodation; (b) medical, nursing and other services required for the purposes of the hospitals; (c) the services of specialists, whether at a hospital, a health centre . . . , or a clinic, or, if necessary on medical grounds at the home of the patient, . . .' However, in Razzel v. Snowball,[2] the Court of Appeal, before whom it was sought to establish that specialists within s. 3 (1) (c) of the 1946 Act were not public servants within the protection of s. 21 of the Limitation Act 1939[3] although other medical practitioners employed by hospital authorities and falling within s. 3 (1) (b) were, firmly rejected that contention. In the course of his judgment Denning, L.J., said:[4]

'An attempt was made to distinguish between doctors and nurses under paragraph (b) and specialists under paragraph (c). It was conceded that doctors and nurses were carrying out the duty of the Minister but it was said that specialists were not. I cannot see any justification for this distinction. All of them, doctors, nurses and specialists, are carrying out the Minister's duty to treat the sick. . . .'

and later,[5]

'. . . whatever may have been the position of a consultant in former times, nowadays, since the National Health Service Act 1946, the term consultant does not denote a particular relationship between a doctor and a hospital. It is simply a title denoting his place in the hierarchy of the hospital staff. He is a senior member of the staff but nevertheless just as much a member of the staff as the house surgeon. Whether he is called specialist or consultant makes no difference. He, like all the others, is just carrying out the duties of the Minister. . . .'

Birkett, L.J., in a concurring judgment, was no less emphatic. He said that the Minister's duty was not merely to provide the men but also the services. Of the defendant in the case, he said:

[1] Now 1977 Act s. 3 (1).   [2] [1954] 1 W.L.R. 1382; 3 All E.R. 429.
[3] S. 21 has since been repealed.
[4] [1954] 1 W.L.R. 1382, 1385; [1954] 3 All E.R. 429, 432–3.
[5] [1954] 1 W.L.R. 1382, 1386. See also Higgins v. North-West Metropolitan Hospital Board and Bach [1954] 1 W.L.R. 411; 1 All E.R. 414.

'It seems plain that what Mr Snowball was doing was that which the Minister through the Board had appointed him to do. The act that he did, therefore, was done as an agent of the regional board, or the agent of the Minister, and, in so doing, he brought himself entirely within the words of section 21 (1) of the Limitation Act. . . .'[1]

Morris, L.J., said:

'It is clear that the position in this case cannot be affected by the circumstance that Mr Snowball was engaged only as to part of his time; nor can it in any way affect the position that he was exercising his skill in a manner for which he was specially qualified, so that it would be inappropriate for anyone to interfere while he was in the actual course of doing what he thought best in a particular case. He was engaged by the Minister to give certain services which were a part of the hospital and specialist services which it was the duty of the Minister to provide'[2]

Apparently no hospital authority under the National Health Service Act 1946, when sued for the negligent or otherwise wrongful acts of a consultant or other member of its medical staff in the course of his duties has ever pleaded non-responsibility. Indeed the basis of the Minister's agreement with the medical defence societies, embodied in Circular H.M. (54) 32,[3] appears to be his acknowledgment of the fact that hospital authorities are vicariously liable for the acts and omissions of medical staff, including consultants, to the like extent to which they are vicariously liable for the acts and omissions of nurses and other members of the staff of their hospitals who may be concerned with the treatment of patients.

Before leaving the general topic of the basis of vicarious liability, it must be recalled that an inadequate system of working or inadequate rules for correlating the work and responsibilities of different persons may be evidence upon which a finding of negligence may be made against a Health Authority even though no single individual had been demonstrably negligent in carrying out his duties. Moreover it must be appreciated that failure of a Health Authority to take precautions advised by the Secretary of State in an official circular might well invite a finding of negligence.[4]

The question of vicarious liability in respect of injuries to patients making a strictly limited payment towards cost of accommodation in a single room or a small ward — the so-called amenity bed — does not call for special consideration. Such patients do not pay for treatment nor do they, or can they, make a separate contract for medical or surgical attendance as can patients received as private in-patients under s. 65 of the National Health Service Act 1977 or treated as private out-patients under s. 66 of that Act. In all other respects their position is identical with that of the normal Health Service patient.

[1] [1954] 1 W.L.R. at p. 1387.   [2] Ibid at p. 1388.   [3] For text see pp. 725–728.
[4] See above, pp. 250–252.

The position would however be different in the case of a patient paying charges designed to cover full cost of hospital accommodation and services[1] under ss. 65 or 66 of the National Health Service Act 1977, when the possible liability of a hospital for negligence would depend on whether the alleged negligence were that of a medical practitioner — usually a consultant — with whom the patient had made a private contract and for whose acts and omissions the authority was, therefore, not liable, or of some employee or agent of the authority — whether medical or domestic — for whose acts and omissions in the course of duty it was responsible.

In theory, though not usually in practice, it is possible for a patient to have pay-bed accommodation without being attended by a consultant with whom he has made a private contract. In such case the patient would pay the hospital at a higher daily rate than would a patient who was receiving privately arranged specialist treatment, to take into account all necessary medical and surgical services, including the cost of the necessary services of hospital consultants,[2] who would not receive any extra remuneration for attending him. In such circumstances the authority would be undertaking the whole treatment of the patient and doing so for reward. That the authority would then be vicariously liable for the negligence of any of those — including consultants — who actually treated the patient on its behalf is an inescapable conclusion.

But it is usually the case that a private patient is admitted under the care of a consultant on the staff of the hospital with whom the patient has made direct contract to pay for specialist services.[3] But even when a private patient makes his own arrangements with one or more consultants, he still has the services of junior professional medical or surgical staff of the hospital, as well as of nursing staff and of hospital facilities generally. Everything, except what the patient has arranged for his own consultant to do, is nominally taken into account in calculating the charge to be made. The exact charge is determined by the Secretary of State.

In the result it seems clear that the authority will not ordinarily be liable for the negligence of a consultant chosen and employed by the

---

[1] Such patients may still exist despite the passage of the Health Services Act 1976. See above p. 105.

[2] The additional charge made is usually much below what the patient would have had to pay a consultant with whom he made a private contract but it must be borne in mind that such a patient would have no greater right than a general ward patient to the services of any particular consultant and that, not being bound by a private contract, any consultant attending him could delegate responsibility for the care of the patient to such extent as he thought proper. Some degree of delegation is also proper when there is a private contract but then there still remains the contractual obligation on the consultant who, for example, could not properly delegate his obligation to perform an operation.

[3] The patient may, in fact, have contracted privately for the services of more than one consultant, e.g., a surgeon, a radiologist and a pathologist. Alternatively he might rely on the hospital for such supporting services on the hospital staff.

patient or his relatives but it will be liable for the negligence of members of the hospital staff of whatever kind and grade whose services are meant to be covered by the charge made by the Health Authority. Hence the authority would not be liable for the negligence of the consultant surgeon — although a member of its staff — because he would not be treating the patient by virtue of his contract with the authority but by virtue of his contract with the patient. But the authority would be liable for the negligence of a registrar or house surgeon who looked after the patient between visits of the consultant and for whose services the hospital was being paid. Similarly, the hospital would be responsible for the negligence of nurses, physiotherapists and other members of the staff.

But though when a private patient in hospital is attended by a consultant under a separate contract made by him or on his behalf or for his benefit — the distinction between those for whose actions the authority is liable and those for whose actions it is not liable is tolerably clear, the practical possibility of a successful claim against the authority is much smaller than in the case of the normal type of Health Service patient. The reason for this is made clear by reference to *Cassidy's* case.[1] The plaintiff in that case left hospital in a worse state than he entered it. He went in with two crippled fingers and left with four. Making his claim against the hospital authority, he asserted negligence, but could not say who had been negligent. It might have been the specialist, a houseman, a sister, a nurse, or any two or more of them. In these circumstances, he therefore relied on the doctrine *res ipsa loquitur* and won his case against the hospital. But had the consultant been employed, not by the hospital but by the patient, to substantiate his claim against the hospital the patient would ordinarily either have had to prove positively that some one person or more for whom the hospital was responsible had been negligent or, at least, bring evidence to prove that the circumstances were such as to show that someone on the hospital staff other than the consultant — or consultants — had been negligent. In short, where a private patient who has employed his own consultant or consultants, suffers harm as a result of alleged negligent treatment and brings an action for damages, he will as a rule find the doctrine of *res ipsa loquitur* of much less use, his chance of success thereby being correspondingly reduced.

However, even so, the doctrine can be of assistance in a case such as *Urry* v. *Bierer and Another*,[2] where both the operating surgeon and the proprietor of the nursing home were sued on grounds of alleged negligence for harm suffered by a patient through a swab being left in after an operation. The surgeon was sued for his own alleged negligence

---

[1] [1951] 1 T.L.R. 539; 1 All E.R. 574.
[2] (1955) *The Times*, July 15 (C.A.).

in failing to remove the swab and the nursing home on grounds of the alleged negligence of the theatre sister who had miscounted and told the surgeon that all the swabs and packs were accounted for. The action succeeded against both defendants, the plaintiff apparently having the benefit of the doctrine of *res ipsa loquitur* against both. In effect the Court of Appeal held that the surgeon should have known what swabs and packs he had put in and where and was negligent if he failed to remove them but that insofar as the nurse had been at fault in telling him all the swabs and packs were accounted for her negligence had contributed to the mistake and so the nursing home was vicariously liable for her negligence. Each of the defendants were, therefore, made liable for half the damages.

(b) Liability of negligent employee to indemnify his employer

It has in the past been generally accepted that an employer is entitled to indemnity from the employee whose negligence had resulted in damages being awarded against the employer. The decision in *Jones* v. *Manchester Corporation and Others*[1] made the proposition seem doubtful and was some authority for the view that the employer's right of indemnity was restricted to apportionment of liability at the discretion of the Court under the Law Reform (Married Women and Tortfeasors) Act 1935.

In *Jones's* case a patient suffered harm as a result of the negligence of an anaesthetist of house officer status and little experience. On grounds that they had allowed a doctor of such slight experience to administer pentothal, the trial judge ordered the Regional Hospital Board fully to indemnify the doctor against the damages under the Act of 1935. The Board appealed and the appeal was allowed. Singleton and Denning, L.JJ., held that the Hospital Board were negligent not merely vicariously, and that the doctor was negligent not only through inexperience but also in some degree in not carrying out what she had been taught. They apportioned responsibility as to 20 per cent on the doctor and 80 per cent on the Board. Hodson, L.J., who dissented, would have granted full indemnity to the Board. Denning, L.J., referring to the suggestion made on behalf of the Board that an employer who was made liable for the negligence of an employee was entitled to indemnity, said that he knew of no case in which that had actually been decided and he could see no contractual basis for such indemnity. The issue was entirely a matter for the discretion of the Court exercised under the 1935 Act whether it should order any, and if so, what contribution or indemnity between them.

The opinion expressed by Denning, L.J., although important was not binding and indeed the other members of the Court did not indicate

[1] [1952] 2 Q.B. 852.

agreement with it. In *Lister* v. *Romford Ice and Cold Storage Co. Ltd.*[1] the House of Lords rejected Denning, L.J.'s, *dictum* and asserted an implied contractual obligation of an employee to indemnify his employer against the vicarious liability for his negligence. Viscount Simonds and Lord Morton of Henryton said that the employer was also entitled to recover contribution from the servant under the Law Reform (Married Women and Tortfeasors) Act 1935: In the course of their opinions both Viscount Simonds and Lord Somervell of Harrow cited with approval and in support of the proposition that a servant impliedly undertakes to exercise due skill — carrying with it the duty of reasonable care — the judgment of Wiles, J., in *Harmer* v. *Cornelius*:[2]

'When a skilled labourer, artisan or artist is employed, there is on his part an implied warranty that he is of skill reasonably competent to the task he undertakes — *Spondes peretiam artis*. Thus, if an apothecary, a watch-maker or an attorney be employed for reward, they each impliedly undertake to possess *and exercise* reasonable skill in their several arts.'

Lord Somervell of Harrow added by way of gloss that the learned judge was saying that the skilled labourer of the first sentence is under the same contractual obligation to his master as those mentioned in the second sentence are to their customers and clients. This serves to underline the point that it matters not whether a member of the medical or surgical staff of a hospital is employed under a contract of service or a contract for services: he will in either case be liable contractually to the employing Health Authority for any loss occasioned by his failure to use reasonable skill, unless such implied term is expressly excluded.[3]

As regards the policy of the Department on the bringing in of medical practitioners and dentists as co-defendants when a Health Authority under the National Health Service Act 1977, is sued for negligence, reference should be made to Departmental Circular H.M. (54) 32, printed in Appendix D at p. 725. The policy laid down in the circular must make the way of the plaintiff harder as does the questionable device referred to on p. 351 for throwing the cloak of professional privilege over all routine reports of accidents — including injuries to patients — in hospital. The Departmental circular there referred to (H.M. (55) 66) is also set out in an Appendix at p. 743 *et seq.*

(c) *Vicarious liability of nursing home proprietor*

Powel v. *Streatham Manor Nursing Home*[4] is authority for the proposition that the proprietors of a private hospital or nursing home are liable for injury caused to a patient by the negligence of nurses or

---

[1] [1957] A.C. 555. See also the case in the C.A. at [1956] 2 Q.B. 180.
[2] [1858] 5 C.B. (N.S.) 236.
[3] As to the measure of responsibility of the professional man with special reference to the surgeon see *Mahon* v. *Osborne* [1939] 2 K.B. 14, and see above, p. 228 *et seq.*
[4] [1935] A.C. 243.

others employed by the nursing home for the treatment of a patient. In that case a patient's bladder was punctured by the negligence of two trained nurses using a catheter and the proprietors of the nursing home were held liable. Since, however, patients in nursing homes almost almost invariably arrange for their own medical attendant — surgeon, physician, obstetrician or gynaecologist — and also on the advice of their consultant, for the help of ancillary specialists, radiologists, pathologists and the like, an aggrieved patient would find the same limits to reliance on the doctrine *res ipsa loquitur* as would a private patient in hospital, as to which see *Urry* v. *Bierer and Another*.[1]

(*d*) *Vicarious liability when hospital services are provided for the Secretary of State under contractual arrangements*

(i) *In a voluntary hospital.* That a corporate or unincorporated body responsible for the administration of a voluntary hospital[2] is vicariously liable for the negligence of any member of the staff of the hospital in the course of his duties if that negligence causes injury or loss to a N.H.S. patient treated in the hospital under contractual arrangements entered into with it by a Health Authority acting on behalf of the Secretary of State[3] does not seem open to question. Moreover, since the contracting Health Authority is itself responsible on behalf of the Secretary of State for providing hospital care and treatment to N.H.S. patients, that Authority will also be vicariously liable for negligent injury to such a patient suffered in the voluntary hospital.[4] This is so, not because it is directly answerable for the negligence of members of the staff of the voluntary hospital but because it is vicariously liable for the failure of its agent, the voluntary hospital, to provide proper care and treatment, for the injured N.H.S. patient.

If, in respect of such negligent injury to a N.H.S. patient in a voluntary hospital, the contracting Health Authority alone were sued, of course, it would have a right of indemnity against its agent, the voluntary hospital unless any such right were excluded by contract. But it would have no right of indemnity against the negligent member of the staff of the voluntary hospital, there being no contractual nexus between them and so no duty of care owing by him to the Authority. If, however, the Health Authority claimed indemnity from the voluntary

---

[1] *The Times*, July 15, 1955.
[2] As to voluntary hospital governing bodies and the extent of any personal liability of their members, see Chapter 4, p. 54. When in this part of this chapter reference is made to the liability of voluntary hospitals it is shorthand for the liability of trustees, board or committee responsible for the institution.
[3] It is conceivable that, in exceptional circumstances, any such contractual arrangements have been entered into directly by the Secretary of State. In such case any rights and liabilities of the kind discussed in this part of the chapter would be directly those of the Secretary of State.
[4] C.f. *Razzel* v. *Snowball* [1954] 1 W.L.R. 1382; 3 All E.R. 429.

L

hospital, that hospital in turn could seek indemnity from any member of the staff whose negligence had given rise to the claim.[1]

The position would be different if a N.H.S. patient being treated in a voluntary hospital suffered injury in consequence of the negligence of a visiting medical practitioner, say a consultant, in contract with the Health Authority and not with the voluntary hospital. Clearly the Health Authority would be vicariously liable for the consequences of his negligence; but whether the voluntary hospital, with which the negligent practitioner had no contractual nexus, would also be so liable, if sued, is a matter of some uncertainty. On balance it may be suggested that the hospital would be responsible because, so far as the injured patient was concerned, it would have been the voluntary hospital which had taken immediate responsibility for his treatment. If in such circumstances the voluntary hospital were sued, it could look for indemnity not only to the negligent practitioner but also to the Health Authority as being vicariously answerable for him. But should it be that it were held that the voluntary hospital was not vicariously liable for the acts of such a visiting practitioner and the facts were such that, as in *Cassidy* v. *Ministry of Health*,[2] the plaintiff could not establish exactly who had been negligent though seemingly someone must have been and so sought to rely on *res ipsa loquitur* to shift the burden of proof to the defendant, his chance of doing so successfully would be much diminished. The only prudent course would seem to be to make the Health Authority as well as the voluntary hospital a defendant.

(ii) *In a nursing home*.[3] The extent both of vicarious liability and of rights of indemnity of a nursing home proprietor in respect of the negligent injury of any N.H.S. patient received for treatment by virtue of contractual arrangements with a Health Authority is the same as that of a voluntary hospital in like circumstances.

(e) Vicarious liability of agency supplying nurse to hospital

An agency which undertakes to supply nurses — sometimes, not always accurately, called a 'cooperation' — is not as a rule the employer of the nurse supplied and will not ordinarily therefore be liable either to the patient or to the employing Health Authority for her wrongful acts and omissions. But if an agency has agreed either expressly or by implication to supply, say, a state registered nurse, and the nurse

---

[1] Ordinarily a Health Authority desirous of claiming indemnity against a voluntary hospital would bring it in as co-defendant in any action for damages brought against it. If so brought in, the voluntary hospital could similarly bring in any allegedly negligent person the consequences of whose conduct it might be held responsible.

[2] [1951] 2 K.B. 343; 1 T.L.R. 539; 1 All E.R. 574.

[3] In this section *nursing home* means any institution, large or small, receiving patients, not being a charitable institution. (For purposes of registration voluntary hospitals are also classed as nursing homes. See p. 454 *et seq.*)

supplied is not so qualified, it is probable that the cooperation would be held liable for any loss consequent on her not exhibiting the degree of competence and care expected of a state registered nurse. There may be other circumstances, too, in which liability might arise but such possibilities are too speculative for discussion here.

4. Personal Liability of Members of Governing Body or Proprietors

Where it has been stated that there is any liability on a hospital or nursing home under any of the foregoing heads it means, of course, that the liability falls on the proprietors or responsible authority. There may or may not be a *personal* responsibility on the members of the governing body.[1]

The extent of any personal responsibility may be summed up as follows:

A public authority, e.g., a Regional, Area or special Health Authority under the National Health Service Act 1977, is liable in its corporate capacity only; the members, as such, are under no personal liability to the injured party.[1]

If a voluntary hospital or a nursing home is incorporated with limited liability either by Royal Charter, or special Act of Parliament or under the Companies Act 1948, the members of the governing body are under no personal liability unless they have exceeded the powers they are entitled to exercise under the Charter, Act, or memorandum of association of the hospital or nursing home and the injury has arisen therefrom and they are sued personally. Hence any judgment awarding damages against an incorporated hospital or nursing home can be enforced only against the assets of the incorporated body.

If a nursing home is unincorporated, the proprietor or proprietors are personally answerable in damages in any of the aforementioned cases when the employer is under a vicarious liability for the acts of his servants or for the dangerous state of the premises.

If a charitable hospital is unincorporated, the better opinion appears to be that the subscribers, even though they may have voting rights as regards the appointment of the members of the governing body, are under no personal responsibility for the liabilities of the institution. It may, however, be relevant in deciding the question of liability of subscribers in any particular case to consider whether the voting power is conferred only as a result of formal application to become a 'governor' or whether it is a right automatically conferred by virtue of subscription and possibly even without the knowledge of the subscriber. In the latter

[1] The nature and extent of personal responsibility of members of hospital governing bodies is discussed fully under appropriate heads. See p. 37 particularly as to members of Health Authorities under the National Health Service Act 1977 and p. 54 *et seq* as to members of governing bodies of voluntary hospitals.

case it might also be relevant to consider whether the right had ever been exercised and how recently.

The members of the governing body are probably personally responsible for the liabilities of the hospital but if they have acted properly they are entitled to indemnity out of the available assets of the hospital, which can then be used directly to satisfy the liability.

5. Addition of Defendants

If a Health Authority is sued for damages for injury due to alleged negligence of a member of its staff it may have that person joined as co-defendant and, if the plaintiff succeeds, the court will apportion liability for damages or give one or other co-defendant full indemnity under the provisions of the Law Reform (Married Women and Tortfeasors) Act 1935. This is of course without prejudice to the plaintiff's right to recover in full from either co-defendant. Similarly, a member of the hospital staff who is sued personally, if he alleges that the Health Authority or some other member of the staff is blameworthy in the matter, can have the authority or such other person joined as a co-defendant. Then, as in the former case, if damages are awarded the court will either apportion liability or give one co-defendant the right of full indemnity against the other or others.

6. Limitations of Actions

(a) Generally

Under the Limitation Acts 1939–1975, an action must be brought within a specified period from the date of the account of the cause of action.[1] Since the passing of the Law Reform (Limitation of Actions, etc.) Act 1954 actions in tort against public authorities and public officials must be brought within the same period of time as would be applicable in the case of any other defendant. The effect of the expiry of the limitation period is to bar the remedy but not the right to it and accordingly a defendant who wishes to rely on the Limitation Acts must specially plead it in his defence.

The period for actions founded in tort and simple contract is generally six years.[2] However, where the claim is for damages for negligence, nuisance or breach of duty (whether the duty exists by virtue of a contract or of provision made by or under a statute or independently of any contract or any such provision) where the damages claimed by the plaintiff for the negligence, nuisance or breach of duty consist of or include damages in respect of personal injuries to any person, the

---

[1] The day itself on which a cause of action occurs is not included in computing the period of limitation, Kaur v. Russell [1973] 1 All E.R. 617.
[2] Limitation Act 1939 s. 2 (1).

period is reduced to three years.[1] Personal injuries for the purpose of the subsection include any disease and any impairment of a person's physical or mental condition.[2]

In *Letang* v. *Cooper*,[3] the Court of Appeal held that these words were wide enough to include all tortious breaches of duty, including trespass to the person, so that an action in trespass, no less than an action for negligence, was statute barred after three years. Lord Denning said: 'the truth is that the distinction between trespass and case is obsolete. . . . Instead of dividing actions for personal injuries into trespass (direct damage) or case (consequential damage) we divide the causes of action now according as the defendant did the injury intentionally or unintentionally.'[4]

In respect of any claim falling within s. 2A of the Limitation Act 1939, it is important to appreciate that the shorter period of limitation applies whether it is the injured person himself suing or someone else who may have suffered loss through his injury. Moreover, if a plaintiff couples in a single action a claim in respect of personal injuries to himself or another, being an injury caused by negligence, nuisance or breach of duty, and therefore within the section, and also a claim in respect of some other damage suffered as a result of the same negligence, nuisance or breach of duty, the period of limitation in respect of the whole cause of action is three years, not six. As to the possible effect of concealed fraud[5] on the period of limitation and the possibility of an action being commenced out of time where facts of a decisive character were outside the knowledge of the plaintiff, reference should be made to later sections of this chapter.

(b) *Extension of period of limitation; Persons under a disability (including minors)*

For the sake of completeness it may be mentioned that s. 22 of the Limitation Act 1939 which, broadly, provides that when a person to whom a right of action has accrued was under a disability, the period of limitation is extended until six years from the date when the disability ceased or the person died, whichever event first occurred, is amended to reduce the period to three years in those cases of negligence, nuisance or breach of duty for which three years is now the normal period. Under the 1963 Limitation Act the period was not extended at all in such cases unless the plaintiff proved that the person under the disability

---

[1] This provision is now contained in s. 2A of the 1939 Act having been added by s. 1 of the 1975 Act. It was formally contained in s. 2 (6) of the 1954 Act.
[2] See 1939 Act s. 31 as amended by the 1954 and 1975 Acts.
[3] [1965] 1 Q.B. 232 (C.A.). *Letang* v. *Cooper* was a case of direct but accidenta l injury. See also *Long* v. *Hepworth* ([1968] 1 W.L.R. 1299; [1968] 3 All E.R. 248) a case of intentional trespass in which Cooke, J., both agreed with and considered himself bound by *Letang* v. *Cooper*.
[4] [1964] 1 Q.B. 232, 239.   [5] Limitation Act 1939, s. 26.

was not, at the time when the right of action accrued to him, in the custody of a parent. This provision has been abolished by the 1975 Act. Accordingly time does not begin to run against a minor until his eighteenth birthday.

The meaning of *disability* is made clear by s. 31 of the 1939 Limitation Act. Section 31 (2) (as amended) says:

'A person shall be deemed to be under a disability while he is an infant or of unsound mind.'

And s. 31 (3) as amended says that a person is of *unsound mind* if either he is liable to be detained or be subjected to guardianship under the Mental Health Act 1959 or he is still, without a gap, receiving treatment as an in-patient in a hospital or mental nursing home without being liable to be detained after having been liable to be detained.

(c) The period of limitation in personal injury cases

As already stated, the general rule in personal injury cases is to limit the period of limitation to three years.

It was held in *Cartledge* v. *E. Jopling and Sons Ltd.*[1] that where a plaintiff did not know and could not have known even with proper medical advice that he had been injured, nevertheless time ran against him under the 1939 Act. This was generally felt to be an injustice. Accordingly Parliament and the Courts have endevoured to provide a remedy. Parliament has done so in successive Statutes in 1963, 1971 and 1975. The Courts have been busy interpreting these Statutes. This book is not the place to enter into a discussion of the subtle changes of law or of policy which can be discerned throughout these events. It suffices here to set out the law on the basis of the 1975 legislation.

By s. 1 of the Limitation Act 1975 new sections are added to the 1939 Act. The new section 2A of that Act now says:

(1) This section applies to any action for damages for negligence, nuisance or breach of duty (whether the duty exists by virtue of a contract or of provision made by or under a statute or independently of any contract or any such provision) where the damages claimed by the plaintiff for the negligence, nuisance or breach of duty consist of or include damages in respect of personal injuries to the plaintiff or any other person.

(2) Section 2 of this Act shall not apply to an action to which this section applies.

(3) Subject to section 2D below, an action to which this section applies shall not be brought after the expiration of the period specified in subsections (4) and (5) below.

(4) Except where subsection (5) applies, the said period is three years from —

(*a*) the date on which the cause of action accrued, or

(*b*) the date (if later) of the plaintiff's knowledge.

[1] [1963] A.C. 758.

(5) If the person injured dies before the expiration of the period in sub-section (4) above, the period as respects the cause of action surviving for the benefit of the estate of the deceased by virtue of section 1 of the Law Reform (Miscellaneous Provisions) Act 1934 shall be three years from —

(a) the date of death, or

(b) the date of the personal representative's knowledge,

whichever is the later.

(6) In this section, and in section 2B below, references to a person's date of knowledge are references to the date on which he first had knowledge of the following facts —

(a) that the injury in question was significant, and

(b) that that injury was attributable in whole or in part to the act or omission which is alleged to constitute negligence, nuisance or breach of duty, and

(c) the identity of the defendant, and

(d) if it is alleged that the act or omission was that of a person other than the defendant, the identity of that person and the additional facts supporting the bringing of an action against the defendant.

and knowledge that any acts or omissions did or did not, as a matter of law, involve negligence, nuisance or breach of duty is irrelevant.

(7) For the purposes of this section an injury is significant if the plaintiff would reasonably have considered it sufficiently serious to justify his insti-tuting proceedings for damages against a defendant who did not dispute liability and was able to satisfy a judgment.

(8) For the purposes of the said sections a person's knowledge includes knowledge which he might reasonably have been expected to acquire —

(a) from facts observable or ascertainable by him, or

(b) from facts ascertainable by him with the help of medical or other appropriate expert advice which it is reasonable for him to seek,

but a person shall not be fixed under this subsection with knowledge of a fact ascertainable only with the help of expert advice so long as he has taken all reasonable steps to obtain (and, where appropriate, to act on) that advice.

(9) For the purposes of this section 'personal representative' includes any person who is or has been a personal representative of the deceased, including an executor who has not proved the will (whether or not he has renounced probate) but not anyone appointed only as a special personal representative in relation to settled land; and regard shall be had to any knowledge acquired by any such person while a personal representative or previously.

(10) If there is more than one personal representative, and their dates of knowledge are different, subsection (5) (b) above shall be read as referring to the earliest of those dates.

In this way, the section specifies the period of limitation as being three years. The time runs from either the date of the accrual of the cause of action or, if it is later, the date when the plaintiff first had knowledge of the cause of action (see sub-section 4). The section then goes on to define (as best it can) what it means by this (see sub-section (6)). It will be noted that the mischief disclosed in *Cartledge* v. *Jopling*[1] is dealt with by the section. In that case the plaintiff had no reason even to consult medical advisors about any industrial injury until after three

[1] [1963] A.C. 758.

years from the date when by his employers negligence he had in fact been injured. However, even if he had consulted them they would not have been able to link his physical state with damage done to him by dust getting into his lungs. Under this section, first his injury would not have appeared 'significant' (see sub-sections (6) and (7)) and secondly he would not have had knowledge that the injury was attributable to negligence or breach of duty (see sub-sections 6 (b) and 8).

The new sub-section 2D of the 1939 Act, deals with the question of what is to happen to a plaintiff whose delay in bringing an action, apparently barred even by the relatively liberal provisions of s. 2A, is understandable.

It provides:

(1) If it appears to the court that it would be equitable to allow an action to proceed having regard to the degree to which —
(a) the provisions of section 2A or 2B of this Act prejudice the plaintiff or any person whom he represents, and
(b) any decision of the court under this subsection would prejudice the defendant or any person whom he represents,
the court may direct that those provisions shall not apply to the action, or shall not apply to any specified cause of action to which the action relates.

(2) . . .

(3) In acting under this section the court shall have regard to all the circumstances of the case and in particular to —
(a) the length of, and the reasons for, the delay on the part of the plaintiff;
(b) the extent to which, having regard to the delay, the evidence adduced or likely to be adduced by the plaintiff or the defendant is or is likely to be less cogent than if the action had been brought within the time allowed by section 2A or as the case may be 2B;
(c) the conduct of the defendant after the cause of action arose, including the extent if any to which he responded to requests reasonably made by the plaintiff for information or inspection for the purpose of ascertaining facts which were or might be relevant to the plaintiff's cause of action against the defendant;
(d) the duration of any disability of the plaintiff arising after the date of the accrual of the cause of action;
(e) the extent to which the plaintiff acted promptly and reasonably once he knew whether or not the act or omission of the defendant, to which the injury was attributable, might be capable at that time of giving rise to an action for damages;
(f) the steps, if any, taken by the plaintiff to obtain medical, legal or other expert advice and the nature of any such advice he may have received.

(4) In a case where the person injured died when, because of section 2A, he could no longer maintain an action and recover damages in respect of the injury, the court shall have regard in particular to the length of, and the reasons for, the delay on the part of the deceased.

(5) In a case under subsection (4) above, or any other case where the time limit, or one of the time limits, depends on the date of knowledge of a person other than the plaintiff, subsection (3) above shall have effect with appropriate modifications, and shall have effect in particular as if references to the

plaintiff included references to any person whose date of knowledge is or was relevant in determining a time limit.

It will be noted that whereas under the new s. 2A, ignorance that the known facts give rise in law to a cause of action does not prevent time from running, under the new s. 2D bad legal advice is not an absolute ban to bringing an action. Under s. 2D the Court is bound to consider the balance of advantage between plaintiff and defendant and in addition to consider the above named factors.

Perhaps some indication of the way in which the Courts will use the discretion given them by s. 2D is offered by *Buck* v. *English Electric Co.*[1] where the plaintiff realised he might have a claim in 1963 but his condition continued to worsen and, he to work, until 1973. The writ was not issued until 1975. The action was thus barred under s. 2A but, although the delay had been inordinate, the defendant had not, on the facts, been prejudiced thereby and the action was allowed to proceed.

The new ss. 2B and 2C as well as certain sub-sections of 2D deal with the period of limitation in actions for death under the Fatal Accidents Act 1976.[2] Broadly speaking the time is three years from the death or the date of knowledge of the person for whose benefit the action is brought but reference should be had to the sections.

Finally, in this brief discussion of the 1975 legislation, it is still important to note that s. 3 applies the Act to causes of action which accrued before as well as after it came into force and this is extended to cases where leave to bring an action was either given or refused under the 1963 Act.

(*d*) *When the person having the cause of action is unaware of it owing to the concealed fraud of the potential defendant*

If it can be established that the plaintiff could not with reasonable diligence have obtained knowledge of his right of action earlier, due to the fraud of the defendant or to his having done the wrongful act furtively, then the plaintiff's cause of action is deemed to arise when he could with reasonable diligence have become aware of his right.[3]

---

[1] [1977] 1 W.L.R. 806. But compare *Davies* v. *B.I.C.C. The Times*, 15th February 1977.

[2] The Fatal Accidents Act 1976 consolidates the previous Fatal Accidents Acts. It gives a right of action to certain relatives in respect of the death of one of the family. Such a course of action is additional to the right of the deceased to sue — which right is not extinguished by the death (Law Reform (Miscellaneous Provisions) Act 1934). The reader who requires to know more of these matters is referred to standard works on the law of torts.

[3] Limitation Act 1939, s. 26. The word *fraud* does not here imply any degree of moral turpitude (*Beaman* v. *A.R.T.S. Ltd.* [1949] 1 K.B. 550; 65 T.L.R. 389; [1944] 1 All E.R. 465). What is referred to is *equitable fraud* which 'covers conduct which, having regard to some special relationship between the parties concerned, is an unconscionable thing for the one to do towards the other' (Lord Evershead, M.R., in *Kitchen* v. *Royal Air Force Association and Others* [1958] 1 W.L.R. 563, 572, 573). In *Gerber* v. *Pines* (1935) 79 Sol. Jo. 13, du Parq, J., held that as a general rule a doctor who found that he had left some foreign substance in a patient's body should tell the patient at once, though there were exceptions Concealment, unless justified, would, therefore, amount to equitable fraud.

But what is the position when a surgeon has injured a patient by his negligence in performing an operation or has done the patient harm by performing the wrong operation (*e.g.*, through two patients getting mixed up and the wrong one taken to the operating theatre) and the patient is not told what has happened, although it is known to the surgeon and, possibly, to other hospital officers, the injury being one of which the patient could not be aware unless informed? As an example, an incident of which Dr Speller was credibly informed may be taken. Two female patients were mixed up and one, who needed but minor surgical treatment, was subjected to a major gynaecological operation which inevitably resulted in her being unable to have children, this without preventing sexual intercourse, so that she would have been unaware of what had happened. She was not told of the wrongful act, apparently on the ground that the surgeon, having consulted her family doctor, reached the conclusion that it was not desirable that she should be told because of the possible ill effect on her mental and physical health. In such case, is a claim to damages statute barred after the normal period of three years?

The answer seems to be that if the surgeon had no valid and special reason for his reticence the patient would have her right of action on grounds of concealed fraud at any time within three years of the time when, with reasonable diligence, she could have discovered the wrong. This seems to be the conclusion to be derived from s. 26 of the Limitation Act 1939 and *Gerber* v. *Pines*.[1] Accordingly it appears that the scope for s. 26 in personal injury cases has been considerably cut down by the amendments to the 1939 Act in the 1975 legislation, since a similar result could be obtained by applying s. 2A if or need be s. 2D. However, s. 26 still stands and the discussion of it is included in this book since there are differences between it and the new sections in the 1939 Act added in 1975.

(e) Time-limit for claiming contribution between joint tortfeasors

It is beyond the scope of this work to make any close examination of the rules relating to contribution between joint tortfeasors but it may here be noted that under s. 4 of the Limitation Act 1963,[2] a tortfeasor who has become entitled to a right to recover contribution from a joint tortfeasor, must bring his action within two years from the date on which the right accrued to him, being either the date on which the tortfeasor had judgment given against him or an award made on any arbitration, or, he having admitted liability, the date on which the amount to be paid to discharge that liability was agreed. This could be relevant in a hospital case.

[1] [1935] 79 Sol. Jo. 13; see also footnote 3 on p. 271.
[2] This section is amended in one minor respect but not repealed by the 1975 Limitation Act.

(f) Dismissal of action for want of prosecution

Detailed discussion of the circumstances in which the court will dismiss, for want of prosecution, an action which — although commenced in time — has since gone to sleep for an unreasonable time is outside the scope of this book. It fits badly into a section on limitation of actions. Nevertheless, attention may be directed to *Allen* v. *Sir Alfred McAlpine & Sons Ltd.; Bostock* v. *Bermondsey and Southwark Group Hospital Management Committee;* and *Sternberg and Another* v. *Hammond and Others*,[1] all three cases being applications by defendants for dismissal of an action for want of prosecution and in respect of all of which judgment was delivered at the same time. The second action, the only one in which the defendant's application was not successful was by a nurse who alleged injury through the negligence of her employers. One of the factors in the decision of the court in that case was that the hospital authority had itself failed to deliver a defence.

In *Birkett* v. *James*[2] the House of Lords discussed the question of dismissal during the currency of the limitation period. They held that this should only apply where there was a breach of an order as to the time for taking a step in the action.

7. The Congenital Disabilities (Civil Liability) Act 1976

This statute was passed after this chapter had gone to press. It is however too important to be omitted from this edition and its provisions are noted in Appendix G on pages 783–786.

[1] [1968] 2 Q.B. 229; [1968] 1 All E.R. 366 (C.A.). *Trotter* v. *Lambeth, Southwark and Lewisham A.H.A.* (T.), *The Times,* 6th November 1976 (action brought just within limitation period but undue delay in serving statement of claim. Held a fair trial no longer possible); *British Insulated Callender's Cables* v. *Keir, The Times,* 9th November 1976 (delay before the issue of the writ is as material as the delay thereafter and the court should consider the totality of the delay); *Pryer* v. *Smith,* [1977] 1 All E.R. 218. (court has power to fix time limits for the future conduct of an action subjected to delay); and *Towli* v. *Fourth River Property Co., Michaelides* v. *Cormican Properties, The Times,* 24th November 1976 (where there has been 'scandalous' delay, the solicitors responsible may be ordered to pay the costs of the action personally).

[2] [1977] 3 W.L.R. 38. *See also Unsworth* v. *Hill (Probert, Third Party) The Times,* 5th July 1977.

CHAPTER 15

LIABILITY FOR SAFETY OF PREMISES

A. INTRODUCTORY

THE subject of possible liability for harm to person or property caused by the condition of the premises where the accident happens, or by things done or omitted to be done on such premises, is here being dealt separately from other causes of liability for negligence because of the very considerable modification of the common law rules effected by the Occupiers' Liability Act 1957, and the Defective Premises Act 1972.

Broadly the Occupiers' Liability Act 1957 placed upon the occupier of premises the duty to exercise the *common duty of care*[1] for the reasonable safety of all *visitors*,[2] which expression substantially includes all persons lawfully on the premises. Furthermore, the occupier is ordinarily also responsible for the reasonable safety of the personal property of visitors,[2] except so far as he may lawfully have modified or excluded responsibility.[3] The Defective Premises Act 1972 concerns the extent of the responsibility of landlords and contractors for personal injury when the state of the premises which has caused or contributed to injury to a person thereon is attributable to the fault of any such landlord or contractor. The Health and Safety at Work etc. Act 1974 sets out a broad range of duties owed by employers to their employees and to the general public and by the occupiers of premises to those using plant or substances provided for their use there. However, the provisions of these Acts are considered in this chapter only so far as is necessary to understand their application to hospital patients, patients' visitors and similar categories. The position of employees, contractors' men, and the like on hospital premises is no different from what it would have been had they been working elsewhere and is only touched on in this chapter.[4] The next section of the chapter in which is examined the extent of the responsibility of an occupier of premises of the safety of a trespasser, had to be completely rewritten for this edition because of the effect of the application of the 'neighbour principle' by the House of Lords in *British Railways Board* v. *Herrington*[5] in favour of an injured trespasser. Finally, briefly discussed in this chapter as possibly affecting hospitals, are the cognate subjects of injury to persons or property not on the premises where the cause of injury originates from the hospital, and

[1] S. 2 (1).   [2] S. 1 (2).   [3] S. 2 (4).
[4] The Act is further discussed below in the Ch. 23 on Injury at Work.
[5] [1972] A.C. 877; [1972] 1 All E.R. 749.

with interference with the quiet enjoyment and normal use of other premises in the neighbourhood, *i.e.* nuisance, and also interference with easements such as the right of light enjoyed by prescription or agreement.

B. INJURIES TO PERSONS LAWFULLY ON HOSPITAL PREMISES

1. Basic terms: Occupiers and Visitors

Before the coming into force of the Occupiers' Liability Act 1957, and leaving aside questions relating to users of public and private rights of way, as well as the statutory and common law obligations of an employer for the safety of his employees, the extent of the responsibility of the occupier of premises either to warn anyone coming onto those premises of any danger there, or to protect him against such danger, depended on whether that person was an invitee, a licensee or a trespasser. Both invitees and licensees were persons on the premises with the express or implied permission of the occupier: the trespasser was there without permission. The distinction between invitees and licensees, now no longer significant, was that invitees were on the premises for a purpose in which the occupier had a material interest whilst licensees were not.

Now, under the Occupiers' Liability Act 1957, all who would have been either invitees or licensees at common law are included in a single category as *visitors*,[1] the invitee being no longer specially favoured, nor the licensee discriminated against. It is also expressly provided that for the purposes of s. 2, which sets out the duty of an occupier to visitors, that persons who enter premises for any purpose in the exercise of a right conferred by law are to be treated as persons permitted by the occupier to be there for that purpose, whether they in fact have his permission or not.[2] In the Act *occupier* has the same meaning as it has at common law[3] in respect of duties owing to invitees and licensees. Also, the rules laid down in the Act in relation to an occupier of premises and his visitors apply in like manner and to the like extent as the principles applicable at common law to an occupier of premises and his invitees or licensees would apply to regulate:

(*a*) the obligations of a person occupying or having control over any fixed or moveable structure, including any vessel, vehicle or air-craft; and

(*b*) the obligation of a person occupying or having control over any premises or structure in respect of damage to property, including the property of persons who are not themselves his visitors.

[1] S. 1 (2).   [2] S. 2 (6).   [3] S. 1 (2).

2. Extent of Occupier's Ordinary Duty

The occupier's ordinary duty to visitors under the Act of 1957 is laid down in s. 2 (1) as follows:

An occupier of premises owes the same duty, the 'common duty of care' to all his visitors, except in so far as he is free to and does extend, restrict, modify or exclude his duty to any visitor or visitors by agreement or otherwise.[1]

3. Common Duty of Care

The definition of the 'common duty of care' is contained in ss. 2 (2)–(5) of the Act. Section 2 (2) provides:

The common duty of care is a duty to take such care as in all the circumstances of the case is reasonable to see that the visitor will be reasonably safe in using the premises for the purpose for which he is invited or permitted by the occupier to be there.

The above definition, including as it does the expressions *such care as in all the circumstances of the case is reasonable* and also *reasonably safe* means that basically the decision in any particular case will usually turn on matters of fact rather than on points of law.

An example, of particular relevance to hospitals, of failure to exercise 'such care as in all the circumstances of the case is reasonable' is afforded by *Marshall* v. *Lindsey County Council*[2] in which case a patient was negligently admitted to a local authority maternity home when there was danger of infection from puerperal fever and did in fact contract the disease.

A somewhat different example is afforded by *Weigall* v. *Westminster Hospital*,[3] in which a visitor enquiring about a paying patient suffered injury as the result of slipping and falling on an unsecured mat on a polished floor. He was awarded damages because there was a concealed danger of which he was not warned and therefore had no opportunity of avoiding. Whether or not anything turned on *Weigall* having been an invitee rather than a bare licensee would be no longer relevant. In *Slade* v. *Battersea and Putney H.M.C.*,[4] also decided before 1958, the plaintiff was a wife who was invited by the hospital to visit her dangerously ill husband in a general ward at any time. Having visited him out of normal visiting hours, she fell and injured herself whilst leaving the ward, her fall being caused by an area round the door of the ward

---

[1] The precise limits within which a hospital authority might restrict or modify its common law duty of care are further discussed on p. 286 *et seq.*

[2] [1937] A.C. 97.

[3] [1935] 51 T.L.R. 554.

[4] [1955] 1 W.L.R. 207; [1955] 1 All E.R. 429. Following *Dunster* v. *Abbott* [1954] 1 W.L.R. 58. Incidentally, it was also held in this case that the plaintiff had a 'material interest' in being on the premises so as to make her an invitee rather than a licensee. See above, p. 275.

having been rendered dangerous by being covered with floor polish prior to final polishing.[1]

The examples which have been cited — although pre-1958 — are all illustrations of how s. 2 (1)–(2) of the Occupiers' Liability Act 1957 would apply to situations peculiar to hospitals. But it must also be appreciated that a Health Authority is liable to visitors in the same way as other occupiers of premises for more common dangers such as defective or badly lit stairs, defective gutterings and the like.

Moreover, quite apart from the provisions of s. 2 (3) (discussed below) the duty on the occupier of premises to take reasonable care to make the premises '*reasonably safe for the purposes for which* (*the visitor*) *is invited or permitted . . . to be there*' import that in the case of both in-patients and out-patients, it is the duty of the occupier, *e.g.*, the Area Health Authority, to take all reasonable precautions for their safety, taking into account their physical and mental[2] condition. Hence, what precautions it may be necessary for an authority to take for the reasonable safety of patients may well be greater than would be expected of an occupier whose premises were not for the care and treatment of the sick.[3]

Section 2 also provides:

(9) The common duty of care does not impose on an occupier any obligation to a visitor in respect of risks willingly accepted as his by the visitor (the question whether a risk was so accepted to be decided on the same principles as in other cases in which one person owes a duty of care to another).

In other words, wide as the section is, it does not affect the common law rules summed up in the expression *volanti non fit injuria*.

Sub-sections (3) and (4) of the Act offer greater guidance on the meaning of the common duty of care. Sub-section 2 (3) says:

(3) The circumstances relevant for the present purposes include the degree of care, and of want of care, which would ordinarily be looked for in such a visitor, so that (for example) in proper cases:

(*a*) an occupier must be prepared for children to be less careful than adults; and

(*b*) an occupier may expect that a person, in the exercise of his calling, will appreciate and guard against any special risks ordinarily incident to it, so far as the occupier leaves him free to do so.

---

[1] Seemingly, knowledge of the state of the floor and the question of warning were equally immaterial in *Slade's* case. since it was reasonable for someone confronted with such slippery floor and having no other way out, to walk over it, taking reasonable care in so doing. See now s. 2 (4) (*a*) of the Occupiers' Liability Act 1957. *London Graving Dock* v. *Horton* ([1951] A.C. 737) is now no longer law.

[2] But mentally disordered patients and those whose faculties have been impaired by age or illness might also be within s. 2 (3). See below, p. 280.

[3] It seems likely, however, that occupiers of premises generally to which the public may have access, *e.g.* offices and shops, no less than hospitals, must foresee and guard against injury to blind persons through unusual hazards. This is illustrated by *Haley* v. *London Electricity Board* ([1965] A.C. 778) which, though not decided as falling within the provisions of the Occupiers' Liability Act 1957, concerned an ineffectively guarded excavation in a public thoroughfare, resulting in injury to a blind man using that thoroughfare.

Moreover, the duty of an occupier to exercise care to see that the premises are safe for visitors extends not only to the condition of the premises themselves but of things in those premises which may have been provided for the use of visitors, or which visitors might reasonably be expected to use, *e.g.* chairs.[1]

Section 2 (3) says that the relevant circumstances will include the degree of care or lack of care to be expected of the visitor himself, by way of example on the one hand, that an occupier must be prepared for children to be less careful than adults and, on the other, that he may expect that a person, in the exercise of his calling, will appreciate and guard against any special risks ordinarily incident to it. These examples, by being embodied in the definition, have become part of the law. But if other circumstances were relied on, by either plaintiff or defendant, as 'circumstances' within s. 2 (2), the judge would have to consider whether they were circumstances appropriate to be taken into account, having regard to the guidance given in s. 2 (3), which does not restrict the meaning of the term to 'the degree of care of want of care' of which examples are given, but rather puts beyond argument that the expression 'all the circumstances of the case' in the definition in s. 2 (2) is wide enough to bring things mentioned in s. 2 (3) within its scope.

The degree of care for the safety of a child which is to be expected of hospital staff was subject of judicial comment in *Gravestock and Another* v. *Lewisham H.M.C.*[2] The case concerned a child of nine years of age who, when running down the ward and swinging on the doors, tripped on a stud and ran into one of the glass-panelled swing doors, thereby suffering injury from broken glass. What the child had been doing at the time of his injury was contrary to the rules. Streatfield, J., dismissed a claim for damages against the Hospital Authority, not being prepared to hold that there had been any lack of proper supervision, notwithstanding that the accident had happened whilst the orderly was absent for a few minutes to get the pudding course. He said that the duty of the hospital towards a child of nine was no greater than that of a schoolmaster, which is that of an ordinary prudent parent.

In his judgment in *Gravestock's* case, Streatfield, J., also referred to

---

[1] *Baxter* v. *St. Helena Group H.M.C.* (*The Times*, Feb. 15, 1972) is not more than a persuasive authority on this point, since it related to an accident which occurred to a member of the staff and could have been decided solely on the basis of the employer's duty to provide safe plant and equipment. A nurse was injured because a chair in the nurses' changing room had collapsed under her. The collapse had been due to extensive infestation with woodworm which would have been apparent on reasonable examination. It was admitted that the defendant Hospital Authority had no system of inspection of furniture at all. Giving judgment in the Court of Appeal, Davies, L.J., said that it was the duty of every employer to take reasonable care to provide and maintain proper plant and equipment, and it seemed to him that chairs, *whether sat on by nurses or patients* (my italics, J.J.) came within that context and therefore the hospital authorities should have had some system of inspection. They had none.

[2] *The Times*, May 27, 1955.

the judgment of Denning, L.J., in *Cox* v. *Carshalton H.M.C.*[1] and which also had turned on adequacy of supervision in a hospital ward. It concerned a child who, whilst in bed suffering from a certain degree of disability, had been left to manage a jug of hot inhalant on a tray, something which she had done quite successfully before. Unfortunately, whilst the nurse was out of the room attending to another patient, the jug tipped over and the child suffered injury. It was held that there had been no failure in supervision, regard being also had to the fact that it was in the child's own interests to have been encouraged to do things for herself.

Two points have to be made on the judgments in *Gravestock* and *Cox* cases. First, whilst *Gravestock* was one concerning the use of premises; *Cox* was rather more concerned with matters incidental to treatment. Despite the different context, the same considerations applied. secondly, whilst the cases are authority for the statement that the standard of care required in a hospital is that of an ordinary prudent parent, it does not follow that another case where the facts were somewhat similar to those in *Cox* or in *Gravestock* would necessarily be decided the same way. In particular, and with respect, it may be questioned whether in the circumstances of *Cox* a reasonably prudent parent would have left so disabled a child unattended to manipulate a jug of water so hot that injury would result if it overturned, or whether, having regard to the provisions of s. 2 (3) of the Occupiers' Liability Act 1957, the glass in the door of the children's ward in *Gravestock* would be regarded as satisfactory. It is pertinent to refer to two cases decided some years after *Gravestock* — and after the coming into force of the Act of 1957 — cases in which local education authorities have been held liable for injury to a child when the injury was caused by breaking of a thin glass panel in a school door. The ground of liability was that the use of thin glass, instead of re-inforced glass, constituted a forseeable danger. It may be suggested that today, in the circumstances of *Gravestock*, thin glass in the door of a children's ward might also be held to be a no less foreseeable danger, though the naughtiness of an injured child in running about and swinging on the door might be found to constitute contributory negligence.[2] Although having regard to the age of the child even this might be doubted.

Furthermore, it is not only to the extent advisable in anticipation of the exercise by children and persons in the classes mentioned above of less care than is exercised by ordinary adults that a hospital has to guard its patients from risks in respect of the hospital premises and their use. The common duty of care is much wider than that, it is 'to take such care

---

[1] *The Times*, summary for March 24, 1955, published on April 21.
[2] *Lyes* v. *Middlesex County Council* (1963) 61 L.G.R. 448; *Reffell* v. *Surrey County Council* [1964] 1 W.L.R. 358 [1964] 1 All E.R. 743.

as *in all the circumstances of the case* is reasonable. ...'[1] Hence a hospital, through its staff, must have regard to the nature of the physical disabilities of its patients, even of patients exercising ordinary adult care, and make the premises reasonably safe. Thus a patient walking upon a crutch — especially if just learning to use it after an amputation — is much more at risk of a fall than a person who is firm on his legs. So also greater care ought to be taken for a person who, of necessity, is using a stick on the highly polished floor. Moreover, what might not constitute a danger to a person of normal sight might well be a danger to a blind person or to one of feeble sight, a danger which, if it existed on hospital premises, would be likely to render the hospital liable if any person under such disability suffered injury thereby.

Section 2 continues:

(4) In determining whether the occupier of premises has discharged the common duty of care to a visitor, regard is to be had to all the circumstances, so that (for example) —

    (*a*) where damage is caused to a visitor by a danger of which he had been warned by the occupier, the warning is not to be treated without more as absolving the occupier from liability, unless in all the circumstances it was enough to enable the visitor to be reasonably safe; and

    (*b*) where damage is caused to a visitor by a danger due to the faulty execution of work of construction, maintenance or repair by an independent contractor employed by the occupier, the occupier is not to be treated without more as answerable for the danger if in all the circumstances he had acted reasonably in entrusting the work to an independent contractor and had taken such steps (if any) as he reasonably ought in order to satisfy himself that the contractor was competent and that the work had been properly done.

The subsection also uses the drafting technique of examples, and so leaves the door open for judicial extension of the application of underlying principles.

That by s. 2 (4) (*a*), the fact that a warning has been given will not necessarily absolve the occupier from liability, must be read in conjunction with s. 3, below, being designed, in particular, to preserve unmodified the occupier's common duty of care towards employees of persons in contractual relationship with the occupier when those employees are on the premises in pursuance of the contract. Examples are, contractors' men on building jobs at the hospital, and suppliers' deliverymen.

For a Health Authority or other occupier to take advantage of the possibility of escape from liability provided by s. 2 (4) (*b*) it will have to show that the delegation to an independent contractor was reasonable and that it had done whatever it ought to do to satisfy itself that the contractor was competent and that the work had been properly done.

[1] S. 2 (2).

Clayton v. *Woodman & Son (Builders) Ltd.*[1] illustrates this exception for Health Authorities. The facts of the case were as follows: some alterations were being made by a contractor, the first defendant, in an old building of which the South-West Regional Hospital Board were occupiers, the Board having also engaged a firm of architects to supervise the work. In the course of the work the plaintiff, a workman, was injured as the result of the fall of a gable wall rendered unsafe by reason of a chase having been cut in the gable on the instructions of the architect. On the facts, the Board, who were the second defendants, were held not liable either under the Occupiers' Liability Act 1957 or for the negligence of the architects whom they rightly believed to be of high repute and who were independent contractors.

4. Effect of Contract on Occupier's Liability to Third Party

Section 3 of the Act reads as follows:

(1) Where an occupier of premises is bound by contract to permit persons who are strangers to the contract to enter or use the premises, the duty of care which he owes to them as his visitors cannot be restricted or excluded by that contract, but (subject to any provision of the contract to the contrary) shall include the duty to perform his obligations under the contract, whether undertaken for their protection or not, in so far as those obligations go beyond the obligations otherwise involved in that duty.

(2) A contract shall not by virtue of this section have the effect, unless it expressly so provides, of making an occupier who has taken all reasonable care answerable to strangers to the contract for dangers due to the faulty execution of any work of construction, maintenance or repair or other like operation by persons other than himself, his servants and persons acting under his direction and control.

(3) In this section 'stranger to the contract' means a person not for the time being entitled to the benefit of the contract as a party to it or as the successor by assignment or otherwise of a party to it, and accordingly includes a party to the contract who has ceased to be so entitled.

(4) Where by the terms or conditions governing any tenancy (including a statutory tenancy which does not in law amount to a tenancy) either the landlord or the tenant is bound, though not by contract, to permit persons to enter or use premises of which he is the occupier, this section shall apply as if the tenancy were a contract between the landlord and the tenant.

(9) This section, in so far as it prevents the common duty of care from being restricted or excluded, applies to contracts entered into and tenancies created before the commencement of this Act, as well as to those entered into or created after its commencement; but, in so far as it enlarges the duty owed by an occupier beyond the common duty of care, it shall have effect only in relation to obligations which are undertaken after that commencement or which are renewed by agreement (whether express or implied) after that commencement.

Whilst it should be observed that the primary object of the inclusion of s. 3 was apparently to make landlords liable to visitors for the safety

---

[1] [1962] 2 Q.B. 533. The subsection also reverses the rule in *London Graving Dock Co. Ltd.* v. *Horton* [1951] A.C. 737; *Thomson* v. *Cremin* [1956] 1 W.L.R. 103.

of such parts of the premises (*e.g.*, forecourts, staircases, *etc.*, of blocks of flats) as the landlord might have retained under his own control, it will also — read with s. 2 (4) (*a*) — protect, *inter alia* employees of persons in contractual relations with the occupier. And since by s. 3 it is provided that 'the duty of care . . . shall include the duty to perform his obligations under the contract . . .' an employee of a contractor who is injured on hospital premises as the result of the failure of the hospital to perform its obligations under the contract will have a direct right of action against the hospital even though there has been no failure in respect of the common duty of care as laid down in 2.

5. Implied Terms in Contracts

Broadly the effect of s. 5 is that whenever a contract with the occupier of premises confers on another party to the contract the right to enter or use, or bring or send goods to, the premises, the duty on the occupier implied by the contract will be the common duty of care. This, like s. 2 also applied to fixed and moveable structures but does not affect the obligations imposed by virtue of a contract of carriage or bailment.

There is nothing in the Act which would prevent a Health Authority as is usual, disclaiming liability for safe keeping of a patient's belongings not handed over for the purpose. See further Chapter 16 below and as regards property belonging to members of the staff, see Chapter 22 below.

6. Landlord's Liability

The provisions of s. 4 of the Defective Premises Act 1972 which have replaced those of s. 4 of the Occupier's Liability Act 1957 in essence make a landlord liable in damages if having an obligation or a right to do so, he fails to keep the premises let in a reasonably safe condition and that failure leads to an injury to anyone whom he might reasonably expect to be affected thereby.

The section is not likely to have any relevance to most premises used as hospitals within the National Health Service because such premises are almost invariably owned by the Secretary of State administered for him by the appropriate authority, the relationship between the Secretary of State and the authority not being that of landlord and tenant. An authority might, however, be using property leased from a private landlord, *e.g.*, for accommodation for nurses.

In such cases, the landlord could be made directly liable to anybody injured thereby under s. 4 of the 1972 Act. That section might also impose a liability on a Health Authority as landlord of any property — including property held on charitable trusts — which it might have let by it to a tenant. If, however, circumstances are envisaged in which it would be proper for a lease of part of the hospital premises owned by

the Secretary of State, the lease would seemingly be granted on behalf
of the Secretary of State and in his name. Consequently, any liability
as landlord would be on the Secretary of State and not on the Health
Authority.[1]

7. Patients, Visitors, etc. — How far can Rights under the Occupiers' Liability Act 1957 be Restricted?

(a) National Health Service hospitals

We must now examine to what extent if any Health Authority or a
hospital is free to restrict, or exclude the ordinary common duty of
care in respect of patients, their visitors and other persons properly
visiting a hospital in relation to the affairs of a patient or former
patient, *e.g.*, the personal representative of a deceased patient or his
agent.

The only relevant circumstances in which the Occupiers' Liability
Act 1957 expressly prevents the cutting down of the Occupier's duty to
exercise the common duty of care are (i) in the case of any person who
enters premises for any purpose in the exercise of a right conferred by
law[2] and (ii) in the case of a stranger to a contract who by virtue of the
contract is entitled to enter or use the premises.[3]

It follows in the case of non-paying patients in a National Health
Service hospital that unless it can be argued that he has entered the
premises on the exercise of a right conferred by law within that and
remains on, meaning of s. 2 (6) of the Occupiers' Liability Act 1957
the hospital could cut down its duty towards him.

Dr Speller argued that it did not appear that the patient does enter
and remain on hospital premises in exercise of such a right, because
although it is the duty of the Secretary of State to provide *inter alia*,
hospital accommodation and medical, dental nursing and ambulance
services to such extent as he considers necessary to meet all reasonable
requirements,[4] nowhere in the National Health Service Act 1977 is
any person given a statutory right to receive treatment in case of need
at any particular hospital. Hence, it seemed to Dr Speller that a non-
paying patient does not enter hospital in exercise of a right conferred
by law and that the Secretary of State, or a Health Authority acting
on his behalf by effective notice, could disclaim liability under the Occupiers' Liability Act 1957.

---

[1] Both the Occupiers' Liability Act 1957, s. 6, and the Defective Premises Act 1972, s. 5,
bind the Crown but as regards the Crown's liability in tort neither Act binds the Crown
further than the Crown is made liable in tort by the Crown Proceedings Act 1947. This
means that in most cases the Crown will be liable to the same extent as any other occupier
or landlord under the Acts of 1957 and 1972.
[2] S. 2 (6).   [3] S. 3 (1).
[4] See s. 2 (2) of the 1973 Act for the full range of services to be so provided.

He also said, however, that a first reaction to that conclusion is that the law as applying to N.H.S. patients is harsh and unreasonable, because by effective prior notice, a hospital receiving a patient for medical attention to say, a broken leg, might disclaim liability for such a possibility as his other leg being broken whilst in hospital or even for his being killed, provided such injury or death, were caused by defective state of the building and the defect were known to the hospital or its staff at the time of the patient's admission. Unreasonable as any such disclaimer would appear to be in normal circumstances, it might be reasonable in exceptionable cases as, for example, if a hospital which had suffered war damage continued to run at their own risk patients urgently in need of treatment. But then, as he said, it is questionable whether any disclaimer would be necessary in such cases.

On the other hand, the unattractiveness of this conclusion predisposes the present editor from accepting it. Might it not be argued that although there is no right that a patient could enforce to receive treatment nevertheless the duty on the Secretary of State to provide treatment does provide a corresponding right of a patient to have it. To say otherwise would seem to make nonsense of cases such as *Barnett* v. *Chelsea and Kensington H.M.C.*[1] This case has already been discussed[2] and it will be remembered that it established a duty on a hospital which held itself out as having a casualty department to ensure that everybody presenting themselves there was under a duty to provide the care and skill normally shown in such departments.

It appears that it is absurd for this duty to co-insist with a right of the hospital to disclaim responsibility for defective premises. Although the Health and Safety at Work Act, etc., 1974 does not affect civil liability,[3] s. 3 (1) clearly imposes a duty on an employer, *e.g.*, a Health Authority to ensure 'that persons not in his employment who may be affected [by the running of his undertaking] are not thereby exposed to risks to their health or safety.' Further, might it not be argued that where a patient has been admitted to hospital, the Secretary of State, through the responsible Health Authority has recognised that the patient is thereby a person in need of health care within the meaning of the National Health Service Act 1977 and accordingly is thereby entering and remaining on the premises as of right.

The case of a paying patient and his visitors is subject to different considerations for it seems clear, by reference to s. 65 and s. 66 of the National Health Service Act 1977 that if a paying patient is received under the contractual arrangements with him,[4] the responsibility of the occupier to exercise the common duty of care could be cut down only

---

[1] [1968] 1 Q.B. 428; [1968] 1 All E.R. 1068.   [2] See above, pp. 241–242.   [3] S. 47.
[4] See below as to patients (*e.g.* children) received under contractual arrangements with third parties.

by express terms of the contract that, subject to his health permitting, the patient will be allowed visitors at certain times it seems that the hospital could not, by any means, limit its liability for failure to exercise the common duty of care towards such visitors. But by s. 3 (2) of the 1957 Act the liability of the occupier to persons who are not parties to the contract under which they enter the premises, in respect of injury or damage due to the fault of independent contractors, is possibly somewhat more circumscribed than to other visitors under s. 2 (4) (b).

Section 3 also confers a direct right on any person on premises under a contract to which he is not a party in respect of the occupier's obligations under the contract, whether undertaken for his protection or not. This, seemingly, means that if the breach of any such obligation by the occupier, whether the obligation was entered into for the protection of visitors or not, does in fact lead to injury to a visitor, or damage to his property, he will be able to claim damages from the occupier.

If a patient received in pay-bed accommodation is not himself a party to the contract for the accommodation, e.g., a child under 16 years of age, the contract being between the parent or guardian and the Health Authority, the rules governing liability to the child for the safety of the premises etc. under the Occupiers' Liability Act 1957 would be as described in s. 3 and could not be cut down below the common duty of care.[1] Substantially, the child's position would be the same as that of an authorised visitor or other stranger to the contract entering the hospital premises by virtue of it. *Gravestock*[2] and *Cox*[3] discussed on pp. 278–279 indicate how narrow may be the margin between injuries within the Act of 1957 and injuries caused during treatment. *Gravestock* appears to be on one side of the fence and *Cox* on the other.

(b) Voluntary hospitals and nursing homes

Prima facie, there is nothing in the Occupiers' Liability Act 1957 to prevent either a voluntary (*i.e.* charitable or non-profit) hospital or a private nursing home from modifying or excluding its obligation to exercise the common duty of care towards patients and towards any other *visitor*[4] to the hospital premises save as stated below. In the case of persons, such as patients on the premises under some contract with the occupier, it would seem necessary for any limitation of liability to be incorporated in the agreement made. But if the patient has been received under a contract between the hospital or nursing home and a third party, e.g. a child received under a contract with the parent, or a health service patient by a voluntary hospital under contract with a Health Authority, s. 3 would apparently operate so that the hospital

---

[1] S. 3 (1).   [2] *The Times*, May 27, 1955.
[3] *The Times*, summary for March 29th published on April 21, 1955.
[4] As defined in s. 1 (2) for the Act.

could not restrict or exclude its duty of care except as provided in
s. 3 (2). Similarly, if the contract with a patient carried with it the
express or implied term that the patient — subject only to his health so
permitting — was entitled to have visitors, it would seem that s. 3
would operate to prevent the hospital cutting down its obligation to
use due care in respect of such visitors except as provided in s. 3 (2).

8. Warning Notices

As has been mentioned s. 2 (1) indicates that there may be circumstances in which an occupier might be free to restrict or exclude,
otherwise than by agreement, his obligation to exercise the common
duty of care towards a visitor or visitors. Presumably, this has reference
to such things as warning notices. And, in so far, therefore, as a hospital
— whether public authority or private — might be able to limit its
obligations towards patients and to patients' visitors it could do so by
notices. But if a patient were entitled to have visitors unless his medical
condition made it unadvisable it would appear that the rights of those
visitors could not be cut down.

If, in any case, a hospital relied on a notice disclaiming liability or
warning of a danger as answer to an action for failure to exercise the
common duty of care under s. 2 of the Occupiers' Liability Act 1957,
the question of fact would then arise whether the notice had been seen
by the injured person and if it had not, whether it was adequate to
limit or exclude liability.

Ashdown v. *Samuel Williams & Sons Ltd.*[1] and *White* v. *Blackmore*[2]
indicate the line the courts may take on this point. But it seems this is
less likely since they were cases of voluntary activity and of voluntary
encounter with a risk. In *Burnett* v. *British Waterways Board*[3] the court
said that where a plaintiff was given no choice in the matter, as where he
was earning his living, it could not be said that he had accepted the
risks which purported to be covered by the warning notice. Accordingly,
the additional question in the hospital context both as regards
patients and their visitors is: was the assumption of the risk
genuinely voluntary? It would appear that often it is not: the patient
may not have a real choice of which hospital he enters; and his visitors
who, it may be assumed do so for more substantial reasons than whim
or fancy even if not to earn their livings, may also be able to say that
they had not voluntarily accepted the risk.

9. Fire Precautions Act 1971

In so far as the provisions of the Fire Precautions Act 1971 may be
made applicable to hospital authorities[4] and its requirements are not

---

[1] [1956] 2 Q.B. 580.   [2] [1972] 2 Q.B. 651.   [3] [1973] 1 W.L.R. 700.
[4] See s. 1 and, as to application to the Crown, s. 40. The Act has not yet been so applied.
But see below, p. 446 *et seq.*

met, that would afford strong evidence of negligence in any action for damages arising from injury to or the death of any person, or loss of or damage to personal property consequential on a fire.

10. Position of Negligent Member of Staff

Even if, under the Occupiers' Liability Act 1957 a hospital authority or the proprietor or occupier of a hospital had been able effectively by warning notice or contract, to disclaim liability for the safety of the premises, or if such authority or persons had, by contract, effectively disclaimed liability for injury or loss to persons on the premises arising in other ways, *e.g.* by reason of the negligence of medical, nursing or other staff when performing their respective duties, that would not protect members of the staff from actions for negligence against them personally.

C. TRESPASS

A trespasser is not a *visitor* within the meaning of the Occupiers' Liability Act 1957 and accordingly the liability of an occupier to a trespasser injured on his land is still a matter of the application of common law principles. Until the House of Lords' decision in *British Railways Board* v. *Herrington*,[1] the only duty of an occupier of land owned was not to act with reckless disregard for a trespasser's safety.[2] In that case however, the House of Lords condemned this rule as harsh and outmoded and substituted a new rule. Lord Denning, *i.e.*, in *Pannett* v. *McGuiness and Co.*[3] has summarised the rule in *Herrington* thus:

'The long and short of it is that you have to take into account all the circumstances of the case and see then whether the occupier ought to have done more than he did. (1) You must apply your common sense. You must take into account the gravity and likelihood of the probable injury. Ultra-hazardous activities require a man to be ultra-cautious in carrying them out. The more dangerous the activity, the more he should take steps to see that no one is injured by it. (2) You should take into account also the character of the intrusion by the trespasser. A wandering child or a straying adult stands in a different position from a poacher or burglar. You may expect a child when you may not expect a burglar. (3) You must also have regard to the nature of the place where the trespass occurs. An electrified railway line or a warehouse being demolished may require more precautions to be taken than a private house. (4) You must also take into account the knowledge which the defendant has, or ought to have of the likelihood of trespassers being present. The more likely they are, the more precautions may have to be taken.'

[1] [1972] A.C. 877.
[2] See *Addie and Sons (Collieries) Ltd.* v. *Dumbreck* [1929] A.C. 358.
[3] [1972] 2 Q.B., 599, 606–7.

In the same case Edmond Davies, L.J., warned 'to attempt to catalogue any means would be undesirable to attempt and impossible of attainment.' If however, it is worth noting some of the factors the courts have indicated they will take into account. This in *Herrington* Lord Reid suggested that an impecunious occupier with little assistance at hand would often be excused from doing something which a large organisation with ample staff would be expected to do; Lord Morris of Borth-y-Gest said that it was a matter of what common sense or common humanity would dictate; Lord Pearson said that with the progress of technology there are more and greater dangers and there is considerably more need for occupiers to take reasonable steps to deter persons, especially children, from trespassing in dangerous places.

Accordingly where in *Herrington*[1] itself a six-year-old child who had trespassed on a railway line by going through a gap in a fence, liability was imposed on the Board because one of their employees (a station-master) knew both of the gap and the general tendency of children to trespass there. In *Pannett*[2] a five-year-old defied both his mother and the employees of the dependants and trespassed on a demolition site. The site, however, was near a children's playground, the time of the trespass was just after school; and perhaps conclusively the danger on the site was enhanced by a fire burning waste. Liability was imposed. So also liability was imposed for injury to a thirteen-year-old in *Southern Portland Cement* v. *Cooper*[3] in which a company, having established an allurement for children, failed to take steps to prevent danger arising from their high-tension electric cable.

In *Harris* v. *Birkenhead Corporation*[4] the dependants were held that to be the occupier of an empty slum dwelling awaiting demolition. The properties were a source of temptation to evil-minded persons intent upon scavenging and looting and of childhood exploration and enjoy-ment. Kilner Brown, J., held :—

'There is of course a difference where there is a live rail or a heap of glowing embers, whereas an open window is a hazard in an ordinarily occupied house. I am firmly of the opinion that a derelict house openly available to a little toddler of four with a gaping window only a few inches above the floor is a potentially dangerous situation, against which any humane and common sense person ought to take precautions.'

Although he thus found there was liability he pointed out that in the tests set out by Lord Denning in *Pannett*[5] perhaps not enough was made of the part that added burdens face even an infant trespasser. An occupier of land does not guarantee the safety of his land for even them. In *Parry* v. *Northampton Borough Council*[6] the plaintiff (aged 9) was injured when an aerosol can was put on fire by another boy when they

---

[1] [1972] A.C. 877.   [2] [1972] 2 Q.B. 599.   [3] [1974] A.C. 623 (P.C.).
[4] [1974] 1 W.L.R. 379.   [5] Quoted above, p. 287.   [6] [1974] 72 L.G.R. 733.

were both trespassing on the dependant's rubbish tip. It was held that although the dependants knew that children trespassed there they were not liable because it would not have been practicable to prevent the trespassing without astronomical expense.

It may also be added that it has been held that a local authority or large corporation which has been warned of the danger on its premises by telephone by a number of the public cannot evade liability merely because of the message failing to find its way through to the appropriate department.[1]

D. NUISANCE

1. Private Nuisance

For an occupier of land wrongfully to allow the escape of deleterious things, such as smells, smoke, noise or vibration, thus interfering with the material enjoyment of other land in the vicinity or thereby causing loss or injury constitutes actionable private nuisance. Other things which have been subject of actions for nuisance are electricity, heat, fumes and noxious vegetation, also pollution of water and apparently 'germs'[2] as well as wild animals and water in an artificial reservoir. Nor is the class of such things closed. Instances that might concern hospitals would be spread of infection or escape of radiation. Roots of trees encroaching on neighbouring property, if they cause damage, e.g., by drying out the soil and so causing cracks in a building on that property, may constitute nuisance.[3] Also actionable as private nuisance is any interference with an easement or other servitude appurtenant to land, e.g., a right of way or right to light.

A hospital or nursing home may be liable for nuisance committed, e.g., if any department such as a maternity block, is inconveniently near residential property so that noises unpleasant either by reason of their nature, volume, continuance, or the time at which they are heard, reach neighbouring residential or business premises. Or again, the risk of disease germs may be a nuisance,[4] though the case in which this was decided, which concerned the erection of a smallpox hospital, might today be decided differently because knowledge of the control of infection has increased.[5] The noise from an engine room may equally be a nuisance,[6] as may the close proximity of a mortuary[7] so that dis-

---

[1] Melvin v. Franklin [1972] 71 L.G.R. 142.

[2] Metropolitan District Asylum Board v. Hill (1881) 6 A.C. 193; 50 L.J. (Q.B.) 353.

[3] Davey v. Harrow Corporation [1958] 1 Q.B. 60.

[4] Metropolitan District Asylum Board v. Hill (1881) 6 A.C. 193; 50 L.J. (Q.B.) 353.

[5] See Marshall v. Lindsey County Council [1937] A.C. 97. This case involved puerperal fever and turned on the safety of the premises.

[6] Allison v. Merton, Sutton and Wandsworth A.H.A. [1975] C.L. 2450. But in Nottingham Area No. 1 H.M.C. v. Owen [1958] 1 Q.B. 50, it was held that an injunction did not lie to order the abatement of a nuisance.

[7] A case on this point is understood to have been settled on terms in 1939.

tressing sights, sounds and obnoxious smells,[1] reach the adjoining property.

What has been said about reasonable standards applies no less to claims for nuisance based on partial obstruction of ancient lights. The occupier of the dominant tenement is entitled only to a reasonable amount of light through the window which, by grant or prescription, has become an ancient light. He is not entitled to continue to receive the same amount of light as at the time the status of an ancient light was acquired, should that exceed what is reasonable judged by ordinary standards. Although the courts have refused to be bound by the 45 degrees formula or by any other, that formula does afford a rough idea of what is likely to be enforceable. There is no prescriptive right to a view, however attractive or however beneficial that might be to the patients of a private nursing home and, therefore, lucrative to the proprietor.

The same kind of standard of reasonableness is applicable in all actions for nuisance. Hence, if a hospital were using delicate electrical apparatus it would not have a remedy in nuisance if vibration from adjoining premises interfered with the use of that apparatus. The test is whether the vibration interferes with normal use or enjoyment not extraordinary use.

2. Public Nuisance

Public nuisances comprise a very heterogenous group of wrongs, some of common law origin some statutory. As examples of the former may be cited obstruction of a highway or of public right of way smoke nuisance and the keeping of a disorderly house.

Generally, public nuisances are not actionable as torts, the appropriate procedure being in the nature of criminal proceedings. But to this rule there is an exception, *viz.*, that anyone who suffers loss or injury beyond the inconvenience suffered by the public at large (*e.g.*, a shopkeeper, access to whose shop is blocked by obstruction such as an unlawful trench in the road) may bring a civil action.

Another example of actionable public nuisance is injury to someone on the public highway caused by the fall of a gutter or overhanging lamp which is out of repair, or of the bough of a tree which has become rotten and the state of which should have been known to the responsible person. Whether the action will lie against the owner or the occupier will depend on the extent of their respective responsibilities for external repairs under the tenancy agreement. That point will usually be academic so far as Health Authorities within the National Health Service are

[1] *Bone* v. *Scale* [1975] 1 W.L.R. 797; [1975] 1 All E.R. 787 (C.A.). The smells came from a pig farm. It was also said in this case that in assessing damages for loss of amenity caused by a nuisance a parallel may be drawn with the loss of amenity caused by personal injury but there is no rigid standard of comparison.

concerned, for hospital premises are usually owned by the Secretary of State and occupied, not by tenants, but by a Health Authority on his behalf. Moreover, so far as hospital houses let on service tenancies are concerned, the standard agreement provides that the Health Authority remains responsible for external repairs and so would be liable for any injury or damage due to failure to carry out the duty.[1] It will, however, be a defence to a claim for damages in such circumstances to show that the accident was due to some latent defect not discoverable by reasonably careful inspection.[2]

3. The Clean Air Acts

The emission of smoke, grit, dust or fumes[3] is subject to the provisions of the Clean Air Acts 1956 and 1968, the purpose of the Acts being to vest in local authorities the power to control and ultimately to forbid the emission of dark smoke, grit or dust into the atmosphere and to forbid the emission of smoke, whether dark or not, in a smoke control area, as well as to control the emission of fumes. Enforcement of the Acts is by way of prosecution of offenders by the local authority in whose area the emission has taken place, save in respect of emission of smoke, grit, dust or fumes from premises which are under the control of any Government department and are occupied for the public service of the Crown or for any of the purposes of any Government department.[4]

The Health and Safety at Work etc. Act 1974[5] created a duty under s. 5 to use the best practicable means for preventing the emission into the atmosphere from any premises of noxious or offensive substances and for rendering harmless and inoffensive such substances as may be so emitted. *Substance* is defined in s. 53 (1) as 'any natural or artificial substance, whether in solid or liquid form or in the form of a gas or vapour'. It is unclear whether noise is included or not. As stated above this Act specifically excludes any civil liability based on its terms[6], but breach of the duties under it is a criminal offence.[7] These provisions apply to N.H.S. hospitals.[8]

In the case of emission of smoke, *etc.*, contrary to the provisions of the Clean Air Acts, from premises, such as a N.H.S. hospital,[9] used for public services of the Crown or for the purposes of any Government department, the local authority for the area in which the premises are

---

[1] See now also Defective Premises Act 1972, s. 4.

[2] *Noble* v. *Harrison* [1926] 2 K.B. 332, a case concerning the bough of a tree which fell on to a motor coach on a public highway.

[3] The emission of fumes is the subject of the 1968 Act, the powers and responsibilities of local authorities under the 1956 Act being widened accordingly.

[4] S. 22 of 1956 Act, which also covers premises in occupation of the Duchy of Cornwall, of the Duchy of Lancaster and of 'visiting forces' as there defined.

[5] The Act is further discussed in Chapter 23 on Injury at Work but it will be noted that many of its provisions apply equally to visitors as well as employees.

[6] S. 47.   [7] S. 33.   [8] S. 48.

[9] *Pfizer Corporation* v. *Ministry of Health* [1965] A.C. 512.

situate, if it seems proper to them to do so, may report the matter to the responsible Minister,[1] who, on receiving any such report, shall inquire into the circumstances and, if the inquiry reveals that there is cause for complaint, shall employ all practicable means for preventing or minimising the emission of the smoke, grit, dust or fumes or for abating the nuisance and preventing a recurrence thereof, as the case may be.[2]

Notwithstanding the passing of the Clean Air Acts 1956 and 1968, the civil remedy of an action for nuisance in respect of emission of smoke, grit, dust or fumes, if such as to constitute actionable nuisance at common law, remains available against Health Authorities constituted under the National Health Service Act 1977, in respect of hospitals under their administration, no less than against occupiers of other hospitals and nursing homes, though one would not expect that an injunction would readily be granted against such authority in any but exceptional circumstances.

In the case of a voluntary hospital the local authority can launch a prosecution under the Clean Air Act 1956, and such hospital may also be made defendant in a civil action for damages for smoke nuisance as for any other common law nuisance.

4. The Control of Pollution Act 1974

Finally, mention must be made of the 1974 Control of Pollution Act. This is a wide ranging measure aimed at improving the environment. It covers the disposal of waste,[3] the pollution of water,[4] the control of noise,[5] and the pollution of the atmosphere.[6] However, the Act apparently does not create any new civil liability[7] and for the most part it does not affect the Crown or its undertakings. For these reasons it is not fully discussed here, since it will have only a marginal impact on the operations of hospitals even if they are outside the health service.

[1] For the Health Service, the Secretary of State for Social Services, or the Secretary of State for Wales. See p. 13.

[2] S. 22. It would seem that he could be compelled by mandamus to carry out his duty under the Act. See also *Nottingham No. 1 Area H.M.C.* v. *Owen* ([1958] 1 Q.B. 50; [1957] decided under the Public Health Act 1936.

[3] See the Act, Part 1.   [4] See the Act, Part II.   [5] See the Act, Part III.
[6] See the Act, Part IV.   [7] But see s. 88.

CHAPTER 16

LOSS OF OR DAMAGE TO PROPERTY
OF PATIENTS AND OTHERS

1 General Principles

BEFORE the Occupiers' Liability Act 1957, a hospital or nursing home proprietor was under no obligation to accept responsibility for property brought in by the patient and, in fact, normally disclaimed such responsibility except for money, valuables or other property handed over for safe custody. Even if property had been so handed over, provided reasonable care had been taken of the goods bailed, the hospital was under no liability if the things deposited were damaged, destroyed or stolen.

Nor does it seem that the position has been altered by s. 1 (3) of the Occupiers' Liability Act 1957,[1] which provides that the rules laid down in that Act in relation to an occupier of premises and his visitors 'apply in like manner and to the like extent as the principles applicable at common law to an occupier of premises and his invitees and licensees would apply to regulate . . . (b) the obligation of a person occupying or having control over any premises or structure in respect of damage to property, including the property of persons who are not themselves his visitors'. But although it is probable that, in any event, a Health Authority would not be liable for loss, damage or destruction of things brought in by a patient and not handed over for safe custody it is advisable that the authority should bring to the notice of the patient its disclaimer of responsibility, and this can conveniently be done when the notice that he can be admitted is sent to him.

All this is provided the hospital took reasonable care of the goods left with it. What is reasonable will depend, of course, on all the circumstances of the case. It is however clear that the lowest duty that might be imposed is to look after the property as if it were the owner. In such a case no liability would be incurred where loss was suffered through the dishonesty of an employee so long as there were not grounds for suspecting him. However where there is a duty to look after the goods it is no excuse for the authority to blame either the carelessness of an employee or even his dishonesty.[2]

---

[1] See further p. 275 et seq.

[2] See *Houghland* v. *R. R. Lowe* (*Luxury Coaches*) *Ltd.* [1962] 1 Q.B. 694, 697–8; *Morris* v. *C. W. Martin and Sons Ltd.* [1966] 1 Q.B. 716; and, *Transmotors* v. *Robertson, Buckley* [1970] 1 Ll. Rep. 224.

In the case of hospitals within the National Health Service it was indicated in a departmental circular[1]:

'. . . Boards and Committees should disclaim responsibility for the loss of personal effects of patients except when property is taken into safe custody on admission of the patient to a hospital.'

which, on the one hand, suggests inviting the patient to deposit an even wider range of property and, on the other, to disclaim liability if he does not.

But, despite any disclaimer of responsibility on the lines indicated in departmental circulars, it is suggested that if, say, a patient's wrist-watch, jewellery, spectacles or dentures, of which he had retained physical control whilst in hospital, had been taken from him when he went to the theatre for an operation, the Hospital Authority at that point in time, and until the patient was again volitional and could exercise effective control, would have to be regarded as having accepted responsibility as bailee. Yet another case in which that would probably be true is that of the out-patient who was not allowed to have personal possessions with him when going for examination or treatment, but was compelled to leave them in a cubicle. It is to be doubted very much whether in such circumstances a notice disclaiming responsibility would be effective, at all events in a hospital within the National Health Service.

Generally it may be said that so far as disclaimer of liability may be necessary, the effectiveness of any notice of disclaimer which might be exhibited in the reception area, whether for in-patients or for out-patients, is doubtful for it seems that unless a patient making a claim for loss of property can be proved to have read the notice he will not be bound by it.[2]

We next have to ask what is the extent of the responsibility of the Hospital Authority for patients' property of which it becomes voluntary, a voluntary bailee. It is probable that even in an accident case, a hospital, at any rate one which made regular provision for accident cases would not be an involuntary bailee.

Since the decision of the Court of Appeal in *Houghland* v. *R. R. Lowe (Luxury Coaches) Ltd.,*[3] it can be said that it matters far less whether the Health Authority is a gratuitous bailee or a bailee for reward, the standard of care necessary to absolve the authority from liability for loss or damage being simply that demanded by the circumstances of the particular case.[4] It is not material whether any action for

---

[1] R.H.B. (49) 127; H.M.C. (49) 107; B.G. (49) 112. See also H.M. (60) 80, (71) 91, (72) 41.

[2] See *Mendelssohn* v *Normand Ltd.* [1970] 1 Q.B. 177 (C.A.).

[3] [1962] 1 Q.B. 694, 697–8. See also Lord Chelmsford in *Giblin* v. *McMullen* (1869) L.R. 2 P.C. 317, 336) and Lord Cranworth in *Wilson* v. *Brett* ((1843) 11 M. & W. 113, 115, 152), whose judgments were followed in *Houghland's* case.

[4] *Martin* v. *London County Council* ([1947] 1 All E.R. 783), a case in which the defendant hospital authority was sued for damages for loss of a patient's property, judgment being given for the plaintiff on the basis of the defendants' having been a bailee for reward.

loss of the thing bailed is brought in detinue or in case, the burden on the defendants being the same either way, *viz.*, that of showing that the loss or damage is not attributable to any negligence on their part.

But although we are thus spared the not always easy task of deciding whether or not in a particular case the handing over of property to the authorities for safe-custody constitutes a bailment for reward[1], we are still left with a practical question, a question of fact to which attention may all too often be directed only when a loss has occurred, *i.e.* as to the standard of care properly to be expected of the authority and its employees in the circumstances of the particular case.

It would seem relevant in considering the degree of care required of a hospital to take account of the Secretary of State's instructions to hospital authorities to take steps to disclaim responsibility for patients' property not handed over for safe custody. That strongly suggests that hospitals hold themselves out as having reasonable facilities for looking after property handed over by patients and that money, unless banked, as well as jewellery and other valuables, would be kept in a safe.[1] Nor must be overlooked the importance of reasonable care during the period before which valuables handed in for safe custody reach the safe and also after they have been taken out of the safe to be handed back to the patient.[2] It may be suggested that the standard of care expected to be taken of a patient's property immediately on reception might well be higher if the patient were not an emergency case, because it is then reasonably practicable to carry out properly whatever precautionary procedure might have been laid down, whereas if the patient were being received in an emergency, say, by the necessarily depleted night staff, the circumstances might well warrant what would otherwise be negligence.

Nor would it seem that if any article, such as a dressing gown, which the patient had kept in the ward for necessary use were stolen, damaged or destroyed in circumstances attributable to the negligence of any member of the hospital staff, the patient would have a good claim against the authority in face of the disclaimer made in accordance with the advice given in departmental circulars.[3] So far as theft is concerned, this view is supported by *Tinsley* v. *Dudley*[4] part of the judgment in which was cited with approval in the Court of Appeal in *Edwards* v. *West Herts. Group H.M.C.*:[5]

[1] See *Martin* v. *London County Council* [1947] 1 All E.R. 783.
[2] The facts of *Houghland*, though in a different field, serve to point that moral, for in *Houghland* there was inadequate supervision of the transfer of luggage after dark from one coach to another, the first coach having broken down.
[3] It does not follow, however, that a member of the hospital staff through whose negligence property was damaged, lost or destroyed which belonged to a patient and had been kept by him in the ward (*e.g.* watch, fountain pen, spectacles) could not be made personally liable. See p. 229 and *Genys* v. *Matthews and Another*, there referred to.
[4] [1951] 2 K.B. 18, 31 *per* Jenkins, J.
[5] [1957] 1 W.L.R. 415. *Edward's* case actually concerned property stolen from the living

'There is no warrant at all on the authorities so far as I know, for holding that an invitor, where the invitation extends to the goods as well as the person of the invitee, thereby by implication of law assumes a liability to protect the invitee and his goods, not merely from physical dangers arising from defects in the premises, but from the risk of the goods being stolen by some third party. That implied liability, so far as I know, is one unknown to the law.'

To that general principle there are exceptions, such as innkeepers and persons keeping guest-houses and boarding-houses, but it is suggested that a hospital is in no such category. And even if, in respect of patients received under ss. 65 or 66 of the National Health Service Act 1977[1] it could be held that the hospital was in the position of a boarding-house keeper, the authority could still, by express notice divest itself of the responsibility for theft by third parties even if facilitated by lack of care on the part of its employees. But unless the common duty of care under the Occupiers' Liability Act 1957, has been expressly disclaimed in respect of the patient's belongings which he keeps in the ward, it is possible that by s. 1 (3) of the Act of 1957, the hospital would be liable for damage to or destruction of such belongings caused by the negligence of its employees.

2. Voluntary Hospitals and Nursing Homes

Except that references to the official circulars and to the Health Service Acts, have no relevance, what has been said in the earlier part of the chapter applies equally to voluntary hospitals and to nursing homes. Such hospitals and homes may make whatever conditions or disclaimers they like concerning patients' property and, provided they do so before the patient is accepted for treatment, any disclaimer of liability is effective. Whether or not a disclaimer made thereafter but before any loss or damage had occurred would be effective would depend on all the circumstances. If, however, no effective disclaimer had been made, paying patients would be entitled to expect of the hospital staff the same degree of care in relation to their property as a prudent owner would take of his own property. Such was the standard of care which, in *Dansey* v. *Richardson*[2] it was held that a boarding-house keeper owed to his guests and there seems no ground on which a lower standard could be postulated in the case of a hospital. Indeed, having regard to the patients' helplessness, the standard might be higher.

3. Deposit of Valuables — Formalities

When valuables are deposited by a patient it is customary, for the

quarters of a resident medical officer and not the property of a patient — but the principle is the same. See further pp. 427–429.
 [1] The sections have been amended on the reorganisation. Previously they were contained in ss. 4 and 5 of the 1946 National Health Service Act and ss. 1 and 2 of the 1968 Act.
 [2] (1854) 3 E. & B. 144.

avoidance of disputes, for a list of the articles deposited be made, acknowledged as correct by the patient's signature. It is a wise precaution to avoid describing any article, e.g., an article of jewellery in such way that the hospital may — possibly after the patient's death — be committed as to its quality or the material of which it is made. It is desirable to include with the list to be signed by the patient, a form of authority to the hospital to dispose of any articles unclaimed within a certain time of the patient's leaving hospital and to be accountable only for the proceeds.[1] If some such expression as 'ceased to be an in-patient at the hospital' were used, the authority might also cover disposal after the patient's death.

If a patient is brought in as an accident or emergency case and therefore cannot sign the form, the correctness of the list made may conveniently be certified by the signature of any accompanying responsible relative or friend, but if there is none such, it is advisable that two members of the staff together remove money and valuables from the patient and both certify the correctness of the list.

If, because a patient is unconscious or too ill to sign when he is received, no form is signed, it is a reasonable assumption that the liability of the hospital is not increased thereby, the only substantial doubt being as to whether the goods could, without express authority, be sold if unclaimed after the patient had left the hospital even though the form of deposit and authority ordinarily in use so authorised. If, in any other case, by inadvertence, no form is signed, the respective rights and duties of the patient and the hospital would have to be determined on the evidence, taking into account any general custom, notices exhibited and any agreement by word of mouth.

4. Handing Over Patient's Property to Third Party

When a patient is admitted in the ordinary way, otherwise than as an emergency case, it is a fairly general custom for him to be accompanied by a friend or relative who, with his knowledge and consent, takes away any valuables and, possibly, clothing not required in hospital. Then no difficulty arises. If, as frequently happens, when a seriously ill patient has been brought into hospital — maybe unconscious as the result of an accident — clothing and even money and valuables may be handed to the accompanying spouse or near relative, there is the risk of an action for conversion against the hospital if the patient loses his property thereby. In practice, however, provided the value of the property handed over is regarded as falling within reasonable limits, that risk is usually taken.

[1] *Beaman* v. *A.R.T.S. Ltd.* [1949] 1 K.B. 550; 65 T.L.R. 389; [1949] 1 All E.R. 465 illustrates the risks of a bailee who disposes of the bailor's property otherwise than in accordance with his authority even after a long interval of time.

5. Property of Deceased Patients

Although, strictly, property of a deceased patient should not be handed over to anyone other than the patient's legal personal representative (*i.e.*, the executor of his will who has obtained probate, or the administrator of his estate under letters of administration), or to a person duly authorised by the personal representative, hospitals do, in fact, exercise some discretion and it is customary to hand over to the deceased patient's widow, widower or next of kin, against a letter of indemnity, property of the deceased patient, provided that property is within a certain limit of value and provided it is not known that there are competing claimants.

If a person dies intestate and without lawful kin[1] his estate passes to the Crown as *bona vacantia* and is administered by the Treasury Solicitor except if the deceased person had been ordinarily resident in the Duchy of Cornwall when it is administered by the Solicitor to the Duchy or, if in the County Palatine, by the Solicitor to the Duchy of Lancaster. If, therefore, a patient dies in hospital leaving in possession of the hospital property (*e.g.*, money or jewellery) of substantial value and he is not known, after reasonable inquiry, to have made a will or to have left any relatives entitled to his estate on intestacy, the Treasury Solicitor or the Solicitor to the Duchy of Cornwall or of Lancaster as appropriate should be informed. Although it is here suggested that the hospital should make reasonable inquiries before communicating with the Treasury Solicitor, that is not a legal obligation and a hospital is under no obligation to go to trouble and expense in pursuing inquiries. The Treasury Solicitor might, however, in any particular case refuse to accept responsibility for the property if he were not satisfied that the patient had died intestate and without lawful next of kin. Then, all that the hospital could do would be to retain the property until claimed by someone having a lawful right to it or until any such claim were statute barred. But a claim by the Crown could not be so barred.

6. Rights of Illegitimate Children on Intestacy of Natural Parent and of Natural Parents on Intestacy of Illegitimate Child

Section 14 (1) and (2) of the Family Law Reform Act 1969 provide as follows:

(1) Where either parent of an illegitimate child dies intestate as respects all or any of his or her real or personal property, the illegitimate child, or, if he is dead, his issue, shall be entitled to take any interest therein to which he or such issue would have been entitled if he had been born legitimate.

[1] See below as to the extension of the meaning of *lawful kin* in this context, to include persons whose claim may be through an illegitimate birth, under s. 14 of the Family Law Reform Act 1969.

(2) Where an illegitimate child dies intestate in respect of all or any of his real or personal property, each of his parents, if surviving, shall be entitled to take any interest therein to which that parent would have been entitled if the child had been born legitimate.

Consequential amendments to Part IV of the Administration of Estates Act 1925 are made by s. 14 (3).[1] The purpose of this brief account is to do no more than to draw attention to the possible effect of the provisions of the Act on the position of a hospital finding itself left in possession of property belonging to a deceased patient, those needing a more exact statement of the changes effected by s. 14 of the 1969 Act must refer to specialist works.

As to the effect on hospitals, it has to be appreciated that where there is near illegitimate kin as well as legitimate kin of a deceased patient who has died intestate, it is unsafe to hand over property without the production of letters of administration in his favour on the rash assumption that his claim to the estate would prevail.[2]

7. Property Left in Hospital

Property left behind by a patient, whether property deposited as valuable or not, presents a special problem unless the patient has given written authority for disposal of any such property. Practically, it is usually reasonable to treat property not deposited as valuables as abandoned by the patient if not speedily claimed after his discharge and to dispose of it accordingly. But if an article left behind in hospital, even though not deposited as valuable, is in fact valuable, precipitate action to dispose of it would be unwise and might lead to an action for conversion — the measure of damages ordinarily being the value of the article at the time of conversion. *Prima facie*, therefore, the measure of damages would be the price obtained, if reasonable, but this is on the assumption that the date of disposal would, in the particular circumstances of the case, be regarded as the date of conversion and that the steps taken to dispose of it were reasonable, having regard to the nature of the article.

Deposited valuables present a more difficult problem for, apart from any authority for disposal contained in the form signed by the patient at the time of deposit, it would seem that such articles could not be treated as abandoned but should, in principle, be held until claimed. Probably, too, the patient's claim would not be barred until six years after his demand for return of the deposited article which would mean

---

[1] There are certain limitations on the rights of illegitimate children, *e.g.* as to entailed interests. Section 14 (5).

[2] Although to take a letter of indemnity from a relative to whom property of moderate value is handed over without production of letters of administration is a sensible precaution, it has to be recognised that the value of such a letter as security against loss is largely dependent on the solvency and integrity of the giver. See also H.M. (62) 2, (71) 90.

that however long after disposal by the hospital such demand were made 'conversion' would be regarded as having taken place only at that date.[1]

8. Property Found on Hospital Premises

Money, valuables or other chattels which have been lost, perhaps by a patient, perhaps by a visitor, perhaps by a member of the staff, are, from time to time, found on hospital premises. Such property may have been found either in a part of the hospital to which the members of the public are admitted or in some other part of the premises and may have been found by any person, possibly a member of the staff or possibly by a 'visitor' within the meaning of the Occupiers' Liability Act 1957 or, possibly by a trespasser. If the owner of any such object so found did not claim it and could not be traced, to whom would it belong?

Prima facie, the finder has good title against all the world except the true owner, and it is suggested that that would apply if the article were found by someone other than a member of the staff in a part of the hospital to which the public had access — even though only at stated times — *e.g.*, in a ward or in the out-patient department. Indeed a member of the public who found a lost article in a part of the hospital in which he was a trespasser might still have a good title except against the rightful owner,[2] though, on the other side, it has to be said that there is a legal presumption that the owner of land is, *prima facie*, the owner of chattels found on the land.[3] But the position of an employee of the hospital who finds an article of value depends on the circumstances of the case and on his conditions of employment. If the finding can fairly be construed as in the course of his duties and on behalf of his employing authority, then the hospital will have good title except against the true owner.[4] A special case would be if among the conditions of employment on which the finder had been appointed was one which imposed on him an obligation to hand over to the hospital any article he might find on the premises. Even so, much would depend on the wording of the relevant term of the agreement, *i.e.*, whether it referred only to things found on hospital premises whilst the employee was on duty, or to whatever he might find there at any time — an important distinction, particularly in the case of a resident officer. Failing any such agreement, the position of an officer who found any money or chattels on hospital premises, otherwise than in the course of his duties,

---

[1] See also *Beaman* v. *A.R.T.S. Ltd.* [1949] 1 K.B. 550.
[2] This would appear to follow from *Bridges* v. *Hawksworth* (1851) 21 L.J. (Q.B.) 75. Reference may also be had to *Hannah* v. *Peel* [1945] K.B. 509.
[3] *City of London Corporation* v. *Appleyard* [1963] 1 W.L.R. 982 and *Moffatt* v. *Kazana* [1969] 2 Q.B. 152.
[4] See *City of London Corporation* v. *Appleyard* [1963] 1 W.L.R. 982 and the cases there referred to.

and otherwise than in a part of the hospital to which he had access only because of his status as an officer, would seem to be indistinguishable from that of a member of the public who did so.

9. Protection of Property of Persons Taken to Hospital or Local Authority home, etc.

Among the provisions of the National Assistance Act 1948, is s. 38 which imposes on local social services authorities the duty of protecting the moveable property[1] of — amongst others — persons admitted as patients to any hospital. The section reads as follows:

48.—(1) Where a person —
    (*a*) is admitted as a patient to any hospital, or
    (*b*) is admitted to accommodation provided under Part III of this Act, or
    (*c*) is removed to any other place under an order made under subsection
        (3) of the last foregoing section,
and it appears to the council that there is danger of loss of, or damage to, any moveable property of his by reason of his temporary or permanent inability to protect or deal with the property, and that no other suitable arrangements have been or are being made for the purposes of this subsection, it shall be the duty of the council to take reasonable steps to prevent or mitigate the loss or damage.

(2) For the purpose of discharging the said duty the council shall have power at all reasonable times to enter any premises which immediately before the person was admitted or removed as aforesaid were his place of residence or usual place of residence, and to deal with any moveable property of his in any way which is reasonably necessary to prevent or mitigate loss thereof or damage thereto.

(3) A council may recover from a person admitted or removed as aforesaid, or from any person who for the purposes of this Act is liable to maintain him, any reasonable expenses incurred by the council in relation to him under the foregoing provisions of this section.

(4) In this section the expression 'council' means in relation to any property *the council which is the local authority for the purposes of the Local Authority Social Services Act* 1970[2] in the area of which the property is for the time being situated.

For the purposes of the provisions of s. 48 of the National Assistance Act 1948, a person is admitted as a patient to a hospital if he is admitted for treatment of mental disorder. Also, as a consequence of the provisions of s. 105 of the Mental Health Act 1959, which allow the holder of an office for the time being to be appointed by the Court of Protection as receiver of the patient's property, it is possible that a mental welfare officer, or other appropriate officer, may be authorised by the local authority to make application to the Court of Protection in appropriate

---

[1] It is suggested that the term *moveable property* is sufficiently wide to include *choses in action* such as banknotes and cheques which, as pieces of paper, at all events are moveable property.
[2] Words in *italics* substituted by Local Government Act 1972.

cases.[1] Moreover, by virtue of s. 49 of the National Assistance Act 1948, as amended, the authority has power to reimburse his expenses. There are no provisions for reimbursement by a hospital of the expenses of an officer of such authority making application or being appointed receiver of a patient's property.

Persons above referred to admitted to accommodation provided under Part III of the Act, are those admitted to accommodation provided by a local authority under s. 21, *viz.* (*a*) residential accommodation for persons who by reason of age, infirmity or any other circumstances including mental disorder are in need of care and attention which is not otherwise available to them, and (*b*) temporary accommodation for persons who are in urgent need thereof, being need arising in circumstances which could not reasonably have been foreseen or in such other circumstances as the authority may in any particular case determine.

The third class of person in respect of whose property s. 48 may apply is those removed under an order made under s. 47 as to which see page 469.

[1] See further below, p. 529.

CHAPTER 17

THE COMPLAINTS MACHINERY

A. GENERALLY

THIS book is concerned with law, not with practice. It has however already been remarked that on occasions it is unreal to discuss the one without at least some reference to the other. Accordingly in this chapter the position of the new Health Service Commissioners will be described, and some reference will be made to other machinery in the field.

In 1971 the Government set up a departmental enquiry under the chairmanship of Sir Michael Davies. That Committee reported in 1973 and offered a wide ranging discussion and some recommendations. At the time of writing,[1] consultations are still proceeding on the report.[2] In due course it is possible that there will be a need to discuss in greater detail the operation of the results of all these new moves. That time has not yet come although it might in the next edition.

Fundamental to any responsible view of the complaints procedure (including litigation) is the philosophy behind the report of the Davies Committee. They said:[3]

In a perfect world, no doubt things never would go wrong in hospitals: no one would ever complain or have cause to do so and there would be no room for any suggestions for improvement. This is a trite observation, but it leads to a point which we want to make. This is that it is absurd — and leads to dissatisfaction, inefficiency or worse — to pretend or persuade oneself that things never do go wrong. We feel that probably in some quarters in the hospital service there has been such a tendency in the past. In extreme cases this has materially contributed to the serious situation which has subsequently been found to have developed in several long stay hospitals, some of which are referred to in our report. We think that some people have felt that to acknowledge that things sometimes do go wrong is detrimental to staff morale and efficiency and fear that to have a well organised complaints procedure will entice many patients to invent or magnify complaints. We believe, on the contrary, that to face up to the realities of life, and to ensure that complaints are fairly and promptly dealt with, can in the long run only improve staff morale and efficiency.

B. THE HEALTH SERVICE COMMISSIONERS

1. Introductory

Health Service Commissioners, one for England and one for

---

[1] July 1976.
[2] It has been announced that the Government has accepted the need to introduce a Code of Practice.
[3] Para. 1.6.

Wales,[1] are appointed under Part V of the National Health Service Act 1977[2] for the investigation of complaints of injustice or hardship allegedly caused by maladministration or by some failure in the provision of health services by a *relevant body*,[3] or by an officer of a relevant body responsible for providing such services, or caused by an action[4] taken by or on behalf of a relevant body.

The terms and conditions under which Health Service Commissioners hold office are dealt with in ss. 106–107 of the 1977 Act. Provision is also made for the appointment of officers[5] who, if so authorised by him, may perform any functions of a Commissioner. A Commissioner may also authorise an officer of another Commissioner to act for him.[6] The duty is placed on the Health Service Commissioner for Wales of including among his officers such persons having a command of the Welsh language as he considers are needed to enable him to investigate complaints in Welsh. To assist him in any investigation a Commissioner may obtain advice from any person who in his opinion is qualified to give it[7] and may pay such fees and allowances to any such person as he may determine with the approval of the Minister for the Civil Service.

2. Matters Subject to Investigation

Matters which may be subject to investigation are to be found in s. 115. This provides:

A Commissioner may investigate—
    (a) an alleged failure in a service provided by a relevant body; or
    (b) an alleged failure of a relevant body to provide a service which it was a function of the body to provide; or
    (c) any other action taken by or on behalf of a relevant body.
in a case where a complaint is duly made by or on behalf of any person that he has sustained injustice or hardship in consequence of maladministration connected with the other action.

With s. 115 must be read s. 120 (2)[8] as follows:

It is hereby declared that nothing in this Part of this Act authorises or requires a Commissioner to question the merits of a decision taken without

---

[1] So far both offices have been held by the same person; when held by different persons, the authority of each to investigate complaints is restricted to matters which are the responsibility of a relevant body within the country for which he had been appointed. As to *relevant bodies* see s. 109, previously 1973 Act s. 34 (1) and footnote 3.
[2] Previously Part III of the Reorganisation Act.
[3] A body against which a complaint to a commissioner may be made is referred to throughout Part V of the Act as a *relevant body*, being a body of a kind within the list contained in s. 109 (s. 120) and, unless the context otherwise requires, includes an officer of such body (s. 120). Although bodies of the kinds mentioned in s. 34 (1) (*a*) to (*d*) the 1973 Act excepting only preserved Boards of Governors, ceased to exist on 1st April, 1974, a Health Service Commissioner has been empowered to investigate or continue to investigate complaints against them after that date. (The Health Service Commissioners (Transitional Provisions) Regulations S.I. 1974 No. 247, *see also* 1977 Act Sch. 14 para. 17).
[4] Section 115.   [5] Section 108 (2).   [6] Section 108 (2).   [7] Section 108 (3).
[8] And also ss. 110, 113, and 116.

maladministration by a relevant body in the exercise of a discretion vested in that body.

Other provisions of the Act limiting the range of matters which may be investigated are, in particular, s. 116 and Schedule 13 which are dealt with below.

3. Matters in Respect of which a Person Aggrieved has or had Some Other Right or Remedy

If the matter complained of is one in respect of which the person aggrieved has or had some other right or remedy within s. 116 (1)[1], a Commissioner may conduct an investigation only if satisfied that in the particular circumstances it is not reasonable to expect him to resort or to have resorted to it. The sub-section says:

Except as hereafter provided, a Commissioner shall not conduct an investigation under this Part of this Act in respect of any of the following matters —
  (a) any action in respect of which the person aggrieved has or had a right of appeal, reference or review to or before a tribunal constituted by or under any enactment or by virtue of Her Majesty's prerogative, or
  (b) any action in respect of which the person aggrieved has or had a remedy by way of proceedings in any court of law;
but a Commissioner may conduct an investigation notwithstanding that the person aggrieved has or had such a right of remedy, if satisfied that in the particular circumstances it is not reasonable to expect him to resort or have resorted to it.

As the Davies Committee point out, many complainants are reluctant to sue but anxious that a similar untoward occurrence happens to nobody else. In such a case they thought the Commissioner should not refuse to investigate since such an attitude, if genuine, was reasonable.[2]

4 Matters Expressly Excluded from Investigation by a Commissioner

By s. 116 (2) and Schedule 13, there are a number of matters which a Commissioner has no authority to investigate. Section 116 (2) reads as follows:

(2) Without prejudice to subsection (1) above—
  (a) a Commissioner shall not conduct an investigation under this Part in respect of any such action as is described in Part II of Schedule 13 to this Act; and
  (b) nothing in sections 110, 113 and 115 above shall be construed as authorising such an investigation in respect of action taken in connection with any general medical services, general dental services, general ophthalmic services or pharmaceutical services by a person providing the services.

[1] Previously 1973 Act s. 34 (4).   [2] The Report, para. 10.7.

The following matters are listed in Schedule 13 as not subject to investigation. They are in addition to those mentioned in section 116. Paragraph 19 says:[1]

(1) Action taken in connection with the diagnosis of illness or the care or treatment of a patient, being action which, in the opinion of the Commissioner in question, was taken solely in consequence of the exercise of clinical judgment, whether formed by the person taking the action or by any other person.

(2) Action taken by a Family Practitioner Committee in the exercise of its functions under the National Health Service (Service Committees and Tribunal) Regulations 1974 or any instrument amending or replacing those regulations.

(3) Action taken in respect of appointments or removals, pay, discipline, superannuation or other personal matters in relation to service under this Act.

(4) Action taken in matters relating to contractual or other commercial transactions, other than in matters arising from arrangements between a relevant body and another body which is not a relevant body for the provision of services for patients by that other body; and in determining what matters arise these shall be disregarded from such arrangements any arrangements for the provision of services at an establishment maintained by a Minister of the Crown for patients who are mainly members of the armed forces of the Crown.

(5) Action which has been or is the subject of an inquiry under section 70 of the principal Act.

A question which here arises for consideration is as to the circumstances in which, if at all, the negligence of medical or other staff leading to injury to a patient may be subject of investigation by a Commissioner.

5 Failure in Treatment of Patient

Because of the limiting provisions of s. 116 (1) and (2) of the Act and of sub-paragraph (1) of paragraph 19 of Schedule 13, it will be but seldom that ill consequences to a patient attributable to the negligence of a medical or dental practitioner or of a nurse or midwife or of others assisting in providing treatment will be accepted for investigation by a Commissioner. First, s. 116 (2) excludes from investigation any action whatever taken or not taken,[2] or thing done in connection with any general medical, general dental etc., services by a person providing those services. If, however, the general practitioner, besides providing general practitioner services for N.H.S. patients, is also in contract with an Area Health Authority for providing services for patients in a local hospital for an agreed number of sessions per week, whatever he does —

---

[1] Sub-paragraphs (3) and (4) of paragraph 19 of Schedule 13 may be excluded by Order in Council (s. 116 (3)).

[2] *Action* in Part V of the Act and in Schedule 13 includes failure to act and other expressions connoting action shall be construed accordingly (s. 120).

or fails to do — in that capacity will not be excluded from investigation under s. 116 (2), though it may be under sub-paragraph (1) of paragraph 19 of Schedule 13. This will be so even though the person aggrieved may also be one of the practitioner's own 'list' patients. Contrariwise, if the general practitioner had been treating a 'list' patient in hospital not because of a contractual obligation to the Health Authority but because the Health Authority provided accommodation and nursing care in a cottage hospital to which general practitioners had the privilege of access to treat their own patients, what the doctor did or did not do would be within s. 116 (2). That too would be the position if a general practitioner attended one of his N.H.S. list patients in a local nursing home.

To ascertain the position with regard to other than general practitioner services, in particular medical *etc.*, care and treatment in a N.H.S. hospital, we have first to take account of the provisions of sub-paragraph (1) of paragraph 19. Despite the wide terms of that sub-paragraph, there are acts and omissions by medical practitioners and by nurses and others assisting them in the care and treatment of the patient which would not be within its scope. The fundamental test in deciding whether any action taken, falls within that paragraph is whether or not that action had been taken solely in consequence of exercise of *clinical judgment*. If the action, or non-action or failure to act had been solely in consequence of an exercise of clinical judgment, it would be within the paragraph: otherwise, it would not. Thus a wrong diagnosis and consequential wrong treatment, however harmful, cannot be subject of investigation by a Commissioner; nor can an otherwise proper operation negligently performed.

A borderline case, which might or might not — according to circumstances — fall within sub-paragraph (1) of paragraph 19, is that of the patient in need of operative or other treatment not believed to be immediately necessary, who — because of a shortage of beds — has been placed on the waiting list.[1] Suppose then that such a patient is not admitted as soon as all the patients before him in the list have been dealt with, patients lower in the list being treated before him. Suppose too, that the extra delay of weeks, maybe months, in obtaining treatment has caused a serious deterioration in his condition so that, either his disease has become inoperable or a much more serious operation is required and one resulting in a greater residual disability than would otherwise have been the case. On the face of it, such a patient, having suffered hardship, would be a person aggrieved. But would sub-paragraph (1) of paragraph 19 prevent his grievance being investigated by a Commissioner? The answer to that question entirely depends

[1] It appears that a number of cases of this sort have been investigated, see 1st Annual Report (1974) H.C. 161.

on the reason for the delay. If it were that the consultant concerned had believed on the basis of his clinical judgment that patients lower in the waiting list had been more urgently in need of treatment than the patient whose operation had been deferred on their account, the matter would not be open to investigation by a Commissioner. But if the failure to call the patient in for treatment at the proper time had been due, say, to his records having been mislaid and overlooked or being misfiled, whether by the consultant himself or by any other member of the hospital staff, the matter would be one which could be subject of such investigation, because the failure to act was not the consequence of the exercise of clinical judgment. The following cases are illustrations of things which are even more clearly outside sub-paragraph (1) of the paragraph and so are open to investigation by a Commissioner.

A wrong operation performed on a patient, not because of faulty diagnosis but because other patient's notes have been referred to, cannot be said to be something done in consequence of the exercise of clinical judgment and is therefore not caught by sub-paragraph (1) of the paragraph. Examples of this are — the performance of a total hysterectomy on a woman admitted to hospital for no more than an internal examination under anaesthetic or, similarly, the performance of a sterilising operation on a patient of either sex in hospital for examination only; or an appendicectomy performed on a child patient admitted to hospital overnight for no more than attention to a whitlow. All the above are cases of operations without consent and usually the consequence of the patient not being properly identified as being the person to whom the accompanying medical notes relate.

Another type of case which would fall outside sub-paragraph (1) of the paragraph is the operation on the wrong limb or digit or organ, where there are a pair or more. A patient may have been advised to have his right leg amputated and accepted the advice. But then, possibly because — owing to someone's mistake in the ward — the patient had been prepared for the theatre as though for the left leg to be removed, the surgeon falls into the trap and removes the wrong limb. He has, thereby, done something harmful to which the patient had not consented.

Ordinarily, in the cases of the kind mentioned above as being outside the ambit of sub-paragraph (1) of the paragraph, the patient or, if he is dead, his personal representatives and dependants are likely to have grounds for claiming damages for negligence or for trespass to the person against both the person who committed the wrong and, vicariously, against the employing Health Authority. If so, investigation of the matter by a Commissioner would still be barred, unless the Commissioner were satisfied that in the particular circumstances it would not have been reasonable to expect the aggrieved person to resort or to have resorted to his right of action.[1]

6. Commissioners' Discretion in Dealing with Complaints

Section 113 provides as follows:

(1) In determining whether to initiate, continue or discontinue an investigation under this Part of this Act, a Commissioner shall, subject to section 110 above and sections 115 and 116 below, act in accordance with his own discretion.

Any question whether a complaint is duly made to a Commissioner under this Part of this Act shall be determined by the Commissioner.

7. The Davies Committee's View of the Limitations on the Commissioners' Jurisdiction

Writing before the Commissioner had been appointed, the Davies Committee said:[2]

From the outset, hopes and expectations of the office of Health Service Commissioner[3] have been pitched high, so the limits to his jurisdiction have brought some disappointment, criticism and even cynicism. We hope that this is too pessimistic a view. Of course the Health Service Commissioner will only be able to act within his statutory powers, but in several important respects he will be required to exercise individual discretion and we believe that his powers will permit him, if he thinks fit, to develop a wide jurisdiction of his own. From the evidence submitted to us, and our own experience, we are satisfied that the need for a Health Service Commissioner is acknowledged; we believe that the general public — and many people in the hospital services — will expect the Commissioner to go to the limit of his jurisdiction and to take such steps as may be necessary to provide or secure the independent review of complaints brought to his attention.

To this end we hope he will:
  (i) interpret his own powers liberally and widely, extending his jurisdiction to its statutory limit;
 (ii) be prepared to review and comment upon the procedures followed by health authorities in the course of investigating a complaint, whether or not the substantive point complained of comes within his jurisdiction;
(iii) in appropriate circumstances be prepared to recommend the type of investigation which in his opinion ought to take place of matters outside his jurisdiction.

In brief, if the Health Service Commissioner is not to disappoint the legitimate expectations of the public and many people in the hospital services he should not be predisposed to present complainants with a blank wall.

The question of what is and what is not a question of clinical judgment is left undefined by the statute.[4] Plainly, however, there will be

---

[1] S. 116(1).   [2] Paragraphs 10.3, 10.4.

[3] They used the singular for 'convenience' when referring to both the English and Welsh Health Service Commissioners.

[4] The Commissioner is the judge of it. His decisions as to whether he has jurisdiction are probably subject to review by the courts using the prerogative orders of mandamus and prohibition.

'mixed cases'. Here the Committee thought the Commissioners should be able with professional assistance to investigate most mixed complaints satisfactorily. They also thought he could comment on the review procedures followed by a Health Authority in dealing with mixed or even purely clinical complaints.[1]

8. Provisions Relating to Complaints

(a) Who may make a complaint

Section 111 (1) says:

A complaint under this Part of this Act may be made by any individual, or by any body of persons whether incorporated or not, not being —
- (a) a local authority or other authority or body constituted for purposes of the public service or of local government or for the purposes of carrying on under national ownership any industry or undertaking or part of an industry or undertaking;
- (b) any other authority or body whose members are appointed by Her Majesty or any Minister of the Crown or government department, or whose revenues consist wholly or mainly of money provided by Parliament.

Although s. 111 (1) provides for complaints not only by natural persons but also by bodies of persons, whether incorporated or not, a complaint must still be made by or on behalf of a person who has suffered injustice or hardship within the provisions of s. 109. In the context in which the word *person* is used in s. 115 it can mean no other than an individual natural person. Hence, a body of persons, whether incorporated or not, cannot themselves have a cause of complaint and their authority to make a complaint can only be on behalf of the person aggrieved.

(b) Complaints on behalf of another person or relating to a deceased person

Section 111 (2) provides:

Where the person by whom a complaint might have been made under the preceding provisions of this Part of this Act has died or is for any reason unable to act for himself, the complaint may be made,
- (a) by his personal representative, or by a member of his family, or
- (b) by some body or individual suitable to represent him

but except as aforesaid and as provided by this section 117 below a complaint shall not be entertained under this Part of this Act unless made by the person aggrieved himself.

It is even possible for an officer of the body against which a complaint may lie to make it to a Commissioner on behalf of the person aggrieved, as to which see s. 112 (b) below. Or the relevant body itself might refer a complaint to a Commissioner under the provisions of s. 117, though not when making a complaint on behalf of the aggrieved person.

[1] Paragraphs 10.9 and 10.10. It appears from the Commissioners' 1st Annual Report 1974 H.C. 161 this is in part happening.

(c) *Complaints to be in writing within one year: Discretion to investigate complaints out of time*

Section 114 (1) provides:

(1) A Commissioner —
(a) shall not be entertained under this Part of this Act unless it is made in writing to him by or on behalf of the person aggrieved not later than one year from the day on which the person aggrieved first had notice of the matters alleged in the complaint, but
(b) may conduct an investigation pursuant to a complaint not made within that period if he considers it reasonable to do so.

(d) *Prior opportunity for investigation by relevant body*

Section 112 provides:

Before proceeding to investigate complaint —
(a) a Commissioner shall satisfy himself that the complaint has been brought by or on behalf of the person aggrieved to the notice of the relevant body in question and that that body has been afforded a reasonable opportunity to investigate and reply to the complaint, but
(b) a Commissioner shall disregard the provisions of paragraph (a) in relation to a complaint made by an officer of the relevant body in question on behalf of the person aggrieved if the officer is authorised by virtue of section 117 (2) above to make the complaint and the Commissioner is satisfied that in the particular circumstances those provisions ought to be disregarded.

(e) *Reference to Commissioner by a relevant body of complaint made to it*

Section 117 says:

Notwithstanding anything in the preceding provision of sections 111 and 112 and section 114 (1) above a relevant body —
(a) may itself (excluding its officers) refer to a Commissioner a complaint that a person has, in consequence of a failure or maladministration for which the body is responsible, sustained such injustice or hardship as is mentioned in section 115 above if the complaint —
  (i) is made in writing to the relevant body by that person or by a person authorised by virtue of section 111 (2) above to make the complaint to the Commissioner on his behalf, and
  (ii) is so made not later than one year from the day mentioned in section 114 (1) above or within such other period as the Commissioner considers appropriate in any particular case; but
(b) shall not be entitled to refer a complaint in pursuance of paragraph (a) after the expiration of three months beginning with the day on which the body received the complaint;
A complaint referred to a Commissioner in pursuance of this section shall, subject to section 113 above, be deemed to be duly made to him under this Part of this Act.

The effect of s. 113, the text of which is on page 309, is to give a Commissioner discretion whether to initiate, continue or discontinue an investigation of a complaint so referred. As a referred complaint is deemed to be a complaint duly made, it follows that all the provisions of Part V of the Act so far as relevant apply to it. Reference of a complaint by a relevant body under s. 117 is to be distinguished from the making of a complaint by one of its officers on behalf of an aggrieved person, as to which see s. 111 (2).

(f) Procedure, evidence, obstruction and contempt; secrecy of information

Section 114 (2) in effect applies the provisions of the Parliamentary Commissioner Act 1967 relating to procedure, evidence, obstruction and contempt and secrecy of information to the Health Service Commissioners. These matters are now contained in Part I of Schedule 13 of the 1977 Act.[1]

[1] The Schedule says —

Procedure in respect of investigations

1. Where the Commissioner proposes to conduct an investigation pursuant to a complaint under Part V of this Act, he shall afford to the relevant body concerned, and to any other person who is alleged in the complaint to have taken or authorised the action complained of, an opportunity to comment on any allegations contained in the complaint.

2. Every such investigation shall be conducted in private, but except as aforesaid the procedure for conducting an investigation shall be such as the Commissioner considers appropriate in the circumstances of the case.

3. Without prejudice to the generality of paragraph 2 above, the Commissioner may obtain information from such persons and in such manner, and make such inquiries, as he thinks fit, and may determine whether any person may be represented, by counsel or solicitor or otherwise, in the investigation.

4. The Commissioner may, if he thinks fit, pay to the person by whom the complaint was made and to any other person who attends or furnishes information for the purposes of an investigation under Part V of this this Act —
   (a) sums in respect of expenses properly incurred by them;
   (b) allowances by way of compensation for the loss of their time,
in accordance with such scales and subject to such conditions as may be determined by the Minister for the Civil Service.

5. The conduct of an investigation under Part V of this Act shall not affect any action taken by the relevant body concerned, or any power or duty of that department or authority to take further action with respect to any matters subject to the investigation.

6. Where the person aggrieved has been removed from the United Kingdom under any Order in force under the Immigration Act 1971, he shall, if the Commissioner so directs, be permitted to re-enter and remain in the United Kingdom, subject to such conditions as the Secretary of State may direct, for the purposes of the investigation.

Evidence

7. For the purposes of an investigation under Part V of this Act the Commissioner may require any employee, officer or members of the relevant body concerned or any other person who in his opinion is able to furnish information or produce documents relevant to the investigation to furnish any such information or produce any such document.

8. For the purposes of any such investigation the Commissioner shall have the same powers as the Court (which in this Schedule means, in relation to England and Wales, the High Court, in relation to Scotland, the Court of Session, and in relation to Northern Ireland, the High Court of Northern Ireland) in respect of the attendance and examination of witnesses (including the administration of oaths or affirmations and the examination of witnesses abroad) and in respect of the production of documents.

9. No obligation to maintain secrecy or other restriction upon the disclosure of information obtained by or furnished to persons in Her Majesty's service, whether imposed by any enactment or by any rule of law, shall apply to the disclosure of information for the purposes of an investigation under this Act; and the Crown shall not be entitled in relation to any such investigation to any such privilege in respect of the production of documents or the giving of evidence as is allowed by law in legal proceedings.

10. No person shall be required or authorised by Part V of this Act and this Schedule

9. Reports and Statements

(a) Reports on completion of investigation

Section 119 (1) requires as follows:

In any case where a Commissioner conducts an investigation under this Part of this Act, he shall send a report of the results of his investigation —

(*a*) to the person who made the complaint;
(*b*) to the relevant body in question;
(*c*) to any person who is alleged in the complaint to have taken or authorised the action complained of;

to furnish any information or answer any question relating to proceedings of the Cabinet or of any committee of the Cabinet or to produce so much of any document as relates to such proceedings.

For the purposes of this paragraph a certificate issued by the Secretary of the Cabinet with the approval of the Prime Minister and certifying that any information, question, document or part of a document so relates shall be conlusive.

11. Subject to paragraph 9, no person shall be compelled for the purposes of an investigation under Part V of this Act to give any evidence or produce any document which he could not be compelled to give or produce in civil proceedings before the Court.

Obstruction and contempt

12. If any person without lawful excuse obstructs the Commissioner or any officer of the Commissioner in the performance of his functions under Part V of this Act, or is guilty of any act or omission in relation to an investigation under that Part and this Schedule which, if that investigation were a proceeding in the Court, would constitute contempt of court, the Commissioner may certify the offence to the Court.

13. Where an offence is certified under paragraph 12, the Court may inquire into the matter and, after hearing any witnesses who may be produced against or on behalf of the person charged with the offence, and after hearing any statement that may be offered in defence, deal with him in any manner in which the Court would deal with him if he had committed the like offence in relation to the Court.

14. Nothing in paragraph 12 above shall be construed as applying to the taking of any such action as is mentioned in paragraphs 5 and 6 above.

Provision for secrecy of information

15. The Commissioner and his officers hold office under Her Majesty within the meaning of the Official Secrets Act 1911.

16. Information obtained by the Commissioner or his officers in the course of or for the purposes of an investigation under Part V of this Act shall not be disclosed except —

(*a*) for the purposes of the investigation and of any report to be made thereon under that Part;
(*b*) for the purposes of any proceedings for an offence under the Official Secrets Acts 1911 to 1939 alleged to have been committed in respect of information obtained by the Commissioner or any of his officers by virtue of that Part or for an offence of perjury alleged to have been committed in the course of an investigation under that Part or for the purposes of an inquiry with a view to the taking of such proceedings; or
(*c*) for the purposes of any proceedings under paragraphs 12 and 13 above,

and the Commissioner and his officers shall not be called upon to give evidence in any proceedings (other than such proceedings as aforesaid) of matters coming to his or their knowledge in the course of an investigation under that Part.

17. A Minister of the Crown may give notice in writing to the Commissioner, with respect to any document or information specified in the notice, or any class of documents or information so specified, that in the opinion of the Minister the disclosure of that document or information, or of documents or information of that class, would be prejudicial to the safety of the State or otherwise contrary to the public interest.

18. Where a notice under paragraph 17 above is given nothing in this Schedule shall be construed as authorising or requiring the Commissioner or any officer of the Commissioner to communicate to any person or for any purpose any document or information specified in the notice, or any document or information of a class so specified.

(*d*) if the relevant body in question is not an Area Health Authority for an area in England, or a Family Practitioner Committee, to the Secretary of State;

(*e*) if that body is an Area Health Authority for an area in England, to the Regional Health Authority of which the region includes that area;

(*f*) if that body is a Family Practitioner Committee, to the Area Health Authority by which the Committee was established.

but paragraph (*d*) does not apply in the case of an investigation conducted in respect of the Health Services Committee unless the Commissioner thinks fit to publish his report under this sub-section.

(*b*) *Report to Secretary of State that injustice or hardship will not be remedied*

Section 119 (3) provides:

If, after conducting an investigation under this Part, it appears to a Commissioner that the person aggrieved has sustained such injustice or hardship as is mentioned in section 115 above and that the injustice or hardship has not been and will not be remedied, he may if he thinks fit —

(*a*) in relation to an investigation conducted in respect, the Health Services Board or the Welsh Committee, lay before each House of Parliament a special report,

(*b*) in relation to any other investigation, make a special report to the Secretary of State who shall, as soon as is reasonably practicable, lay a copy of the report before each House of Parliament.

(*c*) *Decision not to investigate — statement of reasons to complainant and to relevant body*

Section 119 (2) provides:

In any case where a Commissioner decides not to conduct an investigation under this Part of this Act, he shall send a statement of his reasons for doing so to the person who made the complaint and to the relevant body in question.

(*d*) *Annual report to Secretary of State*

Section 119 (4) provides:

Each of the Commissioners shall —

(*a*) annually lay before each House of Parliament a general report on the performance of his functions under this Part in respect of the Health Services Board and the Welsh Committee, and may from time to time lay before each House of Parliament such other reports with respect to those functions as he thinks fit;

(*b*) annually make to the Secretary of State a report on the performance of his functions under this Part and may from time to time make to the Secretary of State such other reports with respect to those functions as the Commissioner thinks fit, and the Secretary of State shall lay a copy of every such report before each House of Parliament.

(e) Privilege for reports and statements

Section 119 (5) provides:

For the purposes of the law of defamation, the publication of any matter by a Commissioner in sending or making a report in pursuance of subsection (1), (3) or (4) above or in sending a statement in pursuance of subsection (2) above shall be absolutely privileged.

C. INFORMAL INVESTIGATIONS

In H.M.(66)15 the Ministry of Health said:

Two general principles apply. First, all complaints should be dealt with as promptly as the circumstances require. Secondly, not only should complaints be investigated, but it should be made evident to complainants that their complaints have been fully and fairly considered.

And that the following procedure should apply:

i. Complaints made orally which cannot be dealt with forthwith to the complainant's satisfaction should be reported for consideration to a senior member of the staff in the department to which they relate, who should make a brief note of the complaint and of the circumstances. Appropriate action should be taken, and the complainant informed of the result. Where the complainant is not satisfied, he should be told that he can take his complaint to a higher level, and if he decides to do so he should be asked to put it in writing or, if necessary and if he agrees, it can be put in writing at his dictation by a member of the staff and signed by him. The complainant should be told to whom the complaint should then be addressed.

ii. Any written complaint should be seen by the Secretary of the Board of Governors or Hospital Management Committee or by a senior member of his staff designated by him, and the action taken or to be taken on the complaint should be agreed by him after consultation with the Head of the Department(s) concerned.

iii. Any complaints which cannot be satisfactorily dealt with by officers in this way should be reported to the Board of Governors or Hospital Management Committee or to an appropriate committee for decision as to further action. Where the Board or Committee consider that further investigation is necessary, they may decide:

   (a) to appoint one or more members of the authority to make an investigation and report back; (Alternatively, a Hospital Management Committee may ask the Regional Hospital Board — or the Board may decide, following a reference [to the Region] to appoint one or more of its members to make such an investigation). In such a case, where it might assist the investigation, or where he so desires, the complainant, accompanied by a friend if he wishes, should be present and allowed to be heard; as also should the person complained against, if he wishes;

   (b) in the small number of cases which are so serious that they cannot be dealt with satisfactorily in this way, that the investigation should be referred for independent enquiry. Action to refer such cases should

be taken by the Board of Governors or the Regional Hospital Board concerned on a reference from the Hospital Management Committee. The general rule should be that an independent lawyer or other competent person from outside the hospital service should conduct the enquiry, or preside over a small committee set up for the purpose, whose membership should be independent of the authority concerned and should include a person or persons competent to advise on any professional or technical matters. The complainant and any persons who are the subject of the complaint should have an opportunity of being present throughout the hearing, and of cross-examining witnesses, and should be allowed to make their own arrangements to be legally represented if they so wish.

Where, however, there are questions of serious discipline reference should be made to the guidance in R.H.B. (51) 80 and H.M. (61) 112. Where there is an accident in the hospital H.M. (55) 66 should continue to be applied so as to preserve legal professional privilege but subject to this, where litigation is thought likely reference should first be made to the hospital's legal advisers. Nevertheless:

Whenever investigation of a complaint may point to action to ensure the proper running of the hospital, however, the authority will wish to take such action without delay, and legal proceedings or the likelihood of legal proceedings should not deter the authority from themselves carrying out whatever investigation is needed to this end.

D. FORMAL INQUIRIES

S. 84 of the National Health Service Act 1977 now provides:

84 — (1) The Secretary of State may cause an inquiry to be held in any case where he deems it advisable to do so in connection with any matter arising under this Act.

(2) For the purpose of any such local inquiry (but subject to subsection (3) below), the person appointed to hold the inquiry —

(a) may by summons require any person to attend, at a time and place stated in the summons, to give evidence or to produce any documents in his custody or under his control which relate to any matter in question at the inquiry; and

(b) may take evidence on oath, and for that purpose administer oaths, or may, instead of administering an oath, require the person examined to make a solemn affirmation:

(3) Nothing in this section —

(a) requires a person, in obedience to summons under the section, to attend to give evidence or to produce any such documents, unless the necessary expenses of his attendance are paid or tendered to him or;

(b) empowers the person holding the inquiry to require the production of the title, or of any instrument relating to the title, of any land not being the property of a local authority.

(4) Any person who refuses or deliberately fails to attend in obedience to a summons issued under this section, or to give evidence, or who deliberately

alters, suppresses, conceals, destroys, or refuses to produce any book or other document which he is required or is liable to be required to produce for the purposes of this section, shall be liable on summary conviction to a fine not exceeding £100 or to imprisonment for a term not exceeding six months, or to both.

(5) Where the Secretary of State causes an inquiry to be held under this section —

(a) the costs incurred by him in relation to the inquiry (including such reasonable sum not exceeding £30 a day as he may determine for the services of any officer engaged in the inquiry) shall be paid by such local authority or party to the inquiry as he may direct, and

(b) may cause the amount of the costs so incurred to be certified, and any amount so certified and directed to be paid by any authority or person shall be recoverable from that authority or person by the Secretary of State summarily as a civil debt.

No local authority shall be ordered to pay costs under subsection (4) of that section in the case of any inquiry unless it is a party to that inquiry.

(6) Where the Secretary of State causes an inquiry to be held under this section may make orders —

(a) as to the costs of the parties at the inquiry, and

(b) as to the parties by whom the costs are to be paid,

and every such order may be made a rule of the High Court on the application of any party named in the order.

CHAPTER 18

BIRTHS AND DEATHS IN HOSPITAL

A. BIRTHS

1. Registration

THE main provisions of the law as to registration of births and deaths in England and Wales are contained in the Births and Deaths Registration Act 1953.[1] By s. 41 of the Act, *house* as referring to the place of a birth or death is defined as including a public institution and *a public institution*, rather inelegantly, as a prison, lock-up or hospital, and such other public or charitable institution as may be prescribed, and *occupier* in relation to a public institution 'includes a governor, keeper, master, matron, superintendent or other chief resident officer'. The substantial result of this is that whenever the responsibility for registering a birth or death is to fall on a hospital officer, the duty is now placed on a resident superintendent or medical superintendent where such there is, and, where there is not such an officer, ordinarily, on the matron.

It is the duty of the father or mother to give information of a birth to the Registrar for the sub-district in which the birth takes place within 42 days, and to sign the register. In the case of the death or inability of the father and mother, the duty is laid on every other qualified informant,[2] *viz.*, the occupier[3] of the house in which the child was, to the knowledge of the occupier, born; any person present at the birth; any person having charge of the child. The giving of information by any one qualified informant discharges the duty of all.[2] In the case of a still-birth,[4] the informant has to deliver to the Registrar a written certificate that the child was not born alive, signed by a registered medical practitioner or a certified midwife who was in attendance at the birth or who has examined the body; or make the prescribed declaration as to the reason for the absence of a certificate and that the child was still-born. Upon registering a still-birth the Registrar, if so required, will give, free of charge, a certificate of having registered a still-birth, either to the informant or to the person who has control over, or who ordinarily effects the disposal of the body, a certificate having to be produced before the body can be buried in a burial ground or church-

[1] The detailed rules made by the Registrar-General under the Act are to be found in the Registration of Births, Deaths, Marriages etc., Regulations S.I. 1968 No. 2049 as amended by S.I. 1969 No. 1811, 1970 No. 1780, 1971 No. 1218, 1974 No. 571 and 1976 Nos. 2081 and 2092.

[2] Section 2. [3] See above definition of *occupier* in the case of a hospital.

[4] For definition of still-birth see p. 332.

yard. It is an offence to dispose of the body of a still-born child by burning, except in an authorised crematorium.[1] Should such a certificate have been issued but, for some reason, is not available for the purposes of the enactments relating to the disposal of dead persons, the Registrar may issue a duplicate on payment of the prescribed fee.[2]

The obligation to give information to the Registrar of any new-born child found exposed is laid on the person finding the child and on any person in whose charge the child may be placed. The informant is bound to give such information as he has and to sign the register. There is, in this case, no order of responsibility. Any one qualified informant giving information and signing the register discharges the duty of all.[3] If a foundling is being cared for in hospital it would seem reasonable to regard the senior resident officer, e.g., medical superintendent or matron, as in charge of him.

If, after the expiry of 42 days, a birth has not been registered, the Registrar, by 7 days notice in writing, can compel any qualified informant to attend to give information and to sign the register within three months of the birth or finding.[4] The registration within three months is free unless, in pursuance of a request in writing, the Registrar registers the birth at the residence of the person making the request or at the house in which the birth took place, not being a public institution. No fee is therefore payable when the Registrar attends a hospital to register births. In any case, however, if the informant wants a certificate of the registration, he must pay for it.

After a lapse of three months, if a birth has not been registered, any qualified informant is compellable by notice in writing to attend within a year before the Superintendent Registrar to make a declaration and to sign the register, when he is obliged to pay a statutory fee to the Superintendent Registrar and also to the Registrar, unless the latter was in default.[5] After twelve months, the birth may be registered only with the written authority of the Registrar-General when double fees are payable.[6]

It will be appreciated that the Act does not require the registration of the child's own name (i.e., christian or given name) although provision is made for registration of the name within twelve months of the original entry or for its alteration within that period.[7] Provision made for re-registration of births of persons legitimised by subsequent marriage of their parents is unlikely to concern hospitals.[8] The circumstances in which the name of the father of an illegitimate child may be registered are dealt with in s. 10.

[1] Crematorium Regulations S.I. 1930 No. 1016, Reg. 3. For further information, see Prof. C. J. Polson's *Disposal of the Dead*, 2nd Edn. (1962).
[2] Section 11.   [3] Section 3.
[4] Section 4.   [5] Section 6.
[6] Section 7.   [7] Section 13.   [8] Section 14.

2. Notification of Births to Area Medical Officer

Under s. 124 of the National Health Service Act 1977,[1] a doctor or midwife attending a woman in childbirth is under an obligation to notify the area medical officer[2] of the birth or stillbirth within 36 hours and this whether the birth occurred at home or in an institution or elsewhere.

3. Babies Born in Hospital — Identification of

There is no reported English case in which a hospital or any of its staff have been sought to be made liable on account of alleged confusion of babies due to negligence, but the risk of such action could be a very real one unless a hospital were able to identify infants with reasonable assurance.

B. DEATHS[3]

1. Registration

Before the expiration of five days[4] from the date of the death, the nearest relative, including a relative by marriage and by adoption,[5] of the deceased person, present at the death or in attendance during his last illness is under a duty to give the Registrar the necessary particulars for registration to the best of his knowledge and belief and to sign the register. If there is no such relative, the duty falls on any relative of the deceased residing or being in the sub-district when the death occurred; failing whom, on any person present at the death or on the occupier[6] of the house, if he knew of the death; failing whom, on any inmate of the house who knew of the happening of the death or on the person causing the disposal of the body. The giving of information and signing the register by any one of the above qualified informants acts as a

---

[1] Formerly s. 203 of the Public Health Act 1936.

[2] See s. 124 (4) and (5) of the N.H.S. Act 1977 and the N.H.S. (Notification of Births and Deaths) Regs. 1974 No. 319 naming the area medical officer as the prescribed medical officer for the purposes of the section. It is also to be noted that by s. 124 (2) the registrar of births and deaths is required to furnish to the prescribed medical officer of the Area Health Authority the area of which includes the whole or part of the sub-district of the registrar, the particulars of each birth and death which occurs in the area of the Authority as entered in the register of births and deaths of the district. At present neither the manner nor the time of communication is prescribed. Under s. 203 of the 1936 Act there was no statutory obligation on the former medical officers of health to communicate to the registrar particulars of births notified under that section, nor has any such statutory obligation now been placed on area medical officers, but the Secretary of State has expressed the hope that the common practice of doing this will be continued. By circular H.S.C. (15) 125, the area medical officer is required to give the birth weight to the registrar. Further reference as to administrative detail may be made to circular H.R.C. (74) 3.

[3] For fuller treatment of many of the matters dealt with in this part of the chapter, reference may be made to Prof. C. J. Polson's *Disposal of the Dead*, 2nd Edn. (1962).

[4] Section 16 but see s. 18 for circumstances in which certain particulars may be given up to 14 days.

[5] Section 14.

[6] See p. 318 for definition of *occupier* in relation to hospitals and certain other residential institutions.

discharge of the duty of every other qualified informant.[1] If an inquest is held, there is no obligation to give information under s. 16.

If a person dies elsewhere than in a house, or a dead body is found and no information as to the place of death is available, the duty of giving information to the Registrar within 5 days[2] is placed on any relative of the deceased who has knowledge of any of the particulars required to be registered concerning the death; failing whom, on any person present at the death, any person finding or taking charge of the body or any person causing the disposal of the body. In this case, too, the section (s. 17) does not apply if there is an inquest and also any qualified person giving information discharges all.

The provisions of s. 17 would appear to concern a hospital only if the body, brought in dead, were taken charge of by the hospital. And since there is under that section no reference to the occupier of the house, it cannot be said dogmatically that the responsibility of registration would, as in the case of deaths in the hospital, fall on the superintendent or matron, failing responsible relatives. It is presumed, however, that the Registrar would readily take the view that it was the 'occupier' as defined in the Act who would have taken charge of the body and would therefore readily accept information from such person. On the other hand, since the ambulance service is now the responsibility of the Health Authorities, if the patient died in the ambulance, whether or not the hospital was held to have taken charge of the body, the responsibility would still fall on one of its officers — possibly the ambulance officer who was with the patient when he died.

Section 19 contains provisions for compelling any qualified person to attend and give information for registration of a death within 12 months of a death or of a finding of a body. No fee is chargeable for registering a death within 12 months otherwise than for the attendance of the Registrar at the residence of a person making a request or at the place where the deceased died, not being a hospital or other public institution. Hence, if a person dies in hospital and the Registrar attends to register the death, no charge is payable. After 12 months, a death can be registered only with the authority of the Registrar-General when a fee of $37\frac{1}{2}$p[3] is payable to the Superintendent Registrar, and, unless he was at fault, a similar fee to the Registrar.

Under s. 24, the Registrar is required to issue to the informant, free of charge, a certificate of registration of the death save when the coroner's disposal order has been issued. If the Registrar does not subsequently in due time receive notice of the disposal of the body, he

[1] Section 16.
[2] Section 17 but see s. 18 for circumstances in which certain particulars may be given up to 14 days.
[3] This figure has been substituted by s. 10 of the Decimal Currency Act 1969.

is to make inquiries of the person to whom he delivered the certificate, who is under the duty of giving information to the best of his knowledge and belief.

Section 22 lays on a registered medical practitioner who has attended a person in his last illness the responsibility of delivering forthwith a certificate of death to the Registrar and, to a qualified informant, of a notice of having done so. Unless there is an inquest or a post-mortem examination under the Coroners (Amendment) Act 1926, the cause of death as shown in the doctor's certificate will be entered in the register.[1] Section 23 provides for information to be sent to the Registrar by the coroner of findings at an inquest or of the result of a coroner's post-mortem.

In the case of a person dying in hospital the duty of issuing a death certificate ordinarily devolves on the resident medical or surgical officer who attended the patient regularly in between visits of the consultant though, technically, it might be argued that the physician or surgeon actually in charge of the case should be responsible. If the cause of death is known, even though it is such as clearly to call for an inquest, it does not appear to be a legal obligation on the medical practitioner who attended the patient in his last illness to do more than to complete the certificate for the Registrar in the normal way and to deliver the usual notice of having done so to the appropriate person. And the position is the same if, for any reason, a medical practitioner is unable to certify the cause of death; likewise if he is called in to an accident or other case not his own, dying or dead, for which he is unable properly to issue a certificate. But it is now the established practice for medical practitioners to advise the coroner direct of cases in which he is likely to be concerned and this, although not obligatory, is generally to be recommended not only in the interests of justice but as limiting the delay inevitably consequent upon reference of a death to the coroner. Moreover, with the coming into force of the Human Tissue Act 1961, which, subject to the provisions of the Act, authorises unofficial post-mortem examinations *inter alia*, for the purpose of establishing or confirming the cause of death,[2] close co-operation between hospital staff and the coroner is more than ever desirable since no such unofficial post-mortem examination may be carried out without the consent of the coroner if there is reason to believe than an inquest may be necessary or that the coroner may require a post-mortem examination.[3]

---

[1] The Registrar is indeed bound to accept the doctor's certificate as to the last illness where there is no inquest or post-mortem. Decision of the National Insurance Commission N.I. Decision No. R. (1) 4/74. For details as to the matters to be entered on the certificate see *Medical Certification of Cause of Death* published by World Health Organization (1968) (available from H.M.S.O.).

[2] Section 2 (1).

[3] Section 2 (2) and see p. 324 *et seq* further as to effect of Human Tissue Act 1961.

2. Notification by the Registrar to the Area Medical Officer of Particulars of Deaths Registered

Under s. 124 (2) of the National Health Service Act 1977, the Registrar is required to notify the prescribed medical officer of the area Health Authority, *i.e.* the area medical officer of the particulars of all deaths within the area of that authority furnished to him for registration.

3. Disposal of Body

(a) Responsibility and expenses

In default of other responsible person such as an executor, husband or parent,[1] the occupier[2] of the premises on which the death took place is responsible for the disposal of the body.

Under the National Assistance Act 1948, the local authorities named in s. 50 (2) as amended[3] are under an obligation, to dispose of the body by burial or cremation[4] of any person dying or found dead in their area and those authorities referred to in s. 50 (3) as amended[5] have permissive power to do so in the case of any deceased person who immediately before his death was being provided with accommodation under Part III of the Act by or by agreement with the Council, or was living in a hostel provided by the Council under s. 29 of the Act.

A local authority may recover the cost of burial or cremation within the provisions of s. 50 (4) of the National Assistance Act 1948 which provides:

(4) An authority may recover from the estate of the deceased person or from any person who for the purposes of this Act was liable to maintain the deceased person immediately before his death, expenses incurred under subsection (1) or subsection (3) of this section and not reimbursed under the next following subsection.

The right given to a social services authority which disposes of the body of a deceased person in accordance with the provisions of s. 50 of the National Assistance Act 1948 to claim reimbursement from any person liable to maintain the deceased[6] does not extend to a Health

[1] The class of responsible persons is nowhere clearly defined.
[2] It will be appreciated that the special definition of *occupier* for the purposes of the 1953 Births and Deaths Registration Act has no application.
[3] *i.e.* districts and London boroughs and the Common Council of the City of London. (Local Government Act 1972, Sched. 29, para. 44.)
[4] Section 50 (6) provides as follows —
(6) Nothing in the foregoing provisions of this section shall affect any enactment regulating or authorising the burial, cremation or anatomical examination of the body of a deceased person; and an authority shall not cause a body to be cremated under this section when they have reason to believe that cremation would be contrary to the wishes of the deceased.
[5] *i.e.* 'any such Council as is referred to in s. 48 (4)' which, following amendments made by the Local Government Act 1972, is 'any council which is a local authority for the purposes of the Local Authority Social Services Act 1970'.
[6] See footnote 1 on page 324.

Authority or preserved Board of Governors under the Health Service Acts which disposes of the body of a patient dying in a hospital which it administers. If, however, at the request of the hospital, responsibility for disposing of the body is undertaken by the local social services authority, that authority can claim repayment of the cost from any relative liable to maintain the deceased.[1]

A hospital, whether administered under the National Health Service Act or voluntary which has incurred expenses in disposing of the body of a deceased patient, as a creditor of the estate of the deceased, may claim reimbursement directly out of any death grant payable out of the National Insurance system. Such a claim has to be made to the Department. Any claim must be limited to the amount spent but if the death grant did not cover the cost, the hospital would remain a creditor of the estate for the balance.

Reference should also be made to the provisions of the Public Health Act 1936, ss. 161 and 163–5,[2] which make further provision for prevention of spread of infection from dead bodies of persons dying of infectious diseases. *Inter alia*, the proper officer of the Local Authority for the district in which a dead body lies[3] can forbid the body of a person who died of a notifiable disease to be removed from hospital otherwise than to a mortuary or to be forthwith buried or cremated.

(b) Duties of the Registrar

It is the duty of the Registrar who issues a certificate for burial or cremation to make inquiry if he does not receive a notification of disposal within a period of 14 days and to report all cases of delayed disposal (except under the Anatomy Acts) to the proper officer of the Local Authority for the district in which the body is lying, whilst in the case of bodies for dissection under the Anatomy Acts he must be notified of disposal within twelve months. (If part of the body of a deceased person has been retained under s. 1 of the Human Tissue Act 1961, the rules as to burial or cremation would apply only to the remainder of the body.)

In addition to burial or cremation, it is lawful to dispose of the body of a deceased person in such other manner as may be authorised by regulations made by the Secretary of State for Social Services under s. 9

---

[1] It is suggested in a departmental circular to N.H.S. hospital authorities (H.M. (72) 41) that if relatives who are thought to be able to afford to do so refuse to undertake responsibility for burial or cremation, the local social services authority should be asked to do so. It must, however, be appreciated that generally liability to maintain, and therefore to be responsible for burial or cremation in case of death, is limited to spouses, each for the other, and to parents for children who have not yet attained the age of 16 but not *vice versa see* R. v. *West London S.B.A.T., ex p. Clarke* [1975] 1 W.L.R. 1396.

[2] In Greater London, the duty is placed on the London boroughs. London Government Act 1963, s. 50 (1).

[3] Local Government Act 1972. He has taken over this function from the former medical officer of health.

(*b*) of the Births and Deaths Registration Act 1926, which procedure offers an interesting possibility should the powers under the Anatomy Acts and the Human Tissue Act 1961, ever appear inadequate.[1]

4. Post-mortem Examinations, etc.

(*a*) *Generally*

Post-mortem examination of the body of a deceased person other than by way of purely external examination, whether to ascertain the cause of death or for any other purpose, is lawful only if it is carried out on the instructions or at the request of the coroner, or is within the provisions of the Human Tissue Act 1961, or of the Anatomy Act 1832.

The Human Tissue Act 1961, also authorises — subject to the provisions of that Act — the removal of parts of the body of a deceased person either for therapeutic purposes or for purposes of medical education and research. These matters, as well as the law as to post-mortem examination under these Acts, will be dealt with in succeeding paragraphs.

(*b*) *Coroner's cases*

A coroner is required to hold an inquest whenever he is informed that the dead body of a person is lying within his jurisdiction, and there is reasonable cause to suspect that such person has died a violent or an unnatural death, *or* has died a sudden death of which the cause is unknown, *or* that such person has died in prison or in such place or under such circumstances as to require an inquest in pursuance of any Act.[2] If, therefore, there is any reasonable possibility of an inquest being necessary or of the coroner requiring a post-mortem examination in order to decide whether an inquest is necessary, no unofficial post-mortem should be undertaken without the coroner's approval as any unauthorised post-mortem would almost certainly prejudice the inquiry and amount to obstructing the coroner in the course of his duties, a punishable offence.[3]

The coroner himself may order any medical practitioner he may summon as a medical witness to make a post-mortem examination or he may request any other medical practitioner to do so even before deciding to hold an inquest. He may also now allow a medical practitioner to make such an examination, without requesting him to do so.[4]

---

[1] See further p. 327 *et seq.*, as to disposal of a body, or parts of a body under the Anatomy Act 1832, and the Human Tissue Act 1961, and as to unofficial anatomical examinations under the former Acts and unofficial post-mortem examinations under the Act of 1961.

[2] The duty on the coroner applies even if a post-mortem would be contrary to the deceased's religious beliefs. *R.* v. *Westminster City Coroner ex. p. Rainer* (1968) 112 Sol. Jo. 883.

[3] Nor does s. 2 (1) of the Human Tissue Act 1961, alter the position since s. 1 (5), which is made applicable by s. 2 (2), in effect, makes the permission of the coroner essential.

[4] Human Tissue Act 1961, s. 2.

If on result of that examination (*e.g.*, in the case of a sudden death without any suspicious features) the coroner decides that the cause of death has been sufficiently ascertained he may issue his certificate to the Registrar accordingly: otherwise he will proceed to hold an inquest in accordance with the Coroner's Acts 1887–1926. Even then, if he is satisfied that it is proper to do so, he may issue a disposal order without necessarily waiting for the conclusion of the inquest.

The following provisions of the Coroner's Rules 1953,[1] should be noted. Any post-mortem examination ordered or authorised by the coroner is to be made, whenever practicable, by a pathologist with suitable qualifications and experience and having access to laboratory facilities. But if the deceased died in hospital the coroner should not direct or request a pathologist on the staff of, or associated with, that hospital to make a post-mortem examination if (i) that pathologist does not desire to make the examination, or (ii) the conduct of any member of the hospital staff is likely to be called in question, or (iii) any relative of the deceased asks the coroner that the examination be not made by such a pathologist, unless the obtaining of another pathologist with suitable qualifications and experience would cause the examination to be unduly delayed. Also if pneumoconiosis is suspected, no member of the pneumoconiosis panel should make the examination.[2] The rule that a post-mortem examination should, whenever practicable, be made by a suitably qualified pathologist and the other rules above set out, do not apparently apply to a post-mortem examination under the Human Tissue Act 1961, s. 2, which the coroner may have permitted to ascertain the cause of death. It seems likely, however, that a coroner would not readily give his consent to such examination except by a suitably qualified pathologist.

If there is to be a coroner's post-mortem, the coroner must, if practicable without undue delay in the examination, inform *inter alia* the hospital, if the deceased died in hospital, and the hospital may be represented at the post-mortem by a medical practitioner.[3] Apart from those persons listed in the rules[3] the coroner *may* inform any person of a post-mortem and permit him to be present.[4] Hence, any medical practitioner on the hospital staff who was concerned might request to be permitted to attend. But neither a hospital representative, nor anyone else permitted to be present at a post-mortem, may interfere with the performance of the examination.[5] Except on his authority, no copy of the report of post-mortem or special examination is to be supplied to anyone other than the coroner.[6]

If a person dies on hospital premises there being suitable accommoda-

---

[1] S.I. 1953 No. 205.   [2] Rule 3.
[3] Rule 4 (2).   [4] Rule 4 (3).
[5] Rule 5.   [6] Rule 7 (2) and 10.

tion at the hospital, the post-mortem, with consent of the hospital is to be made there, unless the coroner otherwise decides.[1]

(c) *Post-mortem examination and use of parts of a body of a deceased person under the Human Tissue Act 1961*

(i) *Generally.* In the long title of the Human Tissue Act 1961, its purposes are summarised in the following words — 'An Act to make provision with respect to the use of parts of bodies of deceased persons for therapeutic purposes and purposes of medical education and research and with respect to the circumstances in which post-mortem examinations may be carried out; and to permit the cremation of bodies removed for anatomical examination'.[2]

(ii) *Removal of parts of bodies for medical purposes.*[3] The removal and use of parts of bodies for therapeutic purposes or for purposes of medical education or research is now dealt with in s. 1 of the Human Tissue Act 1961, s. 1 (1) of the Act provides as follows:

If any person in writing at any time or orally in the presence of two or more witnesses during his last illness, has expressed a request that his body or any specified part of his body be used after his death for therapeutic purposes or for purposes of medical education or research, the person lawfully in possession of his body after death may, unless he has reason to believe that the request was subsequently withdrawn, authorise the removal from the body of any part of or, as the case may be, the specified part, for use in accordance with the request.

Further, by virtue of s. 1 (2), even if the deceased has not expressed any such request, the person in possession of the body may yet authorise the removal of any part of the body for any of the purposes mentioned in s. 1 (1) if, having made such reasonable enquiry as may be practicable, he has no reason to believe —

(a) that the deceased had expressed an objection to his body being so dealt with after his death, and had not withdrawn it; or
(b) that the surviving spouse or any surviving relative of the deceased objects to the body being so dealt with.

Section 1 (4) provides that the removal of any part of a body under s. 1 (1) or (2) is not to be effected except by a fully registered medical practitioner, who must have satisfied himself by personal examination of the body that life is extinct. The use of the expression *fully registered* excludes not only any provisionally registered practitioner[4] but also,

---

[1] Rule 8 (3).
[2] It has been held that although no specific penalties are set out in the Act, breach of the prohibitions contained in it is a criminal offence corresponding to what used to be called a common law misdemeanour. *R.* v. *Lennox Wright* [1973] Crim. L.R. 529.
[3] See further pp. 331 *et seq.* and, in particular, as to the use of whole bodies under s. 1 of the Human Tissue Act 1961, p. 332.
[4] By s. 17 of the Medical Act 1956, a conditionally registered medical practitioner is deemed to be fully registered so far as is necessary to enable him to be engaged in employment in a resident medical capacity in one or more hospitals or institutions approved for the

N

presumably, any practitioner from overseas temporarily registered for some particular purpose and not free to practise where he likes.

(iii) *Coroner must not be obstructed.* Furthermore, under s. 1 (5) where in England and Wales a person has reason to believe that an inquest may be required to be held on any body or that a post-mortem examination of any body may be required by the coroner, he may not, except with the consent of the coroner, give any authority for a body to be dealt with under s. 1 (1) or (2), nor may he act on such authority given by any other person.[1]

(iv) *Person lawfully in possession of body.* Nowhere in the Act is there any definition of 'the person lawfully in possession of his body', the expression used in s. 1 (1) referring to the person who, under s. 1 (1) or (2) may allow removal of a part of a body. By inference it appears that, as under the Anatomy Act 1832, the expression means anyone who has possession of the body even for a strictly limited purpose, as in the case of an undertaker, or for a limited time, as in the case of a hospital which normally has possession of the body only until an undertaker receives it on the instructions of relatives. That view is clearly borne out by the prohibition of the giving of any authority under the Act by a person entrusted with the body for the purpose only of its interment or cremation,[2] without which prohibition an undertaker could have given such authority.

That the person having the control and management of a hospital, nursing home or other institution has lawful possession of the body of a deceased inmate[3] is implicit in s. 1 (7) which lays down that authority may be given on behalf of that person by any officer or person designated for that purpose by him. It must be appreciated that the expression 'person' here includes a corporate body, so that in the case of a Health Service hospital the person having the management and control is, ordinarily, the Area Health Authority[4] and such Authority should designate an officer to act on its behalf in the matter and can, presumably, designate more than one person. In the case of a Local Authority institution, the 'person' having control and management is the Local Social Services Authority. In the case of a nursing home whilst it could be argued that it is the proprietor, whether a limited company, a partnership or a single natural person who is in possession of the body of a deceased patient, it is perhaps the preferable interpretation to assume it to be the person in immediate day to day charge, usually a

---

purposes of the section, but since the removal of parts of the body of a deceased patient is not a necessary part of a house officer's treatment of patients, it would appear that he is not deemed to be fully registered for the purposes of the Human Tissue Act 1961, which Act itself gives no such entended meaning to the words 'fully registered'.

[1] The circumstances in which a coroner may be concerned are set out on pp. 325–326.
[2] Section 1 (6).   [3] As decided in *R. v. Feist* (1858) Dears & B. 590.
[4] It could perhaps be that the duty of designation could be delegated to the District management team or to the Administrator.

resident medical practitioner or a resident registered nurse or, in the case of a maternity home, possibly a state certified midwife.[1]

(v) *Delegation of authority.* It appears that a Health Authority can delegate its functions to an officer, *e.g.*, its Chief Administrative Officer.[2] It is possible that it may also delegate its power of delegation.[3]

It is important that any delegation by an Authority should be by a minuted resolution, that being the only way such a body can make an effective decision.

(vi) *Saving for existing powers.* Nothing in s. 1 of the Human Tissue Act 1961, is to be construed as rendering unlawful any dealing with, or with any part of, the body of a deceased person which is lawful apart from the Act.[4]

(vii) *Post-mortem examinations under the 1961 Act.* Section 2 (1) provides that without prejudice to s. 15 of the Anatomy Act 1832 (which prevents that Act from being construed as applying to post-mortem examinations directed to be made by a competent legal authority) that Act shall not be construed as applying to any post-mortem examination carried out for the purpose of establishing or confirming the causes of death or of investigating the existence or nature of abnormal conditions. Until now, on a strict interpretation of the Act of 1832, any examination for such purpose, otherwise than on the instruction or at the request of the coroner, has been illegal, since the necessary certificate of cause of death could not have been issued prior to the examination. This, incidentally, could not under the Anatomy Act 1832, have taken place until 48 hours after the death.

But the wider powers given in s. 2 (1), the Human Tissue Act 1961, are themselves subject to substantially the same limitations as are dealings with a body for therapeutic purposes or for purposes of medical education or research under s. 1, since no post-mortem may be carried out otherwise by or in accordance with the instructions of a fully registered medical practitioner[5] and no post-mortem examination which is not directed or requested by the coroner or other competent legal authority is to be carried out without the authority of the person lawfully in possession of the body./Furthermore, s. 1 (2), (5), (6) and (7), with the necessary modifications, apply in respect of the giving of this authority.[6] Of particular significance is s. 1 (5) which forbids such examination without the consent of the coroner when there is reason to believe that an inquest may be necessary or a post-mortem examination may be requested by the coroner. It follows that a post-mortem ex-

---

[1] Registration of a nursing home may be refused on the ground that such a person will not be in charge.

[2] N.H.S. Functions (Administrative Arrangements) Regs. S.I. 1974 No. 36. Regs. 3 and 4.

[3] It would be prudent in the exercise of any such power, for both the delegation and the withdrawal to be done in writing.

[4] Section 1 (7).   [5] See footnote 4, page 327.   [6] Section 2 (2).

amination to ascertain the cause of death or in any other case which is or appears to be within the coroner's jurisdiction can still be done only on his instructions, at his request or with his consent.

(d) Anatomical examination under the Anatomy Act 1832

The principal provisions of the Anatomy Act 1832 regarding anatomical examination of the body of a deceased person are:

  (i) that such examination may be undertaken only by a person duly licensed[1] and at a place duly notified to the Secretary of State for Social Services[2];

  (ii) that the examination is undertaken with the permission or at the request of the person[3] in lawful possession of the body, which permission may not be given or request made if any relative of the deceased has objected to anatomical examination of the body[4];

  (iii) that a certificate of the cause of death[5] given by the medical practitioner who attended the deceased in his last illness or, if he was not so attended, by some other medical practitioner to the best of his knowledge and belief is delivered to the licensed person with the body[6];

  (iv) that the removal for anatomical examination does not take place until 48 hours after death and 24 hours after notice of the intended removal has been given to the inspector for the district or, if there is no inspector, to some other local medical practitioner[7];

  (v) that the licensed person within 24 hours of the removal of the body to the place of examination sends on to the inspector for the district under the Act the certificate of cause of death together with a return stating the day and hour when and the name of the person from whom the body was received, the date and place of death, the sex and, so far as known, the name, age and last place of abode of the deceased[8];

  (vi) that the body is removed in a decent shell or coffin and the person removing it or causing it to be removed makes provision for its decent burial, after dissection, in consecrated ground or in some

---

[1] Section 1.   [2] Section 12.

[3] *Person* here includes societies and incorporated bodies (s. 19). If a person dies in hospital or in a Social Services analogous institution, the person having the management of the hospital or institution is in lawful possession of the body and may permit its removal for anatomical examination, subject to the provisions of the Act (*R*. v. *Feist* (1858) Dears & B. 590).

[4] Section 7 but there is no obligation to seek the consent of the relatives.

[5] Section 9.   [6] Section 10.

[7] Section 9. If a patient died in hospital and the body were removed from the ward or from the mortuary of the hospital to another part of the same institution for anatomical examination, that would constitute removal under the Act.

[8] Section 11

burial ground proper to persons of the deceased's religion,[1] or for its cremation[2];

(vii) that a certificate of interment or cremation of the body is sent to the inspector within twelve months after the day on which the body was received for anatomical examination.[3]

Both the licensed person and the inspector are responsible for keeping records in accordance with the Acts.

(e) Further consideration of the application of the Anatomy Act 1832 and of the Human Tissue Act 1961

Because the provisions of the Human Tissue Act 1961 are very much less rigid than those of the Anatomy Act 1832, recourse is now likely to be made to the 1832 Act only when bodies are needed for dissection by medical students, the use of bodies for other purposes being covered by the 1961 Act. But it seems that when a body is removed for dissection under the Anatomy Act 1832, the person having possession of the body may also authorise the removal and retention of any part of the body under s. 1 (1) or (2) of the 1961 Act. If he does so that part must be removed by a registered medical practitioner.[4]

But what if it is desired to retain a specimen for medical education after removal by way of dissection under the Act of 1832? Possibly the best way of dealing with such situation would be for the person in possession of the body — normally a hospital or institution authority — to give general permission for removal of parts of the body under s. 1 of the Human Tissue Act 1961, at the same time as giving permission for removal of the body under the Anatomy Act 1832. Then, the only problem would be that the Act of 1961 required removal of the part by a registered medical practitioner.[5]

Although under s. 1 of the Human Tissue Act 1961, only the removal and, in effect, the retention of any part of the body of a deceased person is authorised, it seems clear that more than one part may be removed from the same body. But could part after part of the body be removed until nothing remained? On balance it seems that it could, provided each part removed was wanted for an authorised purpose and its removal from the rest of the body undertaken by a registered medical practitioner. In support of this point of view it may be indicated that the skeleton may properly be described as a part of the body. That being so, it could be removed from the body to be kept for the purpose of medical education under s. 1. At that point it becomes somewhat

[1] Section 13.   [2] Human Tissue Act 1961, s 3
[3] S.R. & O. Rev. 1904 1 Anatomy, p. 1 and Human Tissue Act 1961, s. 3.
[4] Section 1 (4).
[5] It is, perhaps, a pity that the opportunity was not taken to amend the Anatomy Act 1832, to allow retention of specimens under that Act. Probably no action would be taken in respect of the *bona fide* retention of part of a body as a museum specimen in circumstances that caused no distress to relatives nor outrage to public feelings.

academic to argue about the fate of the rest of the body and which parts and how much should be retained for burial or cremation.

(*f*) *Specimens retained after operations; stillbirths, etc.*

There are no legal obstacles to the retention as museum specimens or for other purposes of medical education or interest of organs, growths, *etc.*, removed from a patient during an operation except the highly theoretical one of little practical importance that whatever is removed is the property of the patient, though on rare occasion, on religious grounds, a patient may ask that some part of his body being removed in an operation, say a limb being amputated, be disposed of in a particular way or that he, or someone nominated by him, may have the disposal of it. In such case, whilst a hospital would be under no obligation to incur any additional expenditure in order to comply with the patient's request it would be reasonable for it to do so, always provided no risk of infection was foreseeable and no nuisance thereby created.

The position with regard to the retention as a museum specimen of a stillborn child and that in respect of the retention of a complete foetus or part of a foetus are quite different, a distinction having to be drawn between a foetus and a stillborn infant.

A child is stillborn which has issued forth from its mother after the twenty-eighth week of pregnancy and which did not at any time after being expelled from its mother breathe or show any signs of life.[1] Notification of the stillbirth has to be given to the Registrar and the better opinion would seem to be that the body should be disposed of by burial in a burial ground or churchyard or by cremation at an authorised crematorium.[2] The body of a stillborn child is not within the provisions of the Human Tissue Act 1961.

But in the case of delivery of the foetus without sign of life before the end of the twenty-eighth week of pregnancy, no registration is necessary and the foetus may be disposed of without formality in any way which does not constitute a nuisance or an affront to public decency. Hence, its preservation for scientific purposes is in order. No foetus which is thus retained should bear any inscription which would identify the patient from whom it was taken as that would constitute a breach of professional confidence, certainly offensive and possibly actionable.

5. Inquests

(*a*) *Generally*

The *Coroners Rules* 1953[3] made some important changes in respect of procedure at inquests more particularly as to the rights of interested

---

[1] Births and Deaths Registration Act 1953, s. 41.
[2] To dispose of a still-birth by burning it elsewhere is unlawful. See note 1 on p. 319.
[3] S.I. 1953 No. 205.

persons and as to the purpose of the inquiry, the latter being dealt with by placing fairly strict limits on verdicts and riders. Some of the points in the new rules of interest to hospital authorities and their professional staff are set out in the following paragraphs. Reference has already been made to the provisions of the rules as to *post-mortems*.

All inquests are to be held in public, exception to be made only on grounds of national security.[1]

Provision is made for any person whose conduct is likely to be called into question to be summoned to give evidence and for the inquest to be adjourned for him to be summoned if that has not been done,[2] and for witnesses to be examined by anyone who in the opinion of the coroner is a properly interested person or by his counsel or solicitor, subject always to the coroner's discretion to disallow irrelevant or improper questions.[3] This lets in the authority as well as any member of its staff personally concerned since the word 'person' includes a corporate body.

Witnesses are ordinarily to be examined first by the coroner and, if the witness is represented at the inquest, lastly by his own representative. No witness may be asked incriminating questions and it is the duty of the coroner, if such question is asked, to tell him that he need not answer.[4] It must be appreciated, however, that the protection extends only to questions which do tend to incriminate (*e.g.*, establish a charge of manslaughter) and that there is no protection against questions tending to establish civil liability (*e.g.*, for negligence) if otherwise proper.

(b) The purpose of an inquest

The proceedings and evidence at an inquest are to be directed solely to ascertaining (*a*) who the deceased was; (*b*) how, when and where the deceased came by his death; (*c*) the persons, if any, to be charged with murder, manslaughter, infanticide or causing death by dangerous driving, or of being accessories before the fact, should the jury find that the deceased came by his death in any one of those ways other than the last-mentioned[5]; (*d*) the particulars for the time being required by the Registration Acts to be registered concerning the death.[6] Neither the coroner nor the jury are to express any opinion on any matter other than the foregoing but this does not preclude the coroner or the jury from making a recommendation designed to prevent the recurrence of

---

[1] Rule 14.
[2] Rules 19 and 20. By the Coroners (Amendment) Rules 1974 No. 2178 in case of a death following an industrial accident, the inquest must be adjourned unless an inspector appointed under the Health and Safety at Work etc. Act 1974 is present.
[3] Rule 16.   [4] Rule 18.
[5] The inquest is no longer allowed to charge any person with these offences — Criminal Law Act 1977 s. 56 and see also Schedule 20.
[6] Rule 26.

fatalities similar to that in respect of which the inquest is being held, and such recommendation being included in a rider.[1] Furthermore, no verdict is to be framed in such a way as to appear to determine any question of civil liability.[2] This last-mentioned provision would preclude a finding of negligence not amounting to manslaughter, though a permissible recommendation for avoiding similar fatalities in future might by implication, suggest carelessness or negligence.

The rules also contain various other important provisions, though not of special concern to hospitals as, for example, restricting the use of documentary evidence without the attendance of the maker; forbidding any address to the coroner as to the facts; and requiring the police to be represented by counsel or solicitor if desiring to examine witnesses.

---

[1] Rules 27 and 34.   [2] Rule 33.

CHAPTER 19

MEDICAL RECORDS

A. OWNERSHIP OF MEDICAL RECORDS

General Principles

IN general terms, if a professional man in independent private practice makes notes for his own guidance in advising his patient or client or in treating his illness or dealing with his affairs, those notes ordinarily remain the property of the maker. This is not the less true because he may be under a duty to his patient or client as to the confidentiality of the information in those notes or the use he may put them to.[1] Such then is the position of the independent medical practitioner in respect of medical records relating to his patient. However, that simple statement has to be modified to take account of the fact that most doctors, other than specialists in private practice, do not nowadays work single-handed. In the hospital, it must be modified because the specialist who, as a member of the staff, treats patients not in direct contractual relationship with him does not own the medical notes relating to such patients; nor is the position clear cut even in respect of medical notes relating to private patients whom he may treat in hospital.

B. HOSPITAL AND SPECIALIST PRACTICE — OWNERSHIP OF RECORDS

1. General Ward and Amenity Patients in N.H.S. Hospitals

Medical notes taken by a member of the staff in respect of a general ward patient in a hospital, or of a patient in an 'amenity bed'[2] do not become the property of the medical practitioner taking them but remain under the ownership and control of the hospital for use by any medical practitioner who may treat the same patient at the hospital subsequently, but there is ordinarily no legal obligation to make the notes accessible, even at the patient's request, to any medical practitioner outside the hospital save in legal proceedings and then only where the appropriate steps have been taken to compel disclosure. It is, however, the accepted custom on discharge of a patient for a member of the hospital professional staff to communicate to the patient's general

---

[1] See below, Chapter 20.
[2] See above, p. 103.

practitioner such information as is necessary to put him in the picture and to give him advice on such further treatment as might be necessary.[1]

2. Private Patients in N.H.S. Hospitals

The 1st Schedule to the Public Records Act 1958, which makes records generally of National Health Service hospitals public records, excludes records of private patients admitted under s. 5 of the National Health Service Act 1946 — now replaced by ss. 65 and 66 of the National Health Service Act 1977[2] — and this lends some support to the suggestion that all medical records of a private patient belong to the consultant in charge of his treatment. But that is not necessarily so. In the first place it must be remembered that, although it is rare, a private patient might be treated under s. 65 (1) of the Act of 1977, in which case the hospital would provide specialist as well as other services at an inclusive charge and there is no contract between patient and consultant. In that case the records would clearly belong to the hospital no less than would those of a N.H.S. patient but, because of the provisions of the Public Records Act 1958, they would not be public records.

Almost invariably, however, the patient, or a relative of the patient, makes a contract with a consultant for medical or surgical treatment under s. 65 (2) of the National Health Service Act 1977. Then it can properly be argued that that consultant's notes are his own property and not that of the hospital. But what of nursing records or records of tests, X-rays or other treatment provided by the hospital or even records of medical oversight of the patient by a registrar or houseman? Are these not properly to be regarded as belonging to the hospital? The point may well be of importance since the hospital may be sued in respect of alleged negligence of members of its staff in these matters and should have the records necessary to help justify or rebut such allegations. But although these records do belong to the hospital, they are not public records. Moreover, should a radiologist's or other report be made in respect of a private patient by virtue of a private arrangement with the patient or, as likely as not, with the consultant on his behalf, then, even though the radiologist or other specialist concerned is on the staff of the hospital, the hospital is not the owner of the record of such report.[3]

However, in so far as a specialist attending a patient in hospital under a private contract enters information and instructions in the

---

[1] As to failure of such communication as the possible basis of an action for negligence, see pp. 236–241.

[2] Section 66 makes provision for private non-resident patients, *i.e.* private out-patients. The same considerations apply to them as to in-patients under s. 65.

[3] In saying this, it is assumed that the hospital appointment of the radiologist or other consultant concerned is one under which he is permitted to undertake private work.

hospital case notes relating to that patient, as he must surely do in order to give direction and guidance to nursing staff as well as to medical staff having oversight of the patient in his absence, those notes will remain the property of the hospital although not public records.

3. Patients in Voluntary Hospitals

Generally, unless a patient in a voluntary hospital has a contract with an attending medical practitioner[1] for treatment as his private patient, all records of his treatment are hospital records. But if he be a private patient, the notes made by the specialist whose private patient he is will normally[2] be the property of that specialist, excepting only, as in N.H.S. hospitals, notes made for the direction and guidance of hospital medical and nursing staff in respect to the patient's care and treatment and incorporated in the hospital case notes for that patient.

Should a N.H.S. patient be treated at a voluntary hospital under contractual arrangements with a Health Authority, any communication concerning the patient sent to the Authority by the voluntary hospital or by a member of its staff would become a public record. The position in respect of case notes, *etc.*, made by members of the staff of a voluntary hospital concerning a particular patient treated under contract with the Health Authority would depend on the terms of the agreement made for treatment of N.H.S. patients in that hospital, but, in the absence of agreement to the contrary, they would probably be the property of the hospital where the patient had been treated.

4. Patients in Nursing Homes

Since a patient in a nursing home usually has a direct agreement with a medical practitioner for such medical or surgical treatment as he needs, the nursing home providing only nursing care, ancillary services and accommodation, the position as to medical records is substantially the same as in the case of a private patient in a voluntary hospital, save in so far as a voluntary hospital is likely to be providing not only nursing care but also medical oversight between visits of the patient's own doctor. Indeed, such medical support is also provided in some larger nursing homes. When medical support as well as nursing care is provided in a nursing home, the position in respect of ownership of medical records will be indistinguishable from that which obtains when a private patient is treated in a voluntary hospital.

---

[1] The term *medical practitioner* is used rather than *consultant* as, occasionally, it may be that a patient is admitted in the care of a general practitioner.

[2] The word *normally* is here used to qualify the general statement since in every case the position will depend on the conditions under which the practitioner had been afforded facilities for attending private patients in the particular hospital.

C. RADIOLOGISTS' REPORTS; X-RAY FILMS AND PRINTS ETC. — OWNERSHIP

If a patient has paid the radiologist's fee, the ownership of developed X-ray films of a particular patient, and prints taken therefrom, constitutes a much more difficult problem than that of a radiologist's report or medical notes. The better opinion seems to be that what the patient pays for is not a photograph but the expert reading by the radiologist of the film and for his opinion on what he believes to be the facts disclosed, that reading and opinion being communicated to the medical practitioner by whom the patient was referred for his guidance. If, as is customary, the report is accompanied by a print of the film, that does not alter the view taken here provided the radiologist is regarded as an expert giving an opinion.

Further, the most telling argument against the patient's right to claim the film or print is to be found in the general custom of the medical profession in the matter. The one obstacle in the way of this appeal to custom arises from a confusion between the functions of the radiologist or medical specialist who, *inter alia*, directs the taking of the X-ray film and is responsible for its interpretation and for giving his opinion to the doctor in charge of the case, and those of the radiographer or technician who is responsible for handling the X-ray apparatus, for actually taking films and — on medical instructions — giving therapeutic X-ray or similar treatment. If a doctor wishing simply to obtain a film or print of a part of the body of a particular patient tells the patient so and sends him to an institution where he can get the film taken on payment of a fee and the film or print is then sent to the doctor, it is understandable that the patient should feel that the 'picture' was his property and demand its surrender, especially if he changes his doctor. And, unfortunately, owing sometimes to the casual use of words by medical men who may say something to the effect that they want an X-ray done, the patient even being sent to a radiologist for an opinion gets the idea that he is getting 'just a picture' for his doctor's use.

In private practice then, if a consultant radiologist makes or obtains an X-ray film relating to a private patient and sends a print to the patient's general practitioner or to another specialist dealing with the patient, it would appear that whilst the print becomes the property of the recipient doctor, the copyright would ordinarily remain vested in the radiologist who had made the X-ray photograph or had paid for it to be made in accordance with his directions.

The question of the rights and duties in respect of X-ray films and prints is chiefly of interest to hospitals and to their staff in respect of paying patients having a direct contract with the specialist or specialists concerned. Paying patients who elect not to make separate arrangements with specialists will be charged inclusive fees by the hospital.[1] It would not seem that there could be any grounds on which such patient could claim possession of an X-ray photograph taken but, presumably, as well as in the case of part-paying and N.H.S. patients, the photographs and radiologists' reports will be available as a matter of practice for the use of medical practitioners at other hospitals within the service where the patient may later be treated.

In respect of N.H.S. patients the question hardly arises. The continued significance of the problem, as of that of availability of medical notes, is chiefly dependent on the survival of competitive medical practice and of entirely independent hospitals. In any fully co-ordinated national medical service, a patient's medical record, including X-ray films and prints with reports thereon, could presumably be passed on with the patient from one doctor and one hospital to another. The question would still remain, however, as to the making of such notes, reports, *etc.*, available for purposes other than the treatment of the patient or of providing reports based on the medical notes *etc.*, for other purposes, *e.g.* to help the patient's legal advisers decide whether to advise him to commence an action against a third party or in the preparation for the trial of any such action. Who should pay for the work involved and to whom should payment be made?

The hospital owns the property in the notes themselves as pieces of paper or film. It owns the copyright in the notes and the information on them. It follows that where a copy is made for the use of a patient's general practitioner, the hospital will not lose either its copyright or the right to control the use to which information is put. In other words, the patient does not have this right. It follows that the patient is not entitled to see the contents of any letter concerning his condition or treatment received by his doctor from a consultant or from any other practitioner who may have examined or treated him. Nor is that unreasonable since, as a rule, the consultant himself will already have given the patient such information and advice as he thinks should properly come from him, for the test leaving it to the discretion of the family doctor what more to tell him, in the light of the consultant's letter. Moreover there may be things in the letter which, in his own interest, the patient should not be told, but which it is necessary that his doctor should know. And there may be other things which the consultant may feel obliged to say, things which might reflect on the patient, or which he might not accept if he were told. Hence, in many cases, the general practitioner will pass on to his patient only an edited and interpreted version of the specialist's report, though he may well choose to quote verbatim any reassuring passage.

[1] National Health Service Act 1977 s. 65.

Further, however, the ownership of the copyright and the information, resting where it does in the hospital, the recipient doctor should not do, save under compulsion of law, is to make the specialist's report available for any purpose other than that for which it was made. If the patient, or anyone else with the patient's consent, wants a report from the specialist, *e.g.* for insurance purposes, the specialist himself should be asked to provide it and, assuming that he were in private practice, he could properly charge a fee for such extra report, this even though no further examination of the patient had been necessary before making it. Whether a specialist or other practitioner who, under his contract with a hospital had examined or treated a N.H.S. patient, either in hospital or at a domiciliary consultation, could charge for any medical report on the patient other than such report as he might have made in the course of duty, would depend on the terms and conditions of hospital medical and dental staff applicable to him at the time.[1]

D. THE PUBLIC RECORDS ACT 1958

Subject to the overall responsibility of the Lord Chancellor,[2] a duty is now placed by the 1958 Public Records Act on every person responsible for public records of any description which are not in the Public Record Office or a place of deposit appointed by the Lord Chancellor to make arrangements for the selection of those records which ought to be permanently preserved and for their safe-keeping and this duty is to be performed under the guidance of the Keeper of Public Records.[3] After thirty years such records have to be deposited with the Keeper or at other appointed place unless needed for administrative purposes.[4] The Lord Chancellor decides who is responsible for the various classes of record.[5]

In effect that means that each Government department is primarily responsible for its own records and by s. 10 and paragraph 3 (1) of the First Schedule to the Act, and Part I of the Table annexed thereto, it is provided that the departmental and administrative records of the N.H.S. hospitals,[6] whether or not records belonging to Her Majesty should be public records for which the Department of Health and Social Security is responsible. Excepted were records of endowments passing to Boards of Governors under s. 7 of the National Health Service Act

---

[1] Assuming that the practitioner is willing to make such report he is in fact ordinarily permitted to make a charge there for. He is not however bound to make any such report without the consent of the patient save in exceptional circumstances discussed below and indeed should not do so.
[2] Section 1 of the Public Records Act 1958.
[3] Section 3 (1) (2).
[4] Section 3 (3).   [5] Section 3 (4).
[6] Records of other National Health Service authorities, other than local authorities, are also within the provisions of the Act.

1946;[1] records relating to funds held by hospital boards and committees under ss. 59 and 60 of that Act; and records of private patients admitted under s. 5[2] of the Act.[3]

Records of property passing to Regional or Area Health Authorities or to special Health Authorities under ss. 23 to 26 of the National Health Service Reorganisation Act 1973 as well as records of property held by a Regional or Area Health Authority or by a special Health Authority under s. 90 or 91 of the 1977 Act are also public records.[4] Since, between them, it can be said that ss. 21 to 26 of the 1973 Act and 90 and 91 of the 1977 Act cover all the modes by which a Health Authority might become possessed of property substantially corresponding, so far as the hospital side of its work is concerned with acquisitions under ss. 7, 59 and 60 of the National Health Service Act 1946, it follows that records of charitable funds of all kinds at the disposal of any Health Authority are public records for the purposes of the 1958 Act. But where, in the case of an Area Health Authority (Teaching), such property has passed to, or is receivable by Special Trustees under s. 95 of the 1977 Act, records relating thereto are not public records. It would be otherwise in any case in which, pursuant to a request under s. 24 (2) of the 1973 Act, Special Trustees had not been appointed, so that such property would have passed to or be receivable by the Authority itself.

The Ministry of Health in July 1961, sent a circular to hospital authorities[5] giving them instructions as to what records are to be permanently retained and what may be destroyed and after what interval. The point is expressly made that if documents have been selected for permanent preservation the original documents must be preserved; it is not permissible to preserve microfilm copies in their place.

When public records have been deposited permanently in the Public Record Office or other place of deposit appointed under the Act, the Keeper of Public Records may nevertheless authorise their destruction or disposal subject to the approval of the Lord Chancellor and of the Minister or other person who appears to the Lord Chancellor to be primarily concerned.[6]

It is provided in s. 9 that the legal validity of any record shall not be

---

[1] It seems probable that it was by an oversight that records relating to property passing to a hospital management committee under the proviso to s. 7 (4) of the 1946 Act were not excluded from the class of public records under the 1958 Act although similar in nature to teaching hospital endowments so passing under s. 70.

[2] Now see ss. 65 and 66 of the National Health Service Act 1977.

[3] It is not easy to see why records of private patients are excluded from the requirements of the Public Records Act since not only any practitioner with whom the patient might have a private contract is concerned with those records but also the hospital authority in respect of and the services of junior medical staff and of nursing and other supporting services for which the authority is responsible.

[4] They were added to the list in Sch. 1 of the 1958 Act by Sch. 4, para. 82, of the 1973 Reorganisation Act. See now 1977 Act Sch. 15 para. 22.

[5] H.M. (61) 73. Set out in Appendix D.   [6] Section 6.

affected by its removal under the Act or under the Public Record Office Acts of 1838 to 1898 now repealed or by the provisions in those Acts with respect to its legal custody. A copy of or extract from a public record in the Public Record Office purporting to be examined and certified as true and authentic by the proper officer and to be sealed or stamped with the seal of the Public Record Office is admissible as evidence in any proceedings without any further or other proof thereof if the original record would have been admissib e as evidence in those proceedings.[1]

[1] Section 9 (2).

PROFESSIONAL CONFIDENCE AND RELATED MATTERS

A. INTRODUCTORY: NATURE OF OBLIGATION OF PROFESSIONAL CONFIDENCE

PROBABLY since recorded history began it has been accepted by the medical profession that, arising out of the doctor–patient relationship, there is a moral obligation on the doctor to exercise great discretion not only concerning the nature of the patient's illness and the attendant circumstances but also about all else which might come to his knowledge concerning the patient, his family and his affairs in the course of such professional relationship. It is also accepted that the obligation is quite independent of contract and arises whoever may be paying the doctor for his services and, indeed, even though his services may have been rendered gratuitously. However, there may be circumstances in which the patient knows, or should know, that the doctor's medical records are, or may be, available to a third party.[1]

What then is the extent of the doctor's obligation to exercise discretion about the patient, his family and his affairs? To assert, as some have done, that the moral obligation is one of absolute secrecy, so that nothing whatever covered by the veil of professional confidence may in any circumstances whatever be disclosed save with the patient's consent, is to go too far.

Accepting that a doctor is under a moral obligation not improperly to disclose anything which he learns about a patient or his affairs, at least where it is information gained during or arising out of the professional relationship, a question remaining to be answered is whether that moral duty is also a legal obligation. In one sense it certainly is, in so far as any breach of it renders a practitioner liable to disciplinary proceedings by the General Medical Council on a charge of serious professional misconduct, which proceedings, if the charge were substantiated, might result in suspension or erasure of the practitioner's name from the Medical Register kept under the Medical Act 1956.

But is it also a legal obligation in the sense that any improper disclosure to a third party would render the practitioner liable for any consequential loss? Would an injunction lie against threatened dis-

---

[1] *e.g.* A person in one of the armed forces attended by a Service doctor. See also *R.* v. *Kent Police Authority ex. p. Godden* [1971] 2 Q.B. 662. (Decision of medical member of a Police Pension Tribunal is judicial and not medical in nature and must conform to rules of natural justice.) and *Watts* v. *Monmouthshire C.C.* (1967) 66 L.G.R. 171. (A pre-employment medical was confidential to the employers.)

closure? These are much harder questions to answer, since binding authority is lacking. The case sometimes quoted in support, *Kitson* v. *Playfair*[1] is not precisely to the point, the claim against the doctor having been for alleged libel and slander and not for breach of professional confidence. In that case, however, the judge in his summing up did assume that a medical practitioner was under a duty of secrecy concerning his patient's illness and the circumstances surrounding it and summarised the exceptions to the obligation of secrecy. Still less are *A.-G.* v. *Mulholland* and *A.-G* v. *Foster*[2] binding authority, since the defendants in those two cases were journalists. Even so, it is interesting that Lord Denning, M.R., in his judgment referred to the medical practitioner's duty to respect his patient's confidence.[3] Further, in a quite separate area of law in *Saltman Engineering Co. Ltd.* v. *Campbell Engineering Co. Ltd.*[4] Lord Greene, M.R., said:

If a defendant is proved to have used confidential information directly or indirectly obtained from a plaintiff without the consent, express or implied, of the plaintiff, he will be guilty of an infringement of the plaintiff's rights.

This of course only covers the case where information has been obtained from the plaintiff; not where it is merely about the plaintiff. Nevertheless it is a considerable pointer to the court's attitude to confidential information.[5]

Against this background it is a reasonable conclusion that, in a proper case, the courts would not be slow to find that the medical practitioner's obligation not to disclose anything about his patient or his patient's affairs save on proper occasion was a legal duty no less than a moral obligation or to give a remedy — damages, or injunction or both — to a patient who had suffered loss or damage to reputation, or even embarrassment, as a result of a breach of that duty.

B. HOSPITAL AUTHORITIES AND THEIR STAFF

The same obligation to treat information about patients and their affairs as confidential and not to be disclosed except on proper occasion has, over the years, been unquestioningly accepted by hospitals of all types — voluntary and local authority and, now, national. It is no less accepted by private hospitals and nursing homes.

Because of the known attitude of the Secretary of State it seems a fair

---

[1] (1896) *The Times*, March 28.
[2] [1963] Q.B. 477; [1963] 1 All E.R. 767 (C.A.).
[3] Lord Denning's judgment is further discussed on p. 348. See also *Pais* v. *Pais* ([1970,] 3 W.L.R. 830, 832) where Baker, J., dwelt on the lack of privilege of professional people.
[4] (1948) 65 R.P.C. 203. Reported only when its general importance was realised in [1963] 3 All E.R. 413.
[5] See [1969] N.L.J. 133 *Confidential Communications*, Jacob and Jacob, and the Law Commission Working Paper No. 58.

deduction that a patient entering or attending for treatment a hospital within the National Health Service may reasonably assume that the hospital authority does undertake in respect of all its staff that due discretion will be observed concerning the patient's illness and affairs. Although there is no case directly on the point, the readiness of the courts to impose liability for breach of confidence points to the conclusion that the obligation of N.H.S. hospitals and their staff would be enforceable.

Dr Speller used to suggest that the legal obligation might be less clear in the case of junior staff who had not been clearly instructed in their duties. However, it appears that the obligation rests with the Authority and therefore on its employees. Equally breach by an employee can incur the Authority in liability. In any event, some types of staff, *e.g.*, nurses and medical social workers, accept the duty of discretion about patients and their affairs as part of their own professional code and their position would be the same as that of medical practitioners.

As to the position of voluntary hospitals, it may be said that long before 1948 when most of those in existence were embodied in the National Health Service, it had been generally understood and impressed on the members of their staffs, particularly on nurses and others dealing with patients, that the staff of such hospitals, as well as their governing bodies, were under the same duty of observing confidentiality about the illness and affairs of the sick who were treated without charge as were the doctors who attended those patients. The position remains the same today in respect of any voluntary hospital which might accept free patients. It seems, too, that just as a medical practitioner treating a patient without charge would be open to an action for breach of confidence so, no less, would a voluntary or private hospital or nursing home or any member of its staff responsible for any improper disclosure.

C. INFECTIOUS DISEASES

1. Information to Area Medical Officer

There is a statutory obligation on medical practitioners to notify the area medical officer of cases of certain infectious diseases[1] and he may use or disclose information concerning individual patients only so far as is required or authorised by statute. In particular, the Area Medical Officer, as an officer of the Area Health Authority, receives information concerning the identity of persons suffering from sexually transmitted diseases subject to the provisions of Reg. 2 N.H.S. (Venereal Diseases) Regulations 1974,[2] which reads:

[1] Public Health Act 1936, s. 343 (1) as amended by the Public Health (Infectious Diseases) Regulations S.I. 1968 No. 1366 and the National Health Service Reorganisation Act 1973.
[2] S.I. 1974 No. 29.

2. Every Regional Health Authority and every Area Health Authority shall take all necessary steps to secure that any information capable of identifying an individual obtained by officers of the Authority with respect to persons examined or treated for any sexually transmitted disease shall not be disclosed except —

(a) for the purpose of communicating that information to a medical practitioner, or to a person employed under the direction of a medical practitioner in connection with the treatment of persons suffering from such disease or the prevention of the spread thereof, and

(b) for the purpose of such treatment or prevention.

The expression *sexually transmitted disease* used in Reg. 2, being apt to include any disease so transmitted, is wider in scope than the expression *venereal disease*, applied only to syphillis, gonorrhoea and soft chancre.[1]

When the N.H.S. (Venereal Diseases) Regulations 1968[2] were made, Hospital Authorities and their staff were sent a departmental memorandum including the following paragraph:[3]

The Minister is advised that the Regulations do not absolve any person from the existing obligation to give evidence in a court of law if required to do so, or to prevent them (*sic*) from giving information about a patient when asked by that patient preferably in writing.

Seemingly the position of a medical practitioner or other member of the staff of a Health Authority required to give evidence in court or asked by a patient to give information to a third party about him is the same under the 1974 Regulations as under those of 1968.

2. Other Disclosures

Apart from disclosures under compulsion of law, is there anyone, to whom on proper occasion, information about a patient, his illness or his affairs may properly be given without his consent.[4] Broadly, the answer is that there should be no disclosure save when the life or health of some other person or persons is put in jeopardy, or in greater jeopardy, by silence. For example, the case of the patient whom despite warnings, persists in exposing others to the risk of contracting an infectious disease in circumstances which do not give grounds for action by the Area Medical Officer. It is suggested that if danger to the health or life of another or others is sufficiently grave, communication to anyone of information necessary to afford opportunity for steps to be taken to prevent or minimise the danger normally would be justifiable.

---

[1] *Venereal diseases* were thus defined in s. 4 of the Venereal Diseases Act 1904.

[2] S.I. 1968, No. 1624.

[3] Paragraph 26 of departmental memorandum 'Contact Tracing in the Control of Venereal Diseases', sent to hospital authorities under cover of circular H.M. (68) 84. See also H.M. (71) 8. I am less certain that the Minister's advisors are right as to compulsion in a court, see my *Discovery and Public Interest* [1976] P.L. 134.

[4] As to reasonably assumed consent to communications to relatives see p. 360. This would not extend to sexually transmitted diseases.

The position is more complicated if what the patient is suffering from is a sexually transmitted disease, this is because any communication concerning the identity of a patient beyond what is authorised in Reg. 2 of the N.H.S. (Venereal Diseases) Regulations 1974[1] would be contrary to the Regulations. Hence, any medical or other officer of a Health Authority who, say, warned any third person that a patient was suffering from such disease, or who authorised anyone else to do so, would be in breach of duty to his employing Authority and a Health Authority which permitted such disclosure would be in breach of its duty to the Secretary of State. But even if the disclosure were made otherwise than as permitted by the Regulations, would either the officer who made the disclosure or his employing Authority be liable to the patient in damages?

Having regard to the terms of not only the 1974 Regulations but also those of the 1948 and 1968 Regulations and to the fact that it has been publicly advertised that treatment for venereal disease is obtainable in hospitals under conditions of secrecy and against the background of the Regulations, it is on the face of it reasonable that the patient should assume that he has an enforceable right to secrecy about his disease. But it would not be a contractual right — unless, possibly, he were a paying patient. If, therefore, any such right exists, it can only be a variant of the more general obligation of discretion about the patient and his affairs which has already been discussed. The most one can say, therefore, is that probably in this instance the obligation undertaken by the hospital and its staff would be construed more strictly than in others but that, even so, the obligation is not absolute. If, for example, disclosure were made to protect third parties against the risk of infection to which the patient had been wilfully exposing them, it is not conceivable that any court would award him damages. On the other hand, if disclosure had been made for no good reason and the court were satisfied that what had been done constituted an actionable wrong, it is possible that damages would be awarded, but, presumably, only on proof of actual loss or damage. That what had been said was true would be no defence.

D. DISCLOSURE UNDER COMPULSION OF LAW

1. Generally

A medical practitioner or other member of the staff of a hospital is a compellable witness on *subpoena* or witness summons and may be obliged to produce his own or hospital records such as case notes, if in his possession, custody or control.[2] And when in the witness box, a medical practitioner or other member of the staff of a hospital may not refuse to answer a question on grounds of professional privilege. Never-

---

[1] For the text of Reg. 2, see p. 347.
[2] Crown privilege (see p. 354) is not generally relevant.

theless, the court has some discretion and will generally compel a breach of confidence only when it is considered necessary in the interests of justice. The position of the medical witness and the attitude of the court towards him was stated in *A.-G.* v. *Mulholland* and *Foster*[1]. Lord Denning, M.R., in the course of his judgment, said:

'The only profession that I know which is given a privilege from disclosing information to a court of law is the legal profession, and then it is not the privilege of the lawyer but of his client. Take the clergyman, the banker or the medical man. None of these is entitled to refuse to answer when directed to by a judge. Let me not be mistaken. The judge will respect the confidences which each member of these honourable professions receives in the course of it, and will not direct him to answer unless not only it is relevant but also it is a proper and indeed, necessary question in the course of justice to be put and answered. A judge is the person entrusted, on behalf of the community, to weigh these conflicting interests — to weigh on the one hand the respect due to confidence in the profession and on the other hand the ultimate interest of the community in justice being done. . . .'

It must be appreciated, however, that the reference to the position of the medical practitioner as a witness was not the subject of the cases. Consequently this statement is not of binding authority. It was, however, substantially in line with what had for a very long time been understood to be the position. The only doubt left in one's mind is whether Lord Denning did not, perhaps, overemphasise the extent to which the judge could properly protect a medical witness. Certain it is that the court may compel disclosure by a medical practitioner of matters concerning his patient if those matters are regarded as essential to the case.

The 16th Report[2] of the Law Reform Committee dealt with privilege in civil actions. The Committee, having summed up the position of the medical practitioner called as a witness, substantially — but not precisely — in line with what Lord Denning said in *A.-G.* v. *Mulholland* and *Foster*,[3] recommended that no change be made in the existing law.[4]

Perhaps the most controversial statement in the Report is that where its authors say that where a doctor is called not in his capacity as a medical adviser to testify as to the physical or mental condition of his patient, any judge would protect him from being questioned upon information obtained by him from his patient in his capacity of medical adviser.[5] This statement, by inference founded in the judge's present discretion to disallow questions, implies that he has the right to disallow them without paying any regard either to 'all the circumstances of the case' or to 'the overriding claims of the interests of justice', which

---

[1] *A.-G.* v. *Mulholland*, *A.-G.* v. *Foster* [1963] 2 Q.B. 477; [1963] 1 All E.R. 767. See also *Pais* v. *Pais* [1970] 3 All E.R. 991.
[2] Cmmd. 3472.   [3] See footnote 3, p. 344.
[4] Paragraph 52. The 11th Report of the Criminal Law Revision Committee (1972 Cmmd. 4991) recommended that the privilege should remain the same in criminal as in civil proceedings.
[5] Paragraph 51.

elsewhere in the Report is apparently regarded as paramount. Lord Denning's more cautious words on the subject in *Mulholland* and *Foster* would appear to be a more accurate statement of the present law. If the view of the Committee is indeed that a judge would protect a doctor from being questioned upon information obtained by him from his patient, save in exceptional cases that is tantamount to saying that the doctor — on behalf of his patient — has absolute privilege. Yet earlier in the Report the Committee in the statement of what the law is, stopped short of saying any such thing.[1]

By way of contrast when one looks at what they said as to confidences between priest and penitent or between any other minister of religion and a person who seeks his help in exercise of his spiritual duties, the Committee is content rather to rely on the fact that, *ex hypothesi*, a confession is known only to priest and penitent and that it is unlikely that any fishing questions would be put or allowed to be put about such confession. This would seem the reasonable line to take in respect of communications between doctor and patient as well, since only if either the doctor or the patient has already talked about it would there be any solid ground for questioning the doctor on what had passed between them.

The Criminal Law Act 1967, abolished the common law offence of misprision of felony,[2] *i.e.*, of having knowledge of the commission of a felony but failing to inform the police. Hence no member of staff of a hospital will longer be even remotely at risk of prosecution for simply not telling the police about, for example, an illegal abortion or attempted abortion, which may possibly have become known to him because of the woman's account of the matter on admission to hospital — such account amounting in law to a confession. If, however, for some consideration — otherwise than allowed by s. 5 of the Criminal Law Act 1967 — anyone withholds information about the commission or the attempted commission of an arrestable offence, *e.g.*, criminal abortion or attempted abortion, he will be committing an offence. Moreover, irrespective of such considerations, there remains the duty of giving information to the police in specific circumstances, *e.g.*, under the Road Traffic Acts. But apart from such exceptional statutory obligation and subject to the provisions of s. 5 of the Criminal Law Act 1967, there being no legally enforceable obligation voluntarily to tell the police of any offence known to one to do so on being questioned, though it could be an offence to give the police false or misleading information.[3]

---

[1] The House of Lords has left the point open in *D.* v. *N.S.P.C.C.* [1977] 1 All E.R. 589.

[2] Misprision of treason remains an offence.

[3] See *Rice* v. *Connolly* ([1966] 2 Q.B. 414) where it was held that preserving silence alone did not amount to obstructing the police, though undoubtedly it made their duties more difficult. Nor, at common law, is it obstruction to refuse to accompany a policeman to a police station unless arrested. But there are numerous local statutory exceptions. Further,

2. Disclosure of Documents etc., by Likely Party to an Action for Personal Injuries or in Respect of the Death of any Person[1]

Section 31 of the Administration of Justice Act 1970[2] provides:

On the application, in accordance with the rules of court, of a person who appears to the High Court[3] to be likely to be a party to subsequent proceedings in that court in which a claim in respect of personal injuries[4] to a person or in respect of a person's death is likely to be made, the High Court shall, in such circumstances as may be specified in the rules, have power to order a person who appears to the court to be likely to be a party to the proceedings and to be likely to have or to have had in his possession, custody or power and documents which are relevant to an issue arising or likely to arise out of that claim —

(a) to disclose whether those documents are in his possession, custody or power; and

(b) to produce to the applicant such of those documents as are in his possession, custody or power.

Dunning v. *Board of Governors of the United Liverpool Hospitals*[5] was the first case in which the courts considered the meaning of the section, and in particular, interpreted the meaning of the words *to be likely* in the four several places in which they appear in the section. The facts were as follows.

In 1963, Mrs Dunning, who was then suffering from a persistent cough, was admitted to the Liverpool Royal Infirmary — a hospital administered by the prospective defendant's — for investigation. After two or three weeks in hospital she became dramatically worse. When she was discharged from hospital some seventeen weeks after her admission her disastrous illness had not cleared up. In hospital the applicant's illness had been diagnosed as '. . . undulant fever and finally as periarteritis nodosa', but her family had taken the view that it had been caused by one of the drugs given to her in hospital. Even so, no action was commenced within the limitation period. Hence any claim based on negligent injury became statute barred unless the court granted leave to sue out of time because of absence of knowledge of material facts.[6] It has to be added that it seems likely that no action was com-

---

it may be noted there are further exceptions placing a duty on hospital staff including medical practitioners to volunteer information concerning offences of violent injury to the person in Northern Ireland.

[1] This is a new procedure introduced as a result of the Report of the Winn Committee on Personal Injury Litigation (1968 Cmnd. 3691).

[2] This section and indeed s. 32 of the 1970 Act and s. 21 of the 1969 Administration of Justice Act (both of which are discussed below) bind the Crown in so far as they involve claims in respect of injuries to the person or in respect of a person's death. 1970 Act, s. 35.

[3] These provisions also cover the County Court. Section 34.

[4] *Personal Injuries* includes any disease and any impairment of a person's physical or mental condition. Section 33 (3).

[5] [1973] 2 All E.R. 454. The case is also summarised in a departmental letter dated 9th August 1973, ref. H/A227/11 to hospitals within the N.H.S. The letter also contains advice based on the decision.

[6] Under the Limitation Act 1963. The procedure for applying for leave to sue out of time has been abolished under Limitation Act 1975. See above, p. 271.

menced within the normal period of limitation because the applicant's doctor had told the patient that her condition would improve. In 1969 Mrs Dunning, still having not recovered, was granted limited legal aid to ascertain whether there were grounds for applying to the court for consent to bring an action against the Board out of time, under the provisions of the Limitation Act 1963.

Mrs Dunning saw a consultant and he sought access to the hospital case notes and medical records. But the Board was unwilling to make them available unless assured that there would be no action. In May 1970, without having seen the notes, the consultant formed the opinion that the hospital had not acted negligently. So, the opinion expressed in his report having disclosed no real basis for any action, nothing more happened until s. 31 of the Administration of Justice Act 1970 came into force. Then, on an application made under that section, Caulfield, J., ordered the Board to make the notes and records available to the consultant. The Court of Appeal dismissed the Board's appeal.

The decision mainly turned on the meaning of the words *to be likely* as used in the section. Lord Denning found it reasonably clear that Mrs Dunning was likely to be a party if proceedings were started and also that in that event the Board would be likely to be a party. Then, turning to consider the meaning to be given to the word *likely* in the passage 'a claim in respect of personal injury . . . is likely to be made', he concluded that it was proper to construe the word *likely* in the sense of *may or may well be made*. In support of this liberal interpretation Lord Denning referred to the recommendations in the Winn Report which had led to the passing of the Act of 1970. James, L.J., concurred in dismissing the appeal against the order. He said that in order to take advantage of the section the applicant had to disclose the nature of the claim and that there was a reasonable basis for making it. There was the evidence of the sudden dramatic change in Mrs Dunning's health in hospital. There was the possibility that the notes, if available, might add to the existing evidence to support a claim. He would construe *likely* as *a reasonable prospect*. The section would not however allow discovery where there was only a *hope* or a *speculation*.

Stamp, L.J., dissented[1] on the basis that in his view, the section only applied where an action would be *likely* even apart from the material disclosed on discovery. However, the majority in the Court of Appeal took the view that the court is not precluded from directing disclosure where the only basis for saying a claim is not likely is the absence of the documents to be disclosed.

Also in *Dunning* it was held that the disclosure could be limited to the prospective plaintiff's medical adviser. In *Deistung* v. *South-West*

---

[1] In a draft for this edition, Dr Speller was more impressed with this judgment than he was with those of the majority.

Metropolitan Hospital Board[1] the court said that this should be the usual practice as regards medical records but that the plaintiffs' lawyers were allowed to seek further elucidation of the medical expert's report. The expert was really only in the class of a prospective witness.

3. Order for Discovery of Documents etc., Made on Persons not Themselves Parties to an Action for Personal Injuries

Section 32 (1) of the Administration of Justice Act 1970[2] reads:

On an application, in accordance with the rules of court, of a party to any proceedings in which a claim in respect of personal injuries to a person or in respect of a person's death is made, the High Court[3] shall, in such circumstances as may be specified in the rules, have power to order a person who is not a party to the proceedings and who appears to the court to be likely to have or to have had in his possession, custody or power any documents which are relevant to an issue arising out of the claim:
- (*a*) to disclose whether those documents are in his possession, custody or power; and
- (*b*) to produce to the applicant such of those documents as are in his possession, custody or power.

In *Paterson* v. *Chadwick, Paterson* v. *Northampton and District Hospital Management Committee*[4] the plaintiff, Mrs Paterson, had suffered a serious and permanent disability to her left arm allegedly caused by the negligent injection of an anaesthetic for the purpose of dental treatment at the Northampton and District General Hospital. She consulted solicitors with the object of obtaining damages but before they started proceedings, her claim became statute barred. She alleged this had been due to the fault of the solicitors. She commenced an action alleging professional negligence against them. She needed the hospital notes in support of her claim. Section 32 would only help her if the action against the solicitors was 'in respect of personal injury'. Boreham, J., held that the words *in respect of* in s. 32 (1) conveyed the need for some connection or relation between the plaintiff's claim and the personal injuries sustained. He found also that there was in this case such a connection or relation because the nature and extent of the plaintiff's injuries were an essential element in the proof of her claim against her former solicitors and that accordingly the plaintiff was 'a party to proceedings in which a claim in respect of personal injuries to a person is made' within the meaning of s. 32 (1), and so entitled to an order for discovery of the medical records.

But where the discovery of hospital medical notes is sought under s. 32 in an action to which the Hospital Authority is not a party, the

[1] [1975] 1 W.L.R. 213. See also *Shaw* v. *Vauxhall Motors Ltd.* [1974] 2 All E.R. 1185'
and *Davidson* v. *Lloyd Aircraft Services Ltd.* [1974] 3 All E.R. 1.
[2] See footnote 2, p. 350, as regards application to the Crown.
[3] The procedure also applies to the County Court. Section 34.
[4] [1974] 1 W.L.R. 891.

purpose of obtaining the notes being to help a doctor make a report on what the patient's personal injuries are mainly attributed to, it is proper to order disclosure to be restricted to the plaintiff's doctor only, and not to the patient or his legal advisers. It would be otherwise in respect of production on a *subpoena*.

In *Davidson* v. *Lloyd Aircraft Services Ltd.*[1] the plaintiff contracted malignant tertiary malaria in 1969 as a result of a short spell in Dar-es-Salam on his job. Subsequently — in 1972 — he suffered from a heart condition which, in making a claim against his employers, he sought to show had been due to the malaria. His solicitors wanted him to be examined by a specialist and the specialist wanted access to all the hospital records and notes made during the plaintiff's illness in 1969. The hospitals where the plaintiff had been a patient were not parties to the proceedings and applications for the release of the complete medical records relative to the plaintiff in the possession, custody or power of the several hospitals — South Middlesex, Hammersmith and Crawley — were made under s. 32. The hospitals, whilst prepared to disclose the records to the specialist, objected to their being disclosed to any other person and, in particular, to the plaintiff's solicitor and to the plaintiff himself. But the Court of Appeal held that, in such circumstances, the court should exercise the power given by s. 32 to order discovery of hospital records, to order discovery only to the medical expert, the documents being confidential records 'in the possession, custody or power of a person not a party to the proceedings' and so should be protected against any disclosure wider than was essential to the determination of the issues arising out of the claim.

So also in *Shaw* v. *Vauxhall Motors Ltd.*[2] the court said that discovery should be ordered in any case (but curiously 'particularly' in a legally aided case) where it would, or would be likely to, assist in disposing fairly of the dispute or would result in the saving of costs.

4. Production, Protection etc., of Property Relevant to Actual or Intended Civil Proceedings

Section 21 (1) of the 1969 Administration of Justice Act[3] provides:

On the application of any person in accordance with the rules of court, the High Court[4] shall, in such circumstances as may be specified in the rules, have power to make an order providing for any or more of the following matters, that is to say,
  (*a*) the inspection, photographing, preservation, custody and detention of property[5] which appears to the court to be property of which may

---

[1] [1974] 1 W.L.R. 1042.   [2] [1974] 2 All E.R. 1185.
[3] See footnote 2, p. 350, as regards application to the Crown.
[4] The procedure also applies to the County Court. Section 21 (3).
[5] *Property* includes any land, chattels or other corporal property of any description. Section 21 (5).

become the subject-matter of subsequent proceedings in the court, or as to which any question may arise in any such proceedings, and

(b) the taking of samples of any such property as is mentioned in the preceding paragraph and the carrying out of any experiment on or with such property.

The section accordingly concerns the court's jurisdiction before the action has actually commenced. For matters after the action has been started s. 32 (2) of the 1970 Administration of Justice Act makes similar provision except that of course only a party to the action may apply and that the property in question should not be in the possession, custody or control of any of the parties.

It has been held that this power does not apply to the taking of a blood sample or to the carrying out of any surgical undertaking on a living body.[1]

5. Crown Privilege[2]

Information is not available either on discovery[3] or as evidence at a trial if it would be injurious to the public interest to allow it. It used to be thought that this only applied to what may be termed *Crown information*[4] and hence non-production of information on this ground became called Crown privilege. However, it is now reasonably clear that the prohibition does not depend on the source of the information but rather on the conclusion of the court[5] that having regard to (a) the public interest in the full disclosure in the interests of the administration of justice and (b) to the damage to the public interest by the disclosure of this information, that on balance the information ought not to be disclosed.[6]

The order for the non-production *etc.* is commonly made on the application of one of the parties and equally commonly it is supported by an affidavit from the head of the relevant Government Department stating what the expected damage to the public interest would be if the court were to order disclosure. However, it is generally accepted that, in a proper case, the court can and should take the point of its own motion. Schedule 5 paragraph 15 (2) of the National Health Service Act 1977 expressly prohibits a Health Authority from making a claim to the privilege. It does however maintain the Crown's right to withhold or process the withholding of a document on the basis of Crown privilege. In short, apparently, where the issue arises, the matter should be referred to the Secretary of State.

[1] *W.* v. *W.* [1964] P. 67 decided under the old R.S.C. Ord. 50 (now R.S.C. Ord. 29).
[2] See my *Discovery and Public Interest* [1976] P.L. 134.
[3] By s. 35 (3) of the 1970 Administration of Justice Act, this also applies to discovery *etc.* under s. 21 of the 1969 Act and to ss. 31 and 32 of the 1970 Act.
[4] *e.g. Broome* v. *Broome* [1955] P. 190.   [5] *Conway* v. *Rimmer* [1968] A.C. 910.
[6] Since the above was written, these propositions have largely been confirmed by the House of Lords in *D.* v. *N.S.P.C.C.* [1977] 1 All E.R. 589.

One is left to speculate on what view the court might take of a claim for Crown privilege in respect of hospital records. It seems unlikely that a claim of Crown privilege would be upheld in respect of most of them. The various views advanced by the judges as to the balance of the public interest are neither the model of clarity nor consistency.[1] However it is clear that where the documents are ordinary documents collected or compiled in the ordinary way and that normally documents of their type are admitted in litigation, the claim will not lie. Where, however, the information has some special confidentiality about it a claim may be allowed. In one case, for example, reports of child welfare officers were protected not only by regulations but also by the court.[2] In another case, the House of Lords allowed a claim made by the National Society for the Prevention of Cruelty to Children to refuse disclosure of the name of an informant.[3] It is thus possible, therefore, that records relating to the treatment of venereal disease might come within Crown privilege protection.

No witness, on a claim of Crown privilege, may refuse to attend court if properly served with a witness summons or *subpoena*. He must attend court and there claim Court privilege in respect of particular matters on which he might be examined or cross-examined. It is then for the court to decide whether the claim has been made out or not.

6. Duty to Give Information to a Police Officer under the Road Traffic Act

By s. 168 of the Road Traffic Act 1972, if the driver of a mechanically propelled vehicle or the rider of a cycle who is alleged to have committed an offence under the Act has not been identified, any person if required to do so by or on behalf of a chief officer of police must give any information which it is in his power to give and which may lead to the identification of the driver. In *Hunter* v. *Mann*[4] it was held that the words 'any . . . person' in s. 168 (2) of the Act had their ordinary unrestricted meaning and that, accordingly, a medical practitioner may be required to give information to the police under the subsection notwithstanding that to give the information otherwise than under compulsion of law might be a breach of professional confidence.[5]

---

[1] Thus compare: *Duncan* v. *Cammell Laird* [1942] A.C. 624; *Conway* v. *Rimmer* [1968] A.C. 910; *Rogers* v. *The Secretary of State for the Home Department* [1973] A.C. 388; *Norwich Pharmacal Co. Ltd.* v. *The Commissioners for Customs and Excise* [1974] A.C. 133, [1973] 2 All E.R. 943; and *Alfred Crompton Amusement Machines Ltd.* v. *The Commissioners for Customs and Excise (No. 2)* [1974] A.C. 405, [1973] 2 All E.R. 1169.

[2] *Re D (Infants)* [1970] 1 W.L.R. 599. The regulations in question were the Boarding Out of Children Regs. S.I. 1955 No. 1377.

[3] *D.* v. *N.S.P.C.C.* [1977] 1 All E.R. 589.

[4] [1974] Q.B. 767 and see Annual Report of M.D.U. 1974 at pp. 18–19.

[5] The facts of *Hunter* were as follows: An accident occurred one day in January 1973 in which a car was involved, the driver of which, together with his passenger had hurried away without disclosing his identity. It was alleged that the driver had been guilty of dangerous

Under the section the information must be 'required by or on behalf of the chief officer of police'. Proof must therefore be offered by a policeman that he requires it in that behalf[1] but this may be implied by his rank.[2]

Although not all offences under the Road Traffic Act 1972 or other relevant statutes are within s. 168 it can be said that it does cover an allegation of any of those offences on the road which are likely to cause the police to suspect that the unidentified driver, or a passenger with him at the time of the incident, might thereafter have sought treatment either from a general practitioner or at the casualty department of a hospital. The section covers *inter alia* an allegation of any of the following — causing death by dangerous driving; careless or inconsiderate driving; driving under age; driving or being in charge whilst under the influence of drink or drugs; taking a car without the owner's consent; or leaving a vehicle in a dangerous position. In the case of a cyclist the alleged offences are, *inter alia*, reckless or dangerous cycling; careless or inconsiderate cycling; and cycling under the influence of drink or drugs. Among the most important offences which are outside the scope of the section and which might concern hospitals are failure to wear protective headgear and driving with uncorrected defective eyesight.

E. JUSTIFIABLE DISCLOSURE

Even when there is no legal compulsion on a medical practitioner, or other member of the staff of a hospital to give information to the police, there may still be a public or social duty to do so. Such public duty would in law be a sufficient justification for disclosure to the police of information which ought normally to remain confidential.[3] Nor could a hospital treat as a breach of discipline such disclosure to the police by one of its staff even though against the hospital rules.

---

driving. On the evening of the same day the man, as well as a girl who was with him and who said she had been involved in a car accident, went to Dr Hunter's surgery and were treated by him. The doctor advised them to see the police but did not seek to obtain their consent to disclose their identity to a police officer. The police later asked the doctor to divulge the names and addresses of both patients or to give information which could lead to the police discovering them. This Dr Hunter declined to do on the ground that information obtained through the doctor–patient relationship was confidential. Dr Hunter was convicted of refusing to give the required information and his conviction was upheld by the Divisional Court.

[1] *Record Tower Cranes Ltd.* v. *Gisbey* [1969] 1 W.L.R. 148.
[2] *Nelms* v. *Roe* [1970] 1 W.L.R. 4.
[3] *Initial Services Ltd.* v. *Putterill* ([1968] 1 Q.B. 396; [1967] 3 All E.R. 145). The court held that there was 'no confidence in an iniquity' but the action was against an ex-employee for publishing complaints of wrong-doing by his employers. It is possible that the situation is different if the 'iniquity' of a patient is not directly related to the doctor–client relationship. Compare *Duchess of Argyll* v. *Duke of Argyll* [1967] Ch. 302. The legal duty of confidence may therefore exist if a patient comes to a doctor having been injured in the course of criminal activities. In any event, damages would not be likely to be more than nominal for breach of such a duty in such circumstances.

However since there is no compulsion to perform the public or social duty of giving information to the police, whether there should be disclosure falls to be decided largely as a matter of conscience and with regard to the balance of social advantage. Into that field no more than pointers can be offered.

Suppose a person attends hospital who, whether as regards injuries from which he is suffering or in appearance, answers the description of some one suspected of being concerned with murder, rape, robbery with violence or other serious crime, Dr Speller asked, can anyone doubt that there is a public duty to tell the police, a duty which should be fulfilled with all practicable speed? But at the other end, would one really feel the same duty in respect of a minor offence? He said in the first example it is not at all clear that the doctor or hospital–patient relationship enters into the matter at all, at all events if what the police are told has been learned from such observation as anyone might have been capable of, irrespective of any professional relationship. But, it may be objected, hospital or at least some of the staff may think their public duty is not the apprehension of criminals but rather the curing of the sick and the alleviation of suffering. In which case they might take the view that it is certainly not their job to volunteer information to the police and possibly not even to answer questions.

The question of the giving of confidential information in order to prevent medical harm to others has already been discussed.[1]

If a Health Authority or members of its staff are sued by the patient, or, after his death, by his personal representatives or relatives, in respect of loss or injury he suffered or is alleged to have suffered by the fault of the authority or its staff, it is proper that all relevant information should be communicated to the solicitors acting for the hospital or its staff. Where a request for information comes from a solicitor acting for the patient in a claim against the hospital or its staff, although production of case notes and similar documents was not obligatory before the stage of discovery in the actual proceedings was reached, the Minister of Health in 1959 advised hospital authorities that he did not feel that boards and committees, especially as they were public authorities, would either wish or be well-advised to maintain their strict rights in this connection except for some good reason bearing on the defence to the particular claim or on the ground that the request was made without substantial justification.[2]

Now following the enactment of s. 31 of the 1970 Administration of Justice Act[3] and such cases as *Dunning*,[4] it would usually be reasonable

[1] See above, p. 346.
[2] H.M. (59) 88 and see W.H.S.C. (15) 71.
[3] See above, p. 350.
[4] *Dunning* v. *Board of Governors of Liverpool United Hospitals* [1973] 2 All E.R. 454, discussed above.

to agree to produce medical notes before an action is commenced limiting the disclosure by agreement to a medical adviser of the person seeking disclosure, leaving him to seek an order of the court if he wants more. A similar restriction might also be imposed if medical notes were voluntarily produced instead of an order under s. 32 of the 1970 Act in an action to which the hospital or the medical practitioner who made the notes was not a party.

Reports by hospital staff made after an accident in hospital has caused some injury to the patient, if they are reports prepared following a request by the solicitor to the hospital that such reports be prepared for his use are less likely to be produced as they are privileged from discovery.[1]

Disclosure about a patient with his consent, express or implied, or reasonably assumed or taken for granted, is also justifiable. A simple example of consent being taken for granted is the customary giving of information to the patient's spouse or to a near relative about his condition, always provided that the patient has not forbidden such communication. But consent to informing even a near relative that a patient was suffering from a sexually transmitted disease could not be assumed.

If a solicitor asks a hospital for information about a patient, stating in writing that he is acting for the patient and has the patient's authority for his request, the hospital — and its staff within the limits of their authority — may properly and without further assurance give such information to the solicitor as they are willing to give, on such terms as to payment for extra work involved as they think proper. But if a solicitor who does not claim to be acting for the patient or his personal representatives, or, perhaps, not a solicitor but an insurance company, seeks information about the patient or deceased patient, even with his or his personal representatives' consent as the case may be, it does not necessarily follow that it is always in the best interests of the patient or of his dependants that the inquiry should be answered especially when it is borne in mind that the circumstances may have been such that the patient or his personal representatives would have found it exceedingly difficult to withhold consent. Then the hospital authority and its staff may consider it more appropriate not to give the required information, being under no legal obligation to do so.

It is made clear in a departmental circular to hospital authorities[2] that the patient's right to have his hospital record treated as confidential is to

---

[1] By legal professional privilege. See *Patch* v. *Bristol United Hospitals* [1959] 1 W.L.R. 955; see also Ministry Circular H.M. (55) 66.

[2] R.H.B. (53) 93. Further advice to hospital authorities on the disclosure of information about patients to solicitors is given in Ministry memoranda H.M. (54) 32, H.M. (59) 88 and H.M. (61) 110. The last-mentioned circular refers to disclosures concerning psychiatric patients.

be respected even as against Ministry of Pensions and National Insurance,[1] Medical Boards and Medical Appeal Tribunals. All these were to be supplied with such records to assist in assessing claims for disablement benefit or war disability pension, only if the Ministry of Pensions and National Insurance had first obtained the consent of the patient in writing. The procedure was that the Department when applying to the hospital for information gives an assurance that the patient's written consent had been obtained. The Department indicated that this would suffice. It is, however, suggested that none the less the hospital might be under a liability for improper disclosure if consent had not in fact been obtained. If not, it is difficult to see how this could fail to be maladministration within the jurisdiction of either the Parliamentary Commissioner for Administration or the Health Service Commissioner. Only such extracts as are essential are to be made and they are to be treated as confidential. They are, however, communicated to the claimant[2] or, if containing information which might be harmful to the claimant, to his doctor or, as appropriate, to his trade union or legal representative.

In the same circular hospital authorities were told that so far as treatment reports on service pensions cases are concerned which, by another circular they are required to furnish to the War Pensions Office of the Ministry, no question of consent arises because they are required only for the clinical records of the medical staff of that Ministry to enable them to act on recommendations from the hospital, to follow up the case and to take such action as is indicated on the pensioner's behalf. Dr Speller and the present writer find that argument quite unconvincing and are of opinion that unless it can be shown that the patient consented to such disclosure or it was a condition of his treatment as a Service pension case that such disclosure was permitted, it would not be proper.

It is understood that the Ministry of Health has given the British Medical Association an assurance that in the event of proceedings for defamation against a doctor arising out of his entries on a hospital patient's case papers by reason of their loan to and use by the Department, the Minister will indemnify the doctor against any damages that may be recovered and against all reasonable costs that he may incur in defending proceedings. The indemnification of medical practitioners called upon to disclose confidential information before tribunals is also covered by this assurance. This indemnity is understood to be subject to the Minister being informed at once of any threatened proceedings and having complete control over the conduct of the defence.[3]

[1] Now the Department of Health and Social Security.
[2] According to a letter from a doctor [Brit. Med. J. (Feb. 11, 1967, p. 367)] case notes lent to the Ministry on request made on Form M.P.A. 378 are photographed and have been made available to a doctor asked to examine the patients.
[3] Brit. Med. J., August 16th, 1952, Suppt. p. 99.

o

F. UNJUSTIFIABLE DISCLOSURE

Broadly, any disclosure of information about a patient and his affairs without the express or implied consent of the patient and not falling within any of the exceptions mentioned above is unjustifiable and, if actual damage could be established, could lead to a claim for damages. But one is left to speculate on the possible measure of damages.

Although in the case of near relatives, the consent of the patient to such disclosures as are normal in the circumstances will readily be implied, it would ordinarily be quite unjustifiable to give information to a spouse or near relative contrary to the express prohibition of the patient. And even though there has been no express prohibition by a married patient on communication of medical information to the other spouse there may still be circumstances in which it should not be given without the patient's express permission, notably if it might be made use of by the other spouse in matrimonial or custody proceedings between the parties. Should it be known to the attendant medical practitioner, or has been recorded by a social worker, in a note or report available to a member of staff of the hospital, that the relationship of the parties is hostile or unusual, that would be an added danger signal.[1] In particular, a doctor having the care of a mentally disordered patient, or who has had the care of such a patient during that patient's stay in hospital, should not disclose information about the patient's condition and treatment to a spouse contemplating divorce proceedings. This applies even though it is with the object of protecting the patient from being unduly bothered about such proceedings.

Even in the case of a minor over 16 years of age it may be appropriate to follow the minor's wish that his — or her — parents be not told, though the hospital or responsible member of its staff would be justified in ignoring the minor's express wish if it was thought to be in his interests to do so. If, however, as has been known to happen in the case of a pregnant young woman, a minor over 16 years of age were willing to enter hospital for necessary treatment only on assurance that her parents would not be communicated with, the responsible member of

[1] An example of this given on p. 21 of the 'Annual Report 1968' of the Medical Defence Union is that of a doctor-husband who asked to be provided with the pathologist's report of the blood group of the foetus, his wife having been admitted to hospital for termination of pregnancy on psychiatric grounds. In the same report (p. 22) it is recorded that a psychiatrist who had treated the estranged wife of a general practitioner for two years, otherwise than under compulsion of law had made an affidavit about the wife's condition for use of the husband's solicitors in custody proceedings between the parties and that his doing so had been subject of complaint to the General Medical Council. The complaint had been dismissed only after the psychiatrist, through his solicitors, had expressed regret. That a similar complaint against the husband's partner, who had also made an affidavit, had been rejected, apparently on the ground that he had used only his general knowledge of the wife, raises alarming possibilities in custody proceedings for wives who do not get on very well with their general practitioner husbands.

the medical staff giving such assurance would doubtless feel obliged to honour his undertaking in any but the gravest emergency, nor can one discover any grounds of liability to the parents for so doing.

G. DISCLOSURE OF INFORMATION CONCERNING THE PATIENT'S WILL, DISPOSAL OF WILL ETC.

Greater caution has to be exercised in discussing a patient's affairs with a relative without his express approval than in so discussing his state of health. For example, should a patient have made a will whilst in hospital, the fact that he has done so should not ordinarily be disclosed to any relative, nor even the fact that he may have requested the attendance of a solicitor for that or any other purpose. Further, if a patient's will is in the possession of the hospital for safe-keeping, it should not, whilst he is alive, be handed over to any other person without his consent, save in the case of one made by a psychiatric patient whose affairs are subject to the Court of Protection, when an order of the Court, or of a receiver appointed by the Court, as to its disposal, must be complied with. If a patient, not being able to take care of his own property, is transferred from one hospital to another, his will should also be passed over to the receiving hospital for safe custody.

If a patient whose will is in possession of the hospital for safe custody dies or if, after the death of a patient in hospital, a will is found with the effects he kept in the ward, it should ordinarily be handed over only to or on the instructions of a person named therein as executor or, if no executor is named or none able and willing to act, then to someone to whom letters of administration *cum testamento annexo* could be granted, *e.g.* a residuary legatee. If, however, the name of a solicitor who prepared it is endorsed on the will, it would be reasonable — especially in case of real doubt — to ascertain whether that solicitor was in a position to accept custody on behalf of whoever might be concerned.

H. PATIENT MAKING WILL[1]

1. Introductory

A will or testamentary disposition is an expression of the maker's wishes as to the disposition of his property after death and may, under the Guardianship of Minors Act 1971, contain an appointment of, testamentary guardians of children under the age of eighteen. Usually,

---

[1] This section of this chapter is included here in the hope that it may prove useful to readers of this book. It and the remaining sections of this chapter are not a part of the law of professional confidence although there is some connection between them and attitudes expected of a professional person.

too, the person or persons the testator desires to carry out the provisions of the will are named as executors.

Any person of full age and of sound mind, memory and understanding may under English law make a will which, under the Wills Act 1837, to be valid must be in writing (including typewriting *etc.*) and must be signed by the testator in the presence of two witnesses who both subscribe their signatures.[1] For a will to be valid it is also necessary that both witnesses should have been present during the whole time that the testator was signing his name. So if, as in *In re Collings, deceased*,[2] one of the witnesses of a patient's will were a ward sister who, after the testator had started signing his name but before he had finished, went to attend to another patient, the will would be invalid, and this even though, before she signed as a witness, both the testator and the other witness had acknowledged to her their respective signatures. If a necessary witness or the husband or wife of a witness is named as a beneficiary under the will, the will is otherwise good but the benefit to witness or the husband or wife of the witness is ordinarily void.[3] If the testator cannot write or is too ill to sign he may make his mark, usually a cross, or in extreme cases when even that is impossible he may, if of full understanding, authorise some third party other than one of the two witnesses to sign for him.[4]

For the sake of completeness it may here be mentioned that it may be possible for a person in contemplation of death to make a gift by handing over a chattel which becomes fully effective only if the donor dies, though any discussion of what, for that purpose, constitutes handing over and of other special features of a *donatio mortis causa* are outside the scope of this book.

The duty of a hospital authority and of its staff to treat as confidential the fact that a patient has made a will and the circumstances in which a patient's will may be given to a third party are discussed at the end of section G of the chapter, at page 361, but see also pages 367–368 concerning wills of psychiatric patients made without approval or professional help.

[1] Soldiers, sailors and airmen on active service and certain prisoners of war are not subject to such strict formalities and may make a will at the age of 14 years. The Wills Act, 1963, also modifies considerably the requirements for wills made by persons domiciled or habitually resident abroad. To discuss such matter is beyond the scope of this work.
[2] *Re Colling* [1972] 1 W.L.R. 1440; [1972] 3 All E.R. 729.
[3] If, disregarding the signature of such beneficiary or spouse as a witness, a will of any person dying after the passing of Wills Act 1968 would still be valid, the gift to such witness or spouse would not now be lost (s. 1).
[4] If a will has been made by a blind, illiterate or disabled person, whether he signs his name or makes his mark or has the will signed for him by another person on his instructions, the registrar, on application for probate, will require proof that the testator had knowledge of the contents of the will at the time of execution. Witnesses of such wills ordinarily subscribe their signatures to an appropriately modified attestation clause which, in the case of a person unable to read, whether from blindness or other cause, would place on record that the will had been read over to him before execution.

2. Patients in Hospitals, other than Mental Cases

(a) Will drafted by patient's solicitor

If a patient in a hospital otherwise than for the treatment of mental disorder expresses the desire to make a will and he has a solicitor of his own, any request he may make to that solicitor should be transmitted with all convenient speed and facilities afforded for the solicitor to visit the patient even outside ordinary visiting hours, subject always to the medical needs of the patient himself.

When the above course can be taken the hospital and its officers are relieved of all moral responsibility in the matter. The only other question arising being as to whether it is proper to allow members of the staff to subscribe as witnesses of a patient's will. There appears to be no good reason forbidding any member of the staff of whatever rank witnessing a will if the patient so desires.[1] It is, however, advisable that no member of the staff of a hospital should witness a will if he has reason to believe that at the time of execution the patient is not of full understanding, as for example, being delirious.[2]

But even to the sound rule of not witnessing a will unless the patient is himself apparently of full understanding when signing it there may be an exception, for there is some authority for suggesting that if a testator is in his full senses when he gives instructions for the drafting of his will he may afterwards validly execute it even if, at the time, he no longer has a perfect understanding of its terms. Consequently, even though the mental capacity of the patient at the time of execution is doubtful, e.g., on account of delirium, it is probably reasonable, especially if the patient is unlikely to attend to business again, for a doctor or senior nurse to witness at the request of the patient's solicitor or his clerk a will drafted by the solicitor on the patient's previous instructions. It must be a matter of personal judgment in each case as to whether before the will is witnessed, the doctor or nurse should advise the solicitor of any doubts as to the full mental capacity of the patient. Even if no member of the hospital staff is allowed or is willing to witness such a will, no obstacle should be placed in the way of the solicitor's arranging for other witnesses.

---

[1] It is perhaps also important to point out that no witness to a will is allowed to take any benefit under it.

[2] The attitude it is appropriate for members of the staff of hospitals and those controlling them to take has been admirably set out in a memorandum 'Legal Documents of Patients: Hospital Staff Responsibilities' (S.H.M. 58/80) issued by the Department of Health for Scotland (now the Scottish Home and Health Department) to Scottish hospital authorities. The text of the memorandum is set out in Appendix D at pp. 735–736. There is nothing whatever in English law which would make the guidance given in S.H.M. 58/80 inapplicable south of the border.

(b) Will drafted otherwise than by patient's solicitor

If a patient, being apparently of full understanding and having apparently prepared a will without the help of a solicitor, simply asks that two members of the hospital staff should witness his will, it will be unreasonable not to comply with his request.

A serious problem is the case of a patient having no solicitor of his own desiring help in making a will in circumstances which brook no delay, e.g., an accident or post-operative patient in a very grave state, or a patient about to undergo a serious major operation which cannot be deferred. Whenever possible it is desirable that hospitals should have an arrangement with local solicitors[1] to be on call, if available, for such emergency cases, subject to its being, understood that the patient and not the hospital would be responsible for his fee. However, there must inevitably be very occasional instances when it is not possible to obtain the help of a solicitor at once and in such circumstances it would seem desirable that some senior member of the administrative staff or failing that, of the medical or senior nursing staff or a medical social worker or, perhaps, the chaplain, should assist the patient if so desired in setting down his wishes for his signature, though this is practicable and should certainly be attempted only when the testator is clear about what he wants and the proposed will is simple and straightforward, e.g., leaving the whole of the testator's property to wife or child or for division among children.[2]

3. Patients of Unsound Mind

(a) Generally

For a will to be valid the testator must be of sound mind, memory and understanding. In an old case[3] it was said:

> To constitute a sound disposing mind, a testator must not only be able to understand that he is by will giving his property to objects of his regard but he must also have capacity to comprehend the extent of his property, and the nature of the claims of others whom by his will he is excluding from participation in that property.

That definition is a purely factual one and its application to a particular person does not depend on legal formalities. The will of a person liable to detention in hospital under the provisions of the Mental Health Act 1959, whether under Part IV or under Part V, may be valid

[1] If the patient is in a condition to choose, he should be given a list of all the local solicitors willing to attend the hospital and asked to select one.

[2] On the face of it, it is ordinarily undesirable that any member of the hospital staff, even at the patient's request, should advise him on his testamentary dispositions. It is however sensible that the will appoints someone to act as executor. Such an executor can also be a beneficiary.

[3] *Harwood* v. *Baker* (1840), 3 Moore P.C. quoted in Heywood and Massey's Court of Protection Practice, 8th Edn. (1961), pp. 177, 178.

and effectual, whilst the will of a person who has either been admitted informally or who has never been under treatment for mental disorder may be upset on grounds of incapacity. In short, the assumption sometimes made that persons liable to detention under the Act can never make a valid will is erroneous. And it is just because that assumption is erroneous that special precautions are taken as far as possible to prevent such persons making a will unless those responsible for their welfare are satisfied that they are really competent to do so.

(b) Technical safeguards

If a patient's affairs are under the jurisdiction of the Court of Protection under Part VIII of the Mental Health Act 1959, it seems that the rule in *Banks* v. *Goodfellow*[1] still applies. The rule is that if a patient is desirous of executing a will whilst he is still under the jurisdiction of the Court, the Master, before granting facilities for doing so, will require to be satisfied that the patient is possessed of full testamentary capacity; that is to say, capacity to understand the nature of the document he is executing, the extent of the property to be disposed of and the claims of those he is benefiting by or excluding from his will. Hence it follows that whenever a mentally disordered patient in hospital expresses the desire to make a will and there is reason to believe that the patient is subject to the jurisdiction of the Court of Protection the Master should be notified of the position so that he can decide whether facilities should be granted.[2]

Apart altogether from any special precautions called for in the case of patients subject to the jurisdiction of the court, it is customarily the rule in psychiatric hospitals, including hospitals for subnormal patients as well as those for patients suffering from other forms of mental disorder, that facilities be not given for any patient to make a will save on the recommendation of the medical practitioner responsible for his treatment. The same rule usually applies to patients in psychiatric wards of other hospitals. Also, it is understood that, if a patient is thought to be capable of executing a will prepared on professional advice, the medical practitioner responsible for his treatment in hospital will normally be willing to be one of the witnesses of its execution.[3] Such medical witness is of value as evidence of the patient's testamentary capacity and this and the preliminary precaution of obtaining the

---

[1] (1870) L.R. 5 Q.B. 549; (1870) L.J. Q.B. 237.

[2] It may here be mentioned that under s. 103A of the Mental Health Act 1959, a section added by ss. 17 to 19 of the Administration of Justice Act 1969, the Court of Protection now has power to authorise the execution of a will or codicil on behalf of a mentally disordered patient who is not himself of testamentary capacity. The use of this power makes irrelevant any discussion of the testamentary capacity of the patient concerned.

[3] In *re Simpson; Schaniel* v. *Simpson* (1977) 121 Sol. Jo. 224 it was said that in the case of an old or infirm testator a medical practitioner ought to be a witness.

approval of the hospital are the best guarantees against the validity of the will being subsequently successfully challenged.

In practice, if a psychiatric patient expresses a serious desire to make a will, the nurse or other member of the staff to whom he expresses his wish should report without undue delay so that the medical practitioner in charge of the treatment of the patient can advise on appropriate action.

Sometimes the patient will himself have communicated with his solicitor who will then doubtless discuss the patient's capacity with the doctor in charge of the treatment and, if necessary, communicate with the Court of Protection. In other cases, where there appears some reasonable possibility of the patient's being competent to make a will, he may properly be advised to consult a solicitor and be given facilities to do so.

(c) Patients admitted informally

Since any mentally disordered patient who does not object to becoming an in-patient may be accepted as an informal patient and it is not necessary that he should be volitional or even of any real understanding, it follows that many informal patients, e.g., patients with severe subnormality, will be quite unfit to make a will. But other patients, not compulsarily detained will be fit.

As has already been indicated, hospital rules against the making of a will by mentally disordered patients otherwise than with the approval of the medical practitioner responsible for his treatment extend to informal patients as well as to those liable to detention. But it has to be appreciated that an informal patient who is volitional may decide to leave the hospital if he is refused facilities to make a will.[1]

Against that background it seems desirable that in the case of a patient admitted informally who might be capable of making a will wishing to see a solicitor about it, obstacles should not ordinarily be put in the way of his doing so, unless he is subject to the jurisdiction of the Court of Protection.[2] The medical practitioner in charge of the patient's treatment should be prepared to advise the solicitor on his client's condition and, if reasonably satisfied as to the patient's testamentary capacity, to be one of the witnesses to the execution of the will.

As to the right of any psychiatric patient to communicate by letter with his solicitor reference should be made to pp. 489.

(d) Will made by mentally disordered patient in hospital without professional advice and without the knowledge of the medical practitioner in charge of his treatment

It sometimes happens that a will is made by a patient in a psychiatric hospital, or in the psychiatric ward of a general hospital, without

[1] See p. 473 .   [2] See pp. 529–530.

professional advice and without the knowledge of the medical practitioner responsible for the treatment of the patient. If later, the existence of such will becomes known it should not be destroyed, however unlikely it is that its validity would be upheld by the court if it were challenged, since the wilful destruction of a will is a criminal offence. The will should be taken into the safekeeping of the appropriate officer on behalf of the managers of the hospital and, if the patient is under the jurisdiction of the Court of Protection, the Master notified. If the patient is not under the jurisdiction of the court it is advisable that the will be retained in the custody of the managers until the patient is discharged or dies. If he were transferred to another hospital it would be convenient that the will be also transferred. It is also most desirable, if possible, that a record be made by the medical practitioner in charge of the treatment of the patient of his opinion of the patient's mental state at the time the will was made or as near to that time as possible.

Except so far as otherwise stated above, the ordinary rules as to the confidentiality of a patient's will apply, as also does the statement on page 361 as to the circumstances in which it is appropriate to hand over a patient's will to a relative or to other third party.

4. Senile Patients and Similar Categories

In any hospital, old people's home or similar institution there may be patients suffering from some degree of mental infirmity or failing memory by reason of old age as well as others whose waning mental capacity is due to chronic disease. Unless such a patient's affairs are subject to the jurisdiction of the Court of Protection, when the Court should be communicated with if the patient desires to make a will, it would not be appropriate for the hospital in any way to obstruct the patient in making a will and, if the patient wishes to consult his solicitor, the solicitor should be told. If, however, the medical practitioner in charge of the treatment of the patient were not satisfied that he was of sufficiently sound mind and understanding to make a will, it would be proper not to permit any member of the staff of the hospital to act as a witness.

I. PATIENTS' EVIDENCE IN LEGAL PROCEEDINGS

Except under a warrant or in pursuit of a criminal or suspect who can be arrested without warrant, a police officer seldom has authority to enter private premises or to remain there without permission.[1] But generally a hospital puts no obstacle in the way of police inquiries, even when there is no legal obligation to afford facilities.

Generally, too, so far as is reasonably practicable hospitals facilitate

[1] The police power to take samples *etc.* from persons suspected of drinking and driving have already been discussed at pp. 189–190.

the task of the police if they desire to be on hand near a patient who has been the victim of a serious crime to try to obtain a statement from him, or wish to remain at the bedside of a criminal or suspect.

When a patient, be he a wrongdoer, a suspect or a witness, is seriously ill the desirability, from the point of view of the patient's possible recovery, of allowing, hindering or facilitating an interview with the police, with a solicitor or with other person concerned must be considered. The ultimate responsibility will be with the surgeon or physician in charge of the case who, in making his decision, may also properly have regard to the distress which questioning may cause the patient who may or may not be beyond hope of recovery. The police or a solicitor interviewing a patient would be no less concerned to know that the responsible medical practitioner believed him to be capable of understanding and answering questions.

Previous editions of this book have contained some outline of the law of evidence as it might affect hospitals. With, on the one side, the book growing in size, and on the other, the law of evidence growing in complicity, the present editor feels that even this must now be omitted.

J. OPENING LETTERS

Under s. 56 of the Post Office Act 1953[1] it is an offence wilfully and maliciously, with intent to injure any other person, to open or cause to be opened any postal packet which ought to have been delivered to that other person, or to do any other act whereby the due delivery of the packet is prevented or impeded. This provision does not, however, apply to a parent or guardian or person in the position of parent or guardian towards the person whose letter has been opened or detained. The consent of the Minister[2] is necessary to a prosecution.

Although therefore the opening of a letter addressed to a patient who was dangerously ill and the holding back of such a letter in the interest of the patient by the matron or other responsible officer is not an offence unless it is done maliciously, it is generally unwise, except in a serious emergency, to open a letter addressed to a patient without his authority, or — except under the Mental Health Act 1959[3] — to withhold it from him. Deliberately and without lawful excuse to withhold a letter or other postal packet from the addressee would be an actionable wrong, detinue, for which the patient could claim damages. The wrongful opening of a letter would also be a trespass to goods. If, however, the medical practitioner in charge of the treatment of a patient had acted reasonably in all the circumstances in authorising the withholding,

---

[1] Section 56 of the 1953 Act is kept in operation despite the creation of the Post Office Corporation by the Post Office Act 1969.
[2] Now the Secretary of State for Industry.
[3] Ss. 36 and 134. See below pp. 478 and 488.

or even the opening, of a patient's letter it seems unlikely that any action would be brought. In the normal event, unless some business or financial transaction were affected by the letter, the damages would only be nominal. However, very considerable caution needs to be exercised before a patient's correspondence is handed over to another person, even to a near relative, unless the patient has given authority for that to be done. Such handing over could well give rise to an action for damages for conversion.

For the special rules relating to mentally disordered patients reference should be made to pp. 478 and 488.

K. ADVICE TO PATIENTS

In the course of their duties, social workers properly give some guidance to patients on such matters as how to make use of the social services, how to obtain Social Security benefit and the like. But if a patient were worried about business affairs, *e.g.*, he were questioning a threatened rent increase or eviction or had an insurance problem or wanted advice on whether he could claim damages for an injury he had suffered, the social worker would ordinarily limit his part in the matter to referring the patient to the appropriate advisory service or, if the patient were manifestly well off, to his professional advisers. If, however, as has been known, the social worker himself gave advice to a patient on any such problem, being on a matter on which he was not competent to advise, and the advice had been bad and led to loss, it seems probable that the social worker would be held liable in an action for negligence[1] as having held himself out as giving advice to patients in the course of his professional duties, the patient probably having no reason to suspect that the advice given was outside the scope of the social worker's duties or that he claimed no expertise in the matter on which the advice was given. Moreover, the social worker's employing authority since 1st April 1974, the local Social Services authority,[2] and not the Health Authority responsible for the administration of the hospital — would, if sued, be vicariously liable for his negligence, unless it was clear to the patient that the social worker had been acting outside the scope of his employment.[3]

L. PATIENT'S VOTING AT ELECTIONS

Under s. 12 of the Representation of the People Act 1949, any person on the electoral register who, although still living in the area to which

[1] See *Hedley, Byrne and Co. Ltd.* v. *Heller and Partners* [1964] A.C. 465.
[2] Local Authority Social Services Act 1970, s. 2 and see, as to transfer of staff, the National Health Service Reorganisation Act 1973, s. 18 (4).
[3] This matter is discussed because of Dr Speller's experience that in at least one case a hospital did have to consult its solicitor.

his registration relates, is unable or likely to be unable, by reason either of blindness or any other physical incapacity, to go to the polling station or, if able to go, to vote unaided, is entitled to apply to vote by post at parliamentary or local government elections. This provision is apt to cover the large majority of hospital in-patients, other than long-stay patients. An in-patient suffering from mental disorder may be entitled to exercise a postal vote in the circumstances outlined above if he is suffering to the requisite degree from blindness or other physical disability.[1] In parliamentary elections only, absent voter facilities are available, *inter alia*, on the grounds that the voter is no longer residing at the qualifying address, providing that his new address is not in the same area as the qualifying address. This applies not only in the case of other long stay hospital patients but also of those received for care and treatment in respect of mental disorder[2] so long as they remain on the register.

The practical question for the hospital authority appears to be whether a patient who is on the register should be allowed out to vote, and this is something for the medical practitioner responsible for the patient's treatment to decide, having regard to what is best for the patient and necessary for the safety of others. The responsibility of accepting or rejecting the patient's vote, if he is allowed out, falls on the returning officer, the hospital and its staff not being concerned. Should an informal patient propose to leave the hospital against advice or contrary to hospital rules whether in order to vote or for any other purpose a report on him may be made under s. 30 (2) of the Mental Health Act 1959.[3] It should go without saying that such a report would be grossly improper if it were made to influence the vote rather than for the reasons set out in the section.

It appears that long-stay patients in mental hospitals might be entitled to have their names entered on the register of electors. This only applies where the patient is not liable to compulsory detention (whatever the original reason for his admission) It thus covers the case of the patient who remains in a hospital merely because there is nowhere else for him to go.

M. BUSINESS INTERVIEWS WITH PATIENTS

Generally speaking, when a patient is received into a hospital for treatment, it seems the hospital does not thereby undertake to allow

---

[1] Practical guidance to hospital authorities on questions relating to patients — including psychiatric patients — voting at elections is contained in departmental circular H.M. (72) 44.

[2] A patient resident in an establishment maintained wholly or mainly for the reception or treatment of persons suffering from mental illness or other form of mental disorder cannot be registered as a voter in respect of his residence at that establishment.

[3] See below, p. 477.

visitors beyond what is ordinarily permitted by the rules made for the conduct of the institution, nor — in particular — does it undertake to provide any special facilities for a patient to enable him to carry on with his business or affairs from the hospital. What actually happens in any particular case is not so much a matter of law as of good sense on both sides. A hospital which placed unnecessary obstacles in the way of a patient seeing his solicitor to make a will or for other urgent affairs would invite serious criticism though, except perhaps in the case of a paying patient under ss. 65 and 66 of the National Health Act 1977 or a private patient[1] in a voluntary hospital or proprietary nursing home, most probably not to any legal liability if loss or damage resulted. On the other hand, refusal of the hospital to permit continual coming and going of business callers would clearly be reasonable. Visiting of private patients is often virtually unrestricted save on medical grounds. When that is so, if callers whom the patient wished to see, even business callers, were unreasonably excluded and the patient suffered any loss in consequence, it would seem that there might be a cause of action. But exclusion of visitors on medical grounds by the medical practitioner in charge of the patient's treatment could be the basis of an action only on grounds of negligence or bad faith, always provided that the patient had understood that despite any arrangement for virtually unrestricted or very liberal visiting hours, any or all visitors could be excluded on such ground.

Particular discretion is needed in dealing with mentally disordered patients. Any such patient may send letters to his solicitor, without those letters being read in the hospital.[2] It would, therefore, be within the spirit of the Act to allow the solicitor to see the patient at any reasonable time, subject only to the patient's own well-being. So also such a patient has a right to be seen by a doctor of his choice with a view to making or providing evidence for appearing before a Mental Health Review Tribunal.[3]

N. MARRIAGE OF MENTALLY DISORDERED PATIENTS

If it were known that a patient liable to detention under the Mental Health Act 1959 might have the intention of getting married and the responsible medical officer were of the opinion that the patient was incapable of understanding the nature of the contract of marriage, it would be appropriate for the Area Health Authority running the hospital[4] where he was liable to be detained to consider whether, as an

---

[1] By a *private patient* here is meant a patient whose admission has been subject of contractual arrangements with him or with a relative or other third party.
[2] See p. 488 below.   [3] See p. 533 below.
[4] *Hospital* here includes mental nursing home. (Mental Health Act 1959, s. 59 (2).)

interested person, to enter a caveat with the Superintendent Registrar,[1] thus ensuring that full inquiries as to the patient's mental capacity would be made before a certificate or licence for his marriage was issued. An authority is, however, under no obligation to enter a caveat, a step which could often more suitably be taken by one of the patient's relatives.

Although it is much less likely that an Authority would consider it appropriate to enter a caveat in the case of a patient not liable to detention who intended to get married, it seems that it could do so.

[1] Under s. 29 of the Marriage Act 1949.

CHAPTER 21

PROFESSIONAL QUALIFICATIONS

IT is proposed in this chapter briefly to outline the qualifications, statutory and otherwise, for medical, dental, nursing and midwifery staff, and for pharmacists, opticians and medical auxiliaries. Although, today, it seems hardly likely that any hospital could escape liability for the negligence of a member of its medical or other professional staff on the grounds that it had done its duty in appointing a properly qualified person, it may be observed that even if circumstances did arise in which such defence could conceivably avail, it would be useless merely to show that a person with, say, the minimum registrable qualification in medicine had been appointed. Nowadays that is not enough and, in making senior hospital appointments, full regard is paid to the applicant's postgraduate experience. Moreover he is expected to have obtained the appropriate higher qualification (M.R.C.P., F.R.C.S., F.F.R., D.P.M., etc.). In these circumstances it is not here proposed to do more than draw attention to the broad features of the relevant legislation.

Strictly, the practice of few callings is limited to those who are on a statutory register, the most notable being veterinary surgery, dentistry, midwifery, pharmacy and, now, practice as an optician. The right to practice medicine is not strictly limited to registered medical practitioners, though the disabilities of the unregistered are such that normal practice is closed to them.

A. MEDICAL PRACTITIONERS

The registration of medical practitioners with appropriate qualifications and experience and their penal removal from and restoration to the register is now dealt with in the Medical Act 1956,[1] the responsible body being the General Medical Council.

1. Conditionally Registered Medical Practitioners

On passing one of the qualifying examinations an applicant is conditionally registered under s. 17 which entitles him to accept an approved resident hospital post. After satisfactory qualifying experience in such medical and surgical posts for the prescribed period, an approved mid-

---

[1] Minor amendments to the Act were made by the Medical Act 1956 (Amendment) Act 1958. *See also* Medical Qualifications (E.E.C. Recognition) Order 1977 No. 827.

wifery post being an acceptable alternative in whole or in part for either a medical or a surgical post, attested as required by the Act, a practitioner may become fully registered under s. 7. A conditionally registered practitioner is deemed to be a fully registered medical practitioner so far as is necessary to enable him to be engaged in employment in a resident medical capacity in one or more approved hospitals or approved institutions.[1]

There are also provisions in the Act relating to the registration of medical practitioners who qualified overseas.

2. Privileges of Fully Registered Medical Practitioners

No one is entitled to recover any charge in any court of law for any medical or surgical advice or attendance, or for the performance of any operation, or for any medicine which he has prescribed and supplied, unless he is fully registered.[2] But this does not permit a fellow of a college of physicians prohibited by the bye-laws of the college from suing for fees to do so.[3]

A fully registered practitioner may claim exemption from serving in corporate and parochial offices[4] and, if in practice, is exempt from jury service.[5]

(a) Appointments not to be held except by Fully Registered Medical Practitioners

No one, not being fully registered, may hold any appointment as physician, surgeon or other medical officer, *inter alia*, in any hospital or other place for the reception of the mentally disordered, or in any other hospital, infirmary or dispensary not supported wholly by voluntary contributions;[6] or in any prison; or in any other public establishment, body or institution. An exception is made in respect of an unregistered medical practitioner who is not a British subject at a hospital exclusively for the relief of foreigners.[7] Also, a conditionally registered practitioner under s. 17 is deemed to be fully registered for the purposes of an approved resident post.

(b) Certificates only to be given by Fully Registered Practitioners

A certificate required by any enactment, whether passed before or after the Medical Act 1956, from any physician, surgeon or other

---

[1] *Approved Institution* covers an approved health centre.
[2] Section 27 (1).   [3] Section 27 (2).
[4] Section 30 (1); s. 30 (2) covers conditionally registered practitioners.
[5] Juries Act 1974.
[6] A voluntary hospital possessing endowments or receiving payments for treating N.H.S. patients would not be supported wholly by voluntary contributions. It is indeed difficult to imagine a voluntary hospital other than one exclusively for the relief of foreigners which could lawfully employ an unregistered practitioner.
[7] Section 28.

medical practitioner, is not valid unless the person signing it is fully registered, or, being conditionally registered, is deemed to be fully registered.[1]

(c) False Claims as to Registration

Anyone who wilfully and falsely pretends to be or takes the name or title of physician, surgeon, . . . , or any name, title or description implying that he is registered commits an offence.[2]

B. DENTISTS AND ANCILLARY DENTAL WORKERS

1. Dentists

The law relating to the training and registration of dentists, restrictions on practice of dentistry and for the control of ancillary dental workers by the General Dental Council are contained in the Dentists Act 1957. It is broadly on the lines of the Medical Act 1956. Disciplinary powers are vested in the Council but, as in the case of the General Medical Council, subject to appeal to the Privy Council.

Only a registered dentist is entitled to take and use the description of dentist, dental surgeon or dental practitioner[3] and it is an offence for anyone other than a registered dentist or registered medical practitioner to practice or hold himself out as practising dentistry.[4]

What constitutes the practice of dentistry for the purposes of the Act is set out in s. 33.

Sections 36–39 deal with the business of dentistry and corporate bodies practising dentistry. They are subject to the control of the General Dental Council.

2. Ancillary Dental Workers

(a) Generally

Under ss. 41–43 of the 1957 Act, provision is made for the establishment of a roll or register of ancillary dental workers by the General Dental Council. Disciplinary authority may be exercised through the Ancillary Dental Workers Committee of the Council.[5]

The Council may not in its regulations authorise any ancillary dental worker to undertake —

   (a) the extraction of teeth other than deciduous teeth,
   (b) except in the course of provision of national and local authority health services, the filling of teeth or the extraction of deciduous teeth,
   (c) the filling or fixing of dentures or artificial teeth.[6]

---

[1] Section 17.   [2] Section 31.   [3] Section 12 (1).
[4] Section 34 (1). See s. 34 (2) for certain limited exceptions.
[5] Section 45.   [6] Section 42.

Under these powers, the General Dental Council has made the Ancillary Dental Workers Regulations 1968,[1] under which separate rolls of dental hygienists and of dental auxiliaries are kept, with provision for penal erasure, as in the case of dentists.

(b) Dental Hygienists

The work which may be undertaken by a dental hygienist and the conditions under which it may be undertaken are laid down in Reg. 23, reading as follows:

(1) Subject to the provisions of this regulation, a dental hygienist shall be permitted to carry out dental work (amounting to the practice of dentistry) of the following kinds:
(a) cleaning and polishing teeth;
(b) scaling teeth (that is to say, the removal of tartar, deposits, accretions and stains from those parts of the teeth which are exposed or which are directly beneath the free margins of the gums, including the application of medicaments appropriate thereto);
(c) the application to the teeth of solutions of sodium or stannous fluoride or such other similar prophylactic solutions as the Council may from time to time determine;
(d) giving advice within the meaning of subsection (1) of section thirty-three of the Act on matters relating to oral hygiene;
but shall not be permitted to carry out dental work amounting to the practice of dentistry of any other kind.

(2) A dental hygienist shall not be permitted to carry out such dental work authorised as aforesaid except under the direction of a registered dentist and after the registered dentist has examined the patient and has indicated to the dental hygienist the course of treatment to be provided for the patient.

(3) Except in the course of providing national or local authority health services, a dental hygienist shall carry out such dental work authorised as aforesaid only under the direct personal supervision of a registered dentist who is on the premises at which the hygienist is carrying out such work at the time at which it is being carried out.[2]

(c) Dental Auxiliaries

The work which may be undertaken by a dental auxiliary, and the conditions under which it may be undertaken, are laid down in Reg. 28, reading as follows:

(1) Subject to the provisions of this regulation, a dental auxiliary shall be permitted to carry out dental work (amounting to the practice of dentistry) of the following kinds:
(a) extracting deciduous teeth under local infiltration anaesthesia;

[1] S.I. 1968 No. 357 as now amended by Ancillary Dental Workers (Amendment) Regulations S.I. 1974 No. 444.
[2] This seems to be a rather unfortunate piece of discriminatory legislation. Either the dentist's personal supervision should be necessary in all cases or it should be left to his discretion whether, in any particular case, such supervision is necessary. The same objection may be made to Reg. 28 (2) below.

(b) undertaking simple dental fillings;

(c) cleaning and polishing teeth;

(d) scaling teeth (that is to say, the removal of tartar, deposits, accretions and stains from those parts of the surfaces of the teeth which are exposed or which are directly beneath the free margins of the gums, including the application of medicaments appropriate thereto);

(e) the application to the teeth of solutions of sodium or stannous fluoride or such other similar prophylactic solutions as the Council may from time to time determine;

(f) giving advice within the meaning of subsection (1) of section thirty-three of the Act, such as may be necessary to the proper performance of the dental work referred to in this regulation, and on matters relating to oral hygiene;

but shall not be permitted to carry out dental work amounting to the practice of dentistry of any other kind.

(2) A dental auxiliary shall not be permitted to carry out such dental work authorised as aforesaid except (a) in the course of providing national or local authority health services, (b) under the direction of a registered dentist, and (c) after the registered dentist has examined the patient and has indicated in writing to the dental auxiliary the specific treatment to be provided for the patient by the said auxiliary.

C. PHARMACISTS

The registration of pharmacists by the Pharmaceutical Society dates back to the Pharmacy Act 1852. Now, however, the powers and responsibilities of the Pharmaceutical Society in the matter are to be found in the Pharmacy Act 1954. The Society itself conducts qualifying examinations, though, under the examination regulations, a candidate who has obtained a degree in pharmacy of a university in Great Britain is deemed to have satisfied the Society's examiners in the subjects taken in his degree examinations. The Society has statutory disciplinary powers.

Restriction on use of Certain Titles

The provisions of s. 78 of the Medicines Act 1968[1] restricting the use of certain titles, such as pharmacy and pharmacist, replace those of s. 19 of the Pharmacy and Poisons Act 1933. To be noted here are (i) that the use of the description *pharmacy* in respect of the pharmaceutical department of a hospital, clinic, nursing home or similar institution, or a health centre, is authorised;[2] and (ii) that, in connection with his work at a hospital, clinic, nursing home or similar institution, or at a health centre, as well as in retail pharmacy, a pharmacist may use any

---

[1] The section is in force, Medicines (Pharmacy) (Appointed Day) Regs., S.I. 1973, No. 1849. Note also the provisions of s. 78 may be modified or extended by order or regulation under s. 79.

[2] Section 78 (4).

of the following titles, *viz.*, pharmaceutical chemist, pharmaceutist, pharmacist, member of the Pharmaceutical Society and, if so entitled, Fellow of the Pharmaceutical Society.[1]

So far as hospitals and similar institutions are concerned the position in law of pharmacists in relation to the control of medicines, poisons and dangerous drugs is set out in Chapter 12.

D. OPTICIANS

1 Registration of Opticians

The qualification and registration of opticians and the keeping of a list of corporate bodies carrying on business as opticians is dealt with in the Opticians Act 1958.[2] Under it the General Optical Council has been established, analogous to the General Medical Council and with substantially similar powers, including the disciplinary powers.

Two registers of ophthalmic opticians are kept, one register of those engaged or proposing to engage both in the testing of sight and in the fitting and supply of optical appliances[3] and the other for the registration of persons engaged or proposing to engage in the testing of sight but not the fitting and supply of optical appliances. There is also a register of dispensing opticians (*i.e.*, those engaging in the fitting and supplying of optical appliances but not the testing of sight).[4]

2 Restrictions on the Testing of Sight

A person who is not a registered medical practitioner or registered ophthalmic optician may not test the sight of another person, the only exceptions to this rule being medical students and, under rules of the General Optical Council, persons training as ophthalmic opticians.[5]

3. Restrictions on Sale and Supply of Optical Appliances

No one may sell any optical appliance unless the sale is effected by or under the supervision of a registered medical practitioner or an optician and this also applies to supply of such appliances under arrangements with the Minister or a Health Authority. It does not, however, apply to sales to medical practitioners, opticians, hospitals and Government departments.[6]

---

[1] Section 78 (5). There are other titles, such as chemist or chemist and druggist, which may be used in connection with retail pharmacy, as to which, and restrictions on the use thereof, reference should be made to s. 78.

[2] And the General Optical Council (Registration and Enrolment Rules) Order S.I. 1977 No. 178.

[3] *i.e.* Appliances designed to correct, remedy or relieve a defect of sight (s. 30).

[4] Section 2.

[5] Section 20 and see General Optical Council (Rules on the Testing of Sight by Persons Training as Ophthalmic Opticians) Order of Council 1974, No. 1329.

[6] Section 21.

E. PROFESSIONS SUPPLEMENTARY TO MEDICINE

1. Generally

The Professions Supplementary to Medicine Act 1960, provided for the establishment of the Council for Professions Supplementary to Medicine with the general function of co-ordinating and supervising the activities of the boards established under the Act and the additional functions assigned to it by the Act.[1] Further, for each of the following professions — chiropodists, dieticians, medical laboratory technicians, occupational therapists, physiotherapists, radiographers, remedial gymnasts and orthoptists[2] there has been established under the Act a body called the Chiropodists Board, the Dieticians Board, and similarly for the other professions, having the general function of promoting high standards of professional education and professional conduct among members of the relevant profession and the additional functions assigned to it by the Act. The Privy Council on the recommendation of the Council and subject to the provisions of s. 10 of the Act may, by order, extend the provisions of the Act to other professions and may order that the provisions of the Act shall cease to apply to any profession. Modification of the list to take account of any amalgamation or proposed amalgamation of professions is also provided for as is any consequential amendment of the constitution of the Council.

2. Registration of Members of the Supplementary Professions

This is the responsibility of the several boards[3] subject to the Registration Rules 1962.[4] Initially, any person qualified in relation to the relevant profession, as mentioned in Reg. 3 of the National Health Service (Medical Auxiliaries) Regulations 1954,[5] was entitled to registration, subject to the provisions of s. 3 (1).[6] Disciplinary powers are vested in the boards substantially similar to those vested in the General Medical Council.[7]

3. Use of Titles

A person who is registered is entitled to use the title state registered chiropodist or state registered dietician (and similarly for the other

[1] Section 1 (1).
[2] Orthoptists Board established under the Professions Supplementary to Medicine (Orthoptists Board) Order in Council, S.I. 1966, No. 990.
[3] Section 2.
[4] Professions Supplementary to Medicine (Registration Rules) S.I. 1962 No. 1765 as amended by S.I. 1966 No. 1111, 1967 No. 266, 1968 No. 1973 and 1975 No. 1691 and (Registration (Appeals) Rules) Orders in Council S.I. 1962 No. 2545.
[5] S.I. 1954, No. 55.   [6] Section 3 (2).
[7] See also Professions Supplementary to Medicine (Disciplinary Committees) (Procedure) Rules Order in Council S.I. 1964 No. 1203 and the Professions Supplementary to Medicine (Disciplinary Proceedings) Legal Assessor Rules S.I. 1964 No. 951.

professions mentioned in s. 1 of the Act or to which the provisions of the Act may subsequently be extended under the provisions of s. 10) according to the profession in respect of which he is registered.[1]

Any person who —

(a) takes or uses either alone or in conjunction with any other words, the title of state registered chiropodist, state chiropodist or registered chiropodist (and similarly as regards the other professions) when his name is not on the register established under the Act in respect of that profession; or

(b) takes or uses any name, title, addition or description falsely implying, or otherwise pretends that his name is on a register established under the Act,

is on summary conviction liable to a fine not exceeding £50 or for a second or subsequent offence £100.[2] The comparatively moderate maximum penalties compared with those under the Acts relating to medical practitioners, pharmacists and opticians is probably related to the fact that whilst those belonging to the last-mentioned three professions have certain exclusive privileges in relation to the practice of their respective professions, persons belonging to professions within the provisions of the Professions Supplementary to Medicine Act 1960, are given no such exclusive privileges. Furthermore, anyone may describe himself as a chiropodist, *etc.*, provided he does not infringe s. 6(2). Hence, a physiotherapist who was not registered under the Act could still call himself a physiotherapist or, if a member of the Chartered Society of Physiotherapists, a chartered physiotherapist in accordance with the rules of that society, but generally unless he is registered he may not be employed by a Health Authority.[3]

4 Approval of Courses, Qualifications and Institutions

The responsibility for the approval of courses, qualifications and institutions, as well as for keeping the register, rests with the relevant board.[4]

F. NURSES

1. Introductory

The principal Act relating to the registration and enrolment of nurses, and to the keeping, as an appendix to the register, of a list of certain other trained nurses, is the Nurses Act 1957.[5] Restrictions on the use of the title or description *nurse*, first imposed by the Nurses Act 1943, are

---

[1] Section (6) 1.   [2] Section 6 (2).
[3] The N.H.S. (Professions Supplementary to Medicine) Regulations S.I. 1974 No. 494.
[4] Section 4.
[5] The 1957 Act together with the amending Acts of 1961, 1964, 1967 and 1969 are cited as the Nurses Acts 1957 to 1969.

continued. The General Nursing Council for England and Wales continues to be the body responsible for the keeping of the register, list and roll of nurses and for prescribing the conditions of admission thereto[1] as well as for disciplinary removal. The Council is also the examining body and responsible for approval and oversight of training institutions. It may also prescribe qualifications for teachers of nursing.[2] In its work it has the assistance of statutory regional nurse-training committees.[3] There is an obligation on the Council to appoint a mental nurses committee[4] to which must be referred:

(a) any matter which wholly or mainly concerns registered or enrolled mental nurses or registered or enrolled nurses for the mentally subnormal (other than a question whether a person shall be registered or enrolled or shall be removed from or restored to the register or the roll or a matter arising out of any such question); and

(b) any matter relating to the training of persons for admission to a part of the register of roll containing the names of nurses trained in the nursing and care of persons suffering from mental disorder.[5]

2 Register of Nurses

(a) Generally

This register is divided into 'parts', *viz.*, a part: (i) for general trained nurses; (ii) for nurses trained in the nursing and care of persons suffering from mental disorder other than severe subnormality or subnormality; (iii) for nurses trained in nursing persons suffering from severe subnormality or subnormality; (iv) containing the names of nurses trained in the nursing of sick children; and (v) such other parts as may be prescribed.[6] Where a person satisfied the conditions of a part of the register other than the general part,[7] her name may be included in that other part notwithstanding that it is also included in the general part.[8] Provision is made for closing parts of the register.[9] Provision is made for admission to the register or roll[10] of persons registered or enrolled in Scotland or Northern Ireland and for securing uniform standards of qualification in all parts of the United Kingdom.[11] Nurses trained abroad may also be registered if their course of training is recognised for the

---

[1] Section 3 as amended by Nurses Act 1964.
[2] Section 17 as substituted by s. 1 of the Teachers of Nursing Act 1967.
[3] Sections 11–16 as amended by the N.H.S. Reorganisation Act and the Nurses (Regional Nurse-Training Committees) Order S.I. 1974 No. 235.
[4] Nurses Act 1957, s. 18 (1) (2) as substituted by the Nurses Act 1969, s. 4 (1).
[5] *Ibid*. s. 18 (3) as substituted by s. 4 (2) of the 1969 Act.
[6] Section 1 (1) of the Nurses Act 1969. *Prescribed* means prescribed by rules made by the Council under the Acts of 1957 to 1969. (1957 Act, s. 33 (1) and 1969 Act, s. 9 Under (v) there is a part of the register for nurses trained in the nursing of infectious diseases. (Nurses Rules S.I. 1969 No. 1675, r. 4 (1).) This part is now closed and accordingly no further names may be added to it.
[7] Female terms are used in the text, although generally they should be taken to include the male.
[8] Section 2 (2).   [9] Section 8.
[10] As to the roll, see p. 382.   [11] Section 3.

purpose by the Council. Nurses trained abroad whose training is not so recognised may be registered after undergoing such further training and passing such further examination as may be specified by the Council.[1]

For the detailed rules relating to qualifications for and admission to the register and matters incidental, reference should be made to the Nurses Rules 1969.[2]

(b) The List

Section 5 (1) provides that the list established under s. 18 of the Nurses Act 1943, of certain trained nurses who are neither registered nor enrolled who completed their training before July 1, 1925, shall continue to be kept, the list consisting of like parts as those of which the register consists. A person on the Northern Ireland 'list' is entitled to be admitted to the corresponding part of the English list.

(c) Registration of Persons who are, or who might have been, on the List

Persons whose names are included on the list and persons who would have been qualified for inclusion on the list had they applied at the proper time, may be admitted to the appropriate part of the register.[3]

(d) The Roll

The roll of nurses kept under the provisions of s. 2 (1) (b) of the Act was originally a roll of assistant nurses but its title was altered by s. 1 of the Nurses (Amendment) Act 1961, though the qualification for admission to the roll remains substantially unaltered. The period of training and experience for a pupil nurse is ordinarily two years as against three for a student nurse preparing for admission to the register.[4] Also, the written examination and practical test for pupil nurses are less demanding.[5]

Since July 25th, 1969 the roll has been divided into parts corresponding with the parts of the register for general nurses, mental nurses and nurses for the mentally subnormal. There is, however, a duty to maintain such other parts as may be prescribed.[6]

(e) Removal from and Restoration to the Register, Roll or List

Rules made under s. 7 of the Nurses Act 1957,[7] and ss. 9, 10 and 11 of the Nurses (Amendment) Act 1961, set out the grounds and procedure for removal and restoration to the register, roll or list. The grounds on which, subject to the prescribed procedure, the Council may remove a

---

[1] Section 4.　　　　　　　　　　[2] S.I. 1969 No. 1675.
[3] Section 6 and the Nurses Rules 1969, r. 28.
[4] A lesser period may be permitted in the case of students already in possession of certain other qualifications.
[5] Anyone desiring further information is referred to the relevant rules.
[6] Section 1 (b) of the 1969 Act. For the meaning of *prescribed*, see footnote 6 on p. 381.
[7] As amended by the Nurses Act 1969.

nurse's name from the register, roll or list are that she has been convicted of a crime or been guilty of misconduct or that the entry of her name has been procured by fraud.[1]

The conduct of proceedings preliminary to and on the hearing of complaints is substantially similar to that of proceedings by the General Medical Council in respect of complaints against medical practitioners. There is now a legal assessor;[2] writs of *subpoena ad testificandum* and *duces tecum* are available and witness may be examined on oath.[3]

On notice of removal of her name from the register, roll or list a person aggrieved may, within three months, appeal to the High Court.[4]

3. Qualification of Teachers of Nurses

Section 17 of the Nurses Act 1957,[5] which gives the Council power to prescribe qualifications for teachers of nurses and to make rules[6] relating thereto reads:

(1) The Council may make rules providing for the giving of certificates by or under the authority of the Council to persons of such classes and descriptions as may be prescribed —

(a) who have undergone the prescribed training (being training carried out in an institution approved by the Council in that behalf) and, if the rules, so provide, passed the prescribed examinations in the teaching of nursing; or

(b) who have such other qualifications for the teaching of nursing as may be prescribed; or

(c) who appear to the Council and the Minister[7] in any particular case, to be qualified for the teaching of nursing otherwise than as mentioned in paragraph (a) or (b) above.

(2) A certificate given in accordance with rules made under this section shall be known as a certificate as a teacher of nurses.

(3) In this section 'qualifications' includes qualifications as to experience and 'qualified' shall be construed accordingly.[8]

4. Restrictions on Use of Title 'Nurse'

Anyone who, not being a duly registered or enrolled nurse or a nurse on the list, uses any such title, or badges or uniform implying that her name is included in the register, roll or list; or, being a person whose name is included in any part or parts of the register or of the role but not in another part, takes or uses any name, title, addition, description, uniform or badge, or otherwise does any act of any kind,

[1] See also Nurses Rules 1969, r. 42 and the Enrolled Nurses Rules S.I. 1969 No. 1674, r. 36, also generally.
[2] Nurses (Amendment) Act 1961, s. 10.
[3] Nurses (Amendment) Act 1961, s. 9. The disciplinary machinery is now as set out in the Nurses Rules 1969 and the Enrolled Nurses Rules 1969.
[4] Nurses Act 1957, s. 7 (4) as amended by the 1969 Act.
[5] As substituted by the Teachers of Nursing Act 1967.
[6] See Nurses Rules 1969, rr. 35 to 40.
[7] *Minister* means the Secretary of State for Social Services (s. 33).
[8] See Nurses Rules 1969.

implying that her name is included in that other part commits an offence.[1] Also, any person who, knowing that some other person is not registered or enrolled, makes any statement or does any act calculated to suggest that that other person is registered or enrolled commits an offence.[2] This last provision might apply, for example, to the matron of a nursing home or manager of a nurses' employment agency who led patients or potential employers to believe a nurse or other person had qualifications she did not possess.

By s. 28 the use of the name or title of nurse whether alone or in combination with any other words or letters is restricted to registered nurses, enrolled nurses and persons authorised by virtue of regulations made by the Secretary of State for Social Services to use such name or title. A person whose avocation is caring for children may still use the title 'nurse' unless the circumstances in which the name or title is taken or used are such as to suggest that she is something other than a children's nurse.

The expression *registered general nurse* is used in the Nurses Rules, 1969, for a nurse on the general part of the register, but the generally accepted title is 'State registered nurse' or S.R.N.[3]

The titles in use for those on the other parts of the register remain as in the rules, *viz.*, registered fever nurse[4] (or R.F.N.), registered mental nurse (or R.M.N.); registered nurse for the mentally subnormal (or R.N.M.S.); and registered sick children's nurse (or R.S.C.N.). The corresponding titles for enrolled nurses are, if on general part of the roll enrolled general nurse (or S.E.N.)[3] or, according to the part of the roll on which entered, enrolled mental nurse (or E.M.N.); and enrolled nurse for the mentally subnormal (or E.N.M.S.).

The Nurses Regulations 1957,[5] as amended by the Nurses (Amendment) Regulations 1960 and 1961,[6] authorise other persons than registered and enrolled nurses to use the name or title of nurse subject to such additions as are there set out. But it is expressly stated[7] that nothing in the regulations entitles anyone who is not a registered or enrolled nurse to use in relation to herself any expression including the word 'registered' or the word 'enrolled'.

The permissive regulation 2 (1) reads:

Subject to the provisions of these regulations, a person who is not a registered nurse or an enrolled[8] nurse may —
   (*a*) if the person, being under the age of twenty-one years has passed the final examination for admission to the part of the register containing

---

[1] Section 27 of the 1957 Act as amended by s. 1 (2) of the 1969 Act.   [2] *Ibid.*, s. 27.
[3] The abbreviation S.R.N. for a registered general nurse is hallowed by custom. It seems that S.E.N. is becoming similarly accepted.
[4] A nurse on the part of the register for those trained in the nursing of patients suffering from infectious diseases.
[5] S.I. 1957 No. 1257.   [6] S.I. 1960 No. 1948, S.I. 1961 No. 1213.
[7] Regulation 2.   [8] Word 'assistant' deleted by the 1961 Regulations.

the names of nurses trained in the nursing of persons suffering from infectious diseases, but cannot because of his or her age be admitted to that part, use the name or title of 'trained fever nurse';

(b) if the person is for the time being on the general part of the list kept under section 5 of the Nurses Act 1957, use the name or title of 'trained nurse';

(c) if the person is for the time being on some other part of the said list, use in relation to himself or herself any expression containing the words 'trained nurse' which sufficiently indicates that he or she is on that part;

(d) *Deleted.*[1]

(e) if the person —

    (i) is certified under the Midwives Act 1951, or

    (ii) is, by virtue of section 6 of the Emergency Laws (Miscellaneous Provisions) Act 1953, for the time being deemed, for the purposes of subsection (2) of section 23 of the National Health Service Act 1946, to be a certified midwife, or

    (iii) is a woman who, before the first day of January 1937, was certified by the authorities of a hospital or other institution, to which the Minister has by order applied proviso (c) to subsection (1) of section 11 of the Midwives Act 1951, to have been trained in obstetric nursing.

use the name or title of 'maternity nurse':

    Provided that a woman may not use that name or title by virtue of sub-paragraph (e) (iii) of this paragraph in an area to which the said subsection (1) has been applied, unless she has given to the authority of the area the notice required by the said proviso (c);

(f) If the person is undergoing training for admission to the register, use the name or title of 'student nurse';

(g) if the person is undergoing training for admission to the roll, use the name or title of 'pupil[2] nurse' during training for the examination prescribed by rules made, or having effect, under section 3 of the Nurses Act 1957, and use the name or title of 'senior pupil[2] nurse' while he or she is undergoing practical experience under trained supervision after passing that examination;

(h) if the person —

    (i) is for the time being employed in a hospital mental nursing home or other institution only in nursing persons suffering from mental disorder within the meaning of the Mental Health Act 1959, or

    (ii) holds the certificate of proficiency in mental nursing or the certificate of proficiency in the nursing of mental defectives granted by the Royal Medico-Psychological Association,

use in relation to himself or herself an expression containing the word 'nurse' which sufficiently indicates that he or she is a nurse only of patients suffering from mental disorder as so defined;[3]

(i) if the person holds the tuberculosis nursing certificate granted by the British Tuberculosis Association, or is in training for that certificate, use in relation to himself or herself any expression containing the word 'nurse' which sufficiently indicates that he or she is a nurse, or, as the case may be, is in training to become a nurse, of tuberculous patients only;

---

[1] By the 1961 Regulations.   [2] Word 'assistant' deleted by the 1961 Regulations.
[3] Substantially amended by the 1960 Regulations.

(*j*) if the person holds the orthopaedic nursing certificate granted by the Central Council for the Care of Cripples or the Joint Examination Board of the British Orthopaedic Association and the said Central Council, or is in training for that certificate, use in relation to himself or herself any expression containing the word 'nurse' which sufficiently indicates that he or she is a nurse, or, as the case may be, in training to become a nurse, only of persons suffering from some orthopaedic disability;

(*k*) if the person has in a country or territory, other than England and Wales, successfully completed his or her training as a nurse in accordance with a scheme of training in force in that country or territory, use in relation to himself or herself any expression containing the word 'nurse' which sufficiently indicates the country or territory in which his or her training was received;

(*l*) if, being a person who is serving in Her Majesty's military or air forces (otherwise than as a member of the Army reserve or the Air Force reserve not for the time being called out on permanent service or as a member of the territorial army or auxiliary air force not for the time being embodied), he or she is qualified therein as a trained nurse, use the name or title of 'trained nurse';

(*m*) if, being a person —

  (i) who has at any time been entitled under the preceding subparagraph to use the name or title of 'trained nurse', or would at any time have been so entitled if these regulations, or the regulations revoked by these regulations had then been in force, or

  (ii) who has, while serving in Her Majesty's naval forces, passed for leading sick berth attendant,

  he or she is no longer serving in Her Majesty's forces (otherwise than as aforesaid or as a member of a naval reserve force not for the time being called out for service or called into actual service) use the name or title of 'service-trained nurse';

(*n*) if, being a person to whom none of the preceding sub-paragraphs of this paragraph applies, he or she is a person to whom any provision of regulations made under proviso (*b*) to subsection (2) of section 12 of the Nurses (Scotland) Act 1951, or under paragraph (*c*) of subsection (2) of section 19 of the Nurses and Midwives Act (Northern Ireland) 1959,[1] applies, use any name or title, or use in relation to himself or herself any expression containing the word 'nurse', which he or she would be authorised to use if that provision extended to England and Wales.

5. Training Institutions — Refusal or Withdrawal of Approval

As a condition of admission to the register or roll, the Council may require that the prescribed training shall be carried out either in an institution approved by the Council or in the service of the Defence Council.[2]

The persons responsible for the management of institutions approved by the Council for the purpose of the training rules and the persons

[1] Amended by S.I. 1961 No. 1213.

[2] Section 3 (1) (*b*) as amended by the Defence (Transfer of Functions) Act 1964 and orders made thereunder.

responsible for the management of institutions who are seeking approval by the Council, not being in either case institutions vested in the Secretary of State for Social Services, may be charged by the Council, such fees by way of contribution towards the expenses of the Council in inspecting and approving institutions for those purposes as may be prescribed.[1] The Secretary of State makes a contribution in respect of inspection and approval of institutions vested in him.[2] As to refusal or withdrawal of approval, s. 21 provides as follows:

(1) If the Council are of opinion that they would be justified in refusing to approve an institution for the purposes of the training rules or in withdrawing approval given by them for those purposes to an institution, they shall give to the persons responsible for the management of the institution a written notice of that fact, stating the grounds on which they have formed their opinion, and shall not proceed to a final determination of the question whether or not to refuse to approve the institution or to withdraw their approval thereof, as the case may be, until they have afforded to those persons an opportunity to make representations in writing to the Council and, if so required by those persons, to be heard by the Council.

(2) A person aggrieved by the refusal of the Council to approve an institution for the purposes of the training rules or by the withdrawal of approval given by them for those purposes to an institution may, by notice in writing served on the Permanent Secretary to the Lord Chancellor before the expiration of the period of twenty-eight days beginning with the day on which notification of the determination of the Council to refuse or withdraw their approval, as the case may be, is received by the persons responsible for the management of the institution, appeal against the refusal or withdrawal, and, upon receipt of the notice, the Lord Chancellor shall nominate two persons, or more, to determine the matter of the appeal and the persons nominated shall, after considering the matter, give such directions therein to the Council as they think proper and the Council shall comply with them.

It shall be the duty of a person who serves a notice under this subsection on the Permanent Secretary to the Lord Chancellor to serve at the same time a copy thereof on the Council.

The Revised Conditions for Approval of Hospitals as Training Schools for Student Nurses for Admission to the General Part of the Register of Nurses which the Council laid down as becoming operative on January 1st, 1964, not having been made by statutory instrument, are not binding on a Tribunal hearing an appeal from refusal or withdrawal of approval. There is, however, no reason why the Council should not announce in advance the general conditions by which they propose to be guided in granting or withholding approval of nurse training institutions, provided that applications are considered individually, that an individual discretion is exercised, and that the conditions are not treated as inflexible requirements. Indeed it is probably an advantage to applicants to know in advance the standards at which they should

[1] Section 22 (1); *prescribed* here means prescribed by rules made by the Council under the Act.
[2] Section 22 (2).

aim. Such was the ruling of the Tribunal nominated by the Lord Chancellor under s. 21 (2) of the Nurses Act 1957, to hear an appeal of the St. Helier Group Hospital Management Committee against a decision of the Council to withdraw approval from the Nelson Hospital and the Wimbledon Hospital.[1]

6. Regional Nurse-Training Committees

A regional nurse-training committee has been established for each of the regions of the Regional Health Authorities. The constitution, functions and finance of regional nurse-training committees and their relations with health service management authorities are dealt with in ss. 11 and 13–16 and the Second Schedule of the Act of 1957.[2]

7. Experimental Training of Nurses

Under s. 12 the Council may authorise a trial to be made of any scheme of training and examination for admission to the register or the roll which appears to the Council no less efficient than the training and examinations required by the rules.

G. MIDWIVES

1. State Certified Midwife

A state certified midwife is a woman authorised to attend on women in childbirth and to undertake responsibility for delivery without the direction and personal supervision of a medical practitioner, being on the roll or certified midwives kept by the Central Midwives Board[3] and, having given notice to the local supervising authority of the area in which she resides or carries on her practice as required by s. 15 of the Midwives Act 1951.[4] A midwife proposing to practise as a maternity nurse also has to give notice to the local supervising authority. (The forms, and others for the use of midwives are given as a schedule to the Rules of the Central Midwives Board.)[5]

2. Restriction in Practice of Midwifery

Any person not certified under the Act, except a medical student or pupil midwife as part of the practical training, attending a woman in

---

[1] The tribunal, which sat in public, gave its determination on March 23rd, 1961.

[2] As amended, and see the Nurses (Regional Nurse-Training Committees) Order S.I. 1974 No. 235.

[3] Midwives Act 1951, s. 2.

[4] The Regional Health Authority in England and Area Authority in Wales, is the local supervising authority for the purpose. Provision is also made for the renewal of the notice each year in January and for notice within 48 hours if a midwife practises or acts as a midwife outside the area for which she has already given notice.

[5] The rules are contained in the schedule to the Midwives Rules, Approval Instrument S.I. 1955 No. 120 as amended by S.I. 1959 No. 162, 1961 No. 810, 1962 No. 766, 1969 No. 1440 and 1974 No. 496.

childbirth, otherwise than under the direction and personal supervision of a registered medical practitioner, and except in case of sudden and urgent necessity, commits an offence.[1]

It is, however, provided by s. 34 (4) of the Midwives Act 1951, that nothing in the Act is to be construed as revoking Reg. 33 of the Defence (General) Regulations 1939,[2] which provides for granting to certain women temporary exemption from the enactments relating to midwives.

By the Sex Discrimination Act 1975, s. 20, men may qualify as midwives but the section expressly allows discrimination against them in the employment, promotion, transfer and training as a midwife. It is said that this effects a compromise between the principle of equality between the sexes and preserving midwifery as a female profession.

3. Midwifery and Maternity Nursing Distinguished

Maternity nursing means attendance *as a nurse* on a woman in childbirth or, for the purposes of the Act, at any time within ten days immediately after childbirth without undertaking responsibility for delivery. The classes of persons entitled to act as maternity nurses *for reward* are laid down in the Midwives Act 1951, s. 11, referred to below, but the restrictions apply only in districts to which the Secretary of State has, by order, brought the section into force. To sum up. Save as mentioned below:

(a) Only a State Certified Midwife may ordinarily attend a woman in childbirth without medical help. (Midwives Act 1951, s. 9.)

(b) Only a State Certified Midwife or a State Registered Nurse may act as a maternity nurse attending a woman at childbirth or within ten days thereafter *for reward* in districts where s. 11 of the Midwives Act 1951, has become operative.

The above rules are subject to exceptions mentioned in the sections of the 1951 Act referred to, viz.:

(i) pupil midwives and medical students as part of their training;

(ii) the staffs of registered nursing homes and of exempt hospitals and institutions, so far as maternity nursing is concerned.

(iii) a woman who before January 1st, 1937, was certified by the authorities of a hospital or institution approved by the Minister of Health as trained in obstetric nursing may, if she has given notice to the local supervising authority, practise as a maternity nurse but not as a midwife.

An important distinction should be observed. The prohibition under s. 9 on unqualified persons acting as midwives is absolute, except in the case of pressing emergency, whilst the prohibition under s. 11 on un-

[1] Midwives Act 1951, s. 9.
[2] See now, Emergency Laws (Miscellaneous Provisions) Act 1953, s. 6; see also s. 10 (4) of the Health Services and Public Health Act 1968.

qualified persons acting as maternity nurses is not absolute but only on their doing so for reward. Thus it is in no circumstances an offence for a relative, a friend, or a person actuated by charitable motives to act as a maternity nurse without payment or other reward but it is an offence for an unqualified relative or friend to act as a midwife except in an emergency, and the absence of payment is no defence.

4. Removal from Roll and other Disciplinary Procedures

A State Certified Midwife is under the disciplinary control of the Central Midwives Board and also, to the extent provided in the Act of 1951, of the local supervising authority.

Rules regulating the course of training for midwives; approval of institutions, lecturers and teachers

These matters are dealt with in section B of the Rules.

5. Protection of Titles

In the Midwives Act 1951, *certified midwife* means a woman who is for the time being certified under the Act,[1] and a woman who, not being a certified midwife, takes or uses the name or title of midwife, either alone or in combination with any other word or words, or any name, title, addition, description, uniform or badge implying that she is a certified midwife or is a person specially qualified to practise midwifery or is recognised by law as a midwife is liable on summary conviction to a fine not exceeding £5.[2] In the Midwives Rules 1955 to 1974, it is laid down that the proper designation of a midwife is 'State Certified Midwife' and that the letters S.C.M. but no other initial letters may be used to indicate that a midwife is certified under the Act. If, however, a midwife has been successful at the examination for the diploma in the teaching of midwifery she may add the letters M.T.D. after the letters S.C.M. Any midwife to whom the description is appropriate may also add the words 'Municipal Midwife' or 'County Midwife'.

H. JURY SERVICE

The following, if actually practising their profession and registered (including provisionally or temporarily registered) enrolled or certified under the enactments relating to that profession, *viz.* medical practitioners, dentists, nurses, midwives, veterinary surgeons and veterinary practitioners, and pharmaceutical chemists are excusable from jury service as of right.[3]

---

[1] Section 32.
[2] Section 8. The maximum penalties under this section and under ss. 9 and 11 which relate to practice of midwifery and maternity nursing are surprisingly light.
[3] Juries Act 1974, s. 9 and Part III of Sch. 1.

CHAPTER 22

LABOUR LAW AS AFFECTING HOSPITAL STAFF

A. INTRODUCTORY

1. General

ORDINARY employment law applies in its entirety to the relationship between voluntary hospital authorities or nursing home proprietors and those they employ. But it is modified in respect of the relationship between statutory Health Authorities under the National Health Service Act and those they employ and also that between the Secretary of State for Social Services and those Crown servants working under him for the purposes of special hospitals.[1] The main purpose of this chapter is to direct attention to the modifications in those two cases, and the ordinary labour law will mostly be set out only in the barest outline, being amplified here and there so far as may be necessary to make the nature of the modifications reasonably intelligible, or to bring out a point of special interest to Health Authorities. It is important to note that the Crown and consequently Health Service Authorities are governed by the principal provision of the Trade Union and Labour Relations Act 1974[2] and its Amendment Act of 1976, the Employment Protection Act 1975[3] and the Sex Discrimination Act 1975.[4]

2. Collective Rights

These Acts not merely make important modifications to the common law contract of employment, but they create new concepts, machinery and rights relating to collective bargaining.[5]

Central to collective bargaining lies the concept of an *independent trade union*.[6] Under s. 8 of the Act of 1974 as amended a list is maintained of trade unions by an officer now known as the 'Certification Officer'. Under s. 8 of the Employment Protection Act trade unions may apply for a certificate that they are *independent*.[7] Unions so certified as independent have many important new legal rights enforceable against the employer. Some of these are discussed below.

---

[1] Now under s. 4 of the 1977 Act.   [2] 1st Schedule, para. 33 (4) (*a*).
[3] Section 121.   [4] Section 85.
[5] Further as Professor Lord Wedderburn points out in *The Employment Protection Act 1975 — Collective Aspects* (1976) M.L.R. vol. 39 at p. 168 the Act so improves individual rights as to materially raise the floor from which the bargaining begins.
[6] *Trade Union* is defined in the 1974 Act, s. 28.
[7] *Independent* in s. 8 by s. 126 (1) takes the same meaning as in s. 30 (1) of the 1974 Act as amended by the 1975 Act, Sch. 16, para. 7 (3).

P

Among the machinery created by the Employment Protection Act is the Advisory, Conciliation and Arbitration Service,[1] ACAS is:[2]

... charged with the general duty of promoting the improvement of industrial relations, and in particular of encouraging the extension of collective bargaining and the development and, where necessary, reform of collective bargaining machinery.

Subsequent sections set out its role in greater detail.[3]

Among the rights accorded to an independent trade union, two must be mentioned at this stage. First, such a trade union may make a written reference to ACAS concerning a 'recognition issue' *i.e.*:[4]

... the recognition of the union by an employer or two or more associated employers, to any extent, for the purpose of collective bargaining.

The scope of this provision is unclear. As, has been noted above, employers in the health Service are employed by the Area Health Authority. This is the main executive body and it operates subject to directions of the Regional Health Authority which in turn carries out the directions of the Secretary of State. It is plain therefore that an independent trade union may seek recognition by an Area Health Authority. The question that needs solving is whether such a trade union can seek, by means of the Act, to gain recognition from the Secretary of State. Thus, for example, the National Health Service (Remuneration and Conditions of Service) Regulations 1974[5] provide for negotiations with a *negotiating body* which regulation 2 defines as:

... any body accepted by the Secretary of State as a proper body[6] for negotiating remuneration and other conditions of service for officers or any class of officers.

Some guidance is given to the meaning of s. 11 in its general application by s. 30 (5) of the 1974 Act.[7] However it is phrased in terms which are more suitable to private law. It says:

Any two employers are to be treated as associated if one is a company of which the other (directly or indirectly) has control, or if both are companies of which a third person (directly or indirectly) has control; and ... 'associated employer' shall be construed accordingly.

Company is not defined. The question is therefore is the Secretary of State a *company* within the meaning of the Act? The legal status of the

---

[1] Often known as ACAS. [2] Section 1 (2).
[3] It suffices here to note that normally ACAS works informally and when occasion arises it has the capacity to work with great speed.
[4] Section 11(2) and see s. 11 (3). [5] S.I. 1974 No. 296.
[6] Whether a body is a *proper body* is for the Secretary of State to decide: it is wholly apart from the concept of an independent trade union. See also National Health Service Act 1977, Sch. 5, para. 10.
[7] Made applicable by s. 126 of the 1975 Act.

Secretary of State is that he is a corporation sole.[1] The word *company* has had its meaning explained on numerous occasions by judges but almost invariably in private law matters and in terms that are only suitable to commercial enterprise.[2] The word has however been applied to a municipal corporation[3] and to statutory commissioners.[4] If therefore regard is had to the policy of incorporation, *company* ought to include a corporation sole. If on the other hand regard is had to the ordinary connotation *company* implies more than one individual the word does not include a corporation sole.

Accordingly it is this last choice that determines whether or not an independent trade union can take a recognition issue against the Secretary of State to ACAS.

Even taking the narrow view that a recognition issue against the Secretary of State cannot be taken to ACAS, such an issue can be taken as against an Area Health Authority. There are provisions for ACAS to make broadly such inquiries as it thinks fit including the holding of a ballot but s. 16 relating to powers of the Central Arbitration Committee[5] does not apply. It would seem that even on the narrow view these provisions are considerable advance for unions in the health service since they give rights at least over such matters as the local interpretation of a national agreement.

The second right which must be mentioned is contained in s. 17 and the following sections.[6] Under these sections employers must give to the representatives of an independent recognised trade union, for the purposes of all the stages of collective bargaining:

> . . . all such information relating to his undertaking as is in his possession or that of any associated employer and is both
>
> (a) information without which the trade union representatives would be to a material extent impeded in carrying on with him such collective bargaining, and
> (b) information which it would be in accordance with good industrial relations practice that he should disclose to them for the purposes of collective bargaining.

Section 18 creates a wide range of types of information which an employer is not bound to disclose including 'any information relating specifically to an individual, unless he has consented to its being dis-

---

[1] Secretary of State for Social Services Order S.I. 1968 No. 1699, para. 4 (as amended by the Ministers of the Crown Act 1974) applying Ministers of the Crown Act 1964, Sch. 1, para. 5. And see Ministers of the Crown Act 1975, s. 6 (2) and Sch. 1, para. 5.
[2] See *e.g. Re Stanley* [1906] 1 Ch. 131 *per* Buckley, J.
[3] *Corporation of Wolverhampton* v. *Bilston Commissions* [1891] 1 Ch. 315.
[4] *Caledonian Canal Commissioners* v. *Inverness C.C.* 31 S.L.R. 830.
[5] Known as CAC. It is established by s. 10 of the Employment Protection Act 1975. S. 16 (which applies in the private sector) relates to applications to CAC if conciliation involving ACAS does not result in a settlement.
[6] Section 17 is to come into force when ACAS has issued a Code of Practice.

closed' — words which plainly preserve the duty of confidence discussed in Chapter 20.[1]

Sections 19–21 deal with complaints about non-disclosure of information. Only s. 19 applies to the Crown.[2]

In the description of the general duty to disclose information, s. 17 places the duty only on the employer but the information can relate to that in the hands of an associated employer. It therefore appears that whichever view was taken earlier as regards the question of whether the Secretary of State is 'an associated employer' of the Area Health Authority the request for information can only be made to the Authority. On the other hand, its legal duty to disclose information in the hands of the Department does turn on the same question. But if it has not got the information it cannot disclose it.

3. Individual Rights — Employee and Independent Contractor Distinguished

A person doing a piece of work for another, whether it be painting a picture, building a house or attending a sick person, must ordinarily[3] be acting in one of two capacities. Either he is an independent contractor or he is an employee either of the person on whose order the work is being done or of an independent contractor who has undertaken it. The distinction is important, for the independent contractor is not subject to any control as regards the method of carrying out the work except so far as special terms in the contract may so stipulate. An employee is always subject to some degree of supervision and obliged to obey lawful orders in accordance with his contract of employment and ordinarily at least a certain portion of his time is at the exclusive disposal of his employer. There are other points peculiar to the contract of employment which we shall discuss later.

The physician or surgeon attending a patient in private practice is acting as an independent contractor exercising professional skill in advising and treating his patient. The patient has no control over him. His only remedy if dissatisfied is to call in another medical adviser and, if he thinks he has grounds for it, to bring an action for negligence or failure to exercise due skill. If, however, a medical practitioner is on the salaried staff of a hospital his position is different for, although he

---

[1] Section 121.

[2] Section 18 also provides for the non-disclosure of information whose disclosure would be contrary to national security. Section 19 (7) re-introduces the illiberal procedure abolished generally by *Conway* v. *Rimmer* [1968] A.C. 910, whereby a certificate signed by or on behalf of a Minister of the Crown is conclusive on this point.

[3] It would be only marginally relevant to our present purpose here to consider the position of the volunteer. The position of the medical practitioner who undertakes the treatment of a patient either without reward or without any contract between him and the patient, as is usually the case when the patient is being treated at a N.H.S. hospital, has already been considered in Chapter 14 dealing with injuries to patients.

has discretion as regards treatment of patients, he is subject to rules and regulations imposed by the governing body as regards, *e.g.*, time of attendance, making of returns, *etc.*, and even in his professional work, unless he is of consultant status, may be subject to the general oversight or even the specific instructions of a more senior member of the medical or surgical staff.[1] The medical practitioner in this case is an employee of the hospital. The position of so-called 'honorary staff' in a voluntary hospital is somewhat more obscure, but there is an increasing tendency for such hospitals to give consultants emoluments, and even a purely nominal payment might suffice as evidence that the contract was one of service. On the other hand it might be held to be a contract for services. Elaborate discussion of the point hardly seems called for having regard to the judgments in *Roe* v. *Minister of Health*[2] indicating that a voluntary hospital authority would be liable for the negligence of a part-time consultant working under a contract for services and *Razzel* v. *Snowball*[3] from which the inference may be drawn that the Secretary of State, through his agents, the Regional and Area Health Authorities, is liable for the acts of part-time consultants in the National Health Service.

Without a very detailed analysis far beyond the scope of this work, any more precise definition of the relation of employer and employee than that given above by way of distinguishing him from an independent contractor, is impossible, nor is it necessary.[4]

In the remainder of this chapter attention will be directed exclusively to those features of the relationship of the contract of employment peculiar to the hospital service. For labour law generally, the reader is referred to standard works on the subject.

B. THE CONTRACT OF EMPLOYMENT

1. Generally in the Health Service

Since Health Authorities under the National Health Service Act 1977 are bound by Part III of Schedule 5 of the 1977 Act and regulations made or preserved under it thereunder in respect of most of the terms and conditions of employment of their officers and, except so far as indicated later,[5] by regulations made under s. 67 in respect of super-

---

[1] This is illustrated by the facts of *Junor* v. *McNicol and Others*, a Scottish case in the House of Lords (*The Times*, March 25, 1959). See further, pp.242 –243.

[2] See further, pp. 254–255. Far more difficult questions may arise on the occasion of an 'industrial' dispute. See Trade Union and Labour Relations Act 1974, s. 13. It would appear that a consultant working under a contract for services who withdraws his labour may receive protection if it is a dispute to which s. 29 (2) applies but not otherwise.

[3] See further, pp. 257–258 *et seq.*

[4] As an illustration of the difficulty of definition may be mentioned the case of the hospital chaplain who, for the purpose of contributions under the National Insurance Acts, is regarded as working under a contract of employment. But would he be so regarded for other purposes?

[5] See further, p. 426.

annuation and continued in force under s. 10 of the Superannuation Act 1972,[1] it is desirable not only that all contracts of employment should be in writing but that they should contain a reference over to such national conditions of employment as might be applicable and to the fact that such conditions are subject to alteration from time to time. Whilst as a matter of law the terms of the contract are offered by the employer to the employee, as a matter of practice they are settled by the Whitley machinery including the negotiation over such matters with the trade unions and other bodies representing the staff side.[2] The period of notice to determine a contract of employment not having been approved or fixed by the Secretary of State under the regulations, should be dealt with explicitly.

In *Wood* v. *Leeds A.H.A. (T.)*[3] it was held that the Contracts of Employment Act 1972 did not apply to the contracts made by a Health Authority with its employees.[4] The Employment Protection Act 1975 now provides that the 1972 Act is to be applied 'for the purpose of computing an employee's period of employment, but not for any other purpose'.[5] Thus such matters as unfair dismissal, maternity leave and other individual rights in the 1974 and 1975 Acts *etc.* are applied.

In the hospital situation the right of suspension, with or without pay, is particularly desirable since it is not always practicable to make a prompt decision on summary dismissal.[6] That, too, should therefore be covered in the written particulars of the contract of employment. A reference over to hospital rules and standing orders is desirable. The person being engaged should — both at the time of engagement and afterwards — have access to all terms and conditions of employment including rules and standing orders written into the agreement by reference over. Standard forms of contract are advisable and no variation should be made without being satisfied that the form of agreement as varied will still conform to statutory requirements and not be contrary to any direction from a higher authority under ss. 13–14 of the National Health Service Act 1977.

Before the reorganisation all officers (*i.e.* employees or servants) of any non-teaching health service hospital were officers[7] of the Regional

[1] See bri efly, se ction I of this chapter.   [2] See p. 398 below.

[3] [1974] I.C.R. The Court followed *Pfizer Corporation* v. *Ministry of Health* [1965] A.C. 512. See als o *Hills (Patents) Ltd.* v. *University College Hospital* [1956] 1 Q.B. 90 (C.A.).

[4] But so far as th e application of the Contracts of Employment Act 1972 is concerned, the Minister has taken s teps to see that conditions of employment in the national hospital service are substantially in l ine with the requirements of the Act.

[5] Section 120 (1). It add s a new paragraph, 10A, to the 1st Schedule of the 1972 Act and applies that schedule fo r the purpose stated in the text.

[6] See further below, p. 41 2, for the effects of the recent legislation. It will be noted that even if the dismissal is wit hin the terms of the contract, it may nevertheless be unfair within the meaning of 1st Sch. of the 1974 Trade Union and Labour Relations Act.

[7] The expression *officer* as here used is , in all but the most exceptional circumstances, indistinguishable from *servant*, although s. 79 of the 1 946 Act leaves the point open, stating simply that *officer* includes servant.

Hospital Board. However, now under the 1977 Act, each authority has the direct (*i.e.* non-delegated) power to employ its own staff. The position of the preserved Boards of Governors[1] is maintained as it was before the reorganisation.[2]

By paragraph 10 of Schedule 5 of the 1977 National Health Service Act regulations may be made as regards the terms of employment, the qualifications of persons who may be employed and the manner in which they are to be employed.[3] Paragraph 11 (1) provides that before the regulations are made, the Secretary of State shall consult 'such bodies as he may recognize as representing persons who in his opinion are likely to be affected by the regulations'.

The N.H.S. (Appointment of Consultants) Regulations 1974[4] provide that, with certain exceptions, consultants may be appointed only after advertisement of the vacancy in the manner required by the regulations and that no one may be appointed unless recommended to the appointing authority as suitable by an advisory appointments committee formed *ad hoc* in accordance with the regulations. The duty of the advisory committee is to select from the list of applicants all those they consider suitable and to forward them to the appointing body with any comments they wish to make. They may forward one name only if they consider one applicant only to be suitable, but they would be exceeding their powers if, there being more than one suitable candidate, they forwarded one name only because they considered him best. If the advisory committee considers none of the applicants suitable and so make no recommendation, the appointing authority may not make an appointment without re-advertisement nor until one or more suitable applicants have been approved by the advisory appointments committee. Other medical and dental appointments are made with less formality by the relevant appointing authority.

Further regulations which have been made under paragraph 10 are the N.H.S. (Remuneration and Conditions of Service) Regulations 1974,[5] the N.H.S. (Professions Supplementary to Medicine) Regulations 1974,[6] and the N.H.S. (Speech Therapists) Regulations 1974.[7] The general effect of the N.H.S. (Remuneration and Conditions of Service) Regulations 1974 is to prohibit any Health Authority from

---

[1] Under the N.H.S. (Preservation of Boards of Governors) Order S.I. 1974 No. 281. See above, pp. 23–24.

[2] So that the sections of the 1946 Act which are repealed by the 1973 Act are preserved for the specified Boards. In particular s. 14 (1) of the 1946 Act still applies and the Boards subject to regulations, determine the remuneration and conditions of employment of their officers.

[3] The paragraph sets out other matters that may be dealt with in regulations.

[4] S.I. 1974 No. 361. In Wales the N.H.S. (Appointment of Consultants) (Wales) Regulations S.I. 1974 No. 477 apply. They are broadly to the same effect as the English Regulations. The preserved Boards, of course, still operate under the previous regulations of 1969 (S.I. 1969 No. 163). But these too are to the same broad effect as stated in the text.

[5] S.I. 1974 No. 296.   [6] S.I. 1974 No. 494.   [7] S.I. 1974 No. 495.

paying more or less remuneration to any class of officer than may be laid down for that class of officer in nationally negotiated agreements approved by the Secretary of State.[1] Similarly, if other conditions of service (*e.g.*, hours, sick pay, holidays) have been nationally negotiated for any class of officer and approved by the Secretary of State, 'the conditions of service of any officer belonging to that class shall include the conditions so approved'.[2] The Secretary of State, however, retains the right to vary the remuneration or other conditions of service so approved in the case of an individual officer or of officers of a particular description.[3] This, of course, gives effect to the Whitely Council procedure within the Health Service.

By paragraph 10 (3) of the Schedule to the Act directions may be given to a lower authority to place the services of any of its officers at the disposal of another authority. However, normally before this can be done, the officer or his negotiating body must be consulted.[4] There is, however, a temporary emergency power which allows the Secretary of State or the Regional Health Authority to give effect to previously negotiated procedures.[5] The powers of direction reserved to the Secretary of State by the Schedule and the regulations appear to exclude, in respect of matters covered by them, the general power of direction he has under s. 13 of the 1977 Act.

2. Miscalculations and Remuneration Not in Accordance with the National Health Service (Remuneration and Conditions of Service) Regulations 1974

What would be the effect in law of an engagement not in accordance with the N.H.S. (Remuneration and Conditions of Service) Regulations 1974? First, what is the position if the rate of remuneration agreed is otherwise than as authorised under the regulations? Could either party, discovering before the person engaged had commenced work that the contract was not in accordance with the Regulations, regard it as a nullity and refuse to be bound by it? Or, suppose the mistake were discovered after the employee had commenced work but at or before the end of the first regular period for which, under the agreement, the employee would be entitled to remuneration. Could the employing authority then refuse to pay more than the remuneration authorised under the Regulations if it were that the agreed remuneration had been in excess thereof, or could the employee refuse to accept the agreed remuneration, being less than that to which he would have been entitled under the Regulations? Suppose, finally, that the fact that the agreement had not been in accordance with the Regulations was discovered after the contract of employment had been in force some time,

---

[1] Regulation 3 (1). [2] Regulation 3 (2). [3] Regulation 3 (3).
[4] 1st Schedule, para. 11 (2). [5] *Ibid.*, para. 11 (3).

maybe a month, maybe a year, maybe longer. Could the Health Authority then claim repayment of any remuneration paid under the agreement in excess of that authorised under the Regulations? Or could the employee whose agreed remuneration had been less than that laid down under the Regulations claim as a debt due to him the difference between the remuneration he had received and that which he ought to have received thereunder? In all the foregoing possible cases mistake or oversight has been assumed. The position would be different if one or both parties had wilfully ignored the effect of the Regulations, and is a matter which will be discussed separately.

As a preliminary to consideration of the different situations outlined above it must be observed that a contract entered into, not in accordance with the Regulations, cannot be dismissed as a nullity as being contrary to law. This is because the Regulations do not themselves contain the authorised scales of salary. Those authorised under Reg. 3 (1) are to be found only in agreements entered into in the various Whitley Councils for the Health Services[1] which, on approval by the Secretary of State under the Regulations, are almost invariably transmitted to Health Authorities under cover of a circular signifying that approval and given instructions for action thereon.[2] The Whitley and departmental circulars are not publications purchasable by the public, though there is, in fact, no obstacle to the dissemination of their contents, e.g., in newspapers, staff magazines, etc. From time to time salary scales and conditions are collected into handbooks which, although, so far as available, purchasable from the Department of Health and Social Security — being mainly bought by trade unions and professional societies — are not, in the ordinary sense, freely on sale, as are publications obtainable from Her Majesty's Stationery Office. Consequently, information about the generally authorised rates and scales of remuneration is not very accessible. In practice, persons accepting a first appointment with a Health Authority must, in the nature of things, rely on what they are told by their prospective employer about pay and conditions of service. Further, since the Secretary of State has power under Reg. 3 (3) to authorise a board or committee to vary the nationally agreed and approved remuneration in the case of an individual officer, or of officers of a particular description, and such authorisation may be known only to the particular employing authority and the Department, it can fairly

---

[1] It is neither practicable nor appropriate here to attempt to explain the precise nature and relationship *inter se* of the N.H.S. Whitley Councils but, broadly, it may be said that the General Council deals with matters affecting all staff whilst the functional councils deal with matters affecting only staff within their purview. Anyone wanting a more precise statement on the constitution and functions of the Whitley councils and on agreements reached should refer to the relevant handbooks and circulars published through the Department of Health and Social Security. What is important is to appreciate that any Whitley agreement approved by the Minister becomes a statutorily binding condition of employment of all officers to which it applies.

[2] Otherwise by individual letter.

be argued that even if a person knew of the existence of nationally approved scales of remuneration he would be under no obligation to check that what he was offered was in accordance with those scales since he could fairly assume that, if what he was offered varied from the approved national rate, the variation had been authorised by the Secretary of State. This assumption is the more reasonable since seemingly the Secretary of State is not obliged to give his authorisation to a variation under Reg. 3 (3) in writing.

Moreover, even had any such authorisation been in writing, it would most probably have been in a letter to the Health Authority, the contents of which would not ordinarily be within the knowledge of any candidate for a post or of any officer whose pay or conditions of service had been varied.

Against that background, what is the position in law if the agreed remuneration exceeds the national rate approved by the Secretary of State under Reg. 3 (1) and no approval has been given under Reg. 3 (3) to a variation, the mistake being discovered before the commencement of the relationship of employer and employee? Dr Speller's first and most reluctant inclination was to the opinion that the Health Authority could decline to employ the employee on the agreed terms on the grounds that the agreement had been *ultra vires* and that the employee would have no redress since he must be presumed to be aware of the Regulations and so was put on inquiry. But that is a conclusion which Dr Speller regarded as so manifestly unfair that the courts would not be likely to reach it if there were any escape from doing so, the fault being wholly that of the employing authority. He asked 'Is there any alternative approach?' and suggested that since under the pre-1974 system, the Regional Hospital Boards acted on behalf of the Secretary of State and not only did the hospital management committee's act on behalf of the Regional Boards but the staff working for the committee were employed by the Board for the area a remedy might have been found for the prospective employee in the doctrine of breach of warranty of authority. He considered that the same principles might apply to a teaching hospital which was always expressed to employ its own staff. Under the reorganisation each authority directly employs its own staff and accordingly this second case now applies generally. Now all Health Authorities carry out their tasks 'on behalf of'[1] the Secretary of State. Reluctant, as I am, I do not see how it is possible to maintain an action for breach of warranty of authority against a corporation[2] for doing something *ultra vires*. The same obstacle that prevents the action on the contract also prevents the action for the breach of warranty. It is possible the position is different where the engagement is made by an officer of the Authority rather than its governing body. It is also possible that the

[1] Section 13 of the 1977 Act.   [2] 1977 Act, 5th Sch., para. 8.

contract would only be void as regards the illegal terms in which case the employment could still take place. It is, however, as Dr Speller said, most unlikely that, in practice, any Health Authority would seek to avoid its obligations under a contract of employment in the manner discussed or that the Secretary of State would expect it to do so. What it would certainly be expected to do would be to terminate the agreement by proper notice as soon as the mistake was discovered, offering the employee, as an alternative to dismissal, continued engagement on the proper remuneration. Even this might cause real hardship to an employee who had altered his position on the assurance that in his new employment he would receive a particular rate of pay, but it would not constitute an actionable wrong.[1]

But what if the fact that the rate of remuneration contracted to be paid exceeds that approved or directed under Reg.3 of 1974 Regulations is discovered only after the agreement has been in force for some time and there has in fact been overpayment? Is any part of the remuneration already paid, maybe over a long period, recoverable? If Dr Speller is correct and the Health Authority claimed a refund of remuneration in excess of that approved under the Regulations, the employee could counterclaim for the same amount from the Authority on grounds of breach of warranty of authority. If, however, that view were erroneous, it may, alternatively, be suggested on the authority of *Holt* v. *Markham*[2] that as the employee had received in good faith money paid by mistake by the employing Authority and, by that mistake, had been led to alter his position, the employing Authority would not be able to recover whether the mistake were of law or of fact. There is also the possibility that the court would decide that the payment had been made by reason of a mistake of law and, therefore, irrecoverable on that ground.

A case of overpayment which is much more troublesome and one suspects much more common is in respect of miscalculation of remuneration of an existing officer who is on the right scale, or a mistake in principle in the calculation of overtime payments or rates of deduction for emoluments or, maybe, a miscalculation on the addition of an increment on a scale or on the application of a new scale by approved national agreement. Here we have to face the fact that the officer might have known that he was being overpaid. If he did know, or the overpayment has been so large as to put him on inquiry, he would be liable to repay. If, however, he had received the overpayment innocently and had altered his position on the strength of it, *Holt* v. *Markham*[2] is authority for his retaining the amount overpaid. But it would not be

---

[1] But *Barber* v. *Manchester R.H.B. and Another* [1958] 1 W.L.R. 181 might constitute a formal obstacle to dismissal of a medical practitioner with notice since the practitioner could exercise his right of appeal to the Secretary of State. There would, however, be no obstacle to the Secretary of State's upholding the decision of the employing authority.

[2] [1923] 1 K.B. 504.

easy to prove that an officer had altered his position by reason of a single overpayment, although substantial: indeed his retaining such a payment without inquiry might look suspicious. However, even in that case, it is suggested that the recipient might have received the money in good faith and that, unless repayment were sought promptly, he could have altered his position. A good illustration is the payment in a lump sum of additional remuneration under a back-dated award. An officer might well take without question what he was given and then, on the strength of it, commit himself to a family holiday far more expensive that would otherwise have been practicable, or to alterations or decorations to his house which, without the lump sum, would have been beyond his means.

Here is not the place to embark on a discussion of the weight of evidence necessary to fix an officer with knowledge that he had been or was being overpaid. It is, however, worth reminding ourselves that the expression *officer* includes everyone from consultants and senior administrative staff to porters and kitchen maids. It would be much harder — in law as well as in practice — to obtain a refund from those at the bottom of the ladder than from those at the top, who might more readily be expected to be familiar with their precise terms of service and expected to check any payments received by them. Particularly at the bottom end of the hierarchy, the possibility of recovery of overpayment of remuneration is the more remote if the same miscalculation or misinterpretation of, say, rules as to overtime, has been made in respect of everyone in a particular grade.

Next we have the much easier case of a contract under which an officer has agreed to work, and has worked, for less remuneration than that which, under the Regulations, he should have received. The original mistake having been made by the employing Authority which has misled the employee as to his rights, it seems that the officer who had been underpaid could claim all amounts underpaid within six years of his commencing an action for recovery.[1] An employee who has been paid too little as a result of any miscalculation may, likewise, when he discovers it, claim the balance due to him.

A special case must here be mentioned. Sometimes an officer who has been engaged in a lower grade and on the terms and conditions appropriate to that grade claims that the work he is doing is, in fact, that of a higher grade and that he should be remunerated accordingly. Is he entitled to back pay from the date of his engagement or from the date on which first he undertook the duties of the higher grade, whichever is later? There is no clear cut answer to this. By agreement in the General Council of the Whitley Councils for the Health Services and subject to the conditions of that agreement, grading appeals, as well as

---

[1] Limitation Act 1939, s. 2.

THE CONTRACT OF EMPLOYMENT

other appeals on the application of Whitley agreements on remuneration and conditions of service to individual officers, may be referred, through a trade union or professional society accepted for the purpose as a nationally 'recognised negotiating body', to an appeals committee, the committee being free if it decides an officer should be up-graded to backdate its award or not. Although an officer who alleged that he had not been paid, say, the proper acting allowance or travelling or subsistence allowance or had not received the pay appropriate to his work in the grade in which he had actually been engaged, as an alternative to application to an appeals committee would have the right to pursue his claim in the courts, it is by no means clear that he would have such recourse in respect of alleged underpayment on account of wrong grading.

The difficulty of deciding whether recourse may be had to the courts lies in deciding the precise effect of Reg. 3 (1) of the Regulations, which refers to 'the remuneration of any officer who belongs to a class of officers whose remuneration . . . has been approved by the Secretary of State'. Take then an officer engaged in the clerical grade but doing work, by definition, appropriate to the higher clerical grade. Is he for the purpose of his right to a certain level of remuneration to be regarded as in the clerical grade until his grading is altered or, having regard to the fact that the definitions of the various grades are laid down in Whitley agreements approved by the Secretary of State, can he claim that he is actually entitled to the pay of the higher grade so long as he is undertaking the duties of the higher grade?[1] Only if the latter were the correct hypothesis, which is to be doubted, would he have the right of recourse to the courts.

3. Conditions not in accordance with the 1974 Regulations

The number of possibilities of unauthorised variation of conditions of employment is so great that it is impossible to deal with them exhaustively here. But one or two major problems may usefully be mentioned.

First as to hours of duty. If an officer has been engaged on terms that he is to work for, say, three hours less per week than is required under a relevant, approved[2] national agreement, but for the same pay as for the full number of hours, it seems that it is the duty of the employing Authority on discovering the irregularity, to terminate the agreement by notice and offer new conditions in accordance with those authorised. In an officer is found to have been employed on terms which required him to undertake longer hours than are authorised under the Regulations but for the same pay as for the lesser number of hours to which the standard week's pay is related, and he is in an overtime grade, it is

---

[1] Otherwise than in an acting capacity, for which special provision is made.
[2] *i.e.*, approved by the Secretary of State under the Regulations.

suggested that the excess hours worked should count for overtime payment; and that is probably what would happen. The case is analogous to underpayment of wages, though not precisely the same.

Other conditions which might, by mistake, have varied from those under the Regulations are as to sick-pay and holidays. The factors governing the position regarding the claiming back of overpaid sick-pay, or of the making up sick-pay wrongfully withheld or insufficient in amount, would be the same as in respect of overpayment or under-payment of remuneration generally. The granting, by mistake, of too long a holiday presents no problem. The officer has had it; no court would be likely to entertain a claim by the employing authority in respect thereof. If, on the other hand, owing to a mistake and without protest on his part, an officer had not been granted all holidays to which under the Regulations he was entitled, it is possible that the court might award him damages in respect of the advantage lost, though this is most doubtful. After all, in most cases, an officer of a Health Authority is likely to find out the correct holiday from others working with him and he could, therefore, easily be held to have acquiesced in the wrong which he had suffered.

4. Gifts to Officers on Retirement or Otherwise; Superannuation Payments, or Supplementary Superannuation Payments, by Health Authorities

The questions here posed are whether a Health Authority under the National Health Service Act 1977, may (i) make any gift to an officer in its service; (ii) make a retiring gift to any such officer; (iii) make any periodic or other payment to a former officer by way of super-annuation.

(a) Gifts to or for the Benefit of Serving Officers

A gift to an officer which was in the nature of remuneration for his service beyond what had been authorised under the N.H.S. (Remuneration and Conditions of Service) Regulations 1974, could not be justified whether or not paid out of Exchequer funds, as it would contravene the express terms of those Regulations which forbid payment of remuneration in excess of that authorised, whether or not paid out of moneys provided by Parliament.[1] And this would be so whether it was a single payment or periodic.

But payments to officers for special purposes may nevertheless be justified and, indeed may be authorised by the Secretary of State. For example, subject to conditions set out in the relevant circulars to Health Authorities, officers may be paid expenses of attendances at conferences and residential courses. Also, any officer undertaking a course of study

[1] Regulation 3 (1).

for a qualification likely to increase his usefulness, may receive financial aid within approved limits, in both cases out of Exchequer funds. Similarly, payment by way of *ex gratia* compensation may be made out of Exchequer funds to an officer who, say, has had his spectacles broken or his clothing damaged in an accident on duty for the consequences of which the Health Authority are not responsible in law, *e.g.*, damage caused by a patient having an epileptic fit, there being no question of the damage having been caused or contributed to by inadequate staffing, by the negligence of a fellow employee or by anything else which might import liability.

There is, however, a whole range of gifts for particular purposes which may be made out of non-Exchequer funds which the Secretary of State would not authorise to be made out of Exchequer funds. By way of example may be mentioned financial aid beyond that authorised in departmental circulars for officers studying for approved qualifications or paying for time-off work for trade union activities under s. 58 of the Employment Protection Act[1] or payment of convalescent home charges for a nurse who had been seriously ill. The tests to be applied to ascertain whether a payment to or for the benefit of an officer out of a trust might, *prima facie*, be justifiable are (i) to ask whether, in all the circumstances, the payment proposed is for purposes relating to Health Services or to the functions of the Authority with respect to research; and (ii), if the trusts on which the fund out of which the payment is proposed to be made is held are for more specific purposes, to ask whether the proposed payment can fairly be regarded as for those purposes. Whether a payment can be regarded as 'for purposes relating to Health Services . . .' is a question of fact. If it were of a kind designed, even indirectly, to advance the efficiency of the Authority or to promote research, then it might be so regarded. Payments to assist officers improve their qualifications in particular fields of work clearly would[2]; so would *ex gratia* compensation for, say, spectacles broken in carrying out duty such as restraining an epileptic patient, because it would encourage staff to do their utmost in such circumstances without worrying about possible loss to themselves. In *re White's Will Trust, Tindale* v. *United Sheffield Hospitals and Others*[3] a gift for provision of a rest home for nurses was held to be a charitable trust which a hospital authority could accept, and affords strong evidence that payment for a nurse at a convalescent home would in appropriate circumstances be within the powers of a Health Authority.

But even though a payment to or for the benefit of a serving officer

[1] As to time-off work under s. 57 (which is, unlike s. 58, limited to time-off for industrial activities related to industrial relations of an employee with his employer and which may be normal paid time) see below p. 433.
[2] See also *The Annual Report of the M.D.U.* for 1971, at p. 67.
[3] [1951] 1 All E.R. 528.

may on the face of it be within the powers of a Health Authority as charitable trustees, it must also be reasonable in amount. An excessively large payment would be a breach of trust, because any possible benefit to the Health Service would be so disproportionately small that no prudent trustee could regard the money as spent for the purposes of the service.

A gift for the benefit of officers generally or of a particular class of officer, whether on a single occasion or periodic, *e.g.*, provision of additional amenities for nurses or other resident staff, must be judged on the same principles. The purposes of the Health Service are the provision of care and treatment for the sick and medical and similar reaearch. Extras for the staff out of moneys provided for such purposes generally are justified only if the Authority authorising the expenditure has ground for belief that such expenditure is likely significantly to forward those purposes. To take an example: within common sense limits improvement of accommodation and provision of extra amenities for resident nursing staff, especially in a hospital where the basic accommodation and amenities so far provided out of Exchequer funds are poor, is justifiable because it may be expected to help the Health Authority obtain and keep the nurses it needs. It must, however, be reasonable in amount, having regard to all the circumstances, including the size of the fund available and other calls on it.

(b) Retirement Gifts[1] and Payments in the Nature of Superannuation

The legality of a retirement gift by a Health Authority has to be tested by the same yardstick as a gift to a serving officer. Does it offend against any regulation under the Health Service Acts? If not, is the payment permissible out of Exchequer funds? Or, may it be paid out of trust funds at the disposal of the Health Authority? Let us deal with the first question.

Any payment or payments to an officer on retirement otherwise than payments he has a right to under the Act or regulations, if of substantial amount, must either be regarded as remuneration or as superannuation. If such payment or payments were in the nature of remuneration, they would be unlawful, whether out of Exchequer funds or out of trust moneys, for reasons we have already seen. If regarded as in the nature of superannuation different considerations apply.

On balance, it seems that any lump sum payment to an officer on retirement, as well as any periodic payments to him after retirement, would be in the nature of superannuation rather than remuneration, and that view is strengthened by the fact that superannuation benefits provided for in the N.H.S. (Superannuation) Regulations[2] include not

---

[1] As to comparatively trifling gifts in money or kind, see p. 407.
[2] See below, p. 426.

only a pension but also, and in addition, lump sum retiring allowances.

If, then, one regards either a lump sum payment to an officer on retirement or periodic payments to him thereafter as in the nature of superannuation, such payments would not be rendered unlawful by the N.H.S. (Remuneration and Conditions of Service) Regulations 1974. They could not, however, be made out of Exchequer moneys since the superannuation of officers is provided for in regulations made under s. 10 of the 1972 Superannuation Act and are not a proper purpose for use of Exchequer moneys by a Health Authority.

Would it then be permissible to make such payments out of trust funds not impressed with more than the broad trusts 'for purposes relating to Health Services . . . or in respect of research'? The test is whether such payment, or payments of the particular kind, are designed and likely to advance the efficiency of the hospital or hospitals or other services for which the Authority is responsible or further research. The larger the amount involved, either in one sum or in aggregate, the more clear should the evidence on this point be to a reasonable man if such payment is to be justified. And it must be borne in mind that the provisions of the N.H.S. (Superannuation) Regulations, substantially in line with the provisions for superannuation in public services generally, must ordinarily be regarded as appropriate. It would not on the face of it seem to be designed and likely to further the work of the Authority to make any payments in excess of that to which the retiring officer is entitled. There may however be exceptional circumstances when such payments are reasonable. One example that springs to mind is an officer whose employment was transferred either in 1948 or in 1974 and who would otherwise be worse off than officers in similar grades with similar total length of employment. Of course if at any time an employee had exercised an option and lost, he cannot claim to have been prejudiced in this way.

The limitation on the use of Exchequer moneys or of trust funds for making substantial retirement gifts in money or payments in the nature of superannuation to officers in the Health Service apply with no less force to gifts in kind, although a gift of comparatively small value, especially to someone who had given long and loyal service in one of the lower grades (e.g., hospital porter or kitchen maid), the gift being made either on retirement or on completion of 25 years' employment, might be justifiable if out of trust funds, but not out of Exchequer moneys.

5. Qualifications for Employment Prescribed by Regulations under the National Health Service Act[1]

The N.H.S. (Professions Supplementary to Medicine) Regulations 1974[2], lay down that no officer shall be employed by a Regional or

[1] Made under para. 10 of Sch. 5 of the 1977 Act. [2] S.I. 1974 No. 494.

Area or special Health Authority in the capacity of a chiropodist, dietician, medical laboratory technician, occupational therapist, orthoptist, physiotherapist, radiographer or remedial gymnast unless in effect he is registered under the Professions Supplementary to Medicine Act 1960, in respect of the profession appropriate to the work for which he is employed or was employed in such capacity by a local authority or voluntary organisation immediately before 1st April 1974.[1]

The N.H.S. (Speech Therapists) Regulations 1974,[2] lay down the prescribed qualifications for speech therapists in the service of a Health Authority.

If an Authority engaged a person who, being a member of one of the professions covered by the N.H.S. (Professions Supplementary to Medicine) Regulations 1974, was not registered or, being a speech therapist, was not qualified for employment under the relevant regulations and the Authority had not been deceived by that person as to his qualifications, it could even so be argued that the contract was a nullity because both the employing Authority and that person must be taken to have known the relevant regulations. But so far as services had been rendered there would be no question of obtaining a refund of remuneration paid. If, however, one assumes the contract to be a nullity and the person's employment were terminated summarily on realisation that he was not qualified under the regulations, it seems that the dismissed person would, strictly have no claim to remuneration accruing due nor, possibly, even to that already accrued due under the void contract. But, in practice, no Health Authority would be likely to be so unreasonable as to refuse payment and an authority wishing to act fairly might go further and make an *ex gratia* payment of salary in lieu of notice to the person whose service had been terminated.

If the employing Authority retained the unqualified person longer, allowing him to work his notice under the void agreement, they would continue in breach of the Regulations. That, in itself, would not be a very serious matter unless in flat defiance of a direction from the Secretary of State, since it would constitute neither a criminal offence nor a civil wrong. What could happen if a Health Authority wilfully ignored the Regulations or deliberately disobeyed a direction would be that the Secretary of State might have recourse to his default powers under s. 85[3] of the National Health Service Act 1977. Although, therefore, to retain a person lacking the prescribed qualification either for the appropriate period of notice or, possibly, until a qualified substitute had been found, might thus seem a small matter, it would usually be most inadvisable because the fact that the person lacked a recognised qualification for the work he was doing might make it considerably harder for

---

[1] Under S.I. 1964 No. 940, as amended by S.I. 1968 No. 270.
[2] S.I. 1974 No. 495. [3] Formerly s. 57 of the 1946 Act.

the Health Authority to defend an action for damages based on an allegation of the unqualified person's negligence or incompetence in treating a patient — unless it could be shown that the person was qualified for registration.

Should it be that a person had obtained an appointment by claiming to hold a particular qualification which he did not possess, the employing authority, on discovering the deception, would have the right summarily to dismiss him.

6. Appointments in Excess of Authorised Establishment

If the maximum establishment for a particular grade of staff employed by a Health Authority had been fixed either by itself or by direction of a higher Authority that would not invalidate the contract with a person engaged in excess of establishment since that person could know nothing of the limitation nor, if he did, whether the Authority had a full establishment. Moreover, the fault consists in having in aggregate too large an establishment of, say, physiotherapists, not in having engaged a particular one.

7. Student Nurse and Pupil Nurse Training Agreements

Formerly it was customary in the agreement with a student nurse to bind her for the full three or four years training and to include a clause that an agreed sum was to become payable by her as liquidated damages if she left voluntarily before the completion of training. Today such conditions have vanished, probably never to return and student nurses — and also pupil nurses — like other staff can leave at any time on giving the agreed notice or, if no notice has been agreed, reasonable notice. Although the agreement is expressed to be for training and the remuneration is called a training allowance the contract is, in substance a contract of employment analogous to apprenticeship, though not for a fixed term. What is said elsewhere in this chapter about contracts of employment and national conditions of service therefore applies no less to student and pupil nurses. Indeed, their 'training allowances' and conditions of service are negotiated, as are the salaries and conditions of service of other nursing staff, by the Nurses and Midwives Whitley Council, and observance of the agreed conditions made obligatory on the approval of the Secretary of State being given under Reg. 3 of the N.H.S. (Remuneration and Conditions of Service) Regulations 1974.

8. Contracts of Employment of Persons in Special Hospitals

Special hospitals provided by the Secretary of State under s. 4 of the National Health Service Act 1977 for persons suffering from mental disorder, being persons who, in the opinion of the Secretary of State, require treatment under conditions of special security on account of their dangerous, violent or criminal propensities, are under the control and management of the Secretary of State and not of Health Authorities established under the National Health Service Act. Consequently the staff of those hospitals are civil servants and hold their appointments during the pleasure of the Crown. In practice, as is the case with other civil servants, remuneration and conditions of service of the different grades are subject of negotiation and, in most cases, on disagreement, may be referred to the Civil Service Arbitration Tribunal, though not as of right.

9. Contracts of Employment Outside the National Health Service

This section of the chapter refers to contracts of employment entered into, as employers, by any person or persons, including any corporate body, not being an Authority under the National Health Service Act. It refers therefore to all hospitals and nursing homes outside the national hospital service, whether carried on for private profit or not and whether or not providing accommodation or other services for health service patients under contractual arrangements with a Health Authority.

What has been said above so far as it relates to limitations on the powers of Health Authorities to pay what remuneration they like and engage staff on whatever other conditions they think fit does not apply to these independent employers. But those of them who are responsible for hospitals which are in law charities have to remember their obligations as charity trustees. Any obvious squandering of trust moneys would be a breach of trust.

As the scales of salaries and conditions of service for different grades of health service staff approved or determined under the Regulations are not automatically written into contracts of employment made by those controlling private hospitals or nursing homes it is important that due care should be taken to cover such matters as are there dealt with, holiday entitlement being a case in point. Sometimes an attempt is made to deal with the matter by a statement that National Health Service Whitley conditions[1] shall apply to the post. This may not, however, always be entirely appropriate and may even be ambiguous. As an example of this it may be said that what past service in the grade may be counted for incremental purposes and what past service is to count for sick leave entitlement may be obscure, because the nationally negotiated terms are being applied without amplification or modification to a situation for which they were not intended. Unless specially exempted by order made by the Secretary of State for Employment,

---

[1] Most scales and conditions being settled in Whitley Councils and approved under Reg. 3 of S.I. 1974 No. 296.

employment in charity hospitals and in nursing homes will be within the Contracts of Employment Act 1972 and the Redundancy Payments Act 1965.

10. Inventions by Hospital Staff

Ownership of inventions made by members of the staff of a hospital, failing anything decisive on the matter in the contract of employment of the person concerned, is outside the scope of this book. It may be noted, however, that the position as seen by the Department in relation to staff employed by Authorities within the N.H.S. has been set out in a circular to hospital authorities.[1] What is said in the circular about the common law position is no less relevant to ownership of inventions by persons in the employment of hospitals outside the N.H.S. than to membership of those made by persons within that service.

C. THE CONTRACTS OF EMPLOYMENT ACT 1972

As noted above, it has been held that the Act does not apply to National Health Service employers.[2] It does, however, apply to voluntary hospitals, nursing homes and the like.

The broad effect of the Contracts of Employment Act 1972 is as follows. It fixes minimum periods of notice for determining contracts of employment,[3] though it none the less remains lawful for the parties to agree on longer notice than the statutory minimum. Also, failing any agreed period of notice, the reasonable notice required at common law to determine a contract of employment may well exceed the minimum under the Act of 1972. If in any particular case no more than the statutory minimum notice is required to determine a hiring, the employee whilst working out the period of notice is entitled to have his remuneration determined in accordance with the provisions of Schedule 2 of the Act.[4] The provisions of the Act as to notice do not affect the right of either party to treat the contract as terminable without notice by reason of such conduct by the other party as would have enabled him so to treat it before the passing of the Act.[5]

The Act also obliges the employer to give an employee written particulars of the terms of employment within four weeks[6] of the commencement of that employment and also written particulars of any change within one month of such change. Alternatively, within such periods,

[1] H.M. (67) 63.

[2] See above, p. 396. For guidance on its application to the Health Service see H.M. (64) 49, (70) 26 (in the 1963 Contracts of Employment Act which is repealed and re-enacted by the 1972 Act) and H.M. (72) 35.

[3] Section 1.

[4] Section 2. Schedule 2, as set out in the 1972 Act is replaced by a new Schedule 2 set out in Sch. 5 of the Employment Protection Act 1975.

[5] Section 1 (6), for example, the employer's common law right of dismissal for dishonesty, etc.

[6] Section 1 as amended by Employment Protection Act 1975, Sch. 16.

the employer may give the employee written notice referring the employee to some document which the employee has reasonable opportunities of reading in the course of his employment, or which is made reasonably accessible to him in some other way.[1] Any claim by an employee that his employer has failed to provide written particulars of the terms of employment as required by the Act is to be determined by the Industrial Tribunal.[2]

D. FAIR AND UNFAIR DISMISSAL

1. Generally

The provisions now contained in the 1st Schedule to the Trade Union and Labour Relations Act 1974[3] make very considerable inroads into the traditional individual contract of employment. In particular, the Schedule gives every employee 'the right not to be unfairly dismissed'.[4] A dismissal may be unfair either because of the way in which it takes place ('procedural unfairness') or because of the reasons for the dismissal ('substantive unfairness').

Paragraph 6 of the 1st Schedule to the Trade Union and Labour Relations Act 1974 gives some guidance on the meaning of fair and unfair dismissal. It is for the employer to show the reason for the dismissal and either that it was a specified reason or it was a substantial reason of a kind such as to justify the dismissal.[5] The specified reasons are that it[6]

(a) related to the capability or qualifications of the employee for performing work of the kind which he was employed by the employer to do, or

(b) related to the conduct of the employee, or

(c) was that the employee was redundant, or

(d) was that the employee could not continue to work in the position which he held without contravention (either on his part or on that of his employer) of a duty or restriction imposed by or under an enactment.

Sub-paragraph 8 of para. 6 says that whether a dismissal was fair or unfair shall depend on whether the employer can satisfy the Tribunal

---

[1] Section 3. This obligation to provide written particulars within one month of any change in conditions of employment does not mean that the employer may change the terms unilaterally. There will, however, be the case in which the employee has agreed to work on nationally or locally negotiated terms which may similarly be altered from time to time, this without formal consent of each separate employee.

[2] Section 8.

[3] As amended by the Employment Protection Act 1975, the Sex Discrimination Act 1975 and the Trade Union and Labour Relations (Amendment) Act 1976.

[4] Paragraph 4. By para. 12. The protection does not apply to a contract for a fixed term of two years or more made before 28th February, 1972, or whenever made if the contract excludes the unfair dismissal provisions and the 'dismissal' is solely due to a non-renewal of the contract. See *B.B.C.* v. *Ioannou* [1975] 3 W.L.R. 63; [1975] 2 All E.R. 999; and *R.* v. *Secretary of State ex p. Khan* [1973] 1 W.L.R. 187. (Where the contract was with a doctor for a two year period 'renewable, subject to confirmation, for an indefinite period'.)

[5] Paragraph 6 (1).　　　　　　　　　　　　　[6] Paragraph 6 (2).

that in the circumstances (having regard to equity and the substantial merits of the case) he acted reasonably in treating it as a sufficient reason for dismissing the employee.[1]

Other paragraphs of the Schedule (as amended) make further provision as to the question of whether the dismissal is fair or unfair. Thus membership of, or activities at an appropriate time in, an independent trade union are described as inadmissible reasons for dismissal.

It is however probable that the Act makes no change to the law as regards Health Service employees as regards procedural unfairness since the procedural safeguards in the Act were probably already a part of the contract of employment.

Thus in *Palmer* v. *Inverness Hospitals Board of Management*[2] which was, in effect, a claim by a house officer who had been dismissed for alleged misconduct to have the resolution of the Board sustaining his dismissal by a senior officer set aside on the ground that the principles of natural justice and fair play had not been observed by the Board when considering the appeal in accordance with the procedure laid down in a circular from the Department of Health to Scottish Hospital Authorities in 1953. In that circular the Department had set down the procedure to be followed by hospital employing authorities when representations were made to them on behalf of an employee who was aggrieved by any disciplinary action including dismissal taken or proposed to be taken against him. The circular further provided that the authority should establish an appeals committee to hear each appeal; that the officer should have the right to appear before the committee; and that the report of the committee should be submitted to the Authority for a final decision on the case.

On December 22nd, 1960, the house officer, Dr Palmer, was told by the deputy medical superintendent that, because of incidents in which he had been involved earlier that day regarded as breaches of duty and proper behaviour, it had been decided to dismiss him. He was paid up to December 24th, 1960, and, early on December 25th, 1960, after a series of incidents, he was removed physically from the hospital.

On December 29th, 1961, the house officer submitted to the defenders an appeal against his dismissal.[3] The Board, purporting to act in accordance with the circular, appointed a special committee to hear the appeal and report to them at a special meeting. The committee held an inquiry and heard statements from various witnesses including the house officer and a friend of his who addressed the committee on his

[1] An employer cannot rely on misconduct of which he did not know when he dismissed the employee. But it might be relevant in ascertaining the damages. *Devis and Sons* v. *Atkins* [1977] 3 W.L.R. 214 (H.L.)

[2] [1963] S.L.T. 124. See also *Barber* v. *Manchester R.H.B.* [1958] 1 W.L.R. 181.

[3] It appears that the notice of appeal to the board was, strictly, well out of time but, seemingly, nothing turned on that since the authority did not on that ground refuse recourse to the appeals machinery.

behalf. The medical superintendent was also heard. The committee reported to the special meeting of the board that their unanimous conclusion was that the dismissal was *not* justified. When the report of the committee came before the Board for consideration the chairman allowed to be present the medical superintendent, his deputy, two representatives of the Regional Board and the legal adviser to the Scottish Hospital Service. A resolution that the dismissal of the house officer was justified was carried by the casting vote of the chairman.

The house officer in his action challenged the resolution on the ground that the principles of natural justice and fair play had not been observed by the Board in considering the appeal. The defenders contended that the circular from the Department of Health was advisory and not obligatory. Lord Wheatley, finding in favour of the pursuer, held that the circular was obligatory and was incorporated in the pursuer's contract of service; that in considering the report of the special committee the Board were acting in a quasi-judicial capacity as the appeals procedure desiderated in the circular was a *unum quid*; that in permitting two senior officers who were involved in the pursuer's dismissal and the legal adviser to the Scottish Hospital Service to be present in the absence of the pursuer or his representative the Board transgressed the basic principles of natural justice, equity and fair play. There is no reason to believe that a different decision would have been reached by an English court on a case concerning the conduct of an appeal under the Ministry of Health circulars.[1]

Of course, any similar cases of procedural unfairness or breach of contract would now come within the jurisdiction of the Industrial Tribunals and not the ordinary courts. A full discussion of the meaning of unfair dismissal under para. 6 of the 1st Schedule to the 1974 Act and the view the Tribunals have taken is outside the scope of this book. It is, however, interesting to note that the Tribunal has upheld a dismissal of a ward sister (after due warnings had been given) for her failure to wear the prescribed uniform, and although in all other respects her work was exemplary.[2]

It is also important to note that a dismissal may be constructive,[3] *i.e.* the conditions of the engagement may be so altered by the employer that the employee may reasonably treat the contract as terminated. If, for example, the employer were to unilaterally alter the hours or place of work[4] or payment this might amount to a constructive dismissal.

A practical problem that apparently remains unsolved is whether a Health Service employer has the right to suspend an employee.[5] It

---

[1] See R.H.B. (51) 80, H.M.C. (51) 73, B.G. (51) 77, (H.M. (61) 112.
[2] *Atkin* v. *Enfield Group H.M.C.* [1975] I.R.L.R. 217 (C.A.)   [3] 1st Schedule, para. 5.
[4] But note that collectively agreed procedures for the loan by one health authority of its officers to another are valid. See 1977 Act 5th Schedule, para. 11.
[5] For a reason other than very special medical grounds as to which now see ss. 29–33 and Sch. 2 of the Employment Protection Act 1975.

seems that suspension with pay, even though not expressly provided for in the agreement or in rules accepted by the officer is probably justified in law and is usually not likely to lead to any difficulty if, in the circumstances, the suspension is reasonable, *e.g.* pending the hearing in court of a charge against the officer, either concerning something criminal alleged to have been done in relation to hospital matters or otherwise being of a nature which, if proved, would be strong evidence of the officer's unfitness for his post.

The sending of an officer off duty, whether by his immediate superior or by some more senior officer, because, for some reason he is unfit for duty, or because he has been guilty of some misconduct, such as insolence or refusal to obey a lawful order, is a particular case of suspension, the validity of which could hardly be open to question, being often the only practicable course to be taken, in the ward situation. On the other hand, the suspension would not be lawful if it were, in all the circumstances, unreasonable. Accordingly in these cases, the suspension might amount to a constructive dismissal and the employee might then be entitled to damages and to an order for reinstatement or re-engagement under s. 71 of the Employment Protection Act 1975.

It is convenient here to note that under s. 34 of the Employment Protection Act 1975 a woman employee is unfairly dismissed if the reason is that she is pregnant or it is connected with her pregnancy.[1] This rule does not apply where, because of her pregnancy, she is or will have become incapable of adequately doing the work which she is employed to do or that she will not be able to do it without contravening a duty or restriction on her or her employer imposed by any statute. However, even this exception does not apply where there is a suitable alternative job for her under the same employer and he does not offer it to her. The question of maternity leave is discussed later in this chapter.[2] Where the dismissal (or the refusal of leave) contravenes the statute, there are rights of re-instatement in the discretion of the industrial tribunal.[3] It is also important to note that where the dismissal is fair within the meaning of s. 34 the woman may give notice that she intends to exercise her rights under s. 35 to maternity pay and to return to her job.[4] It is unclear whether this applies where the dismissal is unfair.

2. Remedies

By para. 17 of the 1st Schedule of the 1974 Trade Union and Labour Relations Act where the dismissal is found to be unfair for any reason and the tribunal considers that it would be practicable and in accordance with equity, for the complainant to be reinstated or re-engaged by

[1] Time-off work for a miscarriage is 'a reason connected with pregnancy' *George* v. *Beecham Group* [1977] I.R.L.R. 43.
[2] See p. 434.   [3] Section 71 of the Employment Protection Act 1975.
[4] Section 35 (3). See below, p. 434.

the employer, the tribunal shall make a recommendation or order to that effect, stating the terms on which it considers that it would be reasonable.

Alternatively where the tribunal does not make such a recommendation or order or the recommendation or order is not complied with, the tribunal shall make an award of compensation.

3. Qualifying Period and Upper Age Limit

None of the provisions of the 1st Schedule of the 1974 Act apply to the dismissal of an employee if the employer[1]

(a) was not continuously employed for a period of not less than 26 weeks ending with the effective date of termination, or

(b) on or before the effective date of termination attained the age which, in the undertaking in which he was employed, was the normal retiring age[2] for an employee holding the position which he held, or if a man, attained the age of 65, or, if a woman, attained the age of 60.

These rules do not apply if the reason for the dismissal was one of the inadmissible reasons'[3] (i.e. relating to trade union activities).

E. TERMINATION OF EMPLOYMENT

1. Generally

Subject to what has already been said on the subject of a dismissal being unfair and to the consequences of those remarks on disciplinary matters, an ordinary contract of employment, without more, is ordinarily terminable on reasonable notice, subject always to such notice not being less than that which would be required under the Contracts of Employment Act 1972.[4] If, however, the contract itself specifies the notice necessary for its termination, then — subject to the Contracts of Employment Act — that is the notice required. But, notwithstanding that notice is ordinarily necessary to determine a contract of employment otherwise than one for a fixed time, either party has a right at common law to treat the contract as at an end without notice on any fundamental breach of contract by the other, a right expressly preserved in the Contracts of Employment Act 1972. The most common example of exercise of that right is the summary dismissal of an employee for dishonesty or other serious misconduct.[5]

2. Permanent and Pensionable Employment

Although a general hiring can ordinarily be terminated by proper notice, it is possible for any public authority, other than the Crown,

---

[1] Paragraph 10.

[2] In Ord. v. Maidstone and District H.M.C. [1974] I.C.R. 369 the court considered what was the normal retiring age when the contractual age could vary between 60 and 70.

[3] Paragraph 11.　　　　　[4] See p. 411.　　　　　[5] See p. 420.

just as it is possible for a private employer to make a binding contract for permanent and pensionable employment.[1] Health Authorities, and other bodies established under the National Health Service Acts, being public authorities whose employees are not civil servants, though paid out of public funds,[2] may be bound by a contract with an officer under which he is entitled to permanent and pensionable employment,[3] subject only to his not committing any fundamental breach of the contract before reaching retiring age.

3. Other Employment

Except so far as the period of notice for determining contracts of employment in respect of any grade of staff may have been laid down nationally under the provisions of the National Health Service (Remuneration and Conditions of Service) Regulations 1974, the notice to be given by either party in the national hospital service, is that which had been agreed between them. If no period of notice had been agreed then reasonable notice must be given. The Contracts of Employment Act 1972 does not bind the Crown and therefore the minimum periods of notice there laid down do not apply.

The employer may at common law discharge his obligation to give the proper notice to determine the contract by giving the employee salary or wages in lieu. Moreover, apart from special agreement, a domestic servant who receives board and lodgings as an emolument is not entitled to any compensation in respect of the loss of such emolu, ment if paid off with wages in lieu of notice.[4] It might well be, however, that the old case on which this rests would not apply to domestic service in a hospital or institution where such emoluments as were given were valued for superannuation purposes at an agreed figure. The point is now academic so far as the National Health Service is concerned since domestic staff in the Secretary of State's hospitals now have a fixed cash remuneration from which is deducted an agreed sum for board and

---

[1] *McClelland* v. *Northern Ireland General Health Services Board* ([1957] 1 W.L.R. 594) in which case the House of Lords held that, applications having been invited for appointments expressed to be 'permanent and pensionable' and the terms of conditions of service shown to the officer on appointment having provided for dismissal for gross misconduct or inefficiency or in certain other defined circumstances, the Board could not validly terminate the officer's service otherwise than for one of the reasons stated in the terms and conditions of service. Incidentally, in this case which had been decided by Curran, J., in the Chancery Division of Northern Ireland on the basis that the appellant was a civil servant, it was conceded that she was not a civil servant, so that although the contract of service was on the lines of a civil service contract it was not subject to the paramount right of the Crown to determine it at will. Also, as Lord Goddard pointed out in the House of Lords, although strictly *obiter*, an established civil servant is in practice secure in his employment till he reaches retiring age, apart, of course, from misconduct or complete inefficiency.
[2] In *Pfizer Corporation* v. *Minister of Health* [1965] A.C. 512 it was held that the National Hospital Service was a service of the Crown.
[3] That such a contract would be made, seems highly improbable, and is mentioned as a possibility only because of *McClelland's* case.
[4] *Gordon* v. *Potter* (1859), 1 F. & F. 644.

lodging. Hence the amount of wages in lieu of notice would be the wages before deduction of board and lodging charge.

The old case cited is certainly no authority so far as resident staff other than domestic staff, are concerned, e.g., nurses. Their emoluments in hospitals outside the National Health Service are generally taken into account for superannuation purposes and so it would appear that they are entitled to have them counted for the purpose also of calculating salary in lieu of notice. In the Health Service nurses, like domestic workers and other resident staff, are today entitled to a gross salary from which a board and lodging charge, or a lodging charge, is deducted.[1]

Failing special agreement the case might also be different with an administrative officer, whose emoluments were specifically agreed to include a house or flat and/or meals, e.g., lunch and tea. If it were desired to terminate such an officer's engagement by payment of salary in lieu of notice, it would be advisable, if no value had been fixed for the emoluments in the first place, to reach a compromise figure or, failing compromise, to tender an amount sufficiently generous to avoid his having any reasonable grounds for action. When the emoluments include a house or flat it would usually be the better plan to allow the officer to continue in occupation for the full period of notice if he so desired. Alternatively, if the employer wished him to leave at once a generous offer of compensation for disturbance should be made.

The common law relating to recovery of possession of a house or other accommodation having been so extensively altered by legislation and the topic not being one special to hospitals, no more will be done here than to draw attention to one or two major considerations and to the special position of National Health Service authorities.

When considering what has to be done in order lawfully to recover possession of a house, flat or other accommodation occupied by an officer in connection with his employment and whose lease, licence or contract of service requires him to leave the accommodation on his employment being lawfully terminated and the officer has failed to vacate the premises in accordance with his undertaking, a distinction has to be made between the case of a person provided with board and lodging, who has not a contract for exclusive possession of particular accommodation, and that of a person who has been given the exclusive occupation of a house or flat.

The employer, on dismissing an employee in the first group, the contract being for lodging and not for specific accommodation, e.g., a

---

[1] What is said here and elsewhere about the conditions of service of staff in N.H.S. hospitals will not necessarily apply in toto to a 'transferred officer', i.e. one who before 5th July, 1948, was in the employment of a voluntary or local government hospital authority and was transferred to the service of a N.H.S. authority on that date. Such an officer would have been given certain options in respect of conditions of service. It is also possible that similar options might be given to officers of any hospitals acquired by the Secretary of State after 1948.

nurse or domestic living in a nurses' home or hostel, may ordinarily insist on the person's leaving the premises immediately on the termination of his employment, allowing only reasonable time for that person to pack his belongings, this always provided that the contract of employment has been properly terminated and that what is done is done peaceably. But if the person has been given exclusive possession of a house or flat, *e.g.*, an officer and his family, occupying a house in the hospital grounds or, probably, a matron occupying a flat within the hospital,[1] the employer would be in breach of the law if he ejected him forcibly, otherwise than in accordance with an order of the county court.[2]

So far as hospitals within the National Health Service are concerned, the practical position has been clarified by the issue of Departmental circulars.[3] It has also been agreed that in the case either of a tenancy agreement or a licence the notice to quit to which an officer is to be entitled thereunder shall be not less than the notice required to terminate his appointment. If, in fact, the Department's undertaking were not in any case honoured by a hospital authority and an officer were held to less favourable terms, the remedy would not be in law but by appeal to the Secretary of State in his administrative capacity. The position is similar as regards assurances given for the protection of officers already occupying accommodation on more favourable terms at the date of issue of the circular.

In the case of occupation of Crown property (*e.g.*, hospital property transferred to or acquired by the Secretary of State under the National Health Service Act 1946) under a tenancy agreement, operation of the Rent Act 1977 is also excluded as that Act does not bind the Crown. The Secretary of State has, however, indicated that legal proceedings should not be brought to recover property occupied under licence or lease without the prior approval of the Regional Authority.

Subject to the above reservations, an employer is justified in certain circumstances in dismissing an employee without notice and without salary in lieu of notice. Indeed when circumstances arise which justify this course, the person dismissed is not even entitled to any payment for services rendered since the end of the last regular pay period. However it will be noted that procedural fairness must still be maintained. The particular grounds for dismissal in this way are:

[1] The case of a matron's flat is more obscure because her position is to be distinguished from that of nurses in a nurses' home only so far as she may know at the time of the contract what quarters are to be made available for her. The flat is, ordinarily, provided furnished and meals, attendance and domestic services supplied. It is safer, however, to regard it as in the second category.

[2] See Rent Act 1977. That the Statute of Forcible Entries 1381 remains unrepealed is a further deterrent to self-help. See *Hemmings* v. *Stoke Poges Golf Club Limited* [1920] 1 K.B. 720.

[3] R.H.B. (50) 43 as subsequently modified by R.H.B. (52) 118 and H.M. (54) 2. *See also* H.M. (55) 115 and H.M. (61) 111. As to rents of houses occupied by persons who are not hospital employees, see H.M. (58) 89.

(a) *Wilful disobedience* to a lawful and reasonable order or neglect of duty in a serious matter, or in less serious matters if habitual. Neglect includes forgetfulness.

(b) *Serious misconduct* whether in the course of employment or not, if of a kind likely to be prejudicial to the employer. The following may be cited as examples; (i) dishonesty which, in some circumstances, may not amount to an offence; (ii) insolence or violence, though here there is a question of degree; (iii) receipt of secret commissions.

When misconduct *outside his employment* justifies dismissal of an employee without notice is not always easy to determine. It is, of course, easy to decide that a man who has to handle money in the course of his duties and has been convicted of theft or misappropriation, even outside the scope of his employment, is liable to dismissal without notice. But what of other forms of misconduct? What of the man or woman who is known to have had improper sexual relations either with a fellow employee or with someone else? In the case of a doctor, nurse or other person engaged by virtue of a registerable qualification, presumably any action which would be grounds for erasure from the register would justify dismissal without notice. A man may be dismissed for immorality with a fellow employee, but apart from express agreement it would be difficult to justify similar action in respect of sexual irregularity with outsiders unless (i) the man's suitability for his employment is seriously diminished by his reputation, *e.g.*, a hospital chaplain, or (ii) his reputation is such that it would be seriously harmful to his employer's interests to retain him.

(c) *Incompetency.* If a person is engaged for a post requiring skill — *e.g.*, on the medical, nursing or administrative staff of a hospital — and, in spite of having held himself out as a skilled man, has proved incompetent the Authority is entitled to dismiss him without notice.[1] Even more clear is the right of dismissal if it is found that the employee had falsely laid claim to a particular qualification, *e.g.*, that of state registered nurse or chartered physiotherapist. If a man is engaged for, entrusted with or promoted to work for which he claims no special competence or qualifications then his incompetency is no grounds for immediate dismissal.[1]

(d) *Illness.* Temporary illness is not generally a ground for dismissal without notice. Indeed in *Hardwick* v. *Leeds A.H.A.*[2] a dismissal was held unfair when a night nurse had exhausted her sick pay entitlement of four months and was dismissed. The Health Service booklet on sick pay only laid down normal practice and since the nurse would probably have been able to return to work ten days later it was unreasonable to apply normal practice as a strict rule.

[1] *Harmer* v. *Cornelius* (1858), 5 C.B. (N.S.) 236.
[2] [1975] I. R.L.R. 319

F. STATUTORY COMPENSATION ON REDUNDANCY

The Redundancy Payments Act 1965, which obliges employers to make lump sum payments to staff dismissed by reasons of redundancy if the conditions laid down in the Act are fulfilled, applies to voluntary hospitals as well as to non-charitable hospitals and nursing homes and to similar institutions not in public ownership. It does not, however, apply to hospital authorities within the National Health Service or to special hospitals[1] administered by the Secretary of State for Social Services, nor to Crown services generally.[2]

The exclusion of hospital authorities was subject to the Government's undertaking to provide a separate and no less favourable scheme. The scheme adopted is to be found in an agreement of the General Council of the Whitley Councils for the Health Services,[3] approved under the N.H.S. (Remuneration and Conditions of Service) Regulations.

Although employees in the National Health Service are entitled to any redundancy payment by virtue of the agreement and not of the Redundancy Payments Act 1965, the conjoint effect of para. 12 of the circular embodying the agreement and of s. 42 of the Act is to give a right in the nature of a right of appeal to an Industrial Tribunal to review by way of rehearing the decision of the employing authority; and to confer on the Tribunal a corresponding jurisdiction. The right to apply does not, however, arise unless and until a decision has been made by the employing authority and the prescribed procedures under the agreement strictly followed.[4]

It may also be noted that under s. 61 of the Employment Protection Act 1975 where an employee is given notice of dismissal by reason of redundancy he may be entitled to reasonable time-off work and to be paid at the appropriate hourly rate[5] in order to look for new employment or make arrangements for training for future employment. The only major restriction on this right is that the employee must have been continuously employed for a period of two years or more.[6] It is also important to note that s. 99 of the Employment Protection Act 1975 (which relates to consultation on redundancy) does not apply within the Health Service.[7]

[1] For definition of *special hospital*, see National Health Service Act 1977. By s. 13A (added by the Employment Protection Act 1975, s. 120) the Act does apply to persons transferred from in effect the private to the public sector. It therefore applies to those staff transferred from local authorities to the Health Service. The effect of this is that rights acquired by them under the 1965 Act are maintained by virtue of the amendment to that Act.

[2] Redundancy Payments Act 1965, s. 16 (4) and Schedule 3.

[3] G.C. Hbk. XXV, see also H.M. (68) 4.

[4] *Pearce (Applicant)* v. *Epsom Group H.M.C.* [1967] I.T.R. 328. In this case the Tribunal also expressed the opinion that the reference to the Tribunal if the employee were dissatisfied had to be made by the employing authority.

[5] Defined in s. 61 (4).   [6] Section 61 (2).

[7] S. 121 (1) and (5). Of course, consultation other than under the section, is allowed.

G. MACHINERY FOR SETTLING DISPUTES

1. Remuneration and Conditions of Employment

Within the limits indicated on pages 398–404, disputes regarding the appropriate rates of pay, grading *etc.*, of individual officers or classes of officers employed by any N.H.S. Authority may be dealt with by way of appeal through machinery established by agreement of the General Council of the Whitley Councils for the Health Services (Great Britain), which provides for regional appeals committees composed of equal numbers appointed by the management and staff sides of the appropriate Whitley Council. Such appeals, however, cannot be taken to a regional appeals committee by the aggrieved officer himself but only by a *nationally recognised negotiating body*[1] on his behalf. The expression *nationally recognised negotiating body* here means those trade unions and professional societies having representation on any of the N.H.S. Whitley Councils and, in special circumstances, a trade union not represented on any N.H.S. Whitley Council but participating in other national negotiating machinery through which the pay and conditions of workers in the relevant grade are settled. Consequently, recourse cannot be had to the appeals machinery by an officer who is not in membership of a trade union or professional society within the above definition, nor by one whose organisation is unwilling to back his claim. Hence the appeals machinery is not a complete alternative to the courts for the enforcement of any legally enforceable claim an officer might have, though, on the other hand, recourse to that machinery may be had, through a trade union or professional society, in respect of matters probably not within the jurisdiction of the courts, *e.g.* certain grading appeals.[2]

If a regional appeals committee is equally divided on a claim and records disagreement, the trade union or professional society sponsoring that appeal may take it to a similarly appointed national appeals committee. If disagreement be recorded there also, the claim on behalf of the officer must fail unless either the parties to the dispute agree to arbitration or it is one enforceable by the courts, or the Secretary of State can be prevailed upon to intervene. That is so because, despite an

---

[1] See pp. 392–393 above for a discussion of the reference to ACAS of a recognition issue under s. 11 of the Employment Protection Act 1975.

[2] Examples of claims which could, and probably would, go to the Courts and not to a Whitley appeal committee, should the employing authority refuse to meet its obligation under the officer's conditions of employment — which include conditions embodied in relevant Whitley agreements approved by the Minister — are failure to pay the salary proper to the officer's grade and seniority; or failure to count paid sick leave due to injury caused by a crime of violence as separate from ordinary sick leave entitlement when mandatory on the employing authority to do so. On the other hand, it seems that an appeal by an officer against his grading, *i.e.* a claim that, having regard to the work he is doing or the responsibilities he has been given, he ought to be in a higher grade and paid accordingly, can be dealt with only through the Whitley machinery, with all its limitations.

agreement in 1948 that arbitration machinery should be established, the two sides of the General Council of the Whitley Councils for the Health Services (Great Britain) have still not been able to reach agreement either on the nature of the arbitration tribunal or on the conditions of reference to it.

That being the position, where there is failure to agree, either in negotiations in a N.H.S. Whitley council or in a national appeals committee, the matter is sometimes referred to the ACAS; but this can be done only if, in the case of disagreement in a Whitley Council, both sides agree to the reference or, in the case of failure of a national appeals committee to reach a decision, both parties to the dispute agree to such reference. If, in the latter case, reference to the ACAS is not agreed, the aggrieved officer is without remedy, save where there are grounds for the claim that there has been a breach of contract or a failure of the employing Authority to observe terms and conditions of service binding under the provisions of the N.H.S. (Remuneration and Conditions of Service) Regulations 1974, when the officer could have recourse to the courts. Indeed, in such case he could have had sought to enforce his rights through the courts without first having had recourse to the Whitley disputes machinery.

What has never been tested in the courts is the effect of a decision of a regional or national appeals committee that an officer is entitled to be upgraded, because of the nature of his duties. One view is that, recourse having been had to the appeals machinery in accordance with the Whitley agreement, the decision of the appeals committee is binding on both parties and could be enforced by the court; the other is that the decision is advisory only and not binding on the respondent Health Authority unless accepted by that Authority or unless it is directed by the Secretary of State. It would only be if on some occasion the Secretary of State refused to see that effect was given to the decision of an appeals committee that this question could become of more than academic interest.

2. Disciplinary Matters

The Whitley Council appeals procedure outlined above does not extend to disputes regarding dismissal on disciplinary grounds or other disciplinary proceedings. The Secretary of State has, however, in a circular[1] instructed hospital authorities, pending the conclusion of a Whitley agreement on the subject, to take steps to ensure that their practice in dealing with disciplinary cases is governed by the principles and procedures set out in the memorandum (*i.e.*, the memorandum accompanying the circular). Broadly the memorandum indicates that there should be a right of appeal by an officer aggrieved by a serious

[1] R.H.B. (51) 80. See below, pp. 736–739.

Q

disciplinary decision to 'the employing authority whose function it is to appoint and dismiss employees of the grade in question', when he may appear personally or with a representative of his professional organisation or trade union or with a friend not appearing in a professional capacity. Although the memorandum does not confer on an aggrieved officer any right of appeal beyond his immediate employing authority, the Regional Authority or the Secretary of State may, none the less, entertain an appeal from the decision of a lower authority, but this is entirely discretionary. An aggrieved officer was thought to have no legal right even to the limited protection given in the Secretary of State's memorandum since the memorandum, with its covering circular, were not issued under the provisions of the N.H.S. (Remuneration and Conditions of Service) Regulations 1974. But if, in any way, it could be established that the terms of the Departmental memorandum were to be read into the officer's contract of employment, he would have a cause of action if, in the event, the procedure laid down were not observed. That is just what happened in *Palmer's* case.[1] Apart from any protection the court might afford in a particular case, the effective sanction for ensuring that the procedure laid down in the memorandum is carried out is the Secretary of State's power to intervene by way of direction if his agents fail to act in conformity with his wishes and he is satisfied that an injustice has been done. If, however, a Whitley agreement on the subject of disciplinary appeals were concluded and approved by the Secretary of State the terms of the agreement would become legally enforceable in respect of all officers to whom it applied.

If an employee or ex-employee remains aggrieved after hearing by the appeals committee set up by the immediate employing authority, he or his trade union or professional society may make representations to the Regional Authority or to the Secretary of State, as appropriate, and either Authority has discretion to give a direction[2] in respect of any act or omission by an Area Health Authority.

Another circular, H.M. (61) 112[3] set out the procedure for dealing with disciplinary appeals relating to professional conduct of medical and dental practitioners.

For remedies available to an officer entitled to compensation for loss of employment or diminution of emoluments by reason of redundancy or re-organisation see the previous section.

H. THE TRUCK ACTS

1. The Truck Acts 1831–1896

The general purpose and effect of the Truck Acts is — subject to

---

[1] [1963] S.L.T. 124.   [2] R.H.B. (51) 80. For text, see pp. 736–739.
[3] See also pp. 401 and 413–414 where *Palmer's* and *Barber's* cases are discussed.

certain statutory exceptions — to oblige employers to pay workmen[1] their wages in full in legal tender money, this subject to certain statutory exceptions. So far as the National Hospital Service is concerned, it is reasonable to assume *prima facie* that any grades of staff, other than domestic staff, within the purview of the Ancillary Staffs Whitley Council fall within the Truck Acts and that staff within the purview of the other N.H.S. Whitley Councils do not, and to act accordingly, even though, in fact, a few types of staff within the purview of the Ancillary Staffs Council would almost certainly be regarded by the courts as technical or supervisory and so not within the protection of the Truck Acts.[2]

Nurses, physiotherapists and the like are not within the Acts even though, in the course of their duties, they may much of the time be performing tasks requiring the exercise of bodily strength as well as skill. A hospital engineer, in the sense in which the expression is now used in the national hospital service, *i.e.* a professionally qualified engineer in charge of the engineering services of a hospital or group of hospitals, or one of his qualified deputies or assistants[3] is also outside the provisions of the Truck Acts, this notwithstanding the decision in *Cameron* v. *Royal London Ophthalmic Hospital*[4] which, on the face of it, was that a hospital engineer was within the Acts. But in that case the plaintiff, who was successful in recovering from his former employers the amount of deductions made for food *etc.*, supplied to him, as being deductions made contrary to the provisions of the Truck Acts, was a working engineer-stoker who looked after the boilers used for central heating *etc.*, and was presumably capable of undertaking only those maintenance jobs which such a craftsman could reasonably have been expected to tackle.

Although, subject to the agreement in writing of the workman, it is permissible under s. 23 of the Truck Act 1831 to deduct an amount not exceeding the real and true value of meals *etc.*, supplied on the employer's premises, it is illegal to make any deductions from a workman's wages

---

[1] The expression *workmen* here means all persons, other than domestic staff, who are engaged in manual labour.

[2] Although the kinds of staff within a hospital who would be subject to the provisions of the Truck Act is here discussed against the background of the staffing of hospitals within the national hospital service, what is said applies to other hospitals. Moreover, it has to be remembered that since the decision in *Pfizer Corporation* v. *Ministry of Health* it may be that the Acts do not apply to that service, though that question is largely academic as, ever since the inception of the service in 1948, it has been official policy that all such things as board and lodging provided for staff of all grades otherwise than for cash payment should be paid for by way of nationally agreed deductions from gross pay. Hence, all that would be necessary to comply with the Acts would be the acceptance in writing by a workman of the nationally agreed conditions relating to his grade, which is understood to be customary.

[3] Other members of the engineering staff of a hospital might also be outside the Truck Acts, this depending on whether or not the court, looking at all the circumstances, would regard them as primarily manual workers.

[4] [1940] 57 T.L.R. 105.

in respect of purchases made from a shop kept by the employer,[1] whilst s. 6 of that Act makes it unsafe for an employer to sell goods to his workmen otherwise than for cash. Hence, if a Health Authority itself ran a hospital shop, it would be safer not to allow credit to any employee within the Truck Acts.

Section 4 of the Truck Act 1887 expressly legalises, in the case of a servant in husbandry, the provision of food, drink (other than intoxicants), a cottage or other allowance or privilege in addition to money wages as remuneration for his services, whilst the Truck Act 1896 makes strict provision as to deductions from a workman's wages by way of fines on account of misconduct, bad workmanship *etc.*

2. Payment of Wages Act 1960

The Payment of Wages Act 1960, authorises payment of wages of an employee within the Truck Acts by cheque, money order or postal order or to his credit in a bank account in the name of the employee or in an account in his name jointly with another or others in the circumstances there set out and subject to strict compliance with the terms of the Act.

I. SUPERANNUATION

Section 10 of the Superannuation Act 1972 authorises the Secretary of State to make regulations providing a pensions scheme for those employed in the National Health Service and for certain others closely concerned with it. The Regulations were made under s. 67 of the National Health Service Act, 1946 and they continue in force. They are the Superannuation Regulations 1961[2] as amended by S.I.s 1966 No. 1523; 1972 No. 1339 and No. 1537; 1973 No. 242, 731 and 1649; 1974 No. 223 and No. 1047.

Subject to certain limitations it can be broadly said that all officers in the National Health Service are superannuable under the 1961 Regulations as are some others closely concerned therewith, including family doctors providing services under the N.H.S. and employees of some other bodies closely concerned therewith. The scheme is contributory. The provisions are too detailed and complex to be set out here.

J. STAFF TRANSFERS

On the reorganisation of the Health Service on April 1st, 1974, new Authorities were created, old ones abolished and the staff of some

---

[1] If the shop, although on hospital premises, had been let to a tenant who conducted the business for his own profit, or it were run, say, by British Red Cross workers or by members of the local league of hospital friends, not acting as agents of the health authority, the provisions of the Truck Act 1831 as to the giving of credit would be irrelevant.

[2] S.I. 1961 No. 1441.

Authorities were transferred (principally from Local Government to the Health Service). All of this necessitated a fairly complex scheme for the transfer and in some cases the retirement of staff. However, since most of the effect of the scheme will have been in operation for some years before this edition of this book is published, it is not set out here. For those still needing its details, reference may be made to the Re-organisation Act 1973, ss. 18–20 and the Regulations.[1]

K. LOSS OF OR DAMAGE TO STAFF PROPERTY

To the general rule that employers are not ordinarily liable for loss of or damage to property belonging to an employee, even when the employee is in resident quarters,[2] Health Authorities are no exception. Moreover, on the authority of *Edwards* v. *West Herts. Group Hospital Management Committee*[3] it has to be accepted that the employer's freedom from liability extends to the property of a resident officer paying for board and lodging provided by an agreed deduction from his remuneration.

In *Edward's* case the Court of Appeal held that the defendant Hospital Authority owed no duty to the plaintiff, a resident house-physician, in respect of the theft of his goods whilst he was occupying hostel accommodation in accordance with the terms of his contract. The plaintiff had claimed that the Hospital Authority owed him a duty to take reasonable care of his bedroom, clothes and personal effects and of the keys of the door and that that was an implied term of his contract. Hodson, L.J., said that the duty of an employer towards his employees was free from authority, in the sense that there was no case decided on that express ground. Du Parq, L.J., had said in *Deyong* v. *Shenburn* that there had never been a decision that an employer must, merely because of the employment relationship, take reasonable care for the employee's belongings in the sense that he must take steps to ensure, so far as he could, that no wicked person should have an opportunity of stealing the employee's goods; nor any Authority for the existence at any time of any such duty. The county court judge had held that that language applied directly to the case and he, Hodson, L.J., agreed with him and that its application was not confined to what were called domestic servants. The only way in which the plaintiff could have succeeded would have been if he could have shown that there must be a term implied in the contract of employment that the employer should take

---

[1] The N.H.S. Reorganisation (Retirement of Senior Officers) Regs. S.I. 1974 No. 139; the N.H.S. (Staff Transfer Scheme) Order S.I. 1974 No. 35; the N.H.S. (Staff Transfer Appeals and Schemes Order Amendment) Order S.I. 1974 No. 378; the N.H.S. (Transfer of Social Services Staff) Order S.I. 1974 No. 318; and the N.H.S. (Transferred Social Services Staff — Appeals) Order S.I. 1975 No. 1765. *See also* N.H.S. (Compensation) Regs. S.I. 1971 No. 52 considered in *Showell* v. *D.H.S.S.* [1976] I.C.R. 76.

[2] *Deyong* v. *Shenburn* [1946] K.B. 227. [3] [1957] 1 W.L.R. 415.

such care of his employee's goods so as to enable him to have a chance of avoiding such a calamity as had occurred. There was no room on the facts of the case for such an implication.

The decision in *Edward's* case was not surprising, since any other decision would have gone some way towards making employing Authorities insurers of the property of their resident staff, at least unless all liability were expressly disclaimed by the terms of the agreement made.

Hodson, L.J., in *Edward's* case distinguished the position of the plaintiff from that of the guest of a boarding-house keeper, because, on the authorities, there was a duty to take *some* care of the goods of his guests on a boarding-house keeper.[1] Although there had been an agreed deduction at the rate of £125 per annum from the doctor's remuneration in payment for board and lodging in a staff flat outside the main building his lordship held that the doctor was nevertheless in the same position as if in residence in the hospital building itself and getting his food and lodgings free. He said that the doctor did not make separate payment for the board and lodging provided. The money was deducted from his pay each month and he received the net sum in the same way that a domestic servant who lived in was given her net pay.

With respect, Hodson, L.J.'s argument is difficult to follow. Is the position not rather that it is a term of the contract of employment in such a case — indeed in practically all cases of resident staff in the hospital service — that the employee undertakes to take and pay for certain accommodation and board as a condition of employment? The employer could have made the other type of contract, *viz.*, for salary or wages plus emoluments, instead of for salary with an agreed payment for board and lodging which the employee agreed should be deducted from the salary payable, but had not chosen to do so. Had the first alternative been adopted the relationship would have been merely of employment and nothing more but if, as was the case, the second alternative were chosen, it would appear arguable that there were two distinct parts to the agreement, (i) for service by the doctor for which the consideration was the agreed salary; and (ii) for board and lodging against payment.[2] Nor is that a fanciful distinction between the two types of contract but one which has for many years been made for the purposes of the Acts relating to income tax. If a contract provided for wages plus free board and lodging income tax was not usually payable on the value of the board and lodging provided.[3] If, however, the board

[1] See *Dansey* v. *Richardson* ((1854) 3 E. & B. 144) as to the standard of care required of a boarding-house keeper.

[2] There is also the case of the officer who is not obliged to live in staff quarters and to have board and lodging provided, but who is allowed to live in such quarters and is provided with board, he having agreed to pay the appropriate amount, therefor, and to have it deducted from his salary.

[3] That in recent times emoluments do not always escape the tax net is irrelevant to the present discussion, no attempt being made to give an exact statement of the tax position.

and lodging were provided at an agreed charge, then income tax was payable even though the employee never received more than the net wages after deduction of the board and lodging charge.

Despite such inconsistencies, *Edward's* case must be accepted as binding. But if, as sometimes happens, an employing authority accepted for safe-custody, money, valuables, or other goods belonging to the employee, and such property were lost, stolen, destroyed or damaged, through the negligence of a member of the hospital staff, the employing Authority would be liable unless liability had been disclaimed.[1] But the mere fact that drawers that lock are not provided, however desirable that might be, or that a resident member of the staff cannot lock the door of his room, would not alone make the Authority liable. There might, of course, be special circumstances in which the employer might be liable for damage to the employee's property, *e.g.*, damage to clothes he was wearing or to articles he reasonably had on his person in an accident which renders the employer liable at common law or by statute for injury to the employee. Section 1 (3) of the Occupiers' Liability Act 1957,[2] may also be relevant.

L. LETTERS TO MEMBERS OF STAFF

The question of the opening of letters addressed to members of the staff at the hospital is one of some difficulty. Apart from the provisions of the Post Office Act 1969, the opening of a personal letter addressed to a member of the staff would, *prima facie*, constitute a trespass to goods. There are, however, manifest exceptions. First the strict limits of the offence created by the Post Office Act must be appreciated. The opening or impeding of a letter is an offence only if it is done 'with intent to injure the person to whom the letter is addressed'. If there is no intention to injure no offence is committed. Hence, if a letter were addressed to a nursing sister at the hospital with her ward given as part of the address, there would, in my opinion, be no offence committed if, as might happen, she being absent on holiday or other leave, the letter were opened by a chief nursing officer or some other responsible person on the grounds that letters on official business are very frequently addressed to sisters and other officers by name. An example of such a letter would be an enquiry by a patient who had been discharged about property believed to have been left behind at the hospital or about a medical certificate. If a letter addressed to an officer were opened in such circumstances, even though the letter turned out to be a purely private and personal communication no offence would have been committed since there would have been no intent to injure. Nor would it appear

[1] Further as to the position of a hospital as bailee, see pp. 296–297. The same principles apply whether the bailor is a patient or a member of the staff.
[2] See p. 275 *et seq.*

that a civil action for damages, even if it could be successful, would, if the letter were treated with due discretion, give rise to more than nominal damages.

The mention in the above paragraph of the addressing of letters on official business to officers by name brings us to a case in which it is even clearer. Neither the employer nor any officer who in the course of his duties had opened a letter addressed to another member of the staff would be liable to prosecution or liable in damages *viz.*, where there is a clear rule which is known or ought to be known to all members of the staff that all letters addressed to individual officers at the hospital *may* be treated as official letters and, therefore, opened by some other officer. Nor is it unreasonable that non-resident members of the staff who choose to have letters addressed to them at the hospital should be at risk of personal letters addressed to them at the hospital being opened. But what of resident staff? It is unreasonable that their personal correspondence should be at risk of being opened in the hospital, otherwise than by accident. If there were a rule of the kind above-mentioned the point could be met by expressly excepting from it correspondence addressed to officers living in staff quarters. If a nurse lives in the hospital nurses' home then it should be arranged that 'Nurses' Home' should be included in the address. If the member of the staff is living in quarters which are actually part of the hospital, the problem can be got over by the use in the address of *e.g.*, 'Medical Staff Quarters' or 'Domestic Staff Quarters' as the case may be. Even the Chief Nursing Officer's own private correspondence can be addressed to her by name at 'the Chief Nursing Officer's Flat', or otherwise as appropriate.

Except as above indicated there is no justification for any senior officer opening or detaining personal correspondence addressed to a member of the staff, even a student nurse. That might indeed result in litigation.

M. STAFF REPORTS

Reports on staff, whether routine reports, like ward sisters' reports on the progress of student nurses, or special reports, *e.g.*, by a departmental head who is dissatisfied with the work or conduct of one of his staff or who may have been asked to advise on the respective merits of persons being considered for promotion are subject of qualified privilege for the purposes of the law of defamation. Consequently, provided such a report is made in the course of duty and on proper occasion, provided too that care is taken not to publish defamatory matter more widely than is necessary, and that the maker of the report is not actuated by malice, *i.e.*, any improper motive, he will not be liable for libel or slander should anything in the report be false and defamatory. Should the recipient of such a privileged report containing false defamatory statements allow it to be published to any person other than one having an interest or duty to receive the report, he — and not the original maker — may be liable.[1]

N. TESTIMONIALS AND REFERENCES

An employer is under no obligation, apart from express contract, to give an employee a testimonial on leaving his employment, nor can he be compelled to answer inquiries about the character or competency of an employee or ex-employee. Any testimonial which is given, and the answer to any inquiry should be honest and fair. A wilfully false testimonial may render the giver liable to damages in an action for defamation. If a false statement is made in a testimonial or reference through carelessness and the person commented on is thereby employed, it is possible that damages might be obtained from the maker of the statement or his employing authority on the basis of *Hedley Byrne & Co. Ltd.* v. *Heller & Partners Ltd.*[2] applying *Donoghue* v. *Stevenson.*[3]

A reference or testimonial[4] is subject of qualified privilege. Consequently, if what is said is said honestly and without malice on a proper occasion, care being taken to communicate the defamatory matter to no more persons than is reasonably necessary, the person making the defamatory statement, even though that statement is false, will not be liable in an action for defamation.

What is a proper occasion? Generally, for the maker of a false defamatory statement, as in a reference, to be able to shelter behind qualified privilege, there must have been a moral, social or legal obligation for his making the statement and the recipient must have had an interest in receiving it. This duty and interest is recognised where a prospective employer refers to the prospective employee's present or past employer for an opinion about him. If no such reference had been made but an opinion were volunteered it would usually be much more difficult to substantiate a claim to privilege. However, if both the employer, or former employer, giving the opinion and the prospective employer receiving it were authorities within the National Health Service it seemed to Dr Speller justifiable and indeed entirely proper for the former to volunteer information or an opinion to the latter with the object of safeguarding the efficiency of the service or of preventing

---

[1] Where the report is dictated to a secretary, that too may in effect be privileged. *Bryanston Finance Co. Ltd.* v. *de Vries* [1975] 2 All E.R. 609.
[2] [1964] A.C. 465.   [3] [1932] A.C. 562.
[4] No distinction is here made between testimonials and references because even testimonials are usually communicated to third persons, such as typists, so that even the giver of a testimonial may, on occasion, have to fall back on the defence of qualified privilege. Also, it is not necessary to our present purpose to distinguish libel and slander since even slander in respect of a person's suitability for his office or calling is actionable without proof of special damage.

possible loss of public moneys. The basis of this view is that all such Authorities are agents of the Secretary of State for the management and administration of the health service so that there is sufficient community of interest and duty to justify one such Authority, acting through an appropriate officer in the course of his duties, communicating unasked, with another such Authority or with its appropriate officer concerning the suitability of an employee or ex-employee for a particular post or for employment generally. Whilst the present editor agrees with this view, it is not, to him, quite so obvious.

Another case when it would seem that — even though the statement were volunteered — the employing, or former employing, Authority might claim qualified privilege for a defamatory statement about a person, is when the statement is made in the circumstances referred to in a memorandum from the Department to Hospital Authorities[1] reading as follows:

In order that the statutory bodies responsible for professional discipline may be aware of convictions in the courts leading to dismissal or resignation of members of the professions concerned, the Minister asks that in every case the hospital authority should send a factual report of the charge and sentence to the disciplinary body. A list of the principal disciplinary bodies is appended.[2] A hospital authority is, of course, still free to report to the appropriate body the facts of any other dismissal or resignation where, in the authority's view, these facts should be made known to the body, even though there has been no conviction in the courts. It is for the professional body concerned to decide what action, if any, to take on a report.

O. THE SHOPS ACTS[3]

It is not practicable here to include even a summary of the Shops Acts but it must be remembered that any part of a hospital premises where a retail trade or business is carried on is subject to these Acts and that persons working in the *shop* can be employed only under the conditions as to hours, holidays, *etc.*, laid down in the Acts. There could in theory be a conflict between the provisions of these Acts and of regulations made by the Secretary of State for Social Services under paras. 10 and 11 of the 5th Schedule of the National Health Service Act 1977, but, in practice, such conflict is unlikely. It is very doubtful whether these paragraphs would be interpreted as giving the Secretary of State power to over-ride the provisions of the Shops Acts and,

---

[1] H.M. (61) 37.

[2] The list, not here reproduced, gives the addresses of the registration authorities for medical practitioners; dentists and enrolled dental hygienists; midwives and pupil midwives; registered and enrolled nurses and student and pupil nurses; pharmacists and opticians. Statutory disciplinary machinery has also been set up by the several boards under the umbrella of the Council for the Professions Supplementary to Medicine. What is said in H.M. (61) 37 now therefore also applies to persons on any registers kept under the provisions of the Professions Supplementary to Medicine Act 1960.

[3] See also pp. 444–446 as to the Offices, Shops and Railway Premises Act 1963.

certainly, no regulation he made would be read in that sense unless it were impossible reasonably to interpret it otherwise.

There is also the question to what extent a Health Service Authority is itself entitled to carry on retail trade. It would seem that it is entitled to do so only to the extent reasonably necessary for its main purpose. Hence, it may properly provide a canteen for light refreshments for out-patients. But whether it could lawfully carry on a shop for sale of a wide range of commodities for the convenience of patients, staff and visitors, *e.g.*, for sale of stationery, books, periodicals, confectionery and tobacco and cigarettes, is more doubtful. Usually such shops on hospital premises are carried on either by some trading concern in premises for which rent is paid to the Health Authority, or by a voluntary organisation.

P. TIME OFF WORK

Probably no practical change has been made in this field because the statute has broadly placed what used to be good employment practice on a statutory footing. Briefly, s. 57 of the Employment Protection Act 1975 requires an employer to permit an employee of his who is an official of an independent trade union a reasonable amount of time off[1] during working hours to enable him to carry out his duties or to undergo relevant training in industrial relations with the employer. The employee is to be paid during this time off.[2] By s. 58 of the Act, any employee who is a member of an appropriate trade union[3] is entitled to reasonable time off[4] work but without pay for trade union activities that do not constitute industrial action.

Under s. 59 the employer must permit an employee to take reasonable time off work for specified public duties. The duties include those of a justice of the peace, a member of a local authority, or any statutory tribunal or the managing or governing body of an educational establishment maintained by a local authority or a water authority. Of particular interest in the field of hospital law the duties also include those of the members of a Regional or Area Health Authority but apparently not at the moment those of the members of a special Health Authority or the Board of Governors of a preserved Board. The Secretary of State for Employment has power by order to add to or subtract from this list of offices and bodies.[5]

Q. MATERNITY

The provisions relating to dismissal because a woman employee is pregnant or for some other reasons connected with the pregnancy under

---

[1] ACAS is to issue a Code of Practice under the section.   [2] Section 57 (4).
[3] Defined in s. 58 (2).   [4] Again ACAS is to issue a Code of Practice.   [5] Section 59 (5).

s. 34 of the Employment Protection Act 1975 has already been noted.[1] Section 35 and subsequent sections make provision for maternity leave. She must have been employed for not less than two years and she must give the required notice in writing to her employer.[2] The leave may commence at the beginning of the 11th week before the expected date of confinement. During the leave she is entitled to six weeks maternity pay[3] calculated in accordance with the Act.[4] (The pay generally is recoverable by the employer from the Maternity Pay Fund.) Where the employee's notice has specified an intention to return to work, she is entitled to exercise the right granted by s. 35 within 29 weeks beginning with the week in which the date of confinement falls.[5] On returning to work she is entitled to be employed on terms and conditions not less favourable than if she had not been absent and this includes seniority, pension rights and other similar rights.

Of course an employer may engage a replacement for an employee who exercises these rights. If, however, the employer gives notice to the replacement employee that she (or he) is a replacement, then the second employee may be fairly dismissed[6] when the first employee returns to work.

R. SEX DISCRIMINATION

The Sex Discrimination Act 1975 has outlawed discrimination against women (and also generally[7] against men) on the grounds of sex. The Act applies to a wider field than merely employment. Discrimination is defined in s. 1 as treating on the grounds of sex a person less favourably than another of a different sex or applying a discriminatory condition. Part II of the Act deals with discrimination in the employment field. By s. 3 discrimination in this field on the grounds of marital status is also outlawed. Section 6 (1) outlaws discrimination on the grounds of who shall be offered employment or the terms of the employment. Section 6 (2) provides for equality in the provision by an employer of the opportunities for promotion, transfer or training or to any other benefits, facilities or services so long as they are concerned with the employment.[8] Despite this, discrimination is lawful where being a man is 'a genuine occupational qualification' for a job and one of the following grounds applies:[9] its essential nature calls for a man for reasons of physiology (excluding physical strength or stamina);[10] or it needs to be held by a man to preserve decency or privacy;[11] or the nature

---

[1] See above, p. 415.   [2] Section 35 (3).   [3] Section 36.   [4] Section 37.
[5] Section 48. Section 49 makes provision for the way in which the right shall be exeercisd.
[6] Within the meaning of para. 6 (1) (b) of Sch. 1 to the 1974 Trade Union and Labour Relations Act.
[7] Section 2. But the compromise relating to midwives have already been described on p. 389.
[8] Section 6 (7).   [9] Section 7 (1) and (2).   [10] Section 7 (2) (a).   [11] Section 7 (2) (b).

or location of the establishment makes it impractical for the holder of the job to live elsewhere than in premises provided by the employer and the only such premises are not equipped with separate sleeping accommodation for women or sanitary facilities (and it would not be reasonable to provide them);[1] or the nature of the establishment requires the job to be held by a man because it is, or is part of, a hospital, prison or other establishment for persons requiring special care, supervision or attention and those persons are all men and it is reasonable that the job should not be held by a woman;[2] or the job involves the provision for individuals with personal services promoting their welfare or education or similar personal service and those services can most effectively be provided by a man;[3] or the job needs to be held by a man because of restrictions imposed by the laws regulating the employment of women;[4] or the job is one of two to be held by a married couple.[5]

The provisions of the Act are applied to contract workers as regards discrimination by the principal[6] and to employment agencies,[7] to those bodies which provide authorisation or qualification for a particular profession or trade,[8] to vocational training bodies,[9] and to all educational establishments including universities (and accordingly their medical schools)[10] as regards both their employment and admissions policies.

The 1975 Act compliments the Equal Pay Act 1970 which broadly requires that there shall be equal pay for comparable work.

Although not strictly within the confines of this chapter, it is convenient to note that although s. 29 of the Act generally prohibits discrimination on the grounds of sex in the provision of goods, facilities or services and it expressly includes the provision of the services of any profession, s. 35 (1) (a) says that the section is not to apply to the provision of facilities or services at a hospital or other establishment for persons requiring special care, supervision or attention. This means that hospitals and similar institutions for one sex only are still lawful.

The Act clarifies a number of other points, for example it is an unlawful discriminatory practice to publish an advertisement for an act which would be unlawful under Parts II or III and it is made clear that a job description with a sexual connotation shall be taken to indicate an intention to discriminate unless the advertisement contains an indication to the contrary.[11] It is also made clear that sexual discrimination clauses in charitable instruments remain valid.[12]

---

[1] Section 7 (2) (c).   [2] Section 7 (2) (d).   [3] Section 7 (2) (e).
[4] Section 7 (2) (f).   [5] Section 7 (2) (h).   [6] Section 9.
[7] Section 15 defined in s. 82 (1).   [8] Section 13.   [9] Section 14.
[10] Section 22.   [11] Section 38 (3).
[12] Section 43. Now amended by the Sex Discrimination Act 1975 (Amendment of Section 43) Order S.I. 1977 No. 528. The order substitute new subs. (3) and (4).

CHAPTER 23

INJURY AT WORK

A. LIABILITY OF HEALTH AUTHORITY OR OF PATIENT

1. Generally

The employer's common law liability for injury to members of his staff (as expanded by statute[1]) covers the employer's negligence in failing to take reasonable care to provide and maintain proper tools[2] and equipment,[3] a safe system of working and the negligence of any fellow employee of the injured person. Further, where a statute or regulations impose duties on the employer and provide criminal penalties for their breach, there may also be a civil liability for breach of statutory duty. Moreover, proof of the contributory negligence of the injured person is no longer a complete answer to his claim, though it may reduce the damages awarded.[4] Nor does s. 125 of the National Health Service Act 1977,[5] afford any defence to an action in tort against a Health Authority or one of its officers in respect of injury to a member of the staff. It is not the place here to enter into any greater detail on the subject of liability for injuries to employees except so far as there are features peculiar to hospitals. As regards liability for injuries to employees, reference should also be made to the Occupiers' Liability Act 1957, which deals generally with the obligation of the occupier towards *visitors* for the safety of his premises. *Visitors* in the Act of 1957, includes employees. In particular, regard should be had to the provisions of s. 2.

As is usual with Crown operations, Health Authorities do not insure against the risk of liability for injuries to members of their staff, that risk being carried by the Exchequer. It must be appreciated, however, that if any voluntary organisation such as a league of hospital friends,[6]

---

[1] Law Reform (Personal Injuries) Act 1948.

[2] The defence that a tool having a latent defect had been obtained from a reputable source which prevailed in *Davie* v. *New Merton Board Mills Ltd.* ([1959] A.C. 604) is now no longer open to an employer. See Employer's Liability (Defective Equipment) Act 1969. Section 1 (4) makes the Act applicable to the Crown.

[3] By way of illustration of the extent of the duty of maintenance of equipment may be mentioned *Baxter* v. *St. Helena Group H.M.C.* (*The Times*, Feb. 15, 1972). In that case, the Court of Appeal held the defendants liable for injury caused by a chair in a nurses' changing room collapsing when a nurse sat on it. The collapse was due to extensive infestation with woodworm. The fault attributed to the defendant authority was that it had had no system of inspection of the condition of furniture in use. With such a system, the state of the chair would have been discovered and the accident avoided.

[4] Law Reform (Contributory Negligence) Act 1945.　　　　　[5] Formerly 1946 Act s. 72.

[6] This is a title now frequently adopted by societies for voluntary service to particular hospitals and their patients.

undertakes any activity on hospital premises (*e.g.*, provision of canteen facilities for patients), the risk of liability for injury to an employee or, indeed, to anyone else, would not apparently be carried by the Secretary of State.

It is to be noted that even when an employing Health Authority is under no liability in tort in respect of injury to a member of the staff on duty, the injured person may have a contractual entitlement to sick pay for a limited period in accordance with terms of nationally nego- tiated agreements. He may also have rights under the Superannuation Regulations.[1]

2. Liability in Psychiatric Hospitals

A particular case of injury while on duty here calls for special con- sideration. It is that a member of the staff of a psychiatric hospital who is injured by a violent patient. Can the injured person claim damages from the patient or from the Health Authority ?[2]

The present writer[3] does not know of any reported case in which damages have been claimed by a nurse or similar officer in a psychiatric hospital against the patient in respect of injuries sustained as a result of an attack by that patient. But even, taking into account of *Morriss* v. *Marsden*,[4] and having regard to the relationship of the parties, it seems reasonable to assume that a contractual or quasi-contractual obligation is accepted by the Authority and by the staff to take the risk of damage and injury due to the patient's irresponsible conduct caused by his malady.[5] It is submitted that any other view would make nonsense of the purpose of a psychiatric hospital.[6] But, of course, if it could be shown that a patient's actions, leading, say, to grievous bodily harm to a member of the staff, were wilful and not attributable to his condition, an action in tort would presumably succeed. That most mentally dis- ordered patients have small means and that even those with means are protected against the full rigour of the bankruptcy law must always be something of a disincentive to the bringing of any such action.

But there is another aspect of the risk of injury to a member of the staff by the violence of a patient which is worthy of consideration, *viz.*, the possible common law liability of the employing Authority if reason- able precautions against the more serious consequences of such attacks have not been taken. A Health Authority, like any other employer, is

---

[1] See above p. 426.

[2] What is here said applies no less to injury to the member of the staff of *any* hospital by a mentally disordered patient.

[3] Nor did Dr Speller.

[4] [1952] 1 All E.R. 925. In this case the insanity of the defendant in an action for damages for injury done by him to the plaintiff whom he had attacked was held to be no defence, thus establishing a different basis for civil and for criminal liability.

[5] The defence of *volenti non fit injuria* would appear to be open to a patient who was sued by an officer so injured.

[6] This, at any rate, was Dr Speller's view.

under an obligation, if the work is of a dangerous character, to take all reasonable precautions for the safety of its workers.

Manifestly, a Health Authority cannot by any possible means prevent all attacks on staff nor, therefore, can it — as a matter of course — be held liable to pay damages at common law whenever a member of the staff is injured in an attack by a patient.[1] If, however, the staffing of a ward were inadequate judged by reasonable standards having regard to the type of patient, so that the possibility of attack were thereby increased and also the likelihood of the consequences of an attack being more serious increased because there were not enough capable fellow employees on immediate call, it is suggested that there might well be grounds for liability at common law. Similarly it appears that if a particular patient were known to be violent or of uncertain and dangerous behaviour and such additional precautions for his supervision as were appropriate had not been taken, through the negligence of one or more members of the staff exercising supervisory functions, there would be a common law liability on the employing Authority for consequential injury to any member of the staff. If the injured person was himself in part responsible for the failure in precautions, the degree of his own contributory negligence would be taken into account in assessing damages. It is further suggested that — if the views expressed above are correct — the fact that psychiatric hospital staff might, as at the time of writing, be notoriously hard to obtain, would not constitute an answer to such a claim by an injured officer. It may, however, be observed that the N.H.S. (Superannuation) Regulations do provide in the case of officers within the National Health Service and at discretion of the Secretary of State a fairly generous maximum scale of injury allowances in respect of accidents on duty, and for an enhanced widow's pension if the injury has resulted in an officer's death.[2]

Reference may be made to *Michie* v. *Shenley and Napsbury H.M.C.*[3] In this case an action by a nurse in a psychiatric hospital who had been injured by a patient who attacked him, failed. It seems that the court came to the conclusion that there had been no negligence on the part of the Authority, and, apparently, that the plaintiff, being aware that the patient was likely to become violent, had not taken proper steps for his own safety, *i.e.*, by obtaining help. Although each case must be decided on its own special facts it may be noted that there has been some shift in judicial attitudes since it was decided and today a court might be more willing to infer negligence from an Authority's conduct which in earlier days it might have upheld.

[1] This, at any rate, was Dr Speller's view.
[2] But, in so far as the officer, or his widow may have obtained damages from a third party, the Secretary of State, the Superannuation Act 1972 has power to reduce the pension by an appropriate amount.
[3] *The Times*, March 19th, 1953.

3. Employers' Obligation to Insure against Personal Injury to Employees

The Employer's Liability (Compulsory Insurance) Act 1969, which places an obligation on employers generally to be covered by an approved policy of insurance against liability for bodily injuries or disease sustained by an employee arising out of and in the course of his employment,[1] does not bind the Crown. Nor does it apply, *inter alia* to any body corporate established by or under any enactment for the carrying on ... of any undertaking under national ownership or control.[2] Hence, whether Health Authorities established under the National Health Service Acts are regarded as carrying on a service of the Crown[3] or as a body corporate of the kind above defined, the Act does not apply to such Authorities. Unless exempted by regulations made under s. 3 (1) (*e*) of the Act, its provisions will apply to voluntary hospitals, carried on as charities, and to other private hospitals and nursing homes.[4]

B. INJURY INCURRED OR DISEASE CONTRACTED AT WORK

1. The State Insurance Scheme

Under the Social Security Act 1975[5] cash benefits are payable to persons suffering injury or contracting specified diseases at work. Further benefits are payable under the N.H.S. (Injury Benefits) Regulations 1974[6] in respect of Health Service staff. Space prevents a full description of these schemes in this book.

2. Sick Pay

Any uncertainties of the common law as to the right to pay during sickness when the matter is not covered by express contract, are, in respect of most, if not of all grades of officer within the national hospital service, removed as a result of national agreements approved by the Secretary of State,[7] officers generally having a sick pay entitlement varying with their grade and length of service. This right ordinarily covers accidents as well as illnesses. If a superannuable officer becomes

[1] Section 1.　　　　　　　　　　[2] Section 3 (1).
[3] See *Pfizer's* case, briefly discussed on p. 16.
[4] Other than those within the public sector, no authority providing health care has been exempted, see Employers' Liability (Compulsory Insurance) Exemption Regs. S.I. 1971 No. 1933.
[5] This Act consolidates the law relating to National Insurance. The Social Security Act 1973 made considerable but not fundamental changes to the basic insurance scheme. Those provisions are now to be found in the 1975 Act. Also consolidated in the 1975 Act are the National Insurance (Industrial Injuries) Acts 1965–74.
[6] S.I. 1974 No. 1547 made under ss. 10 and 12 of the Superannuation Act 1972.
[7] N.H.S. (Remuneration and Conditions of Service) Regulations S.I. 1974 No. 296.

permanently incapacitated before reaching retiring age he may qualify for a pension or gratuity.

3. Sick Pay to Victims of Crimes of Violence

Following recommendations by the General Council of the Whitley Councils for the Health Services,[1] provision has been inserted in the sick pay schemes of all the functional Health Service Whitley Councils to the effect that employing authorities in aggregating periods of an officer's absence due to illness, for the purpose of ascertaining his entitlement to whole or half-pay[2] during any period of twelve months, shall not take into account any absence due to an injury resulting from a crime of violence not sustained on duty but connected with or arising from the officer's employment, where the injury has been subject of payment by the Criminal Injuries Compensation Board, or if due to such injury for which the Board has not paid compensation on the ground that it did not give rise to more than three weeks loss of earnings or was not one for which compensation of more than £50 would be given. The Whitley agreements also provide that the employing authority may at its discretion similarly take no account of the whole or part of any periods of absence due to injury — not on duty — resulting from a crime of violence not arising from or connected with the officer's employment.

In a brief explanation of the above arrangements issued by the General Council[3] it was stated that an officer who felt that an employing Authority had decided wrongly that the circumstances[4] were not connected with his employment or profession could appeal through the normal channels (i.e., the normal N.H.S. Whitley appeals machinery.[5]) But there appears to be nothing in the agreement to prevent an aggrieved officer from having such issue determined in the courts.

The right of access to the courts could be important in two cases: (i) where the officer had had recourse to the Whitley appeal machinery and there had been failure to reach an agreed decision first by regional appeal committee and then by a national appeal committee; and (ii) where the officer was not a member of a trade union or professional society represented on an N.H.S. functional Whitley council, through which alone an appeal by an officer may be submitted, or where the body of which he is a member has failed or refused to submit his appeal. But seemingly if an employing Authority had rightly decided that the

[1] See footnote 1, p. 399.

[2] The agreements also provide for adjustments to take account of sickness benefit under National Insurance etc., as well as safeguards against a wrongdoer being able to plead that the officer, having received his pay for the period of illness, could make no claim under that head. It not being my purpose here to set out the Whitley sick pay agreements in extenso but only, and only in respect of this one, to deal with the question of recourse to the courts, it must be appreciated that I have given only such outline of the matter as is relevant to that purpose.

[3] May 10, 1967. See The Hospital, June 1967, 248.   [4] i.e. of his injury.

[5] Further as to Whitley appeals machinery, see p. 422.

circumstances of an officer's injury were not connected with his employment, then, its refusal to allow the officer's sick leave to be aggregated or to allow only part to be disregarded would not be referrable to the courts, being a matter which — by the terms of the agreement — is within the discretion of the Authority.

C. CRIMINAL INJURIES COMPENSATION BOARD — APPLICATION FOR CRIMINAL INJURY OR INJURY CAUSED BY MENTALLY DISORDERED PERSON

A further possibility of obtaining compensation for an injury caused by a mentally disordered person, which may be open to members of the staff of a psychiatric or other hospital in common with other persons, is an application to the Criminal Injuries Compensation Board. The Board may pay compensation to anyone[1] who suffers a criminal injury which for the purposes of the Scheme extends to any personal injury directly due to a crime of violence (including arson and poisoning), any immunity at law of the offender, attributable to his youth or insanity or other condition being left out of account.[2]

A requirement of any application is that the circumstances of the injury have been the subject of criminal proceedings or were reported to the police without delay. The Board may waive this requirement at their discretion.[2] Circumstances in which the Board will waive it in respect of injuries to staff and, more doubtfully, to patients injured by another patient in a mental hospital[3] and steps to be taken by Health Authorities are subject of a circular from the Department of Health and Social Security to hospital administrators in 1971. The specially relevant paragraphs read:

Reports to the police
4. We have been in touch with the Criminal Injuries Compensation Board and explained the complications which would arise, particularly in psychiatuc hospitals, if we were to ask hospital authorities to make it the invariableeyil to report to the police every instance where a member of the staff has been assaulted by a mentally disordered patient under treatment. The Boardcitse that while the Scheme requires that the circumstances of the injury be reprrard to the police without delay they have always recognised that in certain situations different considerations may apply and it would be appropriate in these to waive the requirement of a report to the police. An example is where the full circumstances of an injury inflicted in a prison are reported to the Governor without delay.
5. The Board recognise that a similar situation may exist in mental

---

[1] An award rests at the date when it is made and not at the date when the claimant receives his notification. His estate is therefore entitled to the whole of an award when he dies between the two dates. *R.* v. *Criminal Injuries Compensation Board, ex. p. Tong* [1976] 1 W.L.R. 1237. A widow may also make an application in respect of the death of her husband *Re Lancaster's Application* [1977] 4 C.L. 59.
[2] C.I.C.B. Scheme, para. 5. The Scheme is modified by Home Office Circular 40/1977.
[3] Circular D.S. 166/71 22nd June, 1971.

hospitals[1] and that hospital authorities must have some discretion to decide whether to call the police in or not. They have asked us to make it clear accordingly that it is not their practice to reject applications from staff in mental hospitals simply because the incident has not been reported to the police. Provided the Board are satisfied that the full circumstances of the injury has (*sic*) been reported to the hospital authorities without delay, the Board will waive the requirement. The Board stress, however, that the manner of reporting must be such as to enable a proper decision to be made by the hospital authority whether or not police intervention is appropriate: a mere note in an accident or occurrence book may not, therefore, be sufficient.

Action required by hospital authorities

6. Hospital authorities are asked to take note of this guidance, to review their arrangements for reporting of any assault by a patient involving injury to a member of the staff or to another patient in light of it and to ensure that all such reports are appropriately investigated.

Although there is a reference in para. 6 of the circular to the reporting and investigation of an assault by a patient on a patient, as well as of an assault by a patient on a member of the staff, there is no assurance in para. 5 that waiver of the requirement of prompt report to the police extends to attacks on patients, though it would seem unlikely that the Board would seek to draw any distinction between the two cases.

Whatever may be the understanding between the Department and the Criminal Injuries Compensation Board on waiver of the requirement of prompt report to the police where a proper report has been made within the hospital, that understanding does not take away the right of any injured person, or of any friend or relative of his, or, indeed, of any disinterested observer of reporting the circumstances of the injury to the police. Nor, it is suggested, would a Hospital Authority be within its rights if it sought to enforce by disciplinary action any rule to the effect that injuries caused by patients should not be reported to the police.

D. CONDITIONS AT THE PLACE OF WORK

1. The Factories Act 1961

General Scope and Limits of Application to Hospitals

Section 175 of the Factories Act 1961, contains an exhaustive definition of a *factory* for the purposes of the Act. In the main the provisions of the Act relate mainly to 'factories' carried on by way of trade or for the purpose of gain. However, notwithstanding the references

---

[1] It is assumed that in the circular the expression *mental hospitals* is used in its widest sense, *viz.*, as including psychiatric hospitals for patients suffering from any form of mental disorder, including subnormal and severely subnormal and psychopathic patients, as well as the mentally ill. What is not clear is whether what is said in para. 5 as to waiver will also apply to injuries caused by psychiatric patients being treated in general hospitals or in a psychiatric observation ward of such a hospital.

to *trade* and *gain* in s. 175 (1), subsection (9) expressly extends the Act to any premises belonging to or in the occupation of the Crown or of any municipal or other public authority which would otherwise be excluded because the work carried on thereat is not carried on by way of trade or for purposes of gain.[1]

The principal provisions of s. 175 (1) are as follows:

Subject to the provisions of this section, the expression factory means any premises in which or within the close or curtilage or precincts of which, persons are employed in manual labour in any process for or incidental to any of the following purposes, namely:

(*a*) the making of any article or of part of any article; or

(*b*) the altering, repairing, ornamenting, finishing, cleaning, or washing, or the breaking up or demolition or any article; or

(*c*) the adapting for sale of any article; ...

being premises in which, or within the close or curtilage or precincts of which, the work is carried on by way of trade or for purposes of gain and to or over which the employer of the persons employed therein has the right of access or control.

Moreover, under s. 175 (2) of the Act, whether or not within the foregoing definition, the following, *inter alia*, are also included in the definition of a *factory*.

(*b*) any premises in which the business of sorting any articles is carried on as a preliminary to any work carried on in any factory or incidentally to the purpose of any factory;

(*c*) any premises in which the business of washing or filling bottles or containers or packing articles is carried on incidentally to the purpose of any factory;

(*e*) any laundry carried on as ancillary to another business or incidentally to the purposes of any public institution;

(*g*) any premises in which printing by letterpress, lithography, photogravure, or other similar process, or bookbinding is carried on by way of trade or for purposes of gain or incidentally to another business so carried on;

(*k*) any premises in which mechanical power is used in connection with the making or repair of articles of metal or wood incidentally to any business carried on by way of trade or for the purpose of gain;

(*l*) any premises in which the production of cinematograph films is carried on by way of trade or for purposes of gain, so, however, that the employment at any such premises of theatrical performers within the meaning of the Theatrical Employers Registration Act 1925, and of attenders on such theatrical performers shall not be deemed to be employment in a factory;

(*m*) any premises in which articles are made or prepared incidentally to the carrying on of building operations or works of engineering construction, not being premises in which such operations or works are being carried on;

Hence: (i) *laundries* in all kinds of hospitals and institutions *whether*

---

[1] This would clearly bring in the hospital authorities under the National Health Service Act 1977.

voluntary or public authority are subject to the provisions of the Factories Acts;

(ii) *Any activities* at a *public authority hospital* which if carried on in privately owned premises by way of trade or for purposes of gain would make any part of the premises where they are carried on a *factory* within the meaning of s. 175 (1)–(8) of the Factories Act 1961, render that part of the institution where they are carried on a factory. This would apparently apply, *inter alia*, to such places as the *tailor's shop* in a mental hospital and to the *clerk of works department* of any public authority hospital where articles are made or prepared incidentally to building or engineering operations. Incidentally, any line or siding (not being part of a railway or tramway) and used in connection with a factory is deemed part of that factory. However, it has been decided in the Court of Appeal that a hospital kitchen is not a factory;[1]

(iii) A voluntary hospital being neither controlled by a public authority nor carried on for gain apparently escapes the provisions of the Factories Act 1961, save in respect of the laundry and of any activities carried on for gain, being activities of any of the kinds mentioned in s. 175 (1) of the Act. Also, where in any premises forming part of an institution carried on for charitable or reformatory purposes any manual labour is exercised in or incidental to the making, altering, repairing, ornamenting, finishing, washing, cleaning or adapting for sale, of articles not intended for the use of the institution, but the premises do not constitute a factory, then, nevertheless, the provisions of the Act apply — with certain modifications — to those premises. This might clearly apply to some work done by blind patients, cripples and long-stay patients in some hospitals.

2. Offices, Shops and Railway Premises Act 1963

(a) Generally

The purpose of the Offices, Shops and Railway Premises Act 1963 as set out in the long title is 'to make fresh provision for securing the health, safety and welfare of persons employed to work in office or shop premises . . . to amend certain provisions of the Factories Act 1961; and for purposes connected with the matters aforesaid'.

The premises to which the Act applies are office premises, shop premises and railway premises, being (in each case) premises in the case of which persons are employed to work therein.[2]

In the Act[3]:

(a) 'office premises' means a building or part of a building, being a building or part the sole or principal use of which is as an office or for office purposes;

---

[1] *Wood* v. *London County Council* [1940] 2 K.B. 642.   [2] Section 1 (1).
[3] Section 1 (2). Exceptions in ss. 2 and 3 are not relevant to hospitals.

(b) 'office purposes' includes the purposes of administration, clerical work, handling money and telephone and telegraph operating; and

(c) 'clerical work' includes writing, book-keeping, sorting papers, filing, typing, duplicating, machine calculating, drawing and the editorial preparation of matter for publication;

and for the purposes of this Act premises occupied together with office premises for the purposes of the activities there carried on shall be treated as forming part of the office premises.

In the Act[1]:

(a) 'shop premises' means —

  (i) a shop;

  (ii) a building or part of a building, being a building or part which is not a shop but of which the sole or principal use is the carrying on there of retail trade or business;

  (iii) a building occupied by a wholesale dealer or merchant where goods are kept for sale wholesale or a part of a building so occupied where goods are so kept, but not including a warehouse belonging to the owners, trustees or conservators of a dock, wharf or quay;

  (iv) a building to which members of the public are invited to resort for the purpose of delivering there goods for repair or other treatment or of themselves there carrying out repairs to, or other treatment of, goods, or a part of a building to which members of the public are invited to resort for that purpose;

  (v) any premises (in this Act referred to as 'fuel storage premises') occupied for the purpose of a trade or business which consists of, or includes, the sale of solid fuel, being premises used for the storage of such fuel intended to be sold in the course of that trade or business, but not including dock storage premises or colliery storage premises;

(b) 'retail trade or business' includes the sale to members of the public of food or drink for immediate consumption, retail sales by auction and the business of lending books or periodicals for the purpose of gain;

(c) 'solid fuel' means coal, coke and any solid fuel derived from coal or of which coal or coke is a constituent.

From the foregoing definitions it is clear that any parts of a hospital the main purpose of which is the carrying out of office work is an office within the meaning of the Act, but a ward would not be an office simply because sister did a certain amount of paper work or even if a clerical officer had been assigned to relieve her of that work. Nor, for example, would the pharmacy be an office simply because a considerable amount of paper work were involved in the keeping of records. If, however, a particular part of the pharmacy were given over to clerical staff or even to pharmacists devoting the major part of their time to paper work, it is likely that that part of the pharmacy would be caught by the Act. Besides administrative departments, including matron's office, clearly caught by the Act, there might also be men-

[1] Section 1 (3) (a), (b), (c).

tioned medical records departments and patients' appointments offices as within its provisions.

Hospital shops, including patients' canteens, are also within the Act. But it seems that a hospital staff canteen (unless wholly or mainly for persons employed in office or shop premises), *e.g.* a canteen or dining room mainly for medical, nursing or other professional staff,[1] would not be within its provisions.

The Act is comprehensive in scope and its provisions too detailed for treatment here. Although not as exacting in its requirements as the Factories Act 1961, its provisions follow broadly the same lines.

The Act applies to premises in the occupation of the Crown — including N.H.S. hospitals — only to the extent indicated below. It applies fully to premises in the occupation of other public authorities, *e.g.* welfare institutions under local authorities, as well as to premises in the occupation of charities, *e.g.* voluntary hospitals, except so far as may be otherwise provided in any order made under s. 91 (2) of the Act.

(b) The Application to the Crown

The Act applies to the Crown only so far as is provided in s. 83. The most important and far-reaching provisions of the section are to be found in subsections (1) and (6), which impose a liability in tort in respect of Crown premises, if harm results from failure to comply with certain provisions of the Act.

The effect of s. 83 (1), broadly, is that, whilst the Crown cannot be compelled to comply with the provisions of the Act and of regulations made thereunder as to the safety, cleanliness *etc.* of office and other accommodation within the Act, it will none the less be liable in tort to anyone who suffers harm owing to failure to comply with such provisions as would have been binding on any occupier of the premises other than the Crown or an agent of the Crown.[2]

3. Fire Precautions Act 1971

This Act strengthens and rationalises the law relating to fire precautions. Broadly the Act provides that the local fire authority[3] shall issue fire certificates in respect of those premises governed by the Act. The authority is given the power to restrict the use of the premises to those uses specified in the certificate, to specify the means of escape, the

---

[1] Section 1 (5).

[2] The advice of the Secretary of State to hospital authorities on the observance of such safety *etc.*, precautions in N.H.S. hospitals as would be obligatory under the Act were they not in occupation of the Crown is contained in circulars H.M. (64) and H.M. (65) 17 and 50. As to display of abstract or distribution of books containing it to individual employees, see H.M. (65) 50.

[3] Section 43. Constituted under the Fire Services Act 1947. However, where the premises are occupied by the Crown and the Act applies (see below) the certificate is to be issued by the fire inspector and not the fire authority or a person authorised by the Secretary of State, s. 40 (3) and (4).

means for fighting fire, and the means of giving warning of a fire.[1] It may also impose requirements as to the freedom from obstruction of the means of escape, the number of persons who may be in the premises and similar matters. By s. 1 of the Act the Secretary of State[2] is required to designate by reference to use to which it is put the premises governed by the Act. By subsection 1 (2) he can only do so if the user is at least one of the following classes:[3]

(a) use as, or for any purpose involving the provision of, sleeping accommodation;

(b) use as, or as part of, an institution providing treatment or care;

(c) use for purposes of entertainment, reception or instruction or for purposes of any club, society or association;

(d) use for purposes of teaching, training or research;

(e) use for purpose involving access to the premises by members of the public or otherwise.

The Health and Safety at Work etc. Act 1974 has added:[4]

(f) use as a place of work.

From 1st January 1977, the Act has been applied generally to factories, offices and shops,[5] including those in the occupation of the Crown. It apparently includes those parts of N.H.S. hospital premises coming within each of these descriptions. The reason for this is that by s. 40 the Act[6] applies to premises in the *occupation* of the Crown. The majority view in *Hills (Patents)* v. *University College Hospital Board of Governors*[7] was that although there can only be one person in possession more than one may be in occupation. If this is so, N.H.S. hospital premises generally are premises in the occupation of both the Crown and the Area Health Authority. As far as the preserved Boards[8] are concerned, s. 10A[9] expressly (and probably for the avoidance of doubt) declares that premises in their occupation are to be treated as though they were premises in the occupation of the Crown.

From 1st June 1972, the Act was applied to hotels and boarding houses.[10] It is however probable that a hospital or (less clearly) a nursing

---

[1] Section 6 (1).   [2] *i.e.* the Home Secretary.

[3] There are exceptions relating to single private dwellings which although they may apply to hostel or other accommodation furnished by hospitals for their staff are not further discussed here. See s. 2 (as amended by the Health and Safety at Work Act 1974) and s. 3.

[4] By s. 78.

[5] The Fire Precautions (Factories, Offices, Shops and Railway Premises) Order S.I. 1976 No. 2009 and the Fire Precautions (Non-Certified Factories, Offices, Shops and Railway Premises) Regulations S.I. 1976 No. 2010. These last deal with smaller operations which are not required to have a certificate but which must nevertheless take the specified fire precautions.

[6] Or at least ss. 1, 2, 3 (except subsection (5)), 4, 6 and 12 (1) to (3) and 4 (a) and (b) apply. This broadly includes the regulating sections of the Act, but excludes the enforcement and penalty provisions.

[7] [1956] 1 Q.B. 90. Denning, L.J., made the point expressly and Morris, L.J., appeared to agree. Hodson, L.J., dissented.

[8] Under the N.H.S. Reorganisation Act 1973, s. 15.

[9] Added by s. 78 (8) (d) of the Health and Safety at Work etc. Act. 1974.

[10] The Fire Precautions (Hotels and Boarding Houses) Order S.I. 1972 No. 238.

home is not a hotel or boarding house within the meaning of the regulations.[1] If, however, this is wrong, it will be noted that since 1st January 1977 hospitals, nursing homes and their staff-premises run by the N.H.S. are within the control since on that date s. 40 governing the Act's application to the Crown was brought into force.

By s. 12, the Secretary of State is given power to make regulations governing fire precautions in any of the premises, the uses of which he may designate under s. 1. He need not actually have made an order under s. 1 requiring the premises to have a fire certificate. The regulations under s. 12 may cover broadly similar matters to those which must or may be in a fire certificate under s. 6. As yet the only order under s. 12 is the Fire Precautions (Non-Certified Factory, Offices, Shops and Railway Premises) Regulations 1976.

Fire certificates are not required[2] for any premises constituting or forming part of a prison (which would include the prison hospital), special hospitals run by the Secretary of State for mental patients or any premises occupied solely for purposes of the armed forces of the Crown (which would include any hospital run solely for them).

4. Health and Safety at Work etc. Act 1974

This is a broadly framed measure passed with a view to the creation of a more unified, integrated system to increase the effectiveness of the State's contribution to health and safety at work. In due course, when the appropriate Regulations have been made and the approved Codes of Practice issued, it will replace many of the previous enactments in the field[3] but at present its provisions supplement and do not replace the earlier legislation. As with other enactments of a general nature, a full discussion of its effects cannot be made in this book for reasons of space.

It will however be noted that the main thrust of the Act as regards hospitals is to be found in Part I. Section 1 (1) says:

The provisions of this Part shall have effect with a view to —
 (a) securing the health, safety and welfare of persons at work;
 (b) protecting persons other than persons at work against risks to health or safety arising out of or in connection with the activities of persons at work;[4]
 (c) controlling the keeping and use of explosive or highly flammable or otherwise dangerous substances, and generally preventing the acquisition, possession and use of such substances; and

---

[1] It is also possible, but unlikely, that although a hospital normally has *patients* rather than *guests*, if provision is made for say the parents of a child-patient to stay overnight that might alter the position. This is however unlikely since such a provision is ancilliary to the ordinary business of a hospital or nursing home rather than being itself the business of a hotel or boarding-house keeper.

[2] By s. 40 (2).

[3] Including the Factories Act 1961 and the Offices, Shops and Railway Premises 1963.

[4] The effects of the Act in this regard are noted above, p. 284.

(*d*) controlling the emission into the atmosphere of noxious or offensive substances from premises of a class prescribed for the purposes of this paragraph.

Section 2 provides:

(1) It shall be the duty of every employer to ensure so far as is reasonably practicable the health, safety and welfare at work of all his employees.

Subsection 2 (2) provides for a series of matters included within this general duty. Subsection 2 (3) requires the employer to issue

. . . a written statement of his general policy with respect to health and safety at work of his employees and the organisation and arrangements for the time being in force for carrying out that policy, and to bring the statement and any revision of it to the notice of all his employees.

Subsection 2 (4) provides for regulations[1] to be made for the appointment of safety representatives in prescribed cases by recognised trades unions from amongst the employees. Subsection 2 (6) provides that such representatives shall be consulted and subsection 2 (7) provides that every employer must in prescribed[1] cases establish a safety committee if requested by the safety representatives.

Other sections of the Act deal with the duties to persons other than employees,[2] the duties of persons in control of premises or parts of premises (which would include for example a hospital workshop).[3] Section 7 imposes duties on every employee whilst at work to take reasonable care to look after himself and others and to co-operate with the fulfilment of the statutory duties imposed on his employer and others.

In general, the operation of the Act is supervised by the Health and Safety Commission and the Health and Safety Executive.[4] Inspectors may be appointed.[5] They may enter premises (normally at any reasonable time) with a view to ensuring compliance with the Act and the regulations *etc.* made thereunder and investigating possible breaches.[6] An inspector may generally issue an improvement or prohibition notice and the employer must comply with it.[7] Breach of the duties under the Act can lead to criminal proceedings.[8]

By s. 48 however the provisions as to improvement or prohibition notices *etc.* do not apply to the Crown and consequently not to health service premises. It will be noted that the inspectors may nevertheless enter the premises under s. 20. The Crown (and thus probably health service authorities) is also by s. 48 exempt from possible criminal liability. The section makes it clear however that persons in the service of the Crown can nevertheless be criminally liable.[9] Accordingly a

---

[1] *See now* Safety Representatives and Safety Committee Regs. S.I. 1977 No. 500 which bring these provisions into effect as from 1st August 1978.
[2] Section 3. [3] Section 4. [4] Established under ss. 10–14.
[5] Section 19. [6] Section 20. [7] Sections 21–25. [8] Sections 33–42.
[9] The section refers to 'persons in the service of the Crown'. The view taken here is that

personal responsibility falls upon all Health Service employees and in particular upon those in positions of higher management responsibility. It is unclear whether the individual members of the Authorities themselves are subjected to this potential liability. S. 48 (2) refers to 'persons in the *public*[1] service of the Crown' as it applies the criminal liability provisions. S. 48 (3) refers to 'persons in *the*[1] service of the Crown' being treated 'as employees of the Crown whether or not they would be so treated apart from this subsection'. If 'the service' in subs. (3) is 'the public service' referred to in subs. (2), it appears that individual members of Health Authorities may be in breach of the duty in section 7 (3) to 'co-operate with [the employer] so far as is necessary to enable the [employer's] duty . . . to be performed.' This includes the duties under section 2 and that accordingly they may commit offences under the Act.

this is sufficient to reverse the rule in s. 19 of the Interpretation Act 1889 which provides that normally 'person' includes a corporation. If this view is wrong, there is a potential criminal liability on Regional and Area Health Authorities for their failures under the Act.

[1] My emphasis.

CHAPTER 24

THE NURSES' CONTRACT

A. THE HOSPITAL NURSE

1. The Nurse in Hospital as an Employee

THE nurse working on the staff of a hospital or similar institution is invariably an employee,[1] be she matron or the junior student. The chief nursing officer, or a matron,[2] although in charge of the rest of the nursing staff and empowered to issue orders to them, is herself subject to the general directions of the governing body to which she is responsible and she must attend the hospital in accordance with the terms of her agreement, absenting herself only for agreed holidays at arranged times or on account of sickness or otherwise with the consent of her employers. Her discretion then, although wide, is limited.

Subordinate nurses, including sisters, staff nurses and nursing aides are clearly employees, for besides being under the ultimate control of the governing body of the hospital they are placed under orders of matron and of others to whom matron may be authorised to delegate her authority, e.g., the assistant matron, the home sister and the ward sisters and, as regards the treatment of particular patients, under the directions of the consultant in charge of the case and of other members of the medical or surgical team acting for him.

If a temporary nurse is engaged through an agency for work in a hospital, the usual form of contract between the nurse and the agency and the agency and the Health Authority makes her the employee of that Authority, this even though she may receive her pay, less commission, through the agency. It could be otherwise in a particular case.

2. The Student Nurse, the Pupil Nurse, the Pupil Midwife

The student nurse[3] is ordinarily thought of as a student but in fact in this country she is engaged on a contract of employment analogous to apprenticeship. She undertakes to serve and to obey all lawful orders and the hospital undertakes to teach and to pay a training allowance in consideration of her services. She is therefore an employee and subject to the general employment law, outlined elsewhere in this book. The pupil

---

[1] *Wardell* v. *Kent C.C.* [1938] 3 All E.R. 473.
[2] To maintain some connection with past usage, the usual and femine terms are still used in this chapter. See H.M. (73) 39, H.M.C. Hbk. III.
[3] For definition see p. 385.

nurse[1] is likewise substantially to be regarded as an employee. Nor can the position of the pupil midwife be distinguished.

B. THE NURSE IN A NURSING HOME

The position of the nurse on the staff of a nursing home needs special consideration. If she is not the proprietress of or partner in the home but is engaged at a salary to nurse such patients as may be entrusted to her, she is clearly an employee.

If the proprietress of or partner in a nursing home is herself a nurse and chooses to exercise her skill in the home she is not an employee of the home or of any of the patients since the contract made between the proprietors of a nursing home and the patient is not for service but for services; the contract is not that a particular person will devote any particular time or skill to the individual patient, but that the proprietor of the nursing home will see that the requisite accommodation and skilled nursing and domestic staff will be available to supply the patient's needs, subject always to any special limitations in the contract.

A nursing home may be owned by a company incorporated under the Companies Act 1948. In that case one person may be a shareholder entitled, as such, to share in the profits made, he — or she — may also be a director entrusted with responsibility for oversight of the affairs of the home either alone or in conjunction with other directors *and at the same time* an employee if, for example, employed as a matron or nurse in the home at a salary.

C. THE NURSE AND THE NURSES' CO-OPERATION (OR AGENCY)

Nursing Co-operation is a term loosely used to cover at least four different types of organisation:

(*a*) A number of nurses banded together for the purpose of finding work with rules for sharing profits on an agreed plan. This is rare.

(*b*) A company or partnership finding short-term posts for nurses on terms that the nurse shall pay the co-operation a proportion of her earnings and that she may at the end of each accounting period — usually a year — receive back any amounts paid to the co-operation in excess of her share of the expenses of management computed on an agreed basis or approved by an agreed third party, *e.g.*, a chartered accountant. This, too, is not common.

(*c*) A company or partnership similar to (*b*) but working on a fixed commission and without final profit sharing. This is in fact a type of employment agency and is the most common of the four types of arrangement.

[1] For definition see p. 385.

(*d*) A company or partnership supplying temporary nurses to institutions or individuals needing them, payment being made direct to the company or partnership which in turn employs the nurses.

In none of the first three cases is the nurse the employee of the co-operation or agency although she is under certain contractual obligations to it or in case (*a*) to her fellow-members.[1] Whether she is the employee of a hospital, institution, nursing home or private patient utilising her services depends on the principles enunciated under those several heads.

In the fourth case the nurse is and remains the employee of the company or partnership employing her, and the right of the hospital, *etc.*, engaging her to give her orders is by delegation of authority by the nurse's employer. The hospital would, however, so far as patients, members of the staff and other third parties were concerned, be under all the liabilities of employer, *e.g.*, for negligence causing injury. Whether it would have a claim to indemnity against the company or partnership would depend on the nature of the contract between them.

D. THE NURSE IN PRIVATE PRACTICE

The nurse in private practice may or may not be under a contract of employment with regard to any case she undertakes. In general, however, if she undertakes a whole-time case she is likely to be the employee of the person employing her — usually the patient or the head of the household. But although she may be an employee she cannot be required to undertake duties not within the proper sphere of a nurse unless by chance her contract expressly so provides. There would be a contract for services, not a contract of employment, if a nurse undertook to dress a wound once or twice daily for a patient without undertaking to do it at a particular hour or to give any certain amount of time to the patient.

---

[1] It is not appropriate here to consider the application to co-operation within class (*a*) of the Partnership Act 1890 but anyone called on to advise on the formation of such a co-operation or on the position of an individual member would need to consider the point.

CHAPTER 25

NURSING HOMES AND AGENCIES FOR THE SUPPLY OF NURSES

A. NURSING HOMES

1. Introductory

THE Nursing Homes Act 1975 has consolidated the statute law in this field. The effect of the previous laws remains largely unaltered and previous regulations remain in force.[1]

2. Definitions

By s. 1 of the Act, *nursing home* means:

... subject to subsection (2) below, any premises used, or intended to be used, for the reception of, and the providing of nursing for, persons suffering from any sickness, injury of infirmity.

(2) In this Act 'nursing home' includes a maternity home (that is to say, any premises used, or intended to be used, for the reception of pregnant women, or of women immediately after childbirth), but does not include —

(*a*) any hospital or other premises maintained or controlled by a Government department, a local authority as defined in subsection (3) below, or any other authority or body constituted by special Act of Parliament or incorporated by Royal Charter; or

(*b*) any mental nursing homes as defined in section 2 below.

Section 2 defines a *mental nursing home* and reads:

(1) In this Act 'mental nursing home' means, subject to subsection (2) below, any premises used, or intended to be used, for the reception of, and the provision of nursing or other medical treatment (including care and training under medical supervision) for, one or more mentally disordered patients (meaning persons suffering, or appearing to be suffering, from mental disorder), whether exclusively or in common with other persons.

(2) In this Act 'mental nursing home' does not include any hospital as defined in subsection (3) below, or any other premises managed by a Government department or provided by a Local Authority.

(3) In subsection (2) above 'hospital' means —

(*a*) any hospital vested in the Secretary of State by virtue of the National Health Service Act 1946;

(*b*) any accommodation provided by a Local Authority, and used as a hospital by or on behalf of the Secretary of State under the National Health Service Acts 1946 to 1973; and

[1] See Sch. 2, paras. 3 and 4.

(c) any special hospital within the meaning of s. 40 (1) of the National Health Service Reorganisation Act 1973.

In this book, for convenience the registration and conduct of mental nursing homes is dealt with in Chapter 28 relating to the Mental Health Act 1959 and to the treatment of mentally disordered patients.[1] What is said in the remainder of this part of the chapter applies therefore only to nursing homes which are not for the mentally disordered. It will be noted that the Secretary of State has power to exempt Christian Science nursing homes on condition that any such home to which exemption is given shall be known as a Christian Science house.[2]

3. Registration, Records and Inspection

It is an offence to carry on a nursing home unless it is either registered or exempted under the Act. Although the Secretary of State remains the registration authority,[3] an application is made in writing to the relevant Area Health Authority which may specify that it be given information on any of the matters set out in the Schedule to Nursing Homes (Registration and Records) Regulations 1974.[4] The application must be accompanied by a fee of £1.

The Schedule provides:

Matters on which the Area Health Authority may require information to be furnished by an applicant for registration and on which a medical officer or authorised person may require information to be furnished by a manager.

1. The full name and address, nationality and technical qualifications (if any) of the applicant or manager as the case may be.
2. Where the application is made by, or the manager is, a company, society, association or body, the address of its registered or principal office and the full name and addresses, nationality and technical qualifications (if any) of the directors and officers thereof.
3. The situation of the nursing home and its form of construction.
4. The accommodation available and the equipment provided.
5. The date on which the nursing home was established, or is to be established.
6. Whether any other business is or will be carried on on the same premises as the nursing home.
7. The full names, qualifications and experience of persons employed, or proposed to be employed in the management of the nursing home and whether they are resident in the home.
8. The arrangements for the management and control of the nursing home.
9. The number of patients (excluding staff) who have been received or whom it is proposed to receive, distinguishing between males and females

---

[1] In the previous law, the registration of mental nursing homes was provided for in Part III of the 1959 Act, but this is now repealed.
[2] Nursing Homes Act 1975, s. 18. The exemption may also be applied to a mental nursing home.
[3] Ibid., s. 3.
[4] The Nursing Homes (Registration and Records) Regs. 1974, No. 22. And see Reg. 2 and H.S.C. (15) 106 (powers exercisable by the area administrator).

R

and different categories of patients and indicating the age-range of patients in each category.

10. The full names and qualifications of any resident or visiting physicians or surgeons.

11. The full names and (where appropriate) qualifications of the nursing and other staff employed or proposed to be employed in the home distinguishing between resident and non-resident staff.

12. Whether the nursing home is a maternity home as defined in the Act.

13. The fees charged to patients.

14. The address of any other nursing home or business in which the applicant is interested and the nature and extent of the applicant's interest therein.

By s. 4 of the 1975 Act:[1]

The Secretary of State may refuse to register an applicant in respect of a nursing home or a mental nursing home if he is satisfied —

(a) that the applicant, or any person employed or proposed to be employed by the applicant at the home, is not a fit person (whether by reason of age or otherwise) to carry on or be employed at a home of such a description as that named in the application; or

(b) that, for reasons connected with situation, construction, state of repair, accommodation, staffing or equipment, the home is not, or any premises used in connection therewith are not, fit to be used for such a home; or

(c) that the home is, or any premises used in connection therewith are, used, or proposed to be used, for purposes which are in any way improper or undesirable in the case of such a home; or

(cc) *that the home or any premises to be used in connection therewith consist of or include works executed in contravention of section 12 (1) of the Health Services Act 1976.*[2]

(d) in the case of a home other than a maternity home —
  (i) that the home is not, or will not be, under the charge of a person who is either a registered medical practitioner or a qualified nurse, and is or will be resident in the home; or
  (ii) that there is not, or will not be, a proper proportion of qualified nurses among the persons having the superintendence of, or employed in the nursing of the patients, in the home; or

(e) in the case of a maternity home —
  (i) that the person who has, or will have, the superintendence of the nursing of the patients in the home is not either a qualified nurse or a certified midwife; or
  (ii) that any person employed, or proposed to be employed, in attending any woman in the home in childbirth, or in nursing any patient in the home, is not either a registered medical practitioner, a certified midwife, a pupil midwife, or a qualified nurse.

Where registration is granted, the Certificate of Registration must be affixed in a conspicuous place in the home.[3]

---

[1] The section also applies to a mental nursing home.
[2] Subs. (cc) added by s. 19 of the Health Services Act 1976.
[3] 1975 Act, s. 3 (5) and see s. 13.

4. Cancellation of Registration

By s. 7 of the 1975 Act:[1]

The Secretary of State may at any time cancel the registration of a person in respect of a nursing home or a mental nursing home —

(a) on any ground which would entitle him to refuse an application for the registration of that person in respect of that home;

(b) on the ground that that person has been convicted of an offence against the provisions of this Act relating to nursing homes or mental nursing homes, or on the ground that any other person has been convicted of such an offence in respect of that home;

(c) [relates to mental nursing homes];

(d) on the ground that that person has been convicted of an offence against regulations made under s. 5 or s. 6 above.

Since the effect of paras. 3 and 4 of the 2nd Schedule is to maintain the efficacy of previous (and otherwise unrepealed) regulations, s. 7 (d) is also referring to regulations made under earlier legislation, e.g., the Mental Health (Registration and Inspection of Mental Nursing Homes) Regulations 1960,[2] Conduct of Mental Nursing Homes Regulations 1962[3] and the Conduct of Nursing Homes Regulations 1963.[4]

The 3rd Schedule also maintains by para. 1 the validity of, and subject to, the same requirements and conditions, any registration effected before the 1975 Act came into force[5] and by para. 2 earlier transitional provisions.[6]

5. Notice of Intention to Refuse or Cancel Registration

Before the Secretary of State may refuse to register or cancel the registration of a home, he must give at least 14 days notice that this is his intention and he must give reasons. The applicant (or manager) may then by notice in writing request (and be given) an opportunity of showing cause why the Order should not be made.[7] If despite this, the Order is made, appeal lies to the magistrates court.[8]

6. Records and Inspection

The Nursing Homes (Registration and Records) Regulations 1974[7] provide:

4.—(1) The manager of a nursing home shall maintain a register of patients received into the nursing home which register shall include the following particulars:

[1] The section also applies to a mental nursing home. By H.S.C. (15) 106 the powers are exercisable on behalf of the Secretary of State by the area administrator of the Area Health Authority.

[2] S.I. 1960 No. 1272.   [3] S.I. 1962 No. 1999.   [4] S.I. 1963 No. 1434.

[5] 18th August, 1975. See S.I. 1975 No. 1281.

[6] The effect of the paragraph is that a nursing home which is not a maternity home and which was in existence on the 1st July, 1923 and is still run by the same person maintains its registration unless the nursing is not under the supervision of a resident qualified nurse.

[7] Nursing Homes (Registration and Records) Regs. 1974 No. 22, Reg. 3.   [8] Ibid.

(a) the name and address of the patient;

(b) the date on which the patient entered the nursing home;

(c) the date on which the patient left the nursing home;

(d) if the patient died at the nursing home, the date and hour of death

(2) In the case of a maternity home, the register of patients maintained in accordance with paragraph (1) of this regulation shall include, in addition to the particulars mentioned in that paragraph, the following particulars:

(a) the date and hour of delivery of the patient, the number of children then born, their sex and whether born alive or dead;

(b) the name of the person who delivered the patient;

(c) the method of feeding each child and, if the method is varied, the period or periods during which each method was followed;

(d) the date and hour of any miscarriage occurring in the home;

(e) the date on which any child born to a patient in the nursing home left the nursing home;

(f) if any child born to a patient in the nursing home died at the nursing home, the date and hour of death.

(3) The manager of a nursing home shall maintain a case record in respect of each patient which shall include the following particulars:

(a) in respect of a patient suffering from acute illness, or a patient to whom a child is born in the nursing home, a daily statement of the patient's health;

(b) in respect of any other patient in the nursing home, a periodical statement of the patient's health.

(4) In the case of a maternity home, the manager shall in addition to the case records maintained in accordance with paragraph (3) of this regulation maintain a case record in respect of each child born in the nursing home which shall include a daily statement of the child's health.

Notices

5.—Where any patient, or any child born to a patient, dies at any nursing home, the manager thereof shall send notice in writing of such death to the Area Health Authority not later than twenty-four hours after the death occurs.

Powers of Entry and Inspection

6.—Any medical officer or authorised person shall have power at all reasonable times to enter and inspect any premises which are used, or, which that officer or person has reasonable cause to believe to be used, for the purposes of a nursing home, to inspect any registers or records required to be kept in accordance with the provisions of these regulations and to require the manager to furnish information in relation to the nursing home in respect of any of the matters mentioned in the schedule to these regulations.

Provided that nothing in this regulation shall be deemed to authorise any person who is not a medical officer to inspect any clinical record relating to a patient in a nursing home.

7. Personal Liability of Officers for Offences by Companies

By s. 17 of the 1975 Act, where an offence relating to a nursing home is committed with the consent or connivance or is attributable to any neglect of any senior officer of a company or any person purporting to act in such capacity both he and the company shall be guilty of it.

8. Conduct of Nursing Homes Regulations 1963[1]

(a) Provision of Facilities and Services under Regulation 2

By Reg. 2 of the Conduct of Nursing Homes Regulations 1963, the managers of a nursing home registered under the 1975 Act must:

(a) provide for each patient efficient nursing care and for this purpose employ by day and night suitably qualified and competent staff in numbers which are adequate having regard to the size of the home and the number and condition of the patients received there;

(b) provide for each patient in the home by day and by night reasonable accommodation and space having regard to the age, sex and condition of the patient, including the nature and degree of any illness or disability from which he is suffering;

(c) provide adequate and suitable furniture, bedding, curtains and, where necessary, suitable screens and floor covering in rooms occupied or used by patients;

(d) provide appropriate and suitable medical and nursing equipment and treatment facilities, having regard to the condition of the patients received there;

(e) provide for the use of patients a sufficient number of wash-basins and baths fitted with a hot and cold water supply, a sufficient number of water-closets and any necessary sluicing facilities;

(f) provide adequate light, heating and ventilation in all parts of the home occupied or used by patients;

(g) keep all parts of the home occupied or used by patients in good structural repair, clean and reasonably decorated;

(h) take adequate precautions against the risk of fire and accident, having regard in particular to the condition of such patients as are received there;

(i) provide sufficient and suitable kitchen equipment, crockery and cutlery, together with adequate facilities for the preparation and storage of food;

(j) supply adequate, suitable and properly prepared food for every patient;

(k) arrange for the regular laundering of linen and articles of clothing;

(l) make suitable arrangements for the disposal of soiled dressings and other similar articles;

(m) arrange as may be necessary for the provision for any patient of medical and dental services, whether under Part IV of the National Health Service Act 1946, or otherwise;

(n) make suitable arrangements for the safe keeping and handling of drugs;

(o) permit officers authorised in that behalf by the registration authority to interview in private any person received into the home.

(b) Limitation of Number of Persons in Nursing Homes under Regulation 3

Regulation 3 of the Conduct of Nursing Homes Regulations 1963, provides:

3.—(1) A registration authority may make it a condition of the registration under [The Nursing Homes Act 1975] ... of any nursing home that the number of persons or persons of any description who may be received into

[1] S.I. 1963 No. 1434.

the home shall not exceed such number as may be specified in the certificate of registration.

(2) In the case of any nursing home which has been registered prior to the date of the coming into operation of these regulations, the registration authority may send by post to the person registered in respect of the home notice that, on and after a date not earlier than 30 days from the service of the notice, no persons, or no persons of any description, shall be received into the home so that the total number accommodated in the home exceeds the number specified in the notice.

(3) A registration authority may, upon the application of any person registered in respect of any nursing home or otherwise, vary the number of persons or persons of any description specified under this regulation for that home by giving to the person so registered notice of the variation in the like manner as is mentioned in paragraph (2) of this regulation.

(4) A notice under paragraph (2) or (3) of this regulation shall not prohibit the retention in the home of persons accommodated in the home in excess of the permitted number at the time when the notice has effect.

(c) *Offences under Regulation 4*

By Reg. 4 it is provided:

4.—(1) Where the registration authority consider that the managers of a nursing home have failed or are failing to conduct the home in accordance with the provisions of regulation 2 of these regulations the authority may give written notice by post to the managers, specifying in what respect the managers, in the opinion of the authority, have failed or are failing to comply with the requirements of that regulation and what, in the opinion of the authority, it is necessary for the managers to do so as to comply with the said requirements.

(2) Where notice has been given in accordance with the preceding paragraph of this regulation and a period of 3 months, or such shorter period as may have been specified in the notice, beginning with the date of the notice, has expired, any manager who contravenes or fails to comply with any provision of regulation 2 of these regulations mentioned in the notice shall be guilty of an offence against these regulations.

(3) Any person who receives persons or persons of any description into a nursing home in contravention of any condition or requirement imposed under regulation 3 of these regulations shall be guilty of an offence against these regulations.

(4) The registration authority may prosecute for any offence against these regulations.

Persons concerned with the direction or management of a nursing home owned by a corporate body may be held personally liable for offences against the Conduct of Nursing Homes Regulations 1963.[1]

B. AGENCIES FOR THE SUPPLY OF NURSES

1. Introductory

The Nurses Agencies Act 1957 has replaced Part II of the Nurses Act

---

[1] 1975 Act, s. 17.

1943, regulations made under the earlier Act being expressly saved, until revoked,[1] if within the scope of the Act of 1957.

The different types of agency for the supply of nurses are set out on pp. 452–453, where the relation of the agency with the individual nurse is also examined. Here fall to be noted the provisions of the Nurses Agencies Act 1957, which relate to the licensing and conduct of such agencies.

2. Definition for Purposes of the Act; Exemption in Favour of Certain Hospitals

The term *agency for the supply of nurses* is for the purposes of the Act defined[2] as meaning 'the business (whether or not carried on for gain and whether or not carried on in conjunction with another business) of supplying persons to act as nurses, or of supplying persons to act as nurses and persons to act as midwives but does not include the business carried on by any county or district nursing association or other similar organisation, being an association or organisation established and existing wholly or mainly for the purpose of providing patients with the services of a nurse to visit them in their own homes without herself taking up residence there'.[3] This definition is wide enough to include every type of organisation for the supply of nurses. But by s. 6 (1) of the Act an agency for the supply of nurses carried on in connection with any hospital maintained or controlled by a Government Department or Local Authority or combination of Local Authorities, or by any body constituted by special Act of Parliament or incorporated by Royal Charter is excluded from the operation of the Act. This exclusion thus applies to an agency carried on in connection with a voluntary hospital only if incorporated by *special* Act of Parliament or by Royal Charter but not to such a hospital incorporated under the provisions of some general Act (*e.g.*, the Companies Act 1948). Of course, if a voluntary hospital is incorporated by *special* Act or by Royal Charter the Nurses Agencies Act 1957, does not extend its authorised objects and so the conduct of an agency for the supply of nurses can properly be undertaken only if within the terms of the Act or Charter of incorporation.

3. Conduct of Agencies

A person carrying on an agency for the supply of nurses, in carrying on that agency, may supply only (*a*) registered nurses; (*b*) enrolled nurses; (*c*) certified midwives; and (*d*) such other classes of person as may be prescribed.[4] The intention here is to provide, so far as is considered desirable, for keeping an agency for the supply of nurses separate from any other employment agency business, *e.g.*, supply of domestic

---

[1] Section 9 (2). [2] Section 8.
[3] This does not authorise employment of any but certified midwives as defined by statute.
[4] Section 1 (1).

servants. Class (*d*), however, allows discretion to the Secretary of State, by regulation, to add to the classes of persons or agencies for supply of nurses they supply and he has, in fact, used that discretion in Reg. 3 of the Nurses Agency Regulations 1961,[1] to permit any such agency to supply the following:

(*a*) persons on the list maintained under section 5 of the Nurses Act, 1957;

(*b*) persons who hold the certificate of proficiency in mental nursing or the certificate of proficiency in the nursing of mental defectives formerly granted by the Royal Medico-Psychological Association;

(*c*) persons who hold the tuberculosis nursing certificate granted by the British Tuberculosis Association;

(*d*) persons who hold the orthopaedic nursing certificate granted by the Central Council for the Care of Cripples or the Joint Examination Board of the British Orthopaedic Association and the said Central Council;

(*e*) persons who are entitled, under the Nurses Regulations 1957, to use the name or title of 'service-trained nurse';

(*f*) persons, being persons to whom none of the preceding paragraphs of this regulation applies, of any class prescribed for the purposes of paragraph (*d*) of subsection (1) of section 27 of the Nurses (Scotland) Act 1951, or of paragraph (*d*) of subsection (1) of section 7 of the Nurses Act (Northern Ireland) 1946.

It is, however, clear that the intention of the Act is absolutely to prohibit an agency for supply of nurses acting as an employment agency for classes of employee not falling within s. 1 (1) as expanded by Regulations made under s. 1 (1) (*d*). At first sight the provisions of s. 6 (2) of the Act raise an apparent obstacle to this interpretation, for that sub-section which exempts agencies for supply of nurses from s. 85 of the Public Health Amendment Act 1907,[2] and from any provision relating to employment agencies or employees registries contained in any local Act, expressly excludes from this exemption any other business carried on in conjunction with any agency for the supply of nurses. So it seems that whilst an agency for the supply of nurses is restricted to supply of persons as limited by s. 1 (1) of the Act, there is nothing to prevent the agency being conducted on the same premises as some other type of employment agency carried on by the same person, unless possibly the licensing authority imposes a condition to the contrary 'for securing the proper conduct of the agency' under s. 2 (2). It may be argued, however, that complete separation is nevertheless intended and that the express withholding of exemption from operation of certain Acts in respect of any other types of employment agency is to confirm rights of inspection and control to prevent any breach of the law.

The selection of the person to be supplied for each particular case

---

[1] S.I. 1961 No. 1214.

[2] The section has local application and this is maintained by Local Government Act 1972, Sch. 14, para. 24 (*d*), and see para. 25.

is to be made by or under the supervision of a registered nurse or a registered medical practitioner.[1] By s. 1 (2) a person carrying on an agency for the supply of nurses is obliged, at the prescribed time and in the prescribed manner, to give to every person to whom he supplies a nurse, midwife or other person a statement in writing in the prescribed form as to the qualifications of the person supplied. Regulations may also be made under s. 1 (4) of the Act as to the keeping of records by agencies.[2]

4. Licensing of Agencies

No one is permitted to carry on an agency for the supply of nurses on any premises in the area of any licensing authority without a licence from such authority. The licensing authorities are: for premises within the City of London, the Common Council; in Greater London, the London Borough Council for the area in which the agency is situate, and elsewhere in the country the Social Services Authority.[3]

Any application for a licence to carry on an agency must give the information and be made in the form and manner and at the time prescribed by the Secretary of State, the prescribed fee being payable.[4] Any licence applied for in accordance with the Act must be granted unless statutory grounds for refusal are established to the satisfaction of the licensing authority but the licensing authority when granting a licence may impose such conditions as they think fit for securing the proper conduct of the agency, including conditions as to the fees to be charged by the person carrying on the agency, whether to the nurses or other persons supplied, or to the persons to whom they are supplied.[5]

Ordinarily, but not necessarily, applications for licences will be dealt with at an annual meeting of the licensing authority or an authorised committee of the authority and when granted will be valid until December 31st in the year next following that in which the licence is granted.[6] On the death of the holder of a licence, the licence inures for the benefit of his personal representatives.[7]

5. Refusal or Revocation of Licence

Any application for a licence may be refused, or a licence already granted revoked, on any of the following grounds:[8]

(a) that the applicant or, as the case may be, the holder of the licence is an individual under the age of twenty-one years or is unsuitable to hold a licence; or

(b) that the premises are unsuitable; or

---

[1] Section 1 (3).   [2] See Nurses Agencies Regs. 1961, Reg. 6.
[3] Section 2 (1) as amended by the Local Government Act 1972, Sch. 29, para. 30.
[4] Section 2 (2) and 7; Nurses Agencies Regulations 1961, Reg. 4.
[5] Section 2 (2).   [6] Section 2 (6).   [7] Section 2 (7).   [8] Section 2 (3).

(c) that the agency has been or is being improperly conducted; or

(d) that offences against the Nurses Agencies Act 1957 have been committed.

No licence may be revoked or renewal application refused unless the holder of the licence has been given an opportunity of being heard by the licensing authority or by a committee thereof.[1]

6. Appeals Against Refusal or Revocation of Licence or Conditions Imposed

The applicant for or holder of a licence may within 21 days from receipt by him of notice of the refusal or of the revocation of a licence or of the grant of a licence subject to conditions appeal to a court of summary jurisdiction who may make such order as they think just. The licensing authority must within seven days of demand in writing by the applicant or holder send or deliver to him particulars in writing of the grounds of the refusal, revocation or attachment of conditions.[2]

7. Enforcement of Rules as to the Conduct and Licensing of Agencies

The responsibility for enforcing the provisions of the Nurses Agencies Act 1957, is placed upon the licensing authorities.[3] Any registered nurse *or other officer* duly authorised by the licensing authority may at all reasonable times on producing, if so required, some duly authenticated document showing his authority —

(a) enter the premises specified in any licence or application for a licence or any premises which are used, or which that officer has reasonable cause to believe are used, for the purposes of or in connection with an agency for the supply of nurses; and

(b) inspect those premises and the records kept in connection with such agency as aforesaid carried on at those premises. Obstruction of such officer in the execution of his duty is an offence under the Act.[4]

By s. 4 of the Act penalties are provided for breaches of its provisions. It is further provided that where any such offence by a corporation (which term includes a limited company) is proved to have been committed with the consent or connivance of any director, manager, secretary or other officer of the corporation, he, as well as the corporation, shall be deemed to be guilty of that offence and shall be liable to be proceeded against and punished accordingly.[5]

---

[1] Section 2 (5).   [2] Section 2 (4).   [3] Section 2 (1).
[4] Section 3.   [5] Section 4 (7).

CHAPTER 26

NOTIFIABLE DISEASES

NOTIFIABLE diseases including food poisoning will be discussed in this chapter only so far as the subject is likely in the ordinary way to concern hospital authorities and medical practitioners attending patients in hospitals.[1]

1. Definition

Cholera, plague, relapsing fever, smallpox and typhus are all notifiable diseases to which the full provisions of the Public Health Acts 1936 and 1961 and of the Health Services and Public Health Act 1968 relating to notifiable diseases apply.[2] The following diseases have also been made notifiable by virtue of Reg. 4 of the Public Health (Infectious Diseases) Regulations 1968,[3] viz., acute encephalitis, acute meningitis, acute poliomyelitis, diphtheria, dysentery (amoebic or bacillary), infective jaundice, paratyphoid fever, typhoid fever, anthrax, leprosy, leptospirosis, measles, whooping cough, malaria, tetanus, yellow fever, ophthalmia neonatorum, scarlet fever and tuberculosis. Amendment Regulations of 1976[4] have added lassa fever, rabies, Manberry disease and viral haemorrhagie fever. But in the case of diseases, made notifiable by regulation, the rest of the provisions of the Acts of 1936, 1961 and 1968 apply only to the extent specified in Schedule 2. By an order made by a local authority,[5] other diseases may be made notifiable in its area but there must be specified in the order which of the provisions of the Acts of 1936, 1961 and 1968 apply to each such disease.[5]

2. Cases of Notifiable Disease and Food Poisoning to be Reported to the Local Authority

The duty of reporting cases — or suspected cases — of infectious disease or food poisoning is laid on medical practitioners by s. 48 (1) of the 1968 Act as amended.[6]

(1) If a duly qualified medical practitioner becomes aware, or suspects, that a patient whom he is attending within the district of a local authority is

---

[1] Guidance is given to N.H.S. hospital authorities in Ministry circular H.M. (68) 59. See also for control in the reorganised health service H.R.C. (73) 34, W.H.R.C. (73) 33.
[2] Section 343 (1) of the Public Health Act 1936 as amended by s. 47 of the Health Services and Public Health Act 1968.
[3] S.I. 1968 No. 1366. This consolidates all previous regulations except the Public Health (Prevention of Tuberculosis) Regulations 1925.
[4] S.I. 1976 No. 1226 and No. 1955.   [5] Section 52 of the 1968 Act.
[6] By the N.H.S. (Reorganisation) Act 1973, Sch. 4, para. 122, a new sub-section (2) is substituted.

suffering from a notifiable disease[1] or from food poisoning, he shall unless he believes, and has reasonable grounds for believing, that some other such practitioner has complied with this subsection with respect to the patient, forthwith send to the [proper officer of that district] a certificate stating:

(a) the name, age and sex of the patient and the address of the premises where the patient is;

(b) the disease or, as the case may be, particulars of the poisoning from which the patient is, or is suspected to be, suffering and the date, or approximate date, of its onset; and

(c) if the premises aforesaid are a hospital,[2] the day on which the patient was admitted thereto, the address of the premises from whence he came there and whether or not, in the opinion of the person giving the certificate, the disease or poisoning from which the patient is, or is suspected to be, suffering was contracted in the hospital.

Notification is to be made in the form set out in Schedule 3 to the Public Health (Infectious Diseases) Regulations 1968, or a form substantially to like effect,[3] forms being obtainable from the local authority. The Secretary of State has power, by order, to prescribe the fee payable to medical practitioners making notifications.[4] By the substituted[5] ss 48 (2), the Area Health Authority is to be notified by the officer of the local authority.

The following are provisions of the Public Health Act 1936 which may also be noted:

3. Public Health Act 1936

(a) Disposal of Dead Bodies — Precautions Against Spread of Infection

Section 161 permits the Secretary of State with the concurrence of the Home Secretary to make regulations regarding disposal of dead bodies otherwise than by burial or cremation.

Section 162 provides that if retention of a body would endanger lives of inmates of the building or of adjoining building a justice of the peace may on a certificate to that effect from a medical practitioner in the service of the local authority make an order for its removal to a mortuary and for burial within a limited time or immediately.

Section 163 provides that if a person suffering from a notifiable disease dies in hospital and the local Social Services Authority's proper officer or a registered medical practitioner certifies that in his opinion it is desirable, in order to prevent the spread of infection that the body should not be removed from the hospital except for the purpose of being taken direct to a mortuary or being forthwith buried or cremated it shall be unlawful for any person to remove the body from the hospital except for such purpose.

Sections 164–165 make the person in charge of premises where there is the body of a person who has died of a notifiable disease responsible for preventing anyone from needlessly coming into contact with or the proximity of

[1] For definition of notifiable disease see s. 343 of the Public Health Act 1936 as amended by s. 47 of this Act; see also ss. 56 and 57 of this Act.

[2] For definition of hospital for the purposes of sub-section (1), see s. 48 (5).

[3] Regulation 5.   [4] Regulation 50.

[5] By Sch. 4, para. 122, of the N.H.S. Reorganisation Act 1973.

the body; and no wake is to be held over the body of a person who has died of such a disease.

(b) Compulsory Removal to Hospital of Person Suffering from a Notifiable Disease

Section 169 allows a justice of the peace if satisfied on the application of the local authority that a person is suffering from a notifiable disease and:

(a) that his circumstances are such that proper precautions to prevent the spread of infection cannot be taken, or that such precautions are not being taken, and

(b) that serious risk of infection is thereby caused to other persons; and

(c) *that accommodation for him is available in a suitable hospital vested in the Minister, the justice may, with the consent of the* [Area Health Authority responsible for the administration][1] *of the hospital order him to be removed thereto.*[2]

Section 170 permits a justice to make an order for the detention of a person suffering from a notifiable infectious disease in a hospital after he is already there on the application of a local authority as defined in the Act and including a local health Authority. It is to be observed that the proviso as to cost of maintenance in hospital is deleted from s. 170. See also note to s. 169.

(c) Power of Secretary of State to make Regulations Generally

Under s. 143 the Secretary of State for Social Services may make regulations for England and Wales and for the coastal waters:

(a) With a view to the treatment of persons affected with any epidemic, endemic or infectious disease and for preventing the spread of such diseases.

(b) For preventing danger to public health from vessels or aircraft arriving at any place.

(c) For preventing the spread of infection by means of any vessel or aircraft leaving any place, so far as may be necessary or expedient for the purpose of carrying out any treaty, convention, arrangement or engagement with any other country, and any enactment relating to notifiable diseases may be made applicable to diseases dealt with by such regulations.

[1] Words in brackets substituted by N.H.S. (Reorganisation) Act 1973, Sch. 4, para. 4.

[2] Section 169 (c), shown in italics, was substituted for the previous s. 169 (c) by the 1946 Act, which also provides, in an amended form, that Local Social Service Authorities are included amongst those who may make applications for orders under ss. 169 and 170. As to compulsory removal to hospital of a patient not suffering from a notifiable disease, nor from mental disorder, see s. 47 of the National Assistance Act 1948, referred to on p. 130.

CHAPTER 27

DETENTION OF PATIENT AGAINST HIS WILL

1. Grounds

APART from the right of arrest in respect of certain crimes, a matter entirely irrelevant to our present purpose, a patient may ordinarily be detained against his will only under the provisions of an Act of Parliament authorising such detention. The classes of case may be summarised as follows:

(a) Persons suffering from mental disorder who are liable to be detained in hospital or placed under guardianship if their mental disorder is such as to justify it under the Mental Health Act 1959, and provided that the appropriate steps have been taken under that Act,[1] as to which see the next chapter. If, before a mental welfare officer could be called or other steps taken under the Mental Health Act 1959, it were necessary to restrain a patient in fact suffering from mental disorder where there are reasonable grounds to believe an element of danger exists sufficient to justify apprehension, the patient may possibly, if the old law still applies, be restrained.[2] But since, if it were held that there had been no mental disorder or such reasonable grounds for belief in the danger, the person restrained would be entitled to damages, no one should be subjected to restraint not authorised by the Act except on very clear grounds.[3] Anyone attacking some other person or committing a breach of the peace, as by threatening behaviour, may be arrested in order to be handed over to the police as an offender even though at the time of the arrest there is good reason to believe the offender is suffering from mental disorder.

It should also be noted that a delirious, unconscious or otherwise non-volitional patient may also be held in a hospital. Such a situation is not, of course, a case of detaining a patient against his will since he is in no position to exercise any judgment.

(b) A person suffering from a notifiable infectious disease[4] removed

---

[1] That a person had been made subject of a probation order under s. 4 of the Criminal Justice Act 1948 as amended by the Mental Health Act 1959, with a condition of residence in a psychiatric hospital for treatment does not give the hospital authority the right of detention, though, if the patient were thought likely to leave and his condition warranted it he could temporarily be detained under s. 30 (2) of the Mental Health Act 1959. There is thus no other effective provision for the detention of a drug addict or an alcoholic than a prison sentence.

[2] *Scott* v. *Wakem* (1852) 3 F. & F. 327.

[3] *Sinclair* v. *Broughton* (1882) 47, L.T. 170 (P.C.).

[4] For statutory notifiable infectious diseases see s. 343 (1) of the Public Health Act 1936, as amended by s. 47 of the Health Services and Public Health Act 1968. The Secretary of

to hospital on a justice's order[1] and detained there by a similar order under ss. 169 and 170 of the Public Health Act 1936.

(c) A person who is suffering from grave chronic disease or, being aged, infirm or physically incapacitated, is living in insanitary conditions, or is unable to devote to himself, or to receive from persons with whom he resides, proper care and attention, may be removed to a hospital or to an institution under Part III of the National Assistance Act 1948, on a justice's order[2] under s. 47 of that Act when, in either case, the community physician certifies in writing to the appropriate authority[3] that he is satisfied after thorough inquiry and consideration that in the interests of any such person as aforesaid residing in the area of the authority, or for preventing injury to the health of, or serious nuisance to, other persons, it is necessary to remove any such person as aforesaid from the premises in which he is residing. Section 1 of the National Assistance (Amendment) Act 1951, amends s. 47 of the 1948 Act by providing means of making an *ex parte* order without 7 days notice and other formalities: an *ex parte* order is operative for only three weeks.

Section 47 of the National Assistance Act 1948 does not cover the case of the patient in hospital whose treatment is complete but who has nowhere else to go, *e.g.*, the elderly infirm patient whose relatives refuse to have him back. Such a person cannot be moved from a hospital to Part III accommodation under the Act of 1948 without his consent. If, however, it is practicable for the hospital formally to discharge such a patient, if necessary by ejecting him from the premises, it may well be that if he has nowhere else to go, the Local Authority may be able to take steps which result in his being taken to Part III accommodation.

2. Patient Dangerously Ill or whose Condition is Such that it would be Seriously Detrimental to His Health were He to be Discharged

Unless a patient falls into one of the above classes he may not be detained against his will even though he will run a very grave risk of his illness proving fatal as a result. Equally, there is no power — except as above-mentioned — to detain a person in hospital simply because he is suffering, or reputed to be suffering, from an infectious disease.[4] If,

State for Social Services has power by regulation to add to the list of notifiable diseases and has exercised this power in the Public Health (Infectious Diseases) Regulations S.I. 1968 No. 1366, S.I. 1976 Nos. 1226 and 1955. A Local Authority may, by order, make a disease notifiable within its area and make applicable other provisions of the Acts relating to infectious diseases to the extent permitted by s. 52 of the 1968 Act. Food poisoning is also notifiable under s. 48 of the 1968 Act.

[1] See s. 38 of the Public Health Act 1961 as amended by s. 53 of the Health Services and Public Health Act 1968 for power of justices to order medical examination.

[2] See note 4.

[3] The appropriate Local Authority is defined in the National Assistance Act 1948, s. 47 (12).

[4] In the case of a patient suffering, or suspected to be suffering, from an infectious disease but in respect of whom no justice's order of detention has been obtained, all that can be

however, a patient who is dangerously ill, or who is otherwise in such condition that his departure from hospital would be likely to be detrimental to his health signifies his intention of leaving, it is customary for him to be warned by the physician or surgeon or other medical practitioner on the staff and, if no such practitioner is available, by the matron or other senior member of the nursing staff in the presence of a witness, that he discharges himself against advice and at his own risk. He is then requested to sign a simply worded common form declaration to the effect that the position has been explained to him and that he has elected to take the risk. That a patient refuses to sign the form is no ground for refusing to allow him to depart. It is, however, sensible and customary in that case for the person who gave the explanation to him to record the circumstances. It is desirable that the witness should also sign this record.

A novel point might be made for detaining a patient against his express wish on the grounds either that he was so ill that he did not appreciate the meaning of what he was saying, or the implications of his decision or alternatively that if he did, his decision to leave, if acted upon, would have amounted to attempted suicide. But such defences are best kept in the background and used only as a forlorn hope, especially as attempted suicide is now no longer a crime. If a patient who is seriously ill has to be allowed to go away it is suggested that every means, short of restraint, be used to keep him until he can be handed over to the care of responsible relatives. There would seem to be no obligation on the hospital staff, even at a patient's express request, to take any active part in moving from his bed and from the hospital someone so gravely ill that to move him would be to place his life in immediate danger. It might, however, be otherwise in the case of any other seriously ill patient, even one suffering from a terminal illness, who wanted to go home although, inevitably, his life would be shortened thereby. The same would apply to a patient whose only hope of ultimate recovery was continued hospital treatment. In such cases not only should the patient be afforded the normal facilities for communicating with his friends and for making his own arrangements to leave but, if he has somewhere to go and an ambulance is necessary to take him there, the hospital should arrange through the appropriate department of the Health Authority, for one to be made available. Dr Speller intended to

done, if the patient insists on leaving the hospital, is not only to give him the same warning as is given to other seriously ill patients who discharge themselves, but also to warn him that it is a criminal offence to expose other persons to infection or to enter a public vehicle whilst suffering from a notifiable infectious disease. There is an exception to the rule in the case of cabs, but the conditions of the exception are such that, in practice, it can be disregarded. It is desirable that those responsible for the care in hospitals of patients suffering from such diseases should be instructed to use a set form of words in giving the warning. If there is time the possibility of obtaining a justice's order to detain the patient should be considered. (See generally as to infectious diseases Part V of the Public Health Act 1936 and Part III of the Health Services and Public Health Act 1968.

go further in the draft for this edition by arguing that the refusal to provide an ambulance would be indistinguishable from detaining the patient against his will, because the ambulance service is the responsibility of those same Health Authorities as are responsible for providing hospital services.[1] However, the present editor prefers the view that once a hospital has provided the normal access to friends its responsibilities in this matter are ended.

3. Remedy of Patient Detained Without Justification

If, without justification, a patient is detained against his will those responsible may be sued for wrongful arrest and false imprisonment and, if hands are laid on him, for assault and battery as well. The patient would have a good cause of action against the persons who detained him and also against anyone under whose orders he was detained. Whether he could maintain an action against the governing body of the hospital or nursing home would depend on whether the persons detaining him were acting in the course of their duties as employees or agents of the hospital. The fact, however, that the person was detained by hospital staff on hospital premises would be *some* evidence in support of the liability of the governing body. On the other hand, there would be difficulties in the way of maintaining that the hospital employees *had* been acting in the course of their duties in doing an act the hospital itself was not authorised to do.

The special position of hospital authorities and managers of nursing homes and their staff in respect of the detention of patients under the provisions of the Mental Health Act 1959, is dealt with in the next chapter, as is the position of medical practitioners on whose recommendation or evidence a patient is so detained.

4. Patient in Police Custody

If a person in police custody is admitted to hospital as a patient, *e.g.* a burglar who has met with an accident in the course of his activities, such patient is not in the custody of the hospital but of the police. Sometimes, therefore, by arrangement with the hospital, a police officer will remain at the patient's bedside. Should such officer call for help in frustrating an attempted escape by the prisoner, members of the hospital staff are justified in giving him their assistance in restraining or retaking him.[2]

---

[1] He saw no difference to his argument if the hospital were provided by the Area Health Authority and the ambulance by the Region, since the former acts only on behalf of the latter.

[2] In the case of any such prisoner, or of a suspect whom the police want for questioning as soon as his state permits, who is being treated in hospital under police observation, the hospital would be within its rights if, at the request of the police, it excluded all visitors, or any particular visitors, from the patient's bedside, or admitted them only when a police officer was present.

5. Patient who whilst in Hospital Commits an Offence for which a Person Other than a Police Officer May Arrest

If in circumstances in which a private person has the power of arrest a patient is detained for handing over to the police, *e.g.* on a charge of theft, this is not an instance of detention of a patient as such but of arrest of an alleged wrongdoer.

CHAPTER 28

MENTALLY DISORDERED PATIENTS

In this chapter, unless the context otherwise requires, any references to a section of an Act, are to a section of the Mental Health Act 1959. Also the Mental Health (Hospital and Guardianship) Regulations 1960[1] will be referred to the 1960 Regulations, again unless the context requires otherwise.

A. INTRODUCTORY

THE Mental Health Act of 1959 embodies the law relating to the detention and guardianship of mentally disordered[2] persons and the safeguarding of their property and interests. In the main, it is procedural in character. This chapter outlines those provisions of the Act which most directly concern hospitals[3] and members of their staffs.

1. General Purpose of the Mental Health Act 1959

One of the main purposes of the Act is to provide that any person suffering from mental disorder may be treated as an in-patient without any formality, whether in a hospital or in a registered mental nursing home, provided he is willing to receive such treatment. Only when the patient[4] objects going into hospital[5] may recourse be had to the procedures set out in Part IV of the Act and even then only in highly circumscribed cases. In other words, the old rules as to the necessity for a patient's being able to express himself as willing or unwilling to receive treatment, which bedevilled the procedure for admission as a voluntary patient under the Mental Treatment Act 1930, have been abolished. Part V of the 1959 Act deals with criminal proceedings and persons who are mentally disordered.[6] The Act also establishes an appeal machinery

---

[1] S.I. 1960 No. 1241. These Regulations have been amended by the National Health Service Reorganisation (Consequential Amendments) Ord. 1974 No. 241.

[2] For definition of *mental disorder*, see s. 4.

[3] Dr Speller has dealt with those aspects of the Act not directly concerning hospitals in *The Mental Health Act* 1959 published by the Institute of Health Service Administrators, London. For a brief account reference may also be made to my own *The Mental Health Act Explained* published by MIND (The National Association for Mental Health).

[4] The word *patient* is used in this chapter, unless the context otherwise requires, to mean any mentally disordered person. Terms such as *certified patient, formal patient* are not generally used here for the same reason that they are not used in the Act. The reasons are set out in the Percy Commission Report (The Royal Commission on the Law Relating to Mental Illness and Mental Deficiency 1957) (Cmnd. 169) para. 384, *i.e.* there should be no distinctions of status based on how a patient was admitted to hospital.

[5] The word *hospital* is used in this chapter to include a nursing home registered under provisions described on p. 454 *et seq* below unless the context requires otherwise.

[6] See further, p. 503 *et seq*, for these and related matters.

against unjustified detention. This centres on the Mental Health Review
Tribunals.

2. The Definition of Mental Disorder

Section 4 endeavours to define the term *mental disorder*. Necessarily,
the definitions it sets out entail the legal consequences which follow in
the rest of the Act. However, the doctor's task in deciding in which of
the categories, if any, a patient falls is to relate the diagnosis and the
prognosis to the definitions in the section; he should *not* decide what is
the best means of dealing with patient and then classify the patient by
reference to the legal consequences of each of the definitions classifying
the patient.

Section 4 says:

(1) In this Act 'mental disorder' means mental illness, arrested or incomplete
development of mind, psychopathic disorder, and any other disorder or
disability of mind; and 'mentally disordered' shall be construed accordingly.

(2) In this Act 'severe subnormality' means a state of arrested or incomplete
development of mind which includes subnormality of intelligence and is of
such a nature or degree that the patient is incapable of living an independent
life or of guarding himself against serious exploitation, or will be so incapable
when of an age to do so.

(3) In this Act 'subnormality' means a state of arrested or incomplete
development of mind (not amounting to severe subnormality) which includes
subnormality of intelligence and is of a nature or degree which requires or is
suspectible to medical treatment or other special care or training of the
patient.

(4) In this Act 'psychopathic disorder' means a persistent disorder or
disability of mind (whether or not including subnormality of intelligence)
which results in abnormally aggressive or seriously irresponsible conduct on
the part of the patient, and requires or is susceptible to medical treatment.

(5) Nothing in this section shall be construed as implying that a person
may be dealt with under this Act as suffering from mental disorder, or from
any form of mental disorder described in this section, by reason only of
promiscuity or other immoral conduct.

To avoid an inconvenience that the section creates, reference will be
made in this book to the term *mild subnormality* where the Act speaks of
merely *subnormality*. Plainly under the section the category is in contrast
to *severe subnormality* and it appears helpful in describing the effects of
each of these categories to use in each case a distinguishing adjective.

One further point needs to be made. The Act does not define *mental
illness*. A medical man might say that every type of mental disorder was
either mental illness or arrested or incomplete development of mind.
Such a view is not relevant. What is relevant is the meaning, in law, to be
given to the term for the purposes of the Act. As we shall see, both
mental illness and *severe subnormality* are grounds for the compulsory
admission of an adult to hospital; *mild subnormality* and *psychopathy*
are not.

The Act therefore regards *mental illness* as a serious disability and as opposed to the much broader *mental disorder* which might not be. Further, since the Act defines *psychopathy* as something quite separate from *mental illness* it is to be inferred that, whatever understanding the medical profession may have for these terms, they are for the purposes of the 1959 Act wholly different. It is of course possible that the same person could be suffering from both.[1]

The broad sweep of *mental disorder* is sufficient to bring mild indeterminate mental disorders within paragraph 2 of Schedule 8 of the National Health Service Act 1977[2] so that now local social services authorities have duties with regard to the after-care of patients who were so suffering. Further it brings such mild disorders within the general pattern of health care. The point may be made as usefully here as elsewhere that the definitions of s. 4 are only of relevance when the compulsory powers are being considered.

It may also be noted that the term *patient* means 'a person suffering from or appearing to be suffering from mental disorder'.[3] This definition does not apply to those provisions of the Act dealing with the management and administration of property under Part VIII.

3. Hospitals, Nursing Homes and Residential Homes

The Act divides places for the care of mentally disordered patients into hospitals (including 'special hospitals'), nursing homes and residential homes.

(a) Hospitals

As used in the Act the word *hospital* is defined in s. 147 as meaning:

(a) any hospital vested in the Minister[4] under the National Health Service Act 1946;

(b) any accommodation provided by a local authority and used *as a hospital by or on behalf of the Secretary of State under the National Health Service Act* 1977;[5]

(c) any special hospital.

and 'hospital within the meaning of Part IV of this Act' has the meaning assigned to it by subsection (2) of section 59 of this Act.[6]

Hence, although in practice most mentally disordered patients may be treated in exclusively psychiatric hospitals, any other hospital vested in the Secretary of State, or otherwise within the above definition, may receive a mentally disordered patient, even though such patient is liable

---

[1] *W*. v. *L*. [1974] Q.B. 711.   [2] Formerly s. 12 of the 1968 Act.   [3] Section 147 (1).

[4] In this Act and in instruments made under it, references to the Minister of Health and to the Minister must now read as if they were references to the Secretary of State for Social Services and to the Secretary of State (Secretary of State for Social Services Order 1968, Art. 5 (4)).

[5] Words in italics substituted by National Health Service Acts 1973 and 1977.

[6] As amended, see below, p. 476.

to detention. But a nursing home may receive mentally disordered patients only of the type for reception of which it is registered. So, if it is not registered to receive patients compulsorily detained it may only receive voluntary patients.[1]

Special hospitals for the purposes of the Act are institutions provided by the Secretary of State for Social Services under the provisions of s. 4 of the National Health Service Act 1977 for persons subject to detention under the Mental Health Act 1959, being persons who, in the opinion of the Secretary of State, require treatment under conditions of special security, on account of their dangerous, violent or criminal propensities. These hospitals are controlled and managed directly by the Secretary of State.

(b) Hospitals within the meaning of Part IV

Part IV of the Act is concerned with 'applications for admission', absence of patients with or without leave, continuance of authority for detention, appeals to a tribunal, discharge, *etc.*, of individual patients. For the purposes of that part of the Act, s. 59 (2) provides, in effect, that, except where otherwise expressly provided, Part IV applies to a mental nursing home registered for reception of patients liable to be detained as to a hospital as defined in s. 147 and thus the word *hospital*, as used in Part IV includes a mental nursing home.

(c) Mental nursing homes

In the Mental Health Act, *mental nursing home* takes the same meaning[2] as it now does in the Nursing Homes Act 1975. In that Act, the term means:[3]

... any premises used, or intended to be used, for the reception of, and the provision of nursing or other medical treatment (including care and training under medical supervision) for, one or more mentally disordered patients (meaning persons suffering, or appearing to be suffering, from mental disorder), whether exclusively or in common with other persons.

Expressly excluded from the definition are any premises managed by a Government department or provided by a local authority[4].

It will be noted that a *mental nursing home* need not be exclusively used for mentally disordered patients.

(d) Residential homes

For the purposes of Part III of the Act, relating to registration under the National Assistance Act 1948, 'a residential home for mentally disordered persons' is defined in s. 19 (2)[5] as meaning 'an establishment

---

[1] Section 59 (2) and Nursing Homes Act 1975, s. 3 (2).
[2] Section 147 as amended by the 1975 Act.   [3] Section 2.
[4] See s. 2 (2) and (3).   [5] The section is not repealed.

the sole or main object of which is, or is held out to be, the provision of accommodation whether for reward or not, for persons suffering from mental disorder, not being:

(a) a mental nursing home;
(b) a hospital as defined by this Act; or
(c) any other premises managed by a Government department or provided by a local authority'.

B. ADMISSIONS TO HOSPITALS AND NURSING HOMES

1. Informal Admission, Without Liability to Detention

(a) *Generally*

The Mental Health Act 1959, lays down no rules regarding the reception by hospitals or nursing homes as in-patients of persons suffering from mental disorder, otherwise than where compulsion is necessary either in the interests of the patient or of the public. Consequently, any patient who is willing to receive treatment may be received with no more formality than any other patient. Nor need the patient be volitional. It suffices that he does not refuse to go to hospital or to be taken there by his relatives or friends. And, similarly, if a patient who was volitional when he entered hospital subsequently ceased to be volitional there would be no need to have recourse to the procedure for obtaining compulsory powers to detain him unless he would otherwise insist on leaving and ought not to be allowed to do so.

(b) *In-patient who ought to be made liable to detention*

If the *medical practitioner in charge of the treatment* of an informal patient[1] is of opinion that that patient ought to be made liable to detention, by a report to the managers under s. 30 (2) he may authorise his detention for a period of three days, thus giving time for the completion of the formalities for the making of an application for admission of the patient under s. 26.[2] But as the day on which the report is made counts as one of the three days, this however late in the day the report may have been made, the time for completion of those formalities may be little more than two days.

Since an informal patient is under no obligation to give notice of his intention to leave the hospital, no member of the staff has any statutory right at any time or on any day to hinder his departure, even though such hindrance were with the object of gaining time to advise the

[1] The meaning of the expression *medical practitioner in charge of the treatment of the patient*, is a question of fact.
[2] See further, p. 483 *et seq.*

practitioner in charge of the treatment of the patient so as to give him opportunity of making a report under s. 30 (2) if he thought it necessary so to do. However, if that practitioner were on the premises so that only minutes and not hours, of delay would be involved, some delaying tactics by a member of the staff whilst that practitioner was contacted would hardly be likely to lead to a claim for false imprisonment, even though the consultant concerned decided that there were no sufficient grounds for making a report.

What is most important is that, without a report first having been made under s. 30 (2), no member of the medical staff should authorise the forcible detention of an informal patient or any attempt to interfere with relatives helping him to leave during visiting time.[1] Moreover, even a telephoned instruction from a consultant in charge of the treatment of the patient that that patient should be detained would not be sufficient authority unless the consultant had already delivered a report under s. 30 (2) to an officer entitled to receive it on behalf of the managers.[2] Further, the Act affords no authority for subjecting him to seclusion or restraint of any kind, since that would amount to arrest and detention. Even so, an informal patient — like anyone else — may properly be restrained to prevent his committing a breach of the peace, or to bring to an end a display of violence threatening or causing injury to person — including injury to the patient himself — or damage to property. An alternative possibility to the immediate making of such report would be to call in the police and charge the patient with assault or other breach of the peace, a course which in most cases would have little to commend it.

(c) Correspondence of patients not liable to detention

By s. 134 of the Act, the provisions of s. 36 as to the degree of control over the correspondence of a patient liable to detention which may be exercised by the responsible medical officer[3] are extended to the corre-

[1] It has been known for something in the way of a fracas to develop between nurses attempting to prevent an informal patient departing from a hospital during visiting hours and relatives assisting him to do so. Such interference could leave the nurses concerned open to an action for assault at the hands of both the patient and his relatives. Anyone who gave instructions for such interference would also be liable.

[2] It follows that there should always be someone in a hospital where there are informal patients who is authorised to receive, on behalf of the managers, a report under s. 30 (2). At any time when there may be no administrative officer on duty, e.g. at night and weekends, the senior nursing officer on duty might be so authorised or, if there were more than one medical practitioner on duty, it could be the senior of them. It also follows that there must be a medical practitioner on duty for him to form the opinion that there ought to be compulsory detention. It is understood that in certain hospitals there is a practice when there is no doctor present of the nursing staff being asked to fill in s. 30 (2) forms signed in blank by a doctor. Such forms are wholly invalid and give no legitimacy to the detention. It is dubious if s. 32 could apply since that section allows for rectification of medical recommendations and a blank form under s. 30 does not appear to be a recommendation at all.

[3] The *responsible medical officer* in relation to a patient liable to detention means the medical practitioner in charge of his treatment (s. 59).

spondence of an informal patient, the words 'the medical practitioner in charge of the treatment of the patient' being substituted for 'the responsible medical officer' in s. 36 as applying to such a patient. For the provisions and some discussion of s. 36, see p. 488.

2. Compulsory Admission Otherwise than in Criminal Cases

(a) Generally

Part IV of the Act deals with compulsory admission and detention of non-criminal patients.

All applications for compulsory admission, medical recommendations, etc., referred to below must be in the form prescribed in the 1960 Regulations, or in a form to the like effect. It is, however, a counsel of prudence rigidly to adhere to the prescribed forms[1] and seek to pray in aid the latitude given in the Regulations[2] only when there has been some accidental deviation.

Leaving aside patients concerned in criminal proceedings or otherwise within Part V of the Act, and also patients who appear to be ill-treated, neglected or not under proper control[3] as well as persons apparently suffering from mental disorder who may be found wandering,[4] there are two possible procedures for compulsory admission to hospital[5] of a mentally disordered patient, (a) for observation or (b) for treatment. In either case, the procedure followed is the making of an application for admission in accordance with the provisions of the Act, but no hospital is compellable to receive a patient under such an application. Consequently, before application is made to a particular hospital it should be ascertained that the patient can be received there. If, however, a hospital is willing to receive the patient and the proper formalities in respect of application for admission have been carried out, the application, supported by the required medical recommendations, gives the necessary authority for the conveyance of the patient to the hospital if he is not already there,[6] and for his detention there in accordance with the provisions of the Act.[7]

The application is made to the managers of the particular hospital. This term is defined in s. 59 (as amended). It says:

'
the managers' means:
  (a) in relation to a hospital vested in the Minister under the National Health Service Act 1946, and in relation to any accommodation provided by a

---

[1] As amended in consequence of the N.H.S. Reorganisation.
[2] Regulation 2 (4).   [3] Section 135.   [4] Section 136.
[5] It must be observed that what is laid down in Part IV as relating to the detention of patients applies equally, unless otherwise expressly provided, to their detention in a nursing home registered for the reception of mentally disordered patients liable to be detained. Section 59 (2). See above, p. 476.
[6] Section 30.   [7] Section 31.

local authority and used as a hospital by or on behalf of the Secretary of State under the National Health Service Act 1977, the Area Health Authority or special Health Authority responsible for the administration of the hospital;

(b) in relation to a special hospital, the Minister;

(c) in relation to a mental nursing home registered in pursuance of the Nursing Homes Act 1975, the person or persons registered in respect of the home.

(b) *Who may make an application*

An application for admission of a patient *for observation or for treatment* may be made either by the *nearest relative*[1] of the patient or by a *mental welfare officer*[2] and every application is to be addressed to the managers of the hospital to which admission is sought and must specify the qualification of the applicant to make the application. A mental welfare officer may not, however, make an application for admission for treatment if the nearest relative[1] of the patient has notified the officer, or the local Social Services Authority, that he objects to the application being made. Further, the officer is bound before making the application to endeavour to consult with the person, if any, appearing to be the nearest relative of the patient unless it appears to that officer that in the circumstances such consultation is not reasonably practicable or would involve unreasonable delay.[3] He is also bound to have regard to any wishes expressed by relatives of the patient or any other relevant circumstances.[4] The person making the application must personally have seen the patient within the period of 14 days ending with the date of the application,[5] except in the case of an emergency application when the period is three days.[6] The provisions of s. 27 (2) preserving the right of veto of the nearest relative do not apply in the case of an infant who is a ward of court, in which case the application may be made only with the leave of the court.[7] Otherwise an obstructive nearest relative can be dealt with only under s. 52.

Subject to these rights of the relatives, the Act declares that where the mental welfare officer is satisfied that an application ought to be made and if of opinion that it is necessary or proper, it is his duty to make it. It will be noted that the Act places different but concurrent responsibilities on the doctors and the mental welfare officers. In particular, it is not the duty of the latter to make an application solely because a doctor has made a recommendation.[8]

---

[1] As defined in ss. 49 and 52.

[2] Appointed by the local Social Services Authority (s. 147 (1)). It is the practice in some authorities to designate all their social workers as mental welfare officers. Accordingly it sometimes appears that social workers have taken on these special statutory powers. In this book, however, the statutory term is still used.

[3] Section 27 (2).   [4] Section 54 (1).   [5] Section 27 (3).

[6] Section 29 (4).   [7] Section 58.

[8] *Re Frost* [1936] 2 All E.R. 182; *Buxton* v. *Jayne* [1960] 1 W.L.R. 783.

(c) Admission for observation
   Section 25 provides:

An application for admission for observation may be made in respect of a patient on the grounds:
   (*a*) that he is suffering from mental disorder of a nature or degree which warrants the detention of the patient in a hospital under observation (with or without other medical treatment) for at least a limited period; and
   (*b*) that he ought to be so detained in the interests of his own health or safety or with a view to the protection of other persons.

The application must ordinarily be founded on the written recommendations in the prescribed form[1] of two medical practitioners including in each case a statement that in the opinion of the practitioner the conditions set out in (*a*) and (*b*) above are complied with.
   In any case of urgent necessity, s. 29 provides that an application for admission for observation supported by only one medical recommendation — called *an emergency application* — may be made in respect of a patient either by a mental welfare officer or by *any* relative of the patient and every such application must include a statement that it is of urgent necessity for the patient to be admitted and detained for observation and that compliance with the ordinarily required formalities would involve undesirable delay. It suffices if such an emergency application is in the first instance founded on a single medical recommendation given, if practicable, by a practitioner who has had previous acquaintance with the patient and who is not disqualified under s. 28 from giving a recommendation on that case. If an emergency application is founded on only one medical recommendation, a second must be obtained and received by the managers of the hospital within 72 hours from the time when the patient is admitted. The two recommendations together must comply with the provisions of s. 28.[2]
   An application for admission for observation under s. 25 authorises the conveyance of the patient to the hospital within 14 days beginning with the date on which the patient was last examined by a medical practitioner before giving a medical recommendation. In the case of an emergency application the period is three days beginning with the date on which the practitioner giving the single recommendation examined the patient or with the date of the application, whichever is earlier.[3] A patient admitted on an application for observation may then be detained for a period not exceeding 28 days beginning with the day on which he was admitted, but shall not be detained thereafter unless, before the expiration of that period, he has become liable to be detained under a subsequent application, order or direction under the Act.[4] But

---

[1] See the 1960 Regulations, Forms 3A and 3B, as amended. The medical recommendations are discussed below, at p. 485 *et seq.*
[2] Section 29.   [3] Section 31.   [4] Section 25.

the initial period of 28 days may also be extended under the provisions of s. 52 (4) if, when it is due to expire, there is pending an application to the county court for depriving the nearest relative of his rights on the ground that he has exercised his power to discharge the patient without due regard to the welfare of the patient or the interests of the public, or is likely to do so. In such circumstances the period is extended until the application is disposed of or, if an order is made, until seven days thereafter.[1]

In the case of an emergency application, provided the second medical recommendation is received by the managers of the hospital within 72 hours of the patient's admission, the period of authorised detention will be the same as for any other admission for observation.[2]

(d) Admission of patients ill-treated or neglected

Section 135 (1) provides:

If it appears to a justice of the peace, on information on oath laid by a mental welfare officer, that there is reasonable cause to suspect that a person believed to be suffering from mental disorder:

(a) has been, or is being, ill-treated, neglected or kept otherwise than under proper control, in any place within the jurisdiction of the justice; or

(b) being unable to care for himself, is living alone in any such place, the justice may issue a warrant authorising any constable named therein to enter, if need be by force, any premises specified in the warrant in which that person is believed to be, and, if thought fit, to remove him to a place of safety with a view to the making of an application in respect of him under Part IV of the Act, or of other arrangements for his treatment or care.

It is not necessary to name the patient in the information or warrant.[3] The constable executing the warrant must be accompanied by a mental welfare officer and by a medical practitioner.[4]

A place of safety means residential accommodation provided by a local authority under paragraph 2 of Schedule 8 to the National Health Service Act 1977, Part III of the National Assistance Act 1948, a hospital as defined in the Mental Health Act 1959, a police station, a mental nursing home or residential home for mentally disordered persons or any other suitable place, the occupier of which is willing temporarily to receive the patient.[5]

A patient who is removed to a place of safety in execution of a warrant under s. 135 may be detained there for 72 hours.[6] This period of detention is only allowed if it is undertaken with a view to making an application under Part IV or to making other arrangements for the patient's treatment or care. In no way does it allow either the police to

---

[1] Section 52 (4).   [2] Sections 29 and 25.   [3] Section 135 (5).
[4] Section 135 (4). The extent of any possible liability of the accompanying medical practitioner is discussed in Dr Speller's Law of Doctor and Patient (1973), p. 102.
[5] S. 135 (6).   [6] S. 135 (3).

use the provision as an alternative to the criminal law for certain types of minor offences, *e.g.* drunkenness, nor does it absolve either the mental welfare officer or the doctor of their responsibilities under Part IV.

(e) Admission of mentally disordered persons found in public places

Section 136 provides:

If a constable finds in a place to which the public have access, a person who appears to him to be suffering from mental disorder and to be in immediate need of care or control the constable may, if he thinks it necessary to do so in the interests of that person or for the protection of other persons, remove that person to a place of safety.

A person thus removed to a place of safety may be detained there for a period not exceeding 72 hours for the purpose of enabling him to be examined by a medical practitioner and to be interviewed by a mental welfare officer and of making any necessary arrangements for his treatment or care. The same proviso is to be applied to s. 136 as to s. 135, namely the section merely allows a patient to be held so as to enable the professional people, the mental welfare officer and the doctors, to discharge their statutory responsibilities under Part IV.

(f) Admission for treatment

Section 26 (2) provides:

An application for admission for treatment may be made in respect of a patient on the grounds:
  (a) that he is suffering from mental disorder, being —
    (i) in the case of a patient of any age, mental illness or severe subnormality;
    (ii) in the case of a patient under the age of 21 years, psychopathic disorder or subnormality;
  and that the said disorder is of a nature or degree which warrants the detention of the patient in a hospital for medical treatment under this section; and
  (b) that it is necessary in the interests of the patient's health or safety or for the protection of other persons that the patient should be so detained.

The application[1] must be founded on the written recommendations in the prescribed form of two medical practitioners[2] each stating that, in the opinion of the practitioner, the conditions set out in (a) and (b) above are complied with; Each such recommendation must also include the grounds for the opinion that the above conditions are fulfilled and a statement of the reasons for that opinion; it must specify whether other methods of dealing with the patient are available, and if so why they are not appropriate.[3]

[1] Forms 4A and 4B as amended in the 1960 Regulations.
[2] Forms 5A and 5B as amended in the 1960 Regulations.
[3] Section 26 (1), (2) and (3).

An application for admission for treatment and any recommendation given for the purposes of such an application, may describe the patient as suffering from more than one of the forms of mental disorder referred to in (a) above but the application will be of no effect unless the patient is described in each of the recommendations as suffering from the same one of those forms of mental disorder, whether or not he be also described in either of those recommendations as suffering from another of those forms.[1] Consequently, the detention for treatment must be regarded as by reason of the type or types of mental disorder mentioned in both recommendations.

If an application for admission for treatment is made on the grounds that the patient is suffering from psychopathic disorder or mild subnormality and no other form of mental disorder referred to in (a) above, the age of the patient must be stated, or, if his exact age is not known to the applicant, he must state (if such be the fact) that the patient is believed to be under the age of 21 years.[2] Also regard must be had to the provisions of s. 59 (3) which states that a patient is to be treated as liable to detention (or subject to guardianship) as a psychopathic or subnormal (mild) patient only if the form of disorder specified in the application is psychopathic disorder or subnormality or psychopathic disorder and mild subnormality *and no other form of mental disorder*. Hence, if in both recommendations the additional ground of mental illness or severe subnormality is included, the patient, even though under 21 years of age, cannot be made subject to the special provisions relating to patients suffering from psychopathic disorder or mild subnormality but must be regarded as detained solely on account of mental illness or severe subnormality as the case may be.

(g) *Application for admission of patient already in hospital*

An application for admission of a patient to a hospital whether for observation or for treatment may be made notwithstanding that the patient is already an in-patient in that hospital on a voluntary basis. Similarly, an application for admission for treatment may be made notwithstanding that the patient is for the time being liable to be detained in the hospital in pursuance of his having been admitted for observation. Where an application is so made, the patient is to be treated as if he had been admitted to the hospital at the time when the application was received by the managers.[3]

In the case of a patient not liable to detention in respect of whom an application for admission ought to be made, a report in writing made

---

[1] Section 26 (4).
[2] Section 26 (5). As to the determination of the age of any person whose exact age cannot be ascertained by reference to the registers kept under the Births and Deaths Registration Act 1953, see s. 56 (2) (*f*) and S.I. 1960 No. 1241, Reg. 26.
[3] Section 30 (1).

by the medical practitioner in charge of his treatment that application ought to be made constitutes authority for his detention for up to three days including the day on which the report was made.[1]

Where a patient is admitted to hospital in pursuance of an application for admission for treatment, any previous application under Part IV of the Act by virtue of which he was liable to be detained in a hospital or subject to guardianship ceases to have effect.[2]

(h) Medical recommendations

The medical recommendations supporting any application for admission must be signed on or before the date of application and must be given by practitioners who have personally examined the patient either together or at an interval of not more than seven days.[3] Of the medical recommendations, one must be given by a practitioner approved by the Area Health Authority as having special experience in the diagnosis or treatment of mental disorder;[4] and unless the practitioner has previous acquaintance with the patient, the other such recommendation must, if practicable, be given by a medical practitioner who has such previous acquaintance.[5]

If the application is for admission of the patient to a hospital not being a mental nursing home, one (but not more than one) of the medical recommendations may be given by a practitioner on the staff of that hospital, except where the patient is proposed to be accommodated under ss. 65 and 66 of the National Health Service Act 1977 relating to accommodation for private patients.[6]

None of the following may sign a medical recommendation either for admission to hospital or for guardianship. Section 28 (4) provides.

(a) the applicant;

(b) a partner of the applicant or of a practitioner by whom another medical recommendation is given for the purposes of the same application;

(c) a person employed as an assistant by the applicant or by any such practitioner as aforesaid;

(d) a person who receives or has an interest in the receipt of any payments made on account of the maintenance of the patient; or

(e) except as provided by subsection (3) of this section, a practitioner on the staff of the hospital to which the patient is to be admitted,

[1] More fully explained and discussed above, pp. 477–478.

[2] Section 31 (5). Any previous application for admission would have been for observation.

[3] Section 28 (1).

[4] Section 28 (2) as amended by the N.H.S. Reorganisation Act 1973 speaks of the approval being given by the Secretary of State, but by the N.H.S. Functions (Directions to Authorities) Regulations S.I. 1974 No. 24 this function is delegated to the Area Health Authority.

[5] Section 28 (2).

[6] Section 28 (3) and s. 38 (1) of the Interpretation Act 1889. (The object of this provision is in line with the general policy of not allowing a medical practitioner to sign a recommendation concerning a patient in whose treatment he or his immediate relatives might have a financial interest.)

or the husband, wife, father, father-in-law, mother, mother-in-law, son, son-in-law, daughter, daughter-in-law, brother, brother-in-law, sister, sister-in-law of the patient, or of any such person as aforesaid, or of a practitioner by whom another medical recommendation is given for the purposes of the same application.[1]

For rules as to approval of practitioners under s. 28 and the procedure to be followed reference should be made to the provisions of Reg. 5 of the 1960 as amended Regulations.

(i) Defective applications

Section 31 (3) provides:

Any application for the admission of a patient under [Part IV of this Act] which appears to be duly made and to be founded on the necessary medical recommendations may be acted upon without further proof of the signature or qualification of the person by whom the application or any such medical recommendation is made or given, or of any matter of fact or opinion stated therein.

Section 32 (1) goes on to say:

If within the period of 14 days beginning with the day on which the patient is admitted to hospital in pursuance of an application for observation or treatment the application, or any medical recommendation given for the purposes of the application, is found in any respect to be incorrect or defective, the application or recommendation may, within that period, and, with the consent of the managers of the hospital, be amended by the person by whom it was signed; and upon such amendment being made the application or recommendation shall have effect and shall be deemed to have had effect as if it had been originally made as so amended.

If in the opinion of the managers of the hospital one of the two medical recommendations is insufficient to warrant detention of the patient, the managers may within 14 days of the patient's admission give notice to the applicant, and that recommendation is then disregarded. If within that 14 days a fresh medical recommendation complying with the relevant provisions of the Act is received which together with the remaining recommendation supports the detention, the application is deemed always to have been in order.[2]

Similar power is given to the managers to allow rectification if the two medical recommendations taken together are insufficient to warrant the detention of the patient, save where the defect is that the two practitioners both fail to certify to a single form of mental disorder.[3]

The above procedure for curing defects cannot be used to extend the 72 hours within which a second medical recommendation must be received by the managers in support of an emergency application under

---

[1] Section 28 (4).
[2] Section 32 (2). See also pp. 481–482 as to medical recommendations on applications for admission for observation.
[4] Section 32 (3).

s. 29, but it can be used thereafter to cure any error or defect as though it had been an ordinary application for admission for observation.

The managers of a hospital may in writing authorise an officer on their behalf to exercise functions in relation to amendment of defective applications, the sufficiency of medical recommendations, *etc.*, and the managers of a mental nursing home may likewise authorise one of their number of any other person to exercise such functions on their behalf.[1]

As regards procedure, if it appears to the responsible medical officer that the patient is suffering from a form of mental disorder other than the form or forms specified in the application, see p. 490.

C. PATIENTS IN HOSPITAL

1. Care and Treatment of Patients Generally

The sub-heading in the Act to ss. 35–42 is 'Care and Treatment of Patients'. However, all these sections, other than those relating to guardianship and s. 36 (discussed below) are concerned with matters incidental to compulsory detention. Nowhere in the Act is there any attempt to determine standards of care and treatment otherwise than in the negative sense of laying down that ill-treatment of patients is an offence[2] and that there were rights of inspection in the case of registered mental nursing homes[3] and of residential homes.[4] The Secretary of State may, however, under The Nursing Homes Act 1975 make regulations as to the conduct of mental nursing homes, including provision as to the facilities and services to be provided in such homes, and any contravention of such regulations is an offence. In exercise of those powers the Secretary of State had made the Conduct of Mental Nursing Homes Regulations 1962, the text of which is given on p. 519 *et seq.*

2. The Responsible Medical Officer

The *responsible medical officer* in relation to a patient subject to detention under the provisions of the Act means the medical practitioner in charge of the treatment of that patient.[5] His powers, duties and possible liabilities in respect of various matters concerning that patient, are discussed in this chapter. Who is actually in charge of the treatment appears to be a factual question in each case. Presumably ordinarily it will be the consultant psychiatrist on the staff of the hospital under whose care the patient has been admitted or placed even though that consultant may not himself see the patient frequently. Hence, the Act must be read as placing on the consultant personally the responsibility for performing the various functions of the responsible medical officer

---

[1] Section 59 (2). [2] Section 126.
[3] Section 17. Now see s. 9 of the Nursing Homes Act 1975.
[4] Section 21. [5] Section 59 (1).

S

in respect of every one of the patients of whose treatment he has charge.

The Act is silent as regards who, if anybody, is entitled to carry out the functions of the responsible medical officer during the consultant's temporary absence. However, it appears there is nothing in the Act to prevent someone being temporarily in charge of the treatment of any patient or patients. Hence, if a consultant were absent on annual leave or because of a prolonged bout of illness or for any other cause, it may be assumed that either another consultant or an appropriately qualified senior member of his own medical team would be in charge of the treatment of his patients *pro tem.* and so, in respect of those liable to detention, the responsible medical officer and, as such, qualified to carry out statutory powers and duties under the Act.

3. Correspondence of Patients

As regards incoming postal packets, including letters, s. 36 of the Act provides:

(1) Any postal packet addressed to a patient detained in a hospital under this part of the Act may be withheld from the patient if, in the opinion of the responsible medical officer, the receipt of the packet would be calculated to interfere with the treatment of the patient or to cause him unnecessary distress; and any packet so withheld shall, if the name and address of the sender are sufficiently identified therein, be returned to him by post.

It is to be noted that this statutory authority relates only to the withholding of postal packets and not the withholding of letters or other packets addressed to a patient which may be delivered to a hospital otherwise than by the Post Office. The statutory authority to withhold is required in respect of Post Office deliveries because without it an offence might be committed under the Post Office Act 1969. If the responsible medical officer does not think it advisable for a patient to receive a packet or letter in any other way, his most prudent course is for instructions to be given that any other letter be not accepted at the hospital.[1] For the hospital to accept it and not pass it on may amount to the tort of conversion.

As to the refusal to send duly stamped letters and packets from the patient, s. 36 (2) provides:

(2) Subject to the provisions of this section, any postal packet addressed by a patient so detained and delivered by him for dispatch may be withheld from the Post Office —
    (a) if the addressee has given notice in writing to the managers of the hospital or to the responsible medical officer requesting that communications addressed to him by the patient should be withheld; or
    (b) if it appears to that officer that the packet would be unreasonably

---

[1] He could also give instructions that such letters only be accepted on the terms that he is entitled to open them and only give them to the patient if he considered that they would not interfere with the treatment.

offensive to the addressee, or is defamatory of other persons (other than persons on the staff of the hospital) or would be likely to prejudice the interests of the patient:

provided that this subsection does not apply to any postal packet addressed as follows, that is to say —

    (i) to the Minister;

    (ii) to any Member of the Commons House of Parliament;

    (iii) to the Master or Deputy Master or any other officer of the Court of Protection;

    (iv) to the managers of the hospital;

    (v) to any other authority or person having power to discharge the patient under this part of the Act;

    (vi) at any time when the patient is entitled to make application to a Mental Health Review Tribunal, to that tribunal,

and regulations made by the Minister may except from this subsection, subject to such conditions or limitations (if any) as may be prescribed by the regulations, postal packets addressed to such other classes of persons as may be so prescribed.

(3) Nothing in para. (*b*) of subsection (2) of this section shall be construed as authorising a responsible medical officer to open or examine the contents of any postal packet unless he is of opinion that the patient is suffering from mental disorder of a kind calculated to lead him to send such communications as are referred to in that paragraph.

(4) Except as provided by this section, it shall not be lawful to prevent or impede the delivery to a patient detained as aforesaid of any postal packet addressed to him and delivered by the Post Office, or the delivery to the Post Office of any postal packet addressed by such a patient and delivered by him for dispatch.

(*Subsection* (5) *applies the section, with necessary modifications, to patients under guardianship.*)

(6) In this section 'postal packet' has the same meaning as in the Post Office Act 1953; and the provisions of this section shall have effect notwithstanding anything in s. 56 of that Act.

Under Reg. 23 of the Mental Health (Hospital and Guardianship) Regulations 1960, the list of those to whom a patient may write without restriction and without his letters being subject to any censorship, as set out in the proviso to s. 36 (2) is extended to include:

A solicitor acting or invited to act for the patient, but the regulation applies only (*a*) when the patient has notified the managers of the hospital or the responsible medical officer that the solicitor is so acting or has been so invited and (*b*) where the solicitor has not given a notification to the managers or the responsible medical officer requesting that communications addressed to him by the patient should be withheld.[1]

Having regard to what has already been said about the absence of any provision in the Act for delegation by a responsible medical officer of his statutory functions, the question arises whether he could delegate his power of supervision of correspondence under s. 36. On the face of it,

[1] Without citing authority, Edwards in his *Mental Health Services* (4th Edn. 1975, at p. 114) says that the Secretary of State has added 'under general powers' to the list the European Commission of Human Rights.

he could not. Nevertheless, one would expect that, where practically necessary[1], the delegation of the duty of immediate supervision of the correspondence of named patients by a consultant to a suitable member of his medical team would be unlikely to be challenged, always provided that the consultant had himself first decided that supervision of the correspondence of those patients was necessary and within the terms authorised by the Act.[2] What s. 36 cannot possibly be stretched to permit is the delegation to nursing or other non-medical staff of any power conferred therein, though it would be quite proper that the ward sister or charge nurse or other appropriate officer should be given instructions to withhold *unopened* any incoming postal packet addressed to a named patient for submission to the responsible medical officer for his instructions. But no authority can be conferred on a nurse of any rank to read or censor a patient's correspondence, whether outgoing or incoming.

4. Reclassificaton of Patients

If it appears to the responsible medical officer that the patient is suffering from a mental disorder other than the form or forms specified in the application, he may furnish the managers of the hospital with a report to that effect and the authority to detain will then have effect as if that other form of mental disorder were specified therein.[3] It is now however provided by the Mental Health (Amendment) Act 1975[4] that before he furnishes such a report the officer shall consider whether the patient, if released, would be likely to act in a manner dangerous to other persons or to himself. If he does think the patient would be likely to be dangerous he is bound to include a statement to that effect in the notice and the authority to detain is continued. The Act thus reverses the decision in *re Mental Health Act*[5] in which it was held that where there was a reclassification and if the amended application had been the original one there would have been no authority for the detention, the patient must be released.

If the patient has attained the age of 16, the patient and the nearest relative must be informed of the reclassification and if there is one the barring note and either of them may within 28 days apply to the Review Tribunal. Where there is a barring note the nearest relative cannot order the release of the patient under s. 47[6] for six months.

---

[1] *E.g.* When the consultant is not in daily attendance or is away for a short time.
[2] There is, however, a remote possibility of an action for trespass to goods. If such an action were brought by the patient, it is arguable whether the protection afforded by s. 141 (1) would be available to the defendant practitioner.
[3] Section 38 (1). It will be noted that this power is very different from the rectification power in s. 32: this relates to a different diagnosis; s. 32 is concerned with mistakes.
[4] The 1975 Act also applies to reclassification by a Mental Health Review Tribunal under s. 123.
[5] [1973] 1 Q.B. 452 *sub nom. Re V.E. (A Mental Patient)* [1972] 3 All E.R. 373.
[6] See below, p. 498.

5. Leave of Absence

The responsible medical officer may grant the patient leave to be absent from the hospital subject to such conditions (if any) as he considers necessary in the interests of the patient or for the protection of other persons. Leave of absence may be granted either indefinitely, or on specified occasions, or for any specified period; and leave granted for a specified period may be extended by further leave granted in the absence of the patient. Where it appears necessary in the interests of the patient, the responsible medical officer upon granting leave may order that during the absence the patient remain in custody of an officer on the staff of the hospital, or of any other person authorised in writing by the managers of the hospital.[1]

The responsible medical officer may at any time, in the interests of the patient's health or safety or for the protection of other persons, revoke a patient's leave of absence by notice in writing to the patient or to the person for the time being in charge of the patient.[2]

A patient who has been on leave of absence cannot, however, be recalled after he has ceased to be liable to be detained under Part IV (*e.g.*, by reason of expiry of authority for detention or the patient's discharge)[3] and, without prejudice to other provisions of Part IV, a patient on leave ceases to be liable to recall at the expiry of the period of six months beginning with the first day of his absence, unless either he has returned to the hospital or has been transferred to another meantime; or he is absent without leave at the expiration of the six months.[4]

The purpose of these provisions on leave of absence is to give the opportunity for the hospital and the local social services department to work together towards re-habilitation especially where discharge is the final goal.[5]

6. Patients Absent Without Leave

A patient who is absent without leave or who fails to return on expiration of leave or on recall or who absents himself without permission from any place where he was required to reside as a condition of leave of absence, may be taken into custody and returned to the hospital or place he was supposed to reside at by any mental welfare officer, or by any officer on the staff of the hospital, or by any constable, or by any person authorised in writing by the managers of the hospital.[6] However, a psychopathic patient or one with mild subnormality over the age of 21 may not be so taken into custody after the lapse of a

---

[1] Section 39 (1), (2) and (3).   [2] Section 39 (4).
[3] See further, ss. 43–48.   [4] Section 39 (5).
[5] See Edwards, *Mental Health Services* (4th Edn.) at p. 144 regards it as 'a clinical measure within medical prescription'. This view is narrower than that suggested in the text, and, if right, explains why a Review Tribunal has not got power to order leave of absence.
[6] Section 40 (1).

period of six months starting with the first day of his absence without leave, and any other patient not after the lapse of 28 days. A patient who has not returned or been taken into custody within the relevant period ceases to be liable to be detained.[1]

It will be observed that 'any officer on the staff of the hospital' may take into custody a patient absent without leave. There is no condition that the officer must have been authorised to act nor is the description limited to officers ordinarily in charge of patients. Further, there is no definition of the expression *officer* so as to limit it to any particular class of employee. Seemingly, therefore, as all employees from medical to kitchen staff are officers of their employing Authority under the National Health Service Act 1977,[2] anyone on the staff of a hospital may take into custody a patient absent without leave. As s. 40 also applies to a mental nursing home, could the same liberal interpretation of 'officer' also be applied there? It would seem that the same broad definition could be applied only if all staff had been formally designated officers. Otherwise it is unlikely that the court would regard junior domestic and manual staff as officers. Under Reg. 24 of the 1960 Regulations, the managers of a hospital may authorise in writing any person to retake a patient under s. 40.

7. Responsibility for Acts of Patients Liable to Detention

Is a Health Authority responsible for the acts of a patient liable to detention whilst he is absent with or without leave from hospital? In the *Home Office* v. *Dorset Yacht Club*,[3] the House of Lords held that there was a duty of care owed by those responsible for the custody of borstal boys to take steps to prevent the boys causing damage to the property (and presumably persons in the neighbourhood). In that case, three boys had escaped and damaged a yacht belonging to the Club. Accordingly it would appear that as regards a Health Authority 'a duty of care would be owed to those whose safety, as reasonable foresight would show, might be in jeopardy'.[4] Perhaps pointedly however, the House declined to approve *Holgate* v. *Lancashire Mental Hospitals Board*.[5] There, the defendants, who were responsible for administering an institution under the Mental Deficiency Act 1913, were held liable for negligence in letting out on licence a lunatic with a bad criminal history who committed a savage assault. The House in *Dorset Yacht* followed Lord Blackburn in *Geddis* v. *Proprietors of Bann Reservoir*[6] holding that there was no liability for doing what legislature has authorised but there could be if it were done negligently. If the legislature gave a discretion then liability was not imposed for a mere error of judgment but for the negligent use of the discretion. Where a degree of

---

[1] Section 40 (3).   [2] Section 128.   [3] [1970] A.C. 1004.
[4] *Per* Lord Morris at p. 1041.   [5] [1937] 4 All E.R. 19.   [6] (1878) 3 App. Cos. 430, 455–6.

freedom was given to those in custody with a view to making them better citizens, it neither of itself imposed liability for any damage caused by that freedom nor absolved the authority from exercising due care for the property and persons of others.[1]

Also in *Dorset Yacht*, as regards prisoners but in words that seem at least equally applicable to mental patients Lord Morris said:[2]

'If someone is serving a sentence of imprisonment and consequently is not free to order his own movements I would think it eminently reasonable to hold that those in charge of the prison owe him a duty to take reasonable care to protect him from being assaulted by a fellow-prisoner who may have shown himself to be one who might cause harm (*Ellis* v. *Home Office*[3]; *D'Arcy* v. *Prison Commissioners*[4]). In each of those two cases the defendants had the power to control the persons who caused injury to the respective plaintiffs. The defendants were not under a duty to ensure that no prisoner would be hurt by a fellow-prisoner and the mere occurrence of such an event did not by itself prove that there had been a failure of duty. The circumstances under which the injuries were caused were, however, such as to make it eminently appropriate to hold that a duty of care arose.'

It seems that these principles would apply if a claim were made in respect of injury or damage done by a patient discharged by the responsible medical officer. And likewise[5] if he failed to make a report under s. 43 or s. 44 of the Mental Health Act 1959 extending the period of the patient's liability to detention or, under s. 48, barring the nearest relative's right of discharge or for a failure to consider the dangerousness of the patient as required by the 1975 Amendment Act before reclassifying a patient. Section 43 (3) of the 1959 Act includes 'the protection of other persons' and ss. 44 (2) and 48 (2) '. . . likely to act in a manner dangerous to other persons . . .'. With that background it would not be unreasonable to suggest that negligent failure to make a report might afford ground for an action in respect of injury to a third party but not damage to his property, since the likelihood of damage to property is not one of the criteria.

Possibly the provisions of s. 141 (2) of the 1959 Act,[6] which require leave of the High Court to be obtained before an action in respect of

---

[1] In a series of cases starting with *R.* v. *Croydon Juvenile Court Justices ex p. Croydon, London Borough Council* [1973] 2 W.L.R. 61 the Court has considered the liability for fines that may be imposed on an authority under the Children and Young Persons Act 1933 where a child in the care and control of the authority commits a criminal offence. The definition of *guardian* under the 1933 Act is wide enough to include a Health Authority and so they are potentially liable in the same way as a local authority. The liability is only to be imposed where the authority has shown neglect in any particular case *Somerset C.C.* v. *Kingscott* [1975] 1 W.L.R. 283. This liability is not to be imposed where the child is not under the control of the authority because, *e.g.* he is in an independent institution *Somerset C.C.* v. *Brice* [1973] 1 W.L.R. 1169 or *e.g.* is at home with his parents *Lincoln Corp.* v. *Parker* [1974] 2 All E.R. 949.
[2] At p. 1040.   [3] [1953] 2 All E.R. 149.   [4] *The Times*, 17 November, 1955.
[5] Dr Speller doubted the liability for the failure to make a report though not the negligent discharge.
[6] See below, p. 552.

duties under the Act is brought would apply to all the possible causes of action here discussed.

It is less clear that s. 141 would be applicable in the case of an action by a patient injured by a fellow patient. The principles of such liability would appear to be the same as those outlined above.

8. Transfer of Patients

(a) Generally

In such circumstances and subject to such conditions as may be prescribed by regulations made by the Secretary of State,[1] a patient liable to be detained under Part IV may be transferred to another hospital or into guardianship of a Local Social Services Authority or of a person approved by such authority; and similarly a patient subject to guardianship may be transferred to the guardianship of another Local Social Services Authority or person, or be transferred to a hospital.[2] If, however, a patient who has attained the age of 16 years is transferred from guardianship to a hospital he may apply to a Mental Health Review Tribunal within six months.

Express provision is also made for the transfer of patients liable to detention from one hospital vested in the Secretary of State under the Health Service Acts, to another hospital under what is now the same Area Health Authority (or special Health Authority) and the provisions of Part IV of the 1959 Act apply as though the patient had originally been admitted to the second hospital.[3] Such transfer is not within the regulations referred to in s. 41 (1), except as to conveyance of the patient.[4]

Where a patient, being liable to be detained in hospital under an application for admission for observation or for treatment, is transferred to another hospital, he is treated as though he had originally been admitted to that hospital in pursuance of the application. Similarly, if a patient is transferred from guardianship to hospital, the provisions of Part IV apply to him as though he had been admitted to hospital at the time of the acceptance of the guardianship application. There are analogous provisions in respect of transfer from guardianship of one authority or person to that of another.[5]

(b) Form of authority for transfer

Authority for transfer from hospital to hospital under s. 41 (1) (a) of a patient liable to be detained must be given in Form 16 in the Schedule to the 1960 Regulations, or for transfer to guardianship in Form 17, by the managers of the hospital where the patient is liable to be detained,

---

[1] See Part IV of the 1960 Regulations, the provisions of which are referred to in the appropriate places.
[2] Section 41 (1).   [3] Section 41 (2).   [4] Section 41 (3) and (4).   [5] Section 41 (2).

or by an officer authorised by them. In the case of a patient in a mental nursing home the authority may also be given by the registration authority of the home or, if the patient is maintained under contract with a Regional or Area Health Authority or a special Health Authority, by the board or by an authorised officer of the Authority.[1]

In the case of a patient who, immediately before the commencement of the Act was in custody of a relative or friend under s. 57 of the Lunacy Act 1890, and who is still liable to be detained under para. 7 of the Sixth Schedule to the Act, the managers of the hospital from which he was transferred will have the right to make the transfer.[2]

Authority must not be given for a patient's transfer to hospital unless the person giving the authority is satisfied that arrangements have been made for the admission of the patient to that hospital within 28 days of the giving of the authority.[3]

The completion of Form 16 is not necessary in respect of transfers from one hospital to another under the same Area or special Health Authority[4] nor from one special hospital to another by direction of the Secretary of State under s. 99 (2),[5] nor from one mental nursing home to another where both nursing homes are under the same managers.[6]

Authority for transfer to guardianship will have no effect until confirmed by the Local Social Services Authority which would be the responsible Local Social Services Authority if it took effect. When the proposed guardian is a person other than the Local Social Services Authority, the authority for transfer is not to be confirmed without the agreement of that person. The confirmation must specify the date on which the transfer is to take effect.[7]

9. Duration of Detention

Subject to the provisions of the Act, a patient admitted to hospital on application for treatment may be detained in hospital initially for a period not exceeding one year, beginning with the day of admission.[8] It is, however, the duty of the responsible medical officer to examine any patient detained in hospital within a period of two months ending with the day on which the authority for his detention expires and, if it appears to him that, in the interests of the patient's health or safety or for the protection of other persons, the patient should continue to be liable to be detained he must so report in the prescribed form[9] to the managers of the hospital. When a report is so furnished the authority for detention is thereby renewed for one year in the case of a first renewal, otherwise

[1] The 1960 Regulations, Reg. 13 (1) and (2).
[3] Regulation 13 (3).
[5] Regulation 13 (7).
[7] Regulation 13 (5) and (6).
[9] Section 43 (3), 1960 Regulations, Form 10A.

[2] The proviso to Reg. 13 (2).
[4] Section 41 (3).
[6] Regulation 13 (4).
[8] Section 43 (1).

for two years[1] save in the case of a psychopathic or subnormal patient reaching the age of 25.

A patient liable to be detained under an application for admission for treatment as a psychopathic or as one suffering from mild subnormality ceases to be so liable on attaining the age of 25 unless the responsible medical officer, who must have examined the patient within two months before he attains that age, furnishes a report in the prescribed form[2] to the managers that it appears to him that if the patient were released he would be likely to act in a manner dangerous to other persons or to himself.[3] Where such a report has been furnished the authority for detention continues beyond the age of 25, subject to the provisions of s. 43 as to renewal of authority for detention at two-yearly intervàls.[4] Consequently if a patient had reached the age of 25 at the end of the first six months of a two-year renewal under s. 43, and a report under s. 44 had been made at the proper time authorising his detention beyond that age, he would then be liable to be detained only for a further period of 18 months failing renewal of authority in due time under s. 43 for his detention for another two years. If a patient reaches the age of 25 on the last day of the current authority for his detention reports should be made under both sections of the Act, one to indicate that the conditions for the patient's detention beyond the age of 25 are fulfilled and the other to authorise a two-year renewal. The provisions of s. 44 having been complied with on the single occasion of the patient attaining the age of 25 the psychopathic or mildly subnormal patient can — like any other patient — be detained for any further number of two-year periods, on the broader grounds set out in s. 43 (3) viz., 'that it is necessary in the interests of the patient's health or safety or for the protection of other persons'.

If a report is furnished under s. 43 in respect of a patient who has attained the age of 16, the managers, unless they discharge him, must cause him to be informed, and he may, within the period of renewal, apply to a Mental Health Review Tribunal.[5] Also, if a report is furnished under s. 44 for the detention after the age of 25 of a psychopathic or mildly subnormal patient, the managers of the hospital must cause the patient and the nearest relative of the patient to be informed and the patient or that relative may apply to a Mental Health Review Tribunal within 28 days of the patient's attaining the age of 25.[6] It appears that the right of application under s. 44 (3) is in addition to, and not in substitution for, that given in s. 43 (6) to any patient who has attained the age of 16 in respect of the renewal of authority for detention under s. 43 (3).

[1] Section 43 (2).   [2] Section 44 (1), 1960 Regulations, Form 11.
[3] Section 40 (2).   [4] Section 44 (1) and (2).
[5] Section 43 (6).   [6] Section 44 (3).

10. Patients Absent Without Leave — Renewal of Authority to Detain

If, on the day on which a patient would otherwise cease to be liable to be detained he is absent without leave, he will not then cease to be so liable until the expiry of the period within which he could have been taken into custody under s. 40[1] or until he is returned or returns to the hospital, whichever is earlier and, if he is returned or returns, for a week thereafter. A report under s. 43 (3) or s. 44 (2) may then be furnished within that extended time[2] but for this to be possible the patient must have been duly examined. The period of any renewal of authority under the provisions of s. 45 dates from the day on which the authority renewed would have expired under s. 43.[3]

11. Patients Sentenced to Imprisonment, etc.

If a patient liable to be detained on application for admission for treatment is detained in custody in pursuance of any sentence or order passed or made by a court in the United Kingdom (including an order committing or remanding him in custody), and is so detained for a period exceeding, or for successive periods exceeding in aggregate six months, the application ceases to have effect at the expiration of that period. If, however, a patient is in custody for some shorter period, and would in the ordinary course have ceased to be liable for treatment on or before the day he is discharged from custody, he does not cease to be liable to detention until the end of that day and, for the purpose of ss. 40 and 45 is treated as though he had absented himself without leave on that day.[4]

Seemingly, the effect of s. 46 (2), relating to extensions of authority for detention in hospital of a patient in custody for a period, or successive periods, not exceeding six months, is to allow his being retaken within the appropriate period as laid down in s. 40 (3) dating from his release from custody and not either from what would have been the normal day of expiry of authority for detention or from his being taken into custody. Hence, a person released after not more than six months in prison, the authority for whose detention in hospital would normally have expired when he had been in prison a month, or six months, as the case might be, will still be liable to be retaken within the period of 28 days — or six months, if applicable — from the date of his discharge from custody, whilst the patient but a day longer in prison would be automatically discharged under s. 46 (1). It seems, too, that any renewal of the authority for detention after the patient had returned or been returned to hospital would date from the day of his discharge from

---

[1] See p. 491 et seq.   [2] Section 45 (1) and (2).
[3] Section 45 (3).   [4] Section 46.

prison and not as, under s. 45, from the date of normal expiry of the authority being renewed.

12. Discharge of Patients

By s. 47 and subject to the provisions of s. 48 an order for discharge of a patient liable to be detained on an application for admission must be in writing. Such an order may be made in respect of a patient —

(a) where the patient is liable to be detained in a hospital in pursuance of an application for admission for observation by the responsible medical officer or by the managers of the hospital;

(b) where the patient is liable to be so detained in pursuance of an application for admission for treatment, by the responsible medical officer, by the managers or by the nearest relative of the patient;

and where the patient is liable to be detained in a mental nursing home in pursuance of an application for admission for observation or for treatment, an order for his discharge may also be made by the registration authority or, if he is maintained under a contract with a Regional, Area or special Health Authority, by that Authority.[1] These powers conferred on any Authority or body of persons to discharge a patient may be exercised by any three or more members of that Authority or body authorised by them in that behalf.[2]

Under s. 48 (2) the nearest relative must give 72 hours' notice in writing to the managers of the hospital of his making an order for the discharge of a patient and the order when made will be of no effect if, meantime, the responsible medical officer has furnished to the managers a report that in his opinion the patient, if discharged, would be likely to act in a manner dangerous to other persons or to himself.[3] If such a report is made, the relative can make no further order for discharge for six months beginning with the date of the report. Also, by s. 48 (1), when a report has been furnished under s. 44 for the detention of a psychopathic or subnormal patient beyond the age of 25, the nearest relative may not order the discharge of the patient within six months of the date of the report. The managers must cause the nearest relative to be informed of any barring report under s. 48 (2), and the relative may within 28 days of being so informed apply to a Mental Health Review Tribunal.

D. THE NEAREST RELATIVE

1. Who is the Nearest Relative

The nearest relative of a patient for the purpose of Part IV of the Act

---

[1] Section 47 as amended by the Reorganisation Act 1973.

[2] Section 47 (4). In the case of an Area Health Authority, the Secretary of State has required that a sub-committee be set up (it may include persons who are not members of the Authority) and by resolution of the Authority or of the sub-committee three members of the sub-committee have the power of discharge, H.R.C. (74) 7.

[3] 1960 Regulations, Form 12.

is to be ascertained in accordance with the provisions of ss. 49–51 and subject to the effect of an order of the county court under ss. 52 and 53.

Under s. 49 (1) usually the nearest relative is the person first described in the following list: (*a*) husband or wife, (*b*) son or daughter, (*c*) father, (*d*) mother, (*e*) brother or sister, (*f*) grandparents, (*g*) grandchild, (*h*) uncle or aunt, (*i*) nephew or niece. An adopted[1] person here is treated as a child of the adoptor or adoptors and not of any other person and an illegitimate child is treated as the legitimate child of his mother. Relatives of the half blood rank immediately after relatives description of the whole blood.[2] The elder or eldest of two or more relatives of the same class (*e.g.*, sons and daughters) being preferred to the other or others of their relatives in that class regardless of sex.[3] Hence, the elder child being a daughter would be the nearest relative and not her younger brother.

If the person who would be the nearest relative as thus ascertained by s. 49 (4):

(*a*) is not ordinarily resident within the United Kingdom; or
(*b*) being the husband or wife of the patient, is permanently separated from the patient, either by agreement or under an order of a court, or has deserted or has been deserted by the patient for a period which has not come to an end; or
(*c*) not being the husband, wife, father or mother of the patient, is for the time being under 18[4] years of age;
(*d*) is a man against whom an order divesting him of an authority over the patient has been made under s. 38 of the Sexual Offences Act 1956 (which relates to incest with a girl under 18[4]) and has not been rescinded,

the nearest relative of the patient is ascertained as if he were dead.

If the husband or wife is thus disregarded and some other person is living with the patient as the patient's husband or wife, or was so living until the patient became an in-patient in hospital, and had or has been so living for not less than six months, that person would be treated as husband or wife for the purpose of ascertaining the nearest relative.[5]

In any case in which the rights and powers of a parent of a patient, being a child or young person, are vested in a Local Authority or other person under s. 75 of the Children and Young Persons Act 1933 (which relates to children and young persons committed to the care of fit persons under that Act); s. 79 of the Children and Young Persons (Scotland) Act 1937 (which makes corresponding provision in Scotland); or s. 3 of the Children Act 1948 (which relates to children in respect of whom parental rights have been assumed under s. 2 of that Act), that authority or person is deemed to be the nearest relative of the

---

[1] *i.e.*, validly adopted in England, Scotland or Northern Ireland. See s. 49 (5).
[2] Section 49 (2).   [3] Section 49 (3).
[4] 18 substituted for 21 by s. 1 (3) of the Family Law Reform Act 1969.
[5] Section 49 (6).

patient in preference to any person except the patient's husband or wife (if any) and, except in a case where the said rights and powers are vested in a Local Authority by virtue of subsection (2) of the said section, any parent of the patient, not being the person on whose account the resolution mentioned in that subsection was passed.[1]

Where a patient who has not attained the age of 18[2] years is under guardianship by order of a court or by virtue of a deed or will executed by his father or mother or is under joint guardianship of two persons of whom one is such a person as aforesaid; or is by order of a court in matrimonial or other proceedings or by virtue of a separation agreement in the custody of any such person, the person or persons having guardianship or custody shall, to the exclusion of any other person, be deemed to be his nearest relative.[3] It seems here to be contemplated that two persons, as co-guardians, might have equal powers as 'nearest relative'. This is altogether contrary to the general principle embodied in s. 49 (1) where the father takes precedence of the mother. It seems that if the mother nominated a guardian by deed or will and died, that guardian would have equal powers with the father although the appointing mother would not have done so.

For the purpose of s. 51 *court* includes a court in Scotland or Northern Ireland and a person is treated as being in the custody of another person if he would have been in that person's custody but for s. 34 of the Act (which refers to guardianship of mentally disordered patients).[4]

2. Delegation of Functions by Nearest Relative

The nearest relative of a patient, as defined in s. 49 of the Act and including a person deemed to be the nearest relative under s. 51, may authorise in writing any other person (not being the patient or a person mentioned in s. 49 (4) of the Act)[5] to perform in respect of the patient the functions conferred upon him by or under Part IV of the Act and may revoke any such authority.

Such authority operates to confer the powers to the exclusion of the nearest relative but becomes effective only on its being given in writing to the person named. The nearest relative must also forthwith give notice in writing of the authority or revocation to the managers of the hospital in the case of a patient liable to be detained there, and to the guardian and the responsible Local Social Services Authority in the case of a patient subject to guardianship.

Any revocation of authority becomes operative on receipt of a notice

[1] Section 50. Curiously a custodian under the 1975 Children Act does not become the nearest relative.

[2] 18 substituted for 21 by s. 1 (3) of the Family Law Reform Act 1969.

[3] Section 51.

[4] Section 51 (3) and (4).

[5] *i.e.*, persons who would not themselves be qualified to act as nearest relative despite the necessary relationship.

of revocation by the person to whom the authority was given or by the guardian or any of the authorities above mentioned.[1]

3. Appointment by Court of Acting Nearest Relative

(a) Appointment

On grounds set out hereunder, the county court may, on application by order direct that the functions of the nearest relative of a patient shall, during the continuance in force of the order, be exercisable by the applicant (or by the Local Social Services Authority, if the applicant is a mental welfare officer),[2] or by any other person specified in the application, being a person who, in the opinion of the court, is a proper person to act as the patient's nearest relative and is willing to do so.[3] An application may be made by (a) any relative of the patient; (b) any other person with whom the patient is residing (or, if the patient is then an in-patient in a hospital, was last residing before he was admitted); or (c) a mental welfare officer.

Section 52 (3) provides that the grounds on which an application for an order may be made are as follows:

(a) that the patient has no nearest relative within the meaning of the Act or that it is not reasonably practicable to ascertain whether he has such a relative, or who that relative is;

(b) that the nearest relative of the patient is incapable of acting as such by reason of mental disorder or other illness;

(c) that the nearest relative of the patient unreasonably objects to the making of an application for admission for treatment or a guardianship application in respect of the patient; or

(d) that the nearest relative of the patient has exercised without due regard to the welfare of the patient or the interests of the public his power to discharge the patient from hospital or guardianship under Part IV of the Act, or is likely to do so.

In W. v. L.,[4] the Court of Appeal discussed the meaning of 'unreasonably objects' in paragraph (c). It held that the 'proper test is to ask what a reasonable [relative] in [his] place would do in all the circumstances of the case' and not to ask whether the nearest relative was behaving reasonably from his own point of view or whether his anguish of mind is understandable.

If immediately before the expiry of the period for which a patient is liable to be detained for observation application is made to the county court on grounds (c) or (d) above, the period for which the patient may be detained for observation is extended until the application is finally disposed of and, if an order is made, for a further period of seven days.

---

[1] The 1960 Regulations, Reg. 25. [2] Section 52 (2). [3] Section 52 (1) and (5).
[4] [1974] Q.B. 711 and see also P.T.W. v. G.L. Unreported decided on 24th May, 1973. A copy of the judgment is in the Bar Library at the Royal Courts of Justice.

The application is deemed finally disposed of at the expiration of the time allowed for appeal or when, notice of appeal having been given, the appeal has been heard or withdrawn.[1]

If an order is made it still remains in force notwithstanding that the person who was the patient's nearest relative when the order was made is no longer the nearest relative.[2] But even whilst an order is in force, if the patient is detained for treatment or is under guardianship, the patient's nearest relative, ascertained in accordance with ss. 49–51[3] (*i.e.*, as distinct from the person appointed by the court to exercise his function), may make an application to a Mental Health Review Tribunal within 12 months of the making of the order and within any subsequent 12 months during which the order continues in force.[4] Such a relative is sometimes referred to as the 'displaced relative'.

(b) Discharge or variation of order

The county court may at any time discharge the order on the application of the person having the functions of the nearest relative under it; or, if the order was made on ground (*a*) or (*b*) or where the person who was the nearest relative at the time of the order has ceased to be the nearest relative, on the application of the nearest relative.[5]

An order may be varied on the application of the person exercising functions under it or of a mental welfare officer, by substituting a local Social Services Authority or any other person who, in the opinion of the court, is a proper person to exercise those functions, being an authority or person who is willing to do so.[6] If the person exercising the functions of nearest relative under s. 52 dies, an application for discharge or variation may be made by any relative but, meantime, the functions of nearest relative are not exercisable by any person.[7]

An order for the appointment of a person to exercise the functions of nearest relative ceases to have effect after three months if the patient was not at the time of the making of the order liable to detention for treatment or subject to guardianship and has not become so liable or subject during that period. If the patient was so liable or subject when the order was made or becomes so within three months, the order ceases to have effect when the patient ceases to be so liable or subject. Transfer under the provisions of the Act from guardianship to hospital care or *vice versa* does not affect the order.[8]

The discharge or variation of a county court order does not affect the validity of anything previously done in pursuance of that order.[9]

County court rules may provide for the hearing and determination of applications under ss. 52 and 53 otherwise than in open court; for the

[1] Section 52 (4).
[2] Section 52 (5).
[3] See definition in s. 147 (1).
[4] Section 52 (6).
[5] Section 53 (1).
[6] Section 53 (2) as amended.
[7] Section 53 (3).
[8] Section 53 (4).
[9] Section 53 (5).

admission of evidence of such descriptions as may be specified in the rules notwithstanding anything to the contrary in any enactment or rule of law relating to the admissibility of evidence; and for the visiting and interviewing of patients in private by or under the directions of the court.[1]

E. PATIENTS CONCERNED IN CRIMINAL PROCEEDINGS

Part V of the Act deals with the admission, either to hospital or into guardianship, of patients concerned in criminal proceedings and of patients, being children or young persons before the court as being in need of care and protection or beyond control. It also deals with the classification, transfer, licence, *etc.*, of such patients.

1. Admission to and Detention in Hospital

(a) Hospital orders

(i) *Generally.* A *hospital order* is an order under s. 60 of the Act made by a court of competent jurisdiction for the detention in hospital of an offender suffering from mental illness, psychopathic disorder, mild subnormality or severe subnormality. A magistrates' court may make such an order without recording a conviction. Also under s. 62 a hospital order may be made by a juvenile court in respect of a child or young person brought before the court under s. 62 or s. 64 of the Children and Young Persons Act 1933.

A hospital order may be made only if the court is satisfied that arrangements have been made for the patient's reception into hospital within 28 days beginning with the date of the making of the order.[2] A hospital order must specify the form or forms of mental disorder from which, upon the medical evidence under s. 60 (1), the offender is found by the court to be suffering.[3]

(ii) *Effect of hospital order.* A hospital order is sufficient authority for a constable, a mental welfare officer or any other person directed to do so by the court, to convey the patient to the hospital specified within a period of 28 days[4] and for the managers of the hospital to admit him at any time during that period and thereafter detain him in accordance with the provisions of the Act.[5] The court may also give such directions

---

[1] Section 55. See the County Court (Amendment) Rules 1960, S.I. No. 1275.

[2] Section 60 (3).

[3] There are rules in the Act as to the requisite medical evidence but these do not concern us here (see ss. 60 and 62).

[4] Including the day on which the order is made (s. 60 (3)). The hospital specified may be any hospital with an available vacancy in any part of the country. (*R.* v. *Marsden* (Practice Note) [1968] 1 W.L.R. 785; [1968] 2 All E.R. 341.)

[5] Section 63 (1).

as it thinks fit for the conveyance of the patient to a place of safety[1] and his detention there pending his admission to the hospital within the period of 28 days. If it is impracticable by reason of emergency or other special circumstances for the patient to be received into the named hospital within 28 days, the Secretary of State may direct his admission to some other hospital. The person having custody of the patient is to be so informed and the order is to be read as though the name of that other hospital were substituted for that specified in the order.[2]

A patient admitted to a hospital under a hospital order is to be treated for the purposes of Part IV of the Act, other than ss. 31 and 32,[3] as if he had been so admitted on the date of the order in pursuance of an application for admission for treatment except that by s. 63 (3):

(a) the power to order the discharge of the patient under s. 47 shall not be exercisable by the nearest relative; and

(b) the special provisions relating to the expiration and renewal of authority for detention in the case of psychopathic or [mild] subnormal patients will not apply.

The full effect of these modifications in the case of a patient subject to a hospital order is set out in the second column of the Third Schedule to the Act.

Where a patient is admitted to hospital in pursuance of a hospital order, any previous application or hospital order by virtue of which he was liable to be detained ceases to have effect. If, however, the later order, or the conviction on which it was made, is quashed on appeal, the earlier application or order remains effective.[4] Also, an earlier hospital order, if coupled with an order restricting discharge, remains effective notwithstanding the making of a later order.[5]

(iii) *Re-classification.* Section 38 under which, by report, the responsible medical officer may alter the classification of a patient received under s. 26, also applies to a patient admitted on a hospital order made by the court under s. 60 unless such order be accompanied by a restriction order made under s. 65.[6] It likewise applies to a patient transferred to hospital from a prison or other place of detention on a direction made by the Home Secretary unless he has also given a direction restricting discharge.[7]

---

[1] In s. 80, *a place of safety* is defined for the purposes of Part V to mean 'in relation to a person not being a child or young person, any police station, prison, or remand centre, or any hospital the managers of which are willing temporarily to receive him, and in relation to a child or young person, a place of safety within the meaning of the Children and Young Persons Act 1933'.

[2] Section 64.

[3] Section 31 sets out the effects of an application for admission and s. 32 relates to the curing of defects in an application or in the supporting medical recommendations.

[4] Section 63 (5).   [5] Section 65 (4).

[6] Third Schedule. Similarly as regards a patient in respect of whom a guardianship order or direction has been made. (Sections 63 and 79).

[7] See ss. 72 to 74.

Although, because of the provisions of s. 26 (2) and s. 44 (2), a patient who has been admitted on application under s. 26 as suffering from mental illness or severe subnormality may be detained after re-classification as suffering from psychopathy or mild subnormality provided the application for admission has been made before he attained the age of 21 and the re-classifying report before he reached the age of 25[1] this is not so in the case of a patient who has been admitted on a hospital order or direction and similarly re-classified. His re-classification will not nullify the effect of the order or direction under which he has been admitted. The reason for the difference is that, unlike an application under s. 26, a hospital order or a direction on grounds of psychopathic disorder or mild subnormality may be made whatever may be the age of the patient[2] and s. 44 (2) as to renewal of authority within two months prior to his reaching the age of 25 has no application.[3]

Under s. 60 (2) a magistrates court has power to make a hospital order in respect of a person suffering from mental illness or severe subnormality without in certain circumstances convicting him. Such a patient is re-classifiable. The 1975 Mental Health (Amendment) Act applies.

A patient subject to a hospital order accompanied by a restriction order is not re-classifiable under s. 38; neither is a person in custody who may have been transferred to hospital on the Home Secretary's warrant; nor any person subject to a transfer direction accompanied by a direction restricting his discharge.[4] Furthermore, in the case of such a patient, no reference may be made to a Mental Health Review Tribunal save by the Home Secretary, and by him only for advice.[5] Hence no question of the effect of re-classification by a Tribunal arises.

(iv) *Applications to Mental Health Review Tribunal.* Without prejudice to any provisions of Part IV which may be applicable,[6] a patient admitted to hospital in pursuance of a hospital order, not being coupled with an order restricting discharge, may within six months beginning with the date of the order or with the day on which he attains the age of 16 years, whichever is the later, make application to a Tribunal for discharge. The nearest relative may similarly make application within 12 months and in any subsequent period of 12 months.[7]

(b) *Orders restricting discharge*

(i) *Generally.* Subject to the provisions of the Act, a Crown Court when making a hospital order may also make an order restricting

---

[1] See p. 496.   [2] So can a guardianship order or direction. Section 60.
[3] Nor in fact have any of the provisions in Part IV relating to the expiration and renewal of authority for detention and guardship in the case of s. 26 patients. Section 63 (3). The Mental Health (Amendment) Act 1975 does not therefore apply.
[4] Third Schedule of 1959 Act.   [5] Section 66 (6).   [6] See s. 63 (3).
[7] Section 63 (4). As to patients subject to an order restricting discharge, see ss. 65 and 66.

discharge under s. 65. By s. 65 (3) the special restrictions so long as such an order is in force are:

(a) none of the provisions of Part IV of the Act relating to the duration, renewal and expiration of the authority for the detention of patients applies, and the patient continues to be liable to be detained until he is duly discharged[1] under Part IV or absolutely discharged by the Home Secretary under s. 66 (2);

(b) no application may be made to a Mental Health Review Tribunal either under s. 63 or under any provisions of Part IV of the Act;

(c) the following powers are exercisable only with the consent of the Home Secretary —

    (i) power to grant leave of absence under s. 39 of this Act;

    (ii) power to transfer the patient under s. 41 of this Act;

    (iii) power to order discharge under s. 47 of this Act;

and if leave of absence is granted under the said s. 39 the power to recall the patient under that section shall be vested in the Secretary of State as well as the responsible medical officer.

(d) the power of the Secretary of State and the power to take the patient into custody and return him under s. 40 of this Act, may be exercised at any time.

The provisions of Part IV of the Act described in the first column of the Third Schedule have effect in relation to a patient subject to an order restricting discharge, subject to the exceptions and modifications set out in the third column of that schedule in lieu of those set out in the second column.[2] The remaining provisions of Part IV do not apply.[2]

(ii) *Discharge of restriction order.* If the Home Secretary is satisfied that an order restricting the discharge of a patient is no longer required for the protection of the public, he may direct that the patient shall cease to be subject to the special restrictions set out in s. 65.[3] Where an order restricting discharge of a patient so ceases to have effect while the relevant hospital order continues in force the provisions of s. 63 and the Third Schedule apply to the patient as if he had been admitted to the hospital in pursuance of a hospital order (without an order restricting his discharge) made on the date on which the order restricting his discharge ceased to have effect.[4]

(iii) *Discharge, etc., of patient subject to restriction order.* The Home Secretary may at any time, by warrant, discharge from hospital a patient subject to a restriction order and may do so either absolutely or conditionally. In the case of an absolute discharge the hospital order and the restriction order both cease to have effect.[5]

If a patient subject to a restriction order has been conditionally discharged, the Home Secretary may at any time during the continuance in force of the restriction order, by warrant, recall the patient to such

---

[1] Duly discharged here means discharged under the provisions of s. 47 as modified for the purposes of s. 65, *viz.*, with the consent of the Home Secretary. The references to the nearest relative in s. 47 are omitted in respect of patients subject to the provisions of s. 65.

[2] Section 63 (3).   [3] Section 66 (1).   [4] Section 65 (5).   [5] Section 66 (2).

hospital as may be specified in the warrant. If that hospital is not the hospital from which the patient had been conditionally discharged, the hospital order and the order restricting discharge shall have effect as if the hospital specified in the warrant were substituted for the hospital specified in the hospital order. In any case, the patient shall be treated for the purpose of s. 40[1] as if he had absented himself without leave from the hospital specified in the warrant, and if the order restricting his discharge was made for a specified period, that period will not in any event expire until the patient returns or is returned to the hospital.[2]

If an order restricting discharge of a patient ceases to have effect after the patient has been conditionally discharged under s. 66, the patient, unless he had been previously recalled, will be deemed to be absolutely discharged on the date when the order ceases to have effect, and ceases to be liable to be detained by virtue of the relevant hospital order.[3]

Whilst a patient is subject to a restriction order the Home Secretary may, in the interests of justice or for the purposes of any public inquiry, direct him to be taken to any place in Great Britain, being kept in custody until his return to hospital unless the Home Secretary otherwise directs.[4]

(iv) *Reference of restriction order cases to Tribunal.* Reference to the Mental Health Review Tribunal in the case of a patient subject to an order restricting discharge may be made only by the Home Secretary and only for advice,[5] this matter and also the Home Secretary's power of absolute or conditional discharge being more fully treated above. In practice patients commonly request the Home Secretary to make the reference and about one-third of the cases heard by the Tribunals arise in this way.

2. Persons in Custody During Her Majesty's Pleasure

Any person detained during Her Majesty's pleasure under the Criminal Procedure (Insanity) Act 1964, or under any of the Acts set out in s. 71 (3) of the 1959 Act as amended, being a person found not guilty by reason of insanity or under a disability constituting a bar to his being tried will, by virtue of s. 5 and Schedule 1 of the 1964 Act, be detained in such place of safety[6] as the court may order, being removed to hospital[7] on the Home Secretary's warrant within two months. The effect is as of a hospital order with an order restricting discharge for an unlimited time. The patient is deemed to have been admitted at the date of the warrant.[8] The appeal court on quashing a verdict of not guilty by reason of insanity may make an order for the defendant's admission to hospital for observation within 7 days.

[1] See p. 491.
[2] Section 66 (3).
[3] Section 66 (4).
[4] Section 66 (5).
[5] Section 66.
[6] For definition of *place of safety* see s. 80 (1).
[7] Section 71 (2).
[8] Section 71 (4).

If the Home Secretary, after consultation with the responsible medical officer, is satisfied that a person detained in hospital as under a disability can properly be tried he may remit that person to prison or to a remand centre for trial at the Crown Court and on arrival there the direction for his detention in hospital ceases to have effect.[1]

Under s. 7 and Schedule 2 of the Act of 1964 special verdicts as above, having similar consequences, are now also given by Courts-Marshal where appropriate.

3. Transfer to Hospital, etc., of Prisoners

If in the case of a person serving a sentence of imprisonment[2] the Home Secretary is satisfied, by reports from at least two medical practitioners[3] that that person is suffering from mental illness, psychopathic disorder, mild subnormality or severe subnormality and that the mental disorder is of a nature or degree which warrants the detention of the patient in hospital for medical treatment, the Home Secretary may, if he is of opinion having regard to the public interest and all the circumstances that it is expedient to so do, by warrant, direct that that person be removed to and detained in such hospital (not being a mental nursing home) as may be specified in the direction.[4] Such a transfer direction ceases to have effect at the expiration of the period of 14 days beginning with the date on which it is given unless within that period the person in respect of whom it was given has been received into the hospital specified therein.[5]

A transfer direction with respect to any person has the like effect as a hospital order made in his case.[6] It may also be coupled with 'a direction restricting discharge' which has similar effect to a restriction order under s. 65.[7]

Under s. 73 the Home Secretary also has power of giving transfer directions when, he is satisfied by reports from at least two medical practitioners, persons suffering from mental illness or severe subnormality of a nature or degree which warrant their detention in a hospital for medical treatment and who are committed in custody for trial or sentence by a Crown Court. The section applies to most persons[8] who are in custody who are suffering from the mental disorders described. Again the 1975 Amendment Act applies on a re-classification.

Any transfer direction given under s. 73 in respect of a person committed in custody for trial or to the Crown Court for sentence or remanded in custody by the Crown Court to await judgment or sentence, ceases to have effect when his case has been disposed of by the court

---

[1] Section 5 (4) of 1964 Act.
[2] For precise definition of *person serving a sentence of imprisonment* which includes certain persons detained otherwise than in prison, see s. 72 (6).
[3] See further, s. 72 as to medical reports.   [4] Section 72 (1).
[5] Section 72 (2).   [6] Section 72 (3).   [7] Section 74.   [8] See s. 73 (2).

but without prejudice to the power of that court to make a hospital order or any other order under Part V of the Act.[1] If before his case is dealt with the responsible medical officer[2] notifies the Home Secretary that such person no longer requires treatment for mental disorder, the Home Secretary may by warrant remit him to any place where he might have been detained had he not been removed to hospital. On his arrival there the transfer direction ceases to have effect.[3]

If a transfer direction has been made in respect of any such person and no direction has been made by the Home Secretary for his being remitted to a place of detention, the court dealing with his case may in his absence make a hospital order, with or without a restriction order, and, in the case of a person committed for trial, without convicting him, provided that the court is satisfied on the oral evidence of at least two medical practitioners that the person is suffering from mental illness or severe subnormality of a nature or degree which warrants his detention in hospital for medical treatment and also if the court is of opinion, after considering any depositions or other documents required to be sent to the proper officer of the court that it is proper to make such order.[4]

Where a person has been committed to the Crown Court to be dealt with under s. 67 (1) because the magistrates' court is of opinion that a restriction order should be made and he has been detained in hospital by order of the magistrates' court pending his case being dealt with by the Crown Court, he may be dealt with by that Court in his absence as if he were a person subject to a transfer direction.[5]

If a transfer direction has been given in respect of a person remanded in custody by a magistrates' court it ceases to have effect on the expiry of the remand — including any further remand in custody[6] — unless he is then committed in custody for trial at the Crown Court. If he is so committed the provisions of s. 76 as to remittal to a place of detention and the power of the Court to make a hospital order in his absence and without conviction will apply.[7] If such a transfer direction ceases to have effect under s. 77, unless the Court passes a sentence of imprisonment[8] or makes a hospital or guardianship order, the patient remains liable to be detained in hospital as though in pursuance of an application for admission under Part IV of the Act on the date on which the transfer direction ceased to have effect.[9]

A transfer direction in respect of a civil prisoner[10] ceases to have effect at the expiration of the period for which he would, but for his removal to hospital, be liable to be detained in prison. If the transfer direction ceases to have effect under this provision, the patient is liable

---

[1] Section 76 (1).
[2] *i.e.*, the medical officer in charge of the treatment of the patient (s. 80).
[3] Section 76 (2.)   [4] Section 76 (2) and (3).   [5] Section 76 (4).
[6] Section 77 (3).   [7] Section 77 (1) and (2).   [8] See s. 66.
[9] Section 77 (4).   [10] See s. 73 (2) (*c*).

to continue to be detained in hospital as though on an application for admission under Part IV of the Act.[1]

Where a transfer direction and a direction restricting discharge have been given in respect of a person serving a sentence of imprisonment (other than a person detained in a remand home) and the Home Secretary is notified by the responsible medical officer at any time before the expiration of that person's sentence that that person no longer requires treatment for mental disorder, the Home Secretary may, by warrant, direct that he be remitted to any prison or other institution in which he might have been detained had he not been removed to hospital; or he may exercise, or authorise the Prison Commissioners, or the managers of any approved school to which he may have been remitted to exercise, any power of releasing him on licence or discharging him under supervision which would have been exercisable if he had been remitted to such a prison or institution. The transfer direction and direction restricting discharge cease to have effect on the person's arrival at the prison or institution or on his release or discharge.[2]

A direction restricting discharge of a person serving a sentence of imprisonment (including detention in a remand home under s. 69 of the Children and Young Persons Act 1933) ceases to have effect on the expiration of the sentence. If such a person transferred to a hospital is at large from the hospital in circumstances in which he is liable to be taken into custody under the Mental Health Act 1959, he is treated for the purpose of calculating the expiry of his sentence as having been unlawfully at large and absent from the institution from which he was transferred.[3]

F. REMOVAL AND RETURN OF PATIENTS WITHIN THE UNITED KINGDOM, ETC.

Part VI of the Act provides for the removal to Scotland and to and from Northern Ireland of patients liable to be detained or subject to guardianship. Removal of such patients from Scotland to England and Wales is provided for in the Mental Health (Scotland) Act, 1960.

1. Removal

(a) *Removal to Scotland*

Sections 81 to 84 inclusive of the Mental Health Act 1959, which sections related to the removal of patients to and from Scotland, have been repealed by the Mental Health (Scotland) Act 1960[4] and a new s. 81 substituted dealing only with removal of patients to Scotland, as to which s. 81 (1) provides:

[1] Section 78.   [2] Section 75 (1).   [3] Section 75 (2), (3) and (4).
[4] Section 74 and s. 113 and 4th and 5th Schedules.

If it appears to the responsible Minister in the case of a patient who is for the time being liable to be detained or placed under guardianship under this Act that it is in the interests of the patient to remove him to Scotland or, as the case may be, for receiving him into guardianship there, the responsible Minister[1] may authorise his removal to Scotland and may give any necessary directions for his conveyance to his destination.

Section 81 (2), (3), (4) and (5) in effect provide that where a patient liable to be detained in hospital or subject to guardianship has been removed to Scotland he becomes subject to the corresponding provisions of the Mental Health (Scotland) Act 1960, relating to patients of his category. Similarly, s. 76 of the Act of 1960 continues in effect any order of the County Court directing that the functions of the patient's nearest relative shall be exercisable by some other person, but in Scotland the jurisdiction to discharge or vary the order is vested in the Sheriff.

(b) Removal from Scotland

Section 73 of the Mental Health (Scotland) Act 1960, relating to removal of patients from Scotland to England and Wales provides:

(1) If it appears to the Secretary of State, in the case of a patient who is for the time being liable to be detained or subject to guardianship under this Act, that it is in the interests of the patient to remove him to England and Wales, and that arrangements have been made for admitting him to a hospital or, as the case may be, for receiving him into guardianship there, the Secretary of State may authorise his removal to England and Wales and may give any necessary directions for his conveyance to his destination.

(2) Where a patient who is liable to be detained or subject to guardianship as aforesaid by virtue of an application, order or direction under any enactment in force in Scotland is removed under this section and admitted to a hospital or received into guardianship in England and Wales, he shall be treated —

    (a) where he is admitted to a hospital, as if on the date of his admission he had been so admitted in pursuance of an application made, or an order or direction made or given, on that date under the corresponding enactment in force in England and Wales, and, where he is subject to an order or direction under any enactment in this Act restricting his discharge, as if he were subject to an order or direction under the corresponding enactment in force in England and Wales;

    (b) where he is received into guardianship, as if on the date on which he arrives at the place where he is to reside he had been so received in pursuance of an application, order or direction under the corresponding enactment in force in England and Wales and as if the application had been accepted or, as the case may be, the order or direction had been made or given on that date.

(3) Where a patient removed under this section was immediately before his removal liable to be detained under this Act by virtue of a transfer direction given while he was serving a sentence of imprisonment[2] . . . imposed by a court in Scotland, he shall be treated as if the sentence had been imposed by a court in England and Wales.

---

[1] The Minister of Health or the Home Secretary as may be appropriate (s. 81 (6)).
[2] *Imprisonment* within the meaning of s. 66 (7) of the Mental Health (Scotland) Act 1960.

(4) Where a person so removed as aforesaid was immediately before his removal subject to an order or direction restricting his discharge, being an order or direction of limited duration, that order or direction shall expire on the date on which it would have expired if he had not been so removed.

(5) In this section references to a hospital in England and Wales shall be construed as references to a hospital within the meaning of Part IV of the Mental Health Act 1959.

(c) Removal to Northern Ireland

Section 85 of the 1959 Act provides:

(1) If it appears to the Minister, in the case of a patient who is for the time being liable to be detained or subject to guardianship under this Act, not being a patient subject to an order or direction restricting his discharge, that it is in the patient's interest to remove him to Northern Ireland and that arrangements have been made —

 (a) for his reception into a mental hospital within the meaning of the Mental Health Act (Northern Ireland) 1948; or
 (b) for his reception into an institution within the meaning of that Act or for receiving him into the guardianship of the Northern Ireland Hospitals Authority;

the Minister may authorise the removal of the patient to Northern Ireland and give any necessary directions for his conveyance to his destination.

(2) Where a person is removed under this section to Northern Ireland, and is received in pursuance of the arrangements into a mental hospital, he shall, on his reception, be treated for all purposes as having been so received in pursuance of a judicial order made under Part II of the Mental Health Act (Northern Ireland) 1948, on the date on which he is so received.

(3) Where a person is removed under this section to Northern Ireland, and is received in pursuance of the arrangements into an institution within the meaning of the said Act of 1948, or is received into the guardianship of the Northern Ireland Hospitals Authority, he shall, on being so received, be treated for all purposes as if he had been so received in pursuance of a judicial order made under Part III of that Act on the date on which he is so received.

Section 86 (1) gives corresponding power to the Home Secretary in respect of any patient liable to be detained under an order or direction being a patient who is also subject to an order or direction restricting his discharge if it appears to him that it is in the patient's interests to remove him to Northern Ireland and that arrangements have been made (a) for his reception into a mental hospital within the meaning of the Mental Health Act (Northern Ireland) 1948; or (b) for his reception into an institution within the meaning of that Act, and the Home Secretary may, by warrant, authorise the removal of the patient to Northern Ireland and may give any necessary directions for his conveyance to his destination.

When a patient has been removed to Northern Ireland under s. 86 (1), he becomes subject to the provisions of the Northern Ireland Act corresponding with those of the Mental Health Act 1959, relating to patients subject to an order or direction restricting discharge. In substance this meant that powers exercisable in England and Wales by the Home Secretary pass to the Department for Home Affairs for Northern Ireland and patients detainable during the Queen's pleasure are detainable during the pleasure of the Secretary of State for Northern Ireland.[1]

(d) Removal from Northern Ireland

In s. 87 provision is made for removal to England and Wales of patients, other than criminal patients, whenever it appears to the Department of Health and Local Government that it is in the patient's interests so to remove him and arrangements have been made for his admission to a hospital or for placing him under guardianship. When so removed, the patient is treated as though he had been admitted to hospital or received into guardianship on application on the date on which he is so received.

Criminal patients ('criminal lunatics') may likewise be removed to England and Wales under s. 88 on the authority of the Department of Home Affairs if it appears that such removal is in the patient's interests and that suitable arrangements have been made for his admission to hospital. When so removed to England and Wales, the patient is treated as detained under the provisions of s. 71 (i.e., during Her Majesty's pleasure) or as subject to a transfer direction with a direction restricting discharge under s. 74 corresponding with his classification in Northern Ireland. Also, he is treated as if the sentence or order under which he had been detained before removal had been imposed or made by a court in England and Wales.

(e) Removals from Channel Islands and Isle of Man

The Home Secretary may by warrant direct that any offender found by a court in any of the Channel Islands or in the Isle of Man to be insane or to have been insane at the time of the alleged offence, and ordered to be detained during Her Majesty's pleasure, be removed to a hospital in England and Wales.[2] Such a patient is then treated as though he had been removed to that hospital under s. 71 of the Act.[3]

Any patient so removed may, on the Home Secretary's warrant, be returned to the Island from which he was so removed, to be dealt with there according to law in all respects as if he had not been removed.[4]

(f) Removals to England and Wales

It is provided in s. 96 (3) of the Act that a patient removed to England and Wales in pursuance of arrangements under Part VI of the Act or

[1] Section 86 (2), (3), (4) and (5). As, in effect amended by the Northern Ireland Constitution Act 1973, s. 40 and Sch. 5.
[2] Section 89 (1). [3] Section 89 (2). [4] Section 89 (3).

under Part VI of the Mental Health (Scotland) Act 1960, is to be treated for the purposes of the Act as suffering from such form of mental disorder as may be recorded in his case in pursuance of regulations under the Act. The 1960 Regulations provide that for the purposes of s. 96 (3) of the Act the responsible medical officer, in the case of a patient received into hospital, shall record[1] his opinion as to the form or forms of mental disorder from which the patient is suffering. Such opinion is to be recorded —

(a) where the patient is or becomes at the time of his removal subject to an order or direction restricting his discharge, or is treated as being so subject, as soon as may be after he ceases to be so subject; and

(b) in any other case as soon as may be after the patient's removal.[2]

The managers of the hospital are to cause to be recorded[3] the date on which the patient is admitted to the hospital or arrives at the place where he is to reside on his reception into guardianship in England and Wales.[4]

(g) Removal of alien patients

If it appears to the Home Secretary in the case of any patient, being an alien who is receiving treatment for mental illness as an in-patient in a hospital — including a mental nursing home[5] — in England and Wales or in a mental hospital or institution within the meaning of the Mental Health (Northern Ireland) Act 1948, that proper arrangements have been made for his removal to a country or territory outside the United Kingdom, the Isle of Man and the Channel Islands and for his care and treatment there, the Home Secretary may by warrant authorise such removal and give such directions as he thinks fit for his conveyance to his destination in that country or territory and for his detention in any place or on board any ship or aircraft until his arrival at any specified port or place in such country or territory.[6]

It is to be appreciated that the above provisions as to removal of alien patients extend not only to those detained in hospital but to any patient who is receiving in-patient treatment for mental illness. Consequently even an alien patient who is receiving in-patient treatment of his own volition is within the provisions of the section.

(h) Applications, etc., ceasing to have effect

Once a patient liable to be detained or subject to guardianship under an application, order or direction under Part IV or Part V of the Act has been removed from England and Wales in accordance with the provisions of Part VI of the Act, set out above, and he has been duly received into a hospital or other institution or placed under guardian-

---

[1] In Form 15.   [2] The 1960 Regulations, Reg. 19 (1), (2) and (3).
[3] In Form 21.   [4] Ibid., Reg. 19 (4).   [5] See ss. 96 (1) and 59 (2).   [6] Section 90.

ship in accordance with the arrangements made, the application, order or direction ceases to have effect.[1]

Since in the Act provision was not, and could not be made for disposal of an alien beyond the port of disembarkation, the above provisions for cesser of the authority for detention apply only in respect of transfers to Scotland or Northern Ireland, the Channel Islands or the Isle of Man. In the case of an alien the authority if lapsing under the general provisions of the Act after a fixed period of absence would be determined in that way.

(i) Interpretation and general

In Part VI the expression *hospital* has the same meaning as in Part IV.[2] Hence, by s. 59 (2) it includes a mental nursing home registered for the reception of patients liable to detention unless, as in respect of Part V patients, the context otherwise requires.

Where a patient is treated as if he had been removed to a hospital in England and Wales in pursuance of a direction under Part V, *viz.*, a patient subject to an order or direction restricting discharge under the Mental Health (Scotland) Act 1960; a criminal patient from Northern Ireland under s. 88; a 'Queen's pleasure' patient from the Channel Islands or the Isle of Man under s. 89, the direction is deemed to have been given on the date of his reception into the hospital.[3]

2. Return of Patients Absent Without Leave

(a) Patient absent without leave from a Scottish hospital

Any patient absent without leave from a Scottish hospital may be taken into custody in England and Wales and returned to the hospital by any mental health officer, whether Scottish or English, any constable, any officer on the staff of the hospital from which he is absent without leave, or by any person authorised in writing by the board of management of the hospital within the appropriate period under the Mental Health (Scotland) Act 1960.[4] Those persons do not correspond with those under the Act of 1959. If a patient liable to be detained in hospital undergoes a period of imprisonment not exceeding six months, he is — as under the Act of 1959 — regarded as absent without leave from hospital on the day of his discharge from prison and the foregoing provisions accordingly apply.[5]

(b) Person escaping from legal custody

If any person escapes from Scotland to England or Wales who is required or authorised by or under the Act of 1960 to be conveyed to

[1] Section 95.   [2] Section 96 (1).   [3] Section 96 (2).
[4] See further, s. 36 of the Act of 1960 as applied by s. 83 (1).
[5] Section 42 of the Act of 1960.

any place or to be kept in custody or detained in a place of safety or at any place to which he is taken in the interests of justice under s. 61 (5) of the 1960 Act, he may be retaken by the person in whose custody he was immediately before his escape, by any constable or by any mental health officer. If he was liable to be detained in a hospital he may also be retaken by any of the persons mentioned under the preceding heading.[1]

(c) Patients absent from Northern Ireland institutions

There are similar provisions to the above in respect of Northern Ireland patients absent without leave, and also in respect of criminal lunatics.[2]

(d) Patients absent from hospitals in England and Wales

The effect of s. 93 is that —
  (i) any mentally disordered patient liable to be detained in hospital under the provisions of the Act who absents himself from hospital without leave, or from any place where he is required to reside in accordance with conditions of leave of absence;[3]
  (ii) any person required or authorised by or by virtue of the Act to be conveyed to any place or to be kept in custody or detained in a place of safety[4] escapes; and
  (iii) any person subject to an order restricting discharge who, in the interests of justice or for the purpose of any public inquiry, has been taken from the hospital in which he was detained to any other place on the directions of the Home Secretary[5] escapes;
who may be taken into custody in England and Wales, may be taken into custody in, and returned to, England and Wales from any other part of the United Kingdom or the Channel Islands or the Isle of Man. Those who may retake such patients accordingly include constables or other police officers in other parts of the United Kingdom, the Channel Islands and the Isle of Man. In the application of the section to Scotland 'mental welfare officer' means any mental welfare officer within the meaning of the Mental Health (Scotland) Act 1960, and includes any person, other than a constable, who in Scotland or Northern Ireland, would have power, under the Mental Health (Northern Ireland) Act 1948, to apprehend or retake any person absent without leave when liable to be detained in a hospital or institution under that Act.

G. LOCAL AUTHORITY SERVICES

It is not within the scope of this book to examine in any detail the responsibilities of Local Social Services Authorities. The effect of s. 21

---

[1] Section 106 of the Act of 1960.
[2] Section 92.
[3] Section 40 (1).
[4] Section 139 (1).
[5] Sections 139 (1) and 66 (5).

and Schedule 8 of the National Health Service Act 1977[1]. The relationship between the exercise of the powers of the Secretary of State[2] and the powers of Local Authorities is also outside the scope of this book. It will be noted that under these provisions local authorities appoint mental welfare officers.

It remains to note that on occasions a Local Authority has a duty to take parental responsibility for certain persons in hospitals thus:

Where a mentally disordered patient being —

(a) a child or young person in respect of whom the rights and powers of a parent are vested in a Local Authority by virtue of —

    (i) s. 75 of the Children and Young Persons Act 1933 (which relates to children and young persons committed to the care of fit persons under that Act);

    (ii) s. 79 of the Children and Young Persons (Scotland) Act 1937 (which makes corresponding provision in Scotland); or

    (iii) s. 3 of the Children Act 1948 (which relates to children in respect of whom parental rights have been assumed by a local Authority under s. 2 of that Act);

(b) a person who is subject to the guardianship of a local Social Services Authority under the Mental Health Act 1959; or

(c) a person the functions of whose nearest relative under the Mental Health Act 1959, are for the time being transferred to a local Social Services Authority;

is admitted to a hospital or nursing home in England and Wales (whether for treatment for mental disorder or for any other reason) then, without prejudice to their duties in relation to the patient apart from s. 10 of the Act, the authority must arrange for visits to be made to him on behalf of the Authority and must take such other steps in relation to the patient while in the hospital or nursing home as would be expected to be taken by his parents.[3] Thus is placed on any such local Social Services Authority as a matter of law the duty of visiting and other parental obligations — even though, so far as the parents were concerned, those duties would have been but moral obligations.

H. REGISTRATION AND SUPERVISION OF MENTAL NURSING HOMES, ETC

1. Nursing Homes

(a) Generally

This book has already outlined the law relating to nursing homes in

---

[1] Page 14 above.
[2] By the N.H.S. (Functions–Directions to Authorities) Regulations S.I. 1974 No. 24 the powers are exercisable by Area Health Authorities.
[3] Section 10 (1).

general[1] and defined a mental nursing home.[2] It will be remembered that the law is now governed by the Nursing Homes Act 1975 but that previous Regulations *etc.* remain in force.[3] This part of this chapter seeks to set out the additional provisions relating to mental nursing homes.

Mental nursing home means any premises used or intended to be used for the reception of, and the provision of nursing or other medical treatment for, one or more mentally disordered patients (whether exclusively or in common with other persons), not being a hospital as defined by the Act nor any other premises managed by a Government department or provided by a local Authority. Charitable hospitals and similar institutions are not exempt from registration and are also subject to the Conduct of Mental Nursing Homes Regulations 1962.[4]

(b) The registration authority

The registration authority in relation to a mental hursing home is the Area Health Authority.[5]

(c) The Register — Particulars to be furnished

The registers of mental nursing homes to be kept by registration Authorities must contain the particulars mentioned in the First Schedule to the Mental Health (Registration and Inspection of Mental Nursing Homes) Regulations 1960,[6] and an applicant must supply the following information to the registration authority —

(1) Full name and address of the applicant, including the registered or principal office of any company, society, association or body making the application;

(2) Situation, construction, accommodation for patients and staff and equipment of the home;

(3) Date on which the home was established, or is to be established;

(4) Full names, ages, qualifications and experience of persons employed or proposed to be employed in the management of the home or any part thereof;

(5) Number of patients (excluding staff) who have been received or who are to be received, distinguishing between males and females and different categories of patients and indicating the age-range of patients in each category;

(6) Number and grades of staff (other than staff included under 4 above of this schedule) distinguishing between resident and non-resident, and between males and females;

(7) The arrangements made, or proposed to be made, for medical super-

---

[1] See Chapter 25, pp. 454–460.
[2] Quoting the Nursing Homes Act 1975, s. 2. See above, p. 476.
[3] 2nd Schedule to the 1975 Act, paras. 3 and 4.   [4] S.I. 1962 No. 1999.
[5] Under the 1975 Act, ss. 3 and 4, it is expressed to be the Secretary of State. The Area Authority gets the power under the Nursing Homes (Registration and Records) Regulations S.I. 1974 No. 22. And see N.S.C. (J.S.) 106.
[6] S.I. 1960 No. 1272, s. 14 (5) and Reg. 2.

vision and treatment and for the training or occupation and recreation of patients;

(8) The address of any other mental nursing home or of any residential home for mentally disordered persons in which the applicant is interested, and the nature and extent of the applicant's interest therein;

as well as such other information as the registration Authority may reasonably require.

Further, it is specifically provided in s. 3 (2) (c) that any application for registration in respect of a mental nursing home shall specify whether or not it is proposed to receive therein patients who are liable to be detained under the 1959 Act; and where any person is so registered in pursuance of an application stating that it is proposed to receive such patients, the fact is to be specified in the certificate of registration, and the particulars of the registration entered by the registration Authority in a separate part of the register.[1]

It will be a condition of the registration of any person in respect of a mental nursing home that the number of persons kept at any one time in the home (excluding persons carrying on or employed in the home and their families) does not exceed such number as may be specified in the certificate of registration; and the registration may also be effected subject to such other conditions (to be specified in the certificate) as the registration authority consider appropriate for regulating the age, sex or other category of persons who may be received in the home.[2]

Failure to comply with any condition imposed by the Secretary of State may cancel the registration under his powers under s. 7 (c).

(d) Conduct of mental nursing homes

Under s. 5 (1) the Secretary of State may make regulations as to the conduct of nursing homes and these regulations may make provision for the facilities and services to be provided. As yet he has not done so, but the previous regulations continue in force. The Conduct of Mental Nursing Homes Regulations 1962, provide as follows:

Citation, Commencement and Interpretation
1.—(1) These regulations may be cited as the Conduct of Mental Nursing Homes Regulations 1962, and shall come into operation on 13th September, 1962.

(2) In these regulations unless the context otherwise requires, the following expressions have the meanings hereby assigned to them:
'the Act' means the Mental Health Act 1959;
'the Minister' means the Minister of Health;[3]
'registration authority' has the meaning assigned to it by section 14 (3) or, in the case of London, s. 24 (c) of the Act;
'the managers' means the person or persons registered in respect of a mental nursing home under [The Nursing Homes Act 1975] ...;

---

[1] Section 3 (4).   [2] Section 8 (2).   [3] See footnote 2, p. 14.

T

(3) Any reference in these regulations to the provisions of any enactment or instrument shall be construed, unless the context otherwise requires, as a reference to those provisions as amended by any subsequent enactment or instrument.

(4) The Interpretation Act 1889 applies to the interpretation of these regulations as it applies to the interpretation of an Act of Parliament.

Provision of Facilities and Services

2.—The managers of a mental nursing home registered under [The Nursing Homes Act 1975] shall —

(*a*) provide for each patient efficient nursing care and for this purpose employ by day and night suitably qualified and competent staff in numbers which are adequate having regard to the size of the home and the number and condition of the patients received there;

(*b*) provide for each patient in the home by day and by night reasonable accommodation and space having regard to his age and sex and the nature and degree of the mental disorder or other illness or disability from which he is suffering;

(*c*) provide adequate and suitable furniture, bedding, curtains and, where necessary, screens and floor covering in rooms occupied or used by patients;

(*d*) provide appropriate and suitable medical and nursing equipment, having regard to the condition of the patients received there;

(*e*) provide for the use of patients a sufficient number of wash-basins and baths fitted with a hot and cold water supply, a sufficient number of water-closets and any necessary sluicing facilities;

(*f*) provide adequate light, heating and ventilation in all parts of the home occupied or used by patients;

(*g*) keep all parts of the home occupied or used by patients in good structural repair, clean and reasonably decorated;

(*h*) take adequate precautions against the risk of fire and accident, having regard in particular to the mental and physical condition of such patients as are received there;

(*i*) provide sufficient and suitable kitchen equipment, crockery and cutlery, together with adequate facilities for the preparation and storage of food;

(*j*) supply adequate, suitable and properly prepared food for every patient;

(*k*) arrange for the regular laundering of linen and articles of clothing;

(*l*) arrange as may be necessary for the provision for any patient of medical and dental services, whether under Part IV of the National Health Service Act 1946, or otherwise;

(*m*) Make suitable arrangements for the safe keeping and handling of drugs.

Offences

3.—(1) Where the registration authority consider that the managers of a mental nursing home have failed or are failing to conduct the home in accordance with the provisions of regulation 2 of these regulations the authority may give written notice by post to the managers, specifying in what respect the managers, in the opinion of the authority, have failed or are failing to comply with the requirements of that regulation and what, in the opinion of the authority, it is necessary for the managers to do so as to comply with the said requirements.

(2) Where notice has been given in accordance with the preceding paragraph of this regulation and a period of three months, or such shorter period as may have been specified in the notice, beginning with the date of the notice, has expired, any manager who contravenes or fails to comply with any provision of regulation 2 of these regulations mentioned in the notice shall be guilty of an offence against these regulations.

Inspection of mental nursing homes and visiting of patients

By s. 9 of the Nursing Homes Act 1975 any person authorised by the Secretary of State may, at any time, after producing, if asked to do so, some duly authenticated document showing that he is so authorised, enter and inspect any premises which are used, or which that person has reasonable cause to believe to be used, for the purpose of a mental nursing home, and may inspect any records kept in pursuance of s. 6 (b) of the Act.[1]

By s. 9 (2) a person authorised to inspect a mental nursing home may visit and interview in private any mentally disordered patient residing in the home —

(a) for the purpose of investigating any complaint as to his treatment made by or on behalf of the patient; or

(b) in any case where the person so authorised has reasonable cause to believe that the patient is not receiving proper care;

and where the person so authorised is a medical practitioner, he may examine the patient in private and may require the production of, and inspect, any medical records relating to the treatment of the patient in the nursing home.

The Secretary of State is to cause every mental nursing home to be inspected on such occasions and at such intervals as he may decide but in any case at least once in each successive period of six months commencing 1st May and 1st November.[2] In the case of a mental nursing home, which before the commencement of the 1959 Act was a 'registered hospital' under s. 231 of the Lunacy Act 1890 a person inspecting must be accompanied by a person authorised under s. 9 (2).

(e) Continuance of temporary registration on cancellation or death

By s. 10 of the 1975 Act, in the case of a mental nursing home the particulars of registration of which are entered in the separate part of the register for those mental nursing homes receiving patients liable to be detained under the 1959 Act, the registration is cancelled under s. 7, at a time when any patient is liable to be detained in the home under any of the provisions of the Act, the registration shall, notwithstanding the cancellation, continue in force for two months from the date of

---

[1] Mental Health (Registration and Inspection of Mental Nursing Homes) Regulations 1960, Reg. 4 (1).
[2] Ibid., Reg. 4 (2).

cancellation or until every such patient has ceased to be so liable, whichever first occurs.[1] It will be observed that no extension is given in respect of patients not liable to be detained.

Also if the person registered in respect of a mental nursing home in that part of the register for those receiving patients liable to detention dies at a time when any patient is liable to be detained therein, the registration will continue in force —

(a) as from the grant of representation to the estate of the deceased, for the benefit of the personal representatives of the deceased; and

(b) pending the grant of such representation, for the benefit of any person approved for the purpose by the Secretary of State,

until the expiration of two months beginning with the death, or until every such patient has ceased to be so liable, or until a person other than the deceased has been registered in respect of the home, whichever first occurs, and for the purposes of the 1975 Act, any person for whose benefit the registration continues in force under this provision shall be treated as registered in respect of the home.[2]

2. Residential Homes for Mentally Disordered Persons

(a) Registration under the National Assistance Act 1948

Subject to the provisions of ss. 19 and 20 of the Mental Health Act 1959, ss. 37–40 of the National Assistance Act 1948 (which relate to registration, inspection and conduct of homes for disabled persons and old persons) apply in relation to a residential home for mentally disordered persons[3] as they apply in relation to homes to which those enactments applied immediately before the commencement of the Mental Health Act 1959.[4]

Registration authority, in relation to a residential home for mentally disordered persons, means the local Social Services Authority for the area of which the home is situated.[5]

(b) Special provisions as to registration of residential homes

It is a condition of the registration of any person in respect of a residential home for mentally disordered persons that the number of persons kept at any one time in the home (excluding persons carrying on or employed in the home and their families) does not exceed such number as may be specified in the certificate of registration; and the registration may be effected subject to such conditions (to be specified

---

[1] Section 10 (2). [2] Section 10 (4) and (5).
[3] For definitions of *mentally disordered persons* and *residential home* see pp. 474 and 476.
[4] Section 19 (1).
[5] Section 19 (2) and s. 37 (2) of the National Assistance Act 1948 and s. 46 of the London Government Act 1963.

in the certificate) as the registration authority consider appropriate for regulating the age, sex or other category of persons who may be received in the home.[1] If any such condition is not complied with an offence is committed for which penalties on summary conviction are provided. The registration authority also has the power to cancel the registration under s. 37 of the National Assistance Act 1948, on the ground that any such condition has not been complied with.[2]

The power of the Secretary of State to make regulations under s. 40 of the National Assistance Act 1948, with respect to the conduct of residential homes for mentally disordered persons includes power to make regulations as to the records to be kept and notices to be given in respect of persons received into such homes.[3] The powers of inspection conferred by s. 39 of the Act of 1948 in its application to residential homes for mentally disordered persons, include power to inspect any records required to be kept in accordance with regulations made by virtue of s. 20 (1) of the Mental Health Act 1959, under s. 40 of the Act of 1948.[4]

(c) Residential home not a voluntary home under the Children Acts, etc.

A residential home for mentally disordered persons is deemed not to be a voluntary home within the meaning of Part V of the Children and Young Persons Act 1933, or Part IV of the Children Act 1948; and a child who is resident in a residential home for mentally disordered persons is not a foster child within the meaning of Part I of the Children Act 1948, or a protected child within the meaning of Part IV of the Adoption Act 1958.[5]

(d) Powers of entry and inspection of other premises

A mental welfare officer of a local Social Services Authority may, at all reasonable times, after producing, if asked to do so, some duly authenticated document showing that he is such an officer, enter and inspect any premises (not being a hospital) in the area of that Authority in which a mentally disordered patient is living, if he has reasonable cause to believe that the patient is not under proper care.[6] If, however, there is only reasonable cause to suspect that a person believed to be suffering from mental disorder has been or is being ill-treated, neglected

---

[1] Section 20 (1), which has replaced s. 40 (1) (a) of the National Assistance Act 1948. It has been held in *Retarded Children's Aid Society Ltd.* v. *Barnet London Borough Council* ([1969] 2 Q.B. 22; [1969] 1 All E.R. 300 that justices have no jurisdiction under s. 38 (4) of the National Assistance Act 1948 as applied by s. 19 of the Mental Health Act 1959 to hear an appeal relating to conditions specified by the registration authority in accordance with s. 20 (1) of the 1959 Act since an appeal lay only against refusal to register on the grounds given in s. 37 (3) of the 1948 Act. But the court has power to control a local authority seeking to impose arbitrary or unreasonable conditions. On this see also *Associated Provincial Picture Houses Ltd.* v. *Wednesbury Corporation* ([1948] 1 K.B. 223).
[2] Section 20 (2).   [3] Section 21 (1).   [4] Section 21 (2).
[5] Section 19 (3).   [6] Section 22.

or kept otherwise than under proper control or, being unable to care for himself, is living alone in any such place, the mental welfare officer can act only on a warrant granted by a justice of the peace.[1]

(e) Prosecution of offences

A local Social Services Authority may prosecute for any interference with the right to inspect *etc*. An aggrieved party or the Secretary of State or anybody else with the consent of the Attorney-General may prosecute for failure to register.

I. TRANSITIONAL PROVISIONS

The complete rewriting in the Mental Health Act 1959, of the law relating to treatment and care of persons suffering from mental disorder, made it imperative that there should be some transitional provisions if illegality and chaos, as well as considerable hardship, were to be avoided. Such necessary transitional provisions are contained in the Sixth Schedule. The force of the transitional provisions so far as relating to registration of nursing homes, licensed houses and other institutions receiving mentally disordered patients before the Act came into force is now largely spent. Consequently they are not set out here. They can be found in Part II of the Sixth Schedule to the Act.

1. Patients Liable to be Detained other than 'Transferred' Patients

(a) The initial period

The broad effect of the first part of Part III of the Sixth Schedule was to authorise the continued detention in a hospital or nursing home for a further six months of any patient[2] lawfully detained there because of mental disorder when the Act came into force. During that period, which ended on April 30, 1961, it was the duty of the responsible medical officer to reclassify the patient under the Act of 1959.[3] If the necessary medical record had not been madé during the initial period, with such extension as might have been permitted under the provisions of the Act in respect of a patient absent without leave, the patient could no longer lawfully be detained, otherwise than in accordance with one of the procedures laid down in Part IV of the Act.

(b) Detention after the initial period

If a patient within any of the three classes set out in para. 7 (1) of the schedule[4] had not been previously discharged, he continued to be liable

---

[1] Section 135.
[2] Excluded are such patients as would have fallen within Part V of the Act who are dealt with separately as *'transferred'* patients.
[3] Sixth Schedule, para. 7.
[4] See para. 9. (Broadly, all those liable to detention otherwise than in criminal cases.)

to be detained after the expiry of the initial period if the authority for his detention had been renewed before the expiration of the initial period; or until the expiration of his current period of treatment under the repealed Acts, if that period would expire after the expiration of the initial period under the Act of 1959. But he could be so detained only if —

(i) it had been recorded by the responsible medical officer under para. 7[1] that he was suffering from mental illness or severe subnormality and that his mental disorder was of a nature or degree which warranted the detention of the patient in a hospital for medical treatment; or

(ii) it had been so recorded in Form 13B of the Hospital and Guardianship Regulations 1960 that in the opinion of the responsible medical officer the patient was suffering from mild subnormality or psychopathic disorder, but not from mental illness or severe subnormality, and that his mental disorder was of a nature or degree which warranted his detention in hospital and either — (α) he had been liable to be detained by order under s. 8 (1) or s. 9 of the Mental Deficiency Act 1913, or under s. 30 of the Magistrates' Courts Act 1952; or (β) he was under 21 years of age when first detained and would not attain the age of 25 before the expiration of the initial period; or (γ) in the case of any other patient liable to be detained,[2] if the responsible medical officer before the expiration of the initial period had recorded his opinion in accordance with the following provisions of the schedule that the patient was unfit for discharge.[3]

The grounds on which the responsible medical officer might thus record that the patient was unfit for discharge were that it appeared to him —

(i) that if the patient were released from the hospital he would be likely to act in a manner dangerous to other persons or to himself, or would be likely to resort to criminal activities; or

(ii) that the patient was incapable of caring for himself and that there was no suitable hospital or other establishment into which he could be admitted and where he would be likely to remain voluntarily; and where the responsible medical officer recorded such an opinion he had also to record the grounds for it.[4] The managers of the hospital, or other person in charge, were under an obligation to cause the patient to be informed of any such report. Whereupon he might within 28 days have applied to a Mental Health Review Tribunal which then had to consider whether any of the above conditions had been fulfilled and, if not, would have directed that the patient be discharged. In respect of any such application s. 123 (1) of the Act has effect as if paragraph (b) were omitted.[5]

[1] Paragraph 7 (3).
[2] i.e., any patient concerning whom it has been recorded under para. 7 (3) that he is suffering from subnormality or psychopathic disorder.
[3] Paragraph 9 (2) and (3).   [4] Paragraph 13 (1).   [5] Paragraph 13 (2) and (3).

If a patient continued to be detained under para. 9 after the initial period, Part IV of the Act applies to him as though he had been detained on an application under the Act in respect of the form or forms of disorder recorded by the responsible medical officer under para. 7 in his case, or in respect of any form or forms of mental disorder subsequently recorded under s. 38 of the Act, subject to the provisions of s. 43 being applicable only as modified in para. 11, as to which see p. 527.

Section 44 of the Act, which contains the special provisions relating to detention of psychopathic and subnormal (mild) patients after the age of 25, does not apply to patients within para. 9 (3) of the Schedule, during their detention under the provisions of that paragraph. The patients referred to are those suffering from mild subnormality or psychopathic disorder (i) who were originally detained under order of the court consequent on commission of an offence, or transferred from prison; or (ii) who were under 21 when first detained and who did not reach 25 until after the expiration of the initial period; or (iii) in respect of whom the responsible medical officer has recorded under para. 13 unfitness for discharge. But a patient in the second of the three categories just mentioned could be detained after the age of 25 only if within two months before he reached that age the responsible medical officer had — under para. 13 — recorded in Form 14 that he was unfit for discharge.[1] It must also be appreciated that after the expiry of any period of detention authorised under para. 9 any further period is subject to the more stringent safeguards of para. 11.[2]

So long as a patient who had originally been detained under s. 6, s. 8 (1) or s. 9 of the Mental Deficiency Act 1913 (*i.e.*, by order of a judicial authority on petition or consequent on criminal proceedings or had been transferred from prison) is detained under the provisions of para. 9, the nearest relative will have no power of discharge under s. 47, but may make application to a Mental Health Review Tribunal within 12 months beginning with the expiry of the initial period and in any subsequent period of 12 months.[3]

(c) Period of detention

If, in accordance with the foregoing provisions of paras. 9 and 10 of the schedule, a patient had been detained beyond the initial period, he could, without further renewal of the authority for his detention, be detained for the remainder of his current period of treatment, *i.e.*, under the repealed Acts.[4] Hence he might possibly have been detained considerably longer than would have been permitted in the case of a patient first detained under the 1959 Act. If, however, the current period of treatment continued after the expiration of the period of two years

---

[1] Paragraph 12 (3). For the grounds for such report see (i) and (ii) above.
[2] See p. 527.   [3] Paragraph 12 (4).   [4] Paragraph 10 (1).

beginning with the coming into force of Part IV of the Act, *i.e.*, November 1st, 1960, the patient, between the expiration of the two-year period and the expiration of the current period, could apply to a Mental Health Review Tribunal.[1]

If the patient had not already been discharged on the expiration of the period of detention current when Part IV of the Act came into force or, if that period expired during the initial six months, at the expiry of that initial six months, if the period for which the patient had already been detained was not more than a year, authority for his detention could be renewed for one year and thereafter for two-yearly periods. If the period for which he had already been detained was more than one year then the authority for detention could be renewed for two years and thereafter for two-yearly periods.[2] By para. 11 the procedure for renewal is to be as under s. 43 (3)–(5)[3] of the Act. Consequently any renewal after the expiry of the initial period must be on the grounds set out in s. 43 (3), *viz.*, that in the opinion of the responsible medical officer it is in the interests of the patient's health and safety or for the protection of other persons that he should continue to be detained. This contrasts with the wider grounds for renewal of authority for detention during the initial period or alternatively for continuance of the existing authority beyond that period under para. 9 referred to above.

Renewal of authority for detention in hospital under para. 11 of the Sixth Schedule is to be in Form 10A, and for renewal of guardianship in Form 10B of the Hospital and Guardianship Regulations.

Section 43 (6) as to applications to a Mental Health Review Tribunal applies to renewals under para. 11 of the Schedule.[2]

2. Transferred Patients

Transferred patients includes —

(a) patients who immediately before Part V of the Act came into force were liable to be detained in a hospital or other place as Broadmoor patients;

(b) patients transferred to hospitals (*i.e.*, an institution for mental defectives) from prison or other place of detention under s. 9 of the Mental Deficiency Act 1913 whose sentence or period of detention had not then expired;

(c) Scottish criminal lunatics transferred to a mental hospital in England under s. 63 (3) of the Criminal Justice Act 1948, as Broadmoor patients;

(d) persons removed from prison, *etc.*, to a mental deficiency institution under s. 9 of the Act of 1913 and thence to a mental hospital by warrant of the Home Secretary under s. 64 (3) of the Criminal Justice Act 1948;

[1] Paragraph 10 (2).   [2] Paragraph 11 (1).   [3] Paragraph 11 (2).

(e) patients transferred to England and Wales under s. 64 (2) of the Criminal Justice (Scotland) Act 1949;

(f) patients liable to be detained by virtue of s. 10 of the Colonial Prisoners Removal Act 1884.[1]

Any transferred patient liable to be detained during Her Majesty's pleasure, or until the directions of Her Majesty are known, including similar patients detained under the Colonial Prisoners Removal Act 1884, are treated as detained under s. 71 of the Act of 1959, i.e., as though detained on a hospital order with an order restricting discharge made without limitation of time and otherwise subject to the provisions of that Section. But this does not apply to a patient transferred to England and Wales from Scotland, the Channel Islands or the Isle of Man.[2]

A transferred prisoner subject to a sentence of imprisonment within the meaning of s. 72[3] of the Act of 1959, including a patient detained by virtue of s. 10 of the Colonial Prisoners Removal Act 1884, but who is not within the class of patient referred to in the preceding paragraph, is to be treated as if liable to be detained in a hospital by virtue of a transfer direction under s. 72 and as if a direction restricting his discharge had been given under s. 74.[4]

Section 84 applies to a transferred patient who had been a state mental patient in Scotland and, having been transferred was liable to be detained in a hospital in England and Wales under s. 63 (3) of the Criminal Justice Act 1948, or s. 64 (2) of the Criminal Justice (Scotland) Act 1948, as if he had been removed under the said s. 64 (2). Also, he is treated as if a direction restricting his discharge had been given.[5]

Section 89 applies to 'Queen's pleasure' patients from the Channel Islands as if removed under the provisions of that section.[6]

Any transferred patient within the definition given in para. 15 (1) who is not within any of the categories referred to in the four preceding paragraphs[7] is to be treated for the purposes of the Act, as if he were liable to be detained in a hospital in pursuance of a transfer direction given under s. 73 and as if a direction restricting his discharge had been given under s. 74, and he is to be so treated notwithstanding that he is not suffering from a form of mental disorder mentioned in s. 73.[8]

Any Broadmoor patient conditionally discharged under s. 5 of the Criminal Lunatics Act 1884, before Part V of the Mental Health Act 1959, came into operation, is treated as though he had been conditionally discharged under s. 66 of that Act and any direction given under s. 5 of the Act 1884 — before Part V of the Act of 1959 became operative — for taking any such patient into custody and for his conveyance to

---

[1] Paragraph 15 (1).
[2] Paragraph 15 (2).
[3] See p. 508.
[4] For the effect of these sections, see p. 508 et seq.
[5] Paragraph 15 (4).
[6] Paragraph 15 (5).
[7] i.e., para. 15 (2)–(5).
[8] Paragraph 15 (6).

hospital is to be deemed to have been given under s. 66 of the later Act.[1]

Upon a direction restricting discharge of a transferred patient within para. 15 (1) of the schedule ceasing to have effect, the responsible medical officer is to record his opinion whether the patient is suffering from mental illness, severe subnormality, psychopathic disorder or mild subnormality, and references in the Act to the form or forms of mental disorder specified in the relevant application, order or direction are — in respect of such patient — to be construed as including references to the form or forms of mental disorder so recorded.[2]

J. MANAGEMENT OF PROPERTY AND AFFAIRS OF PATIENTS

1. Court of Protection: Appointment of Receiver

Part VIII of the Mental Health Act 1959 sets out the very wide powers of the Court of Protection over the management of the property and affairs of a person incapable, by reason of mental disorder, of managing and administering his own property and affairs[3] whether or not that person is liable to detention or placed under guardianship under the provisions of the Act. Such a person is called a *patient* in Part VIII.[4] The narrower use of the word in this Part as opposed to the rest of the Act will be noted. Detailed consideration of that part of the Act and of the Court of Protection Rules 1960,[5] are largely outside the scope of this book, but in succeeding paragraphs reference is made to one or two aspects of the subject likely to concern hospitals or nursing homes.

Since it is not within the powers of a Health Authority under the National Health Service Act, to undertake responsibilities in respect of a patient's property, except such property as the patient has brought into hospital with him, and then only doing what is reasonably necessary in the circumstances, it would not normally be a function of any of its officers, as such, to apply for appointment as receiver for a patient, nor is there any statutory authority for reimbursement of the expenses of any such officer if he does so — apart from what he may be authorised to charge against the patient's estate.

But s. 49 of the National Assistance Act 1948, has been amended to authorise payment of the expenses of an officer of a local Social Services Authority who, with the permission of his Authority, applies for appointment under Part VIII of the Act of 1959 as receiver for a patient

---

[1] Paragraph 16 (1).   [2] Paragraph 17.
[3] Section 101. Advice to N.H.S. hospital authorities on Part VIII of the Act and on the circumstances in which the management of a mentally disordered patient's affairs should be referred to the Court of Protection is given in Departmental circular H.M. (60) 80.
[4] Section 101.   [5] S.I. 1960 No. 1146 as later amended.

or as a person otherwise having functions in relation to the property and affairs of a patient.[1] This provision, together with that made in s. 105 of the Mental Health Act 1959, for the appointment of the holder of an office for the time being, points to the possibility of a Local Social Services Authority giving general authority to a particular officer or class of officer to apply *ex officio* in case of need for appointment as receiver or otherwise to safeguard the property or other affairs of a patient in the area of the Authority.

The Court of Protection may act for the benefit of the patient. The term *benefit* is much wider than mere material benefit: it includes divorce proceedings[2] and the making of a gift[3] or a will. The full scope of the powers is set out in s. 103 as amended.

2. Lord Chancellor's Visitors

It is provided in s. 108 of the Act that there shall continue to be medical and legal visitors of patients, being persons qualified as required by the Act, appointed by the Lord Chancellor, to be known as Lord Chancellor's Visitors.

It is the duty of the Lord Chancellor's Visitors to visit patients[4] in accordance with the directions of the judge for the purpose of investigating matters relating to the capacity of any patient to manage and administer his property and affairs or otherwise relating to the exercise, in relation to him, of the functions of the judge under Part VIII of the Act; and the Visitors are to make such reports on their visits as the judge may direct.[5] The Master or Deputy Master of the Court of Protection may also visit any patient for those purposes.[6] For the purposes of s. 109 relating to visitation by Lord Chancellor's Visitors or the Master or Deputy Master the word *patients* includes not only patients within the meaning of s. 101 but also persons *alleged* to be incapable, by reason of mental disorder, of managing and administering their property and affairs.[7]

A Visitor or the Master or Deputy Master, making a visit may interview the patient in private[8] and a medical Visitor may carry out in private a medical examination of the patient and may require the production of and inspect any medical records relating to the patient.[9]

A report made by a Visitor under s. 109 and the information contained in such a report, shall not be disclosed except to the judge and any person authorised by the judge to receive the disclosure.[10] Any wrongful disclosure is a criminal offence.[11]

[1] Section 149 and Seventh Schedule.
[2] *Re W* (E.E.M.) [1971] 1 Ch. 123.
[3] *Re C.M.G.* [1970] 2 All E.R. 740.
[4] See s. 109 (7) for definition.
[5] Section 109 (1).
[6] Section 109 (4).
[7] See section 109 (7) for definition.
[8] Section 109 (2).
[9] Section 109 (3).
[10] Section 109 (5).
[11] Section 109 (6).

K. MENTAL HEALTH REVIEW TRIBUNALS

Under s. 3 of the Mental Health Act 1959 as amended, there has been established for the region of every Regional Health Authority, a Mental Health Review Tribunal (more shortly referred to as a Tribunal) for the purpose of dealing with applications and references to it by and in respect of patients under the provisions of the Act. The constitution of Mental Health Review Tribunals is laid down in the First Schedule to the Act and their procedure and rules, in so far as not provided for in the Act, are set out in the Mental Health Review Tribunal Rules 1960.[1]

1. Applications to a Tribunal

(a) *Generally*

Applications, which must be in writing and addressed to the Tribunal for the region in which the hospital or nursing home in which the patient is detained is situated,[2] are made by the patient or his nearest relative and are with the object of obtaining the patient's discharge or objecting to some decision of the responsible medical officer, such as reclassification.

Except in such cases and at such times as are expressly provided by the Act, no application may be made to a Mental Health Review Tribunal by or in respect of a patient; and where, under any provision of the Act, any person is authorised to make an application to such a Tribunal within a specified period, not more than one such application may be made by that person within that period.[2]

The Secretary of State for Social Services may, however, under s. 57 at any time refer the case of any patient, other than one subject to an order or direction restricting discharge under Part V, to a Tribunal. On such a reference the Tribunal has the same powers as on an application.

(b) *Applications by or on behalf of a patient liable to detention in hospital or under guardianship under Parts IV or V*

(i) *On admission.* A patient who is admitted to hospital[3] in pursuance of an application for admission for treatment[4] or a hospital order without restriction[5] may apply to a Mental Health Review Tribunal within the period of six months beginning with the day on which he is so admitted, or with the day on which he attains the age of 16 years, whichever is the later.[6] In the case of a hospital order without restriction the nearest relative may apply within twelve months beginning with

---

[1] As amended   [2] Section 122 and S.I. 1960 No. 1139.
[3] The term *hospital* throughout this chapter as in Part IV of the Act, unless otherwise indicated includes a mental nursing home, s. 59 (2).
[4] Section 31 (4).   [5] Section 63 (4) (*a*).   [6] Section 31 (4).

the date of the order and in any subsequent period of twelve months.[1]

It will be noted that there is no appeal against an application for admission for observation under s. 25.

A patient who is received into guardianship in pursuance of a guardianship application may apply to a tribunal within the period of six months beginning with the day on which the application is accepted, or with the day on which he attains the age of 16 years, whichever is the later.[2]

(ii) *On reclassification under s. 38 of patient in hospital or under guardianship.* Where a medical report has been furnished under s. 38 (1) reclassifying a patient who has attained the age of 16 years, the managers or guardian are to cause the patient and the nearest relative to be informed, and the patient or that relative may within the period of 28 days beginning with the day on which he is so informed apply to a Tribunal.[3] Where a report is made under s. 38 which contains a barring notice under the Mental Health (Amendment) Act 1975, it is a report under the section and so can be the subject of an appeal. Appeal also lies within the 28 day period in the case of a patient subject to a hospital order or direction under Part V without an order or direction restricting discharge.[4]

(iii) *Patient transferred from guardianship to hospital under s. 41.* A patient who, having attained the age of 16 years, is transferred from guardianship to a hospital in pursuance of regulations made under this section may, within the period of six months beginning with the day on which he was so transferred, apply to a Tribunal.[5] This also applies to a patient transferred from guardianship to hospital by a hospital order or direction under Part V without an order or direction restricting discharge.[6]

(iv) *On renewal of authority for detention or guardianship under s. 43.* Where a medical report is furnished under s. 43 (3) renewing the authority for the detention of the patient in hospital, or under s. 43 (4) renewing the authority for his being under guardianship, and the patient has attained the age of 16 years, the managers of the hospital, or the local Social Services Authority, as the case may be, unless they discharge the patient, cause him to be informed that the Authority has been renewed. So also they must inform him and his nearest relative if the authority is renewed under the Mental Health (Amendment) Act 1975. The patient may, within the period for which the authority for his detention or guardianship is renewed by the report, apply to a Tribunal.[7] This also applies to a patient subject to a hospital order or direction under Part V without an order or direction restricting discharge.[8]

---

[1] Section 63 (4) (*b*).
[2] Section 34 (5).
[3] Section 38 (2).
[4] Section 36 as modified by Third Schedule.
[5] Section 41 (5).
[6] Section 41 as modified by Third Schedule.
[7] Section 43 (6).
[8] Section 43 as modified by Third Schedule.

(v) *Patient suffering from psychopathy or mild subnormality detained in hospital beyond the age of 25 under s. 44.* Where within two months before a subnormal (mild) or psychopathic patient detained in hospital reaches the age of 25, the responsible medical officer furnishes a report under s. 44 (2) that it appears to him that, if released, the patient would be likely to act in a manner dangerous to other persons or to himself, so that the patient remains liable to detention beyond that age, the managers[1] of the hospital are to cause the patient and the nearest relative[2] of the patient to be informed, and the patient and that relative may, at any time before the expiration of the period of 28 days beginning with the day on which the patient attains the age of 25 years, apply to a Tribunal.[3]

(vi) *On report barring discharge by nearest relative under s. 48.* If the responsible medical officer makes a report to the managers of the hospital under s. 48 (2) barring the right of the nearest relative to discharge the patient, the managers must cause that relative to be informed and he may, within 28 days of being so informed, apply to a Tribunal.[4]

(vii) *By displaced relative under s. 52.* If an order has been made by a county court under s. 52, depriving the nearest relative of his powers under Part IV, that relative may make an application to a Tribunal in respect of the patient within the period of 12 months beginning with the date of the order, and in any subsequent period of 12 months during which the order continues in force.[5]

(c) Medical Examination Preliminary to Application

It is provided by s. 37 (1) of the Act for the purpose of advising whether an application to a Tribunal should be made by or in respect of a patient who is liable to be detained or subject to guardianship under Part IV of the Act or of furnishing information as to the condition of a patient for the purposes of such an application, *or of advising as to the exercise by the nearest relative of such a patient of any power to order his discharge,*[6] any medical practitioner authorised by or on behalf of the patient or other person who is entitled to make or has made the application, *or by the nearest relative of the patient, as the case may be,*[6] may, at any reasonable time, visit the patient and examine him in private.

2. Powers of Tribunals

(a) Powers of Tribunals

Section 123 provides:

(1) Where application is made to a Mental Health Review Tribunal by or

---

[1] See pp. 479–480. [2] See ss. 49–53 and p. 498 *et seq* for definition.
[3] Section 44 (3). [4] Section 48 (3). [5] Section 52 (6).
[6] The words in italics do not apply in the case of Part V patients subject to a hospital order or detention without an order or direction restricting discharge. Section 37 (1) does not apply where there is such an order or direction.

in respect of a patient who is liable to be detained under the Act, the tribunal may in any case direct that the patient be discharged, and shall so direct if they are satisfied —

(a) that he is not then suffering from mental illness, psychopathic disorder, subnormality or severe subnormality;

(b) that it is not necessary in the interests of the patient's health or safety or for the protection of other persons that the patient should continue to be liable to be detained; or

(c) in the case of an application under s. 44 (3) or s. 48 (3) of the Act, that the patient, if released, would not be likely to act in a manner dangerous to other persons or to himself.

(2) Where application is made to a Mental Health Review Tribunal by or in respect of a patient who is subject to guardianship under the Act, the tribunal may in any case direct that the patient be discharged, and shall so direct if they are satisfied —

(a) that he is not then suffering from mental illness, psychopathic disorder, subnormality or severe subnormality; or

(b) that it is not necessary in the interests of the patient, or for the protection of other persons, that the patient should remain under such guardianship.

(3) Where application is made to a Mental Health Review Tribunal under any provision of the Act by or in respect of a patient and the tribunal do not direct that the patient be discharged, the tribunal may if satisfied that the patient is suffering from a form of mental disorder other than the form specified in the relevant application, order or direction, direct that that application, order or direction be amended by substituting for the form of mental disorder specified therein such other form of mental disorder as appears to the tribunal to be appropriate.

(4) The above provisions apply in relation to any reference to a Mental Health Review Tribunal made by the Minister under s. 57 of the Act as they apply in relation to an application made to such tribunal by or in respect of a patient, but do not apply in relation to any reference by the Secretary of State[1] under s. 66 (6) of the Act.

(b) The Effect of amendment of an application, order, etc., by a Tribunal

Section 123 (3) gives the Tribunal power to amend an application, order or direction by substituting a different form of disorder when it does not order the discharge of the patient. But since the Tribunal does not and cannot itself order the continued detention or guardianship of the patient, his continued detention must depend on the validity of the application, order or direction as amended by the Tribunal.

This, indeed, was held in *Re The Mental Health Act 1959*.[2] It was the direct consequence of this decision which led to the Mental Health (Amendment) Act 1975. Under that Act, where a Tribunal is minded to re-classify a patient who had been classified as suffering from mental illness or severe subnormality as in fact suffering from psychopathy or mild subnormality[3] shall not do so unless it has first considered whether

---

[1] *i.e.*, the Home Secretary, as to whose powers of reference, see p. 507.   [2] [1973] 1 Q.B. 452.
[3] Like the responsible medical officer considering a re-classification under s. 38. See above, p. 490.

the patient, if released, would be likely to act in a manner dangerous to other persons or to himself.[1] Before coming to a decision on this question, the Tribunal shall cause to make and shall take into consideration a report on it by the responsible medical officer.[2] If it considers the patient would be dangerous, although it may re-classify, the Tribunal's direction will not terminate the authority for the detention. If it decides the patient would not be dangerous it shall record its decision to that effect.

3. References to a Tribunal by the Home Secretary

(a) Patients subject to hospital order with order restricting discharge

It is expressly provided in s. 65 (3) (b) that no application may be made to a Tribunal under s. 63 or any of the provisions of Part IV in respect of a patient subject to a hospital order with an order restricting discharge. Although therefore the Secretary of State for Social Services may not refer the case of such a patient to a Tribunal under s. 57, the Home Secretary under s. 66 (6) has the power at any time of referring such a case to a Tribunal *for advice.* Moreover, in the circumstances set out in the next paragraph he is under a duty to refer to a Tribunal within two months of receiving a request in writing from the patient to do so, unless during that period of two months the patient is discharged absolutely or conditionally under s. 66 (2) or the order restricting his discharge ceases to have effect.

The patient is entitled to make such request obliging the Home Secretary to refer to a Tribunal for advice, after the expiration of one year beginning with the date of the hospital order and, thereafter to make one such request during each period during which he could have made application to a Tribunal if he had been subject to a hospital order without an order restricting discharge and the authority for his detention had been renewed at the requisite intervals.[3] Also, if a patient conditionally discharged is recalled, although the hospital order is regarded as operative from the date of the patient's return, he may have his case referred to the Tribunal between six and twelve months thereafter. The other occasions when the Home Secretary must comply with the patient's request for reference to the Tribunal are (i) within 28 days of reclassification, (ii) on transfer from guardianship to hospital, (iii) at such intervals as the patient would have been able to apply to the Tribunal on renewal of authority had there been no restriction order. The position of the Home Secretary referring a case to a Tribunal under s. 66 (6), whether of his own motion or at the request of the patient, is very different from that of the Secretary of State for Social Services referring

---

[1] 1975 Act section 1 (1).   [2] 1975 Act section 1 (2).   [3] Section 66 (7).

a case under s. 57. The former is not bound by the advice given by the Tribunal; the latter is bound by its decision.

(b) *Persons ordered to be kept in custody during Her Majesty's Pleasure*

Since an order that a person be kept in custody during Her Majesty's pleasure operates as a hospital order with an order restricting discharge,[1] reference to a Tribunal can be made only by the Home Secretary for advice, as explained above.

(c) *Prisoners serving sentences of imprisonment, etc., removed to hospital*

Section 72 of the Act provides for transfer to hospital[2] of any person serving a sentence of imprisonment, or any person ordered to be detained in a remand home, *etc.*,[3] by a transfer direction, by warrant, of the Home Secretary. Such a transfer direction has the same effect as a hospital order.[4] Consequently, the circumstances in which an application or reference can be made to a Tribunal are as set out on p. 531 *et seq* in respect of patients subject to hospital order or guardianship order without restriction, unless the Home Secretary has given a direction restricting discharge.[5] If he has done so, reference may be made to a Tribunal only by the Home Secretary for advice as in the case of a patient subject to a hospital order and a restriction order.

It must be appreciated that even in the case of a prisoner under sentence who has been removed to hospital by a direction given by the Home Secretary without a further direction restricting discharge, the patient is not necessarily entitled to be free of the remainder of his sentence if a Tribunal on application by or in respect of him orders his discharge from hospital. It is provided in s. 75 that if before the expiration of his sentence the prisoner no longer requires treatment for mental disorder — as would be the case if the Tribunal so decided — and the responsible medical officer so notifies the Home Secretary, the Home Secretary may by warrant direct that he be remitted to prison or otherwise dealt with as laid down in that section. It is curious that s. 75 does not, apparently, lay an obligation on the responsible medical officer to make a report.

The added obligation on the Tribunal under the Mental Health (Amendment) Act 1975 to consider whether if released the patient would be dangerous does not affect the operation of s. 75. In other words, apparently if the Tribunal considers that the patient would, in the hypothetical circumstances of his release, be dangerous, they cannot re-classify him. Conversely he is returned to prison and not released if it considers him not to be dangerous.

---

[1] Section 71. [2] See p. 508.
[3] The classes of persons to whom this section applies are set out in s. 72 (6).
[4] Section 72 (3). [5] Section 74.

A direction restricting discharge of a person serving a sentence of imprisonment ceases to have effect on the expiration of the sentence.[1] From that time, therefore, the direction operates as a hospital order without an order restricting discharge and the right of application or reference to the Tribunal is as for persons subject to such order.[2]

(d) Other prisoners removed to hospital

The Home Secretary may also, by warrant, direct the removal to hospital of persons committed or remanded in custody, but if he does so he must also give a direction restricting discharge. The effect is the same as of a hospital order with an order restricting discharge. Consequently reference can be made to a Tribunal only by the Home Secretary for advice as already explained.[3] Since, however, such a transfer direction is effective only until the case has been disposed of by the court,[4] it is hardly likely that the question of reference to a Tribunal would ever be relevant.

The Home Secretary may also, by warrant, give a direction for removal to hospital of civil prisoners[5] and of aliens detained in a prison or other institution to which the Prisons Act 1952, applies, in pursuance of the Aliens Order 1953, or of any order amending or replacing it. But in these cases it is discretionary whether he also gives a direction restricting discharge.[6] If he does not, then reference may be made to a Tribunal as set out on p. 531 in respect of patients subject to hospital order. If the Home Secretary does give a direction restricting discharge only he can refer to a Tribunal for advice.[7]

A transfer direction in respect of a civil prisoner ceases to have effect on the expiration of the period during which he would have been liable to be detained in prison. He is then treated as though admitted on application. Consequently, the ordinary rules as to discharge and applications to a Tribunal under Part IV apply without any of the modifications applicable to Part V patients.

4. Mental Health Review Tribunal Rules 1960

The following is a summary of the Mental Health Review Tribunal Rules 1960,[8] as amended.

Interpretation (Rule 2)

In the Rules, unless the context otherwise requires —

'the Act' means the Mental Health Act 1959;
'applicant' means a person who under the Act is entitled to apply or being

---

[1] Section 75 (2).　　　[2] See p. 531.　　　[3] See p. 507.　　　[4] Sections 76 and 77.
[5] For definition see s. 73 (2) (e).　　　[6] Section 74 (1).　　　[7] See p. 507.
[8] S.I. 1960 No. 1241. Made under s. 59 (1). They have been amended by the N.H.S. (Consequential Amendments) Ord. S.I. 1974 No. 241.

so entitled has applied, as the case may be, to a Mental Health Review Tribunal; and 'application' is to be construed accordingly;

'displaced relative' in relation to a patient means the nearest relative of the patient whose functions under the Act are exercisable by another person in pursuance of an order made under s. 52 or s. 53 of the Act;

'the Minister' means the Minister of Health[1];

'nearest relative' in relation to a patient means the person who has for the time being the functions under the Act of the nearest relative of that patient;

'private guardian' in relation to a patient means a person, other than a local Social Services Authority, who acts as guardian under the Act;

'reference' includes a reference by the Minister under s. 57 of the Act or by the Home Secretary under s. 66 (6);

'responsible authority' means the manager of the hospital or mental nursing home in which the patient is liable to be detained or, as the case may be, the responsible local Social Services Authority if he is subject to guardianship;

'the tribunal' means the members of the Mental Health Review Tribunal for the region appointed to hear the case or over the class or group to which it belongs. If none has been so appointed it means the Mental Health Review Tribunal for the region.

(a) Preliminary Procedure

The Application (Rule 3)

Any application is to be made by the applicant, or by any person authorised by him, on the appropriate form of application set out in the First Schedule and is to be sent to the Tribunal. When the applicant requests a formal hearing that fact is to be stated in his application.

The necessary form is to be supplied to an applicant by the Tribunal or by the responsible authority on request. Form 1 is for the use of a patient when making an application. Form 2 is for use by the nearest relative or displaced relative.

Power to Postpone Consideration (Rule 4)

Where an application by or in respect of a patient has been considered and determined by any Tribunal, the Tribunal or the chairman may postpone the hearing of any further application until such time as they or he direct, not being later than 12 months from the date on which the previous application was determined.[2] The applicant and any other person to whom a copy or notice of the application has been sent are to be informed of any such postponement.[3]

Where a new application is made in respect of a patient and is not postponed under Rule 4, the Tribunal or the chairman may direct that any postponed application shall be dealt with at the same time as the new application.[4]

The power of postponement by Rule 4 (2) does not apply to —
   (a) any application if the previous application was determined before a break or change in the authority for the patient's detention or guardianship, such a break or change being deemed to occur only —
      (i) on admission to hospital on application for treatment or on a

---

[1] Now the Secretary of State.   [2] Rule 4 (1).
[3] Rule 4 (3).   [4] Rule 4 (5).

hospital order without an order restricting discharge;

  (ii) on reception into guardianship in pursuance of a guardianship application or guardianship order;

  (iii) on the application to the patient of the provisions of Part IV or Part V of the Act as if he had been so admitted or received following the making of a transfer direction or following the ceasing of effect of a transfer direction or an order or direction restricting his discharge; or

  (iv) on transfer from guardianship to hospital under s. 41 of the Act;

(b) an application under s. 38 (which relates to reclassification);

(c) an application under s. 43 in respect of a renewal of authority for detention of the patient for a period of one year, unless the previous application was made to the Tribunal more than six months after the patient's admission or reception;

(d) an application under s. 44 (which authorises the continued detention of certain psychopathic and subnormal (mild) patients);

(e) an application under s. 48 (which imposes restriction on discharge by the nearest relative); and

(f) an application under para. 13 of the Sixth Schedule to the Act (which relates to the unfitness for discharge of certain patients).

Notice to and Statement by Responsible Authority (Rules 5 and 6)

On receipt of an application, or at the end of a period of postponement, the Tribunal is to send a copy of the application to the responsible authority. The authority is then as soon as practicable, and in any case within three weeks of receiving the copy, to send to the Tribunal a statement ('the authority's statement') containing the information referred to in the Second Schedule. Any part of the authority's statement which in their opinion should be withheld from the applicant on the grounds that its disclosure would be undesirable in the interests of the patient or for other special reason is to be made in a separate document and the authority must specify their reasons for not wishing the information contained in such document to be disclosed to the patient.

The information required to be included in the authority's statement is as follows:

A. Facts for the information of the Tribunal, so far as known to the authority

1. Patient's full name.

2. Patient's age.

3. Date of patient's admission to hospital or mental nursing home in which now detained, or reception into guardianship.

4. History of present authority for detention or guardianship, *i.e.*, date of admission, section of the Act under which made, and date of any subsequent renewals or transfer, or removal of restriction on discharge.

5. Form or forms of mental disorder from which patient is recorded as suffering in the authority for detention (as amended by any reclassification under s. 38 or s. 123 of the Act).

6. Name and address of patient's nearest relative or, if some other person is exercising functions of nearest relative, that person.

7. If patient is being treated in a mental nursing home under contractual arrangements with a Regional or Area Health Authority or a Special Health Authority, the name of that Authority.

8. If the responsible Authority consider the applicant not entitled under the Act to make the application, reasons for this opinion.

B. Reports

1. Statement of reasons why the responsible authority are not themselves willing to discharge the patient (including a report on the patient's mental condition and an account of the facilities available for care of the patient if the authority for detention or guardianship were discharged) or, in the case of an application under s. 44 or s. 48 or para. 13 of the Sixth Schedule to the Act, the grounds on which the authority consider the special criteria described in those sections or that paragraph to be established.

2. If applicant is the patient and has requested a formal hearing, the opinion of responsible medical officer as to whether this would be detrimental to the patient's health.

3. Any other observations on the application.

The Tribunal on receipt of the authority's statement is to send to the applicant a copy of the statement excluding any part which is contained in a separate document as above-mentioned.[1] They may, however, under the provisions of Rule 13, make available to the applicant any such information which had been withheld from him.

The Tribunal is to inform the responsible authority of any comments on the authority's statement, providing a copy if requested, and giving the authority opportunity of considering such comments.[2]

If any of the above procedure regarding notice to the responsible authority and in respect of its statement had been gone through and the application is subsequently postponed under the provisions of Rule 4, the whole procedure will have to be gone through again when the period of postponement comes to an end.[3]

Notice to Other Persons Interested (Rule 7)

On receipt of the authority's statement the Tribunal is to give notice of the application:
- (a) where patient liable to detention in mental nursing home to the registration authority;
- (b) where patient subject to guardianship of private guardian to that guardian;
- (c) where applicant is the patient or the displaced relative to the person named in the authority's statement as exercising the functions of the nearest relative; and
- (d) where a Health Authority has the right of discharge under s. 47 (3), i.e., where the patient is maintained in a mental nursing home under a contract with that authority.

The Tribunal is also to inform such persons of the arrangements which will be made for determining the application, this being done substantially in the form set out in the Third Schedule to the Rules.

Such notices have to be repeated at the proper time if after they have been given the application is postponed under Rule 4.[3]

Appointment of Tribunal (Rule 8)

On receipt of the authority's statement on an application, or on receipt of a reference from the Home Secretary, the chairman or other member of the

---

[1] Rule 6 (2).   [2] Rule 6 (3).   [3] Rule 4 (4).

Tribunal appointed to act on his behalf[1] is to appoint members of the Tribunal to consider and determine or advise on the application or reference unless it belongs to a class or group of proceedings for which members have already been appointed.[2]

A person is not qualified to serve as a member of a Tribunal to consider an application or reference where —

(a) he has any interest in the patient;

(b) he is a member or officer of the responsible authority or of the registration authority concerned in the proceedings; or

(c) he is a member or headquarters officer of a Regional Health Authority, Area Health Authority or special Health Authority which has the right to discharge the patient under s. 47 (3).[3]

Should an application be postponed under Rule 4 after members have been appointed to deal with it, the appointments will lapse and fresh appointments will have to be made at the expiry of the period of postponement.[4]

Two or more Pending Applications

The Tribunal may consider more than one application in respect of a patient at the same time and may for that purpose adjourn the proceedings relating to any application.[5]

(b) General Provisions as to Procedure

Representation (Rule 10)

The applicant, the responsible authority and any person to whom notice of the application has been given under the provisions of Rule 7 may be represented by any person authorised in that behalf, not being a person liable to be detained or subject to guardianship under the Act or a person receiving treatment for mental disorder at the same hospital or mental nursing home as the patient by or in respect of whom the application is made.

An authorised representative may take all such steps and do all such things relating to the proceedings as the person whom he represents is by these rules required or authorised to take or do.

Unless the Tribunal otherwise direct, a patient or other person appearing before the Tribunal may be accompanied by such other person or persons as he wishes.

Medical Examination (Rule 11)

The medical member of the Tribunal appointed to consider the application shall, or where there is more than one medical member the medical members may and one shall, examine the patient or take such other steps as he or they consider necessary to form an opinion of the patient's mental condition; and for this purpose the patient may be seen in private and his medical records examined.

Interview with Patient (Rule 12)

The Tribunal may at any time before determining the application interview the patient and shall interview him if he so requests, and such interview may take place in private or in the presence of the applicant or any other person as the Tribunal think fit.

Where they think it appropriate the Tribunal may authorise any one or more of their members to visit and interview the patient in private.

[1] Act: First Schedule, para. 4. [2] Rule 8 (1).
[3] See (d) under preceding heading. [4] Rule 9. [5] Rule 4 (4).

Disclosure of Information (Rule 13)

Except in so far as the Tribunal consider it undesirable to do so in the interests of the patient or for other special reasons, they shall make available to the applicant any part of the authority's statement which has been withheld from him under the provisions of Rule 6 and shall on request make available to the applicant and the responsible authority copies of any other documents obtained by or furnished to the Tribunal for the purposes of the application and a statement of the substance of any oral information so obtained or furnished, and shall if so requested adjourn the hearing of the application so far as may in the opinion of the Tribunal be necessary to enable the applicant or the responsible authority to consider any document or information so made available. But the Tribunal may refuse to supply copies of any document, or of any part of any document, or a statement of any oral information which appears to them not to be relevant for the purposes of the application.

The Tribunal may disclose to any person any information withheld under the provisions of these rules on terms that the information shall not be disclosed to the applicant or the patient or to any other person or be used otherwise than in connection with the application.[1]

Evidence (Rule 14)

For the purposes of obtaining information, the Tribunal may take evidence on oath and subpoena any witness to appear before them or to produce documents and the president of the Tribunal shall accordingly have the powers of an arbitrator under s. 12 (3) of the Arbitration Act 1950, and the powers of a party to a reference under an arbitration agreement under s. 12 (4), but no person shall be compelled to give any evidence or produce any document which he could not be compelled to give or produce on the trial of an action.

The Tribunal may receive in evidence any document or information notwithstanding that such document or information would be inadmissible in a court of law.

Adjournment (Rule 15)

The Tribunal may adjourn the hearing of any evidence or representations or the consideration of an application to such date as they may determine.

Withdrawal of Application (Rule 16)

An applicant may withdraw his application at any time by notice in writing to the Tribunal and an application is deemed to be withdrawn if the patient ceases to be liable to be detained or subject to guardianship in England and Wales.

(c) Informal Determinations and References by Secretary of State or Home Secretary

Informal Determinations (Rule 17)

Where the applicant has not requested a formal hearing the Tribunal may determine an application in such manner as they think appropriate.

---

[1] Rule 13 (2).

Before determining the application the Tribunal shall —

(a) take all such steps as they consider proper (including interviewing any person) to ensure that they have before them the information necessary to decide the case;

(b) give to the applicant, the responsible authority and any person to whom notice of the application has been given under the provisions of Rule 7, an opportunity of an interview with the Tribunal, at a time and place of which at least seven days' notice shall be given unless the person concerned has disclaimed any interest in the application; and

(c) consider any written representations made to them with reference to the application. Any person interviewed by the Tribunal shall be given an opportunity of stating his views and drawing the attention of the Tribunal to any evidence or information relevant to the application.

References by the Secretary of State (Rule 18)

The Tribunal is to consider a reference by the Minister as if it were an application by a patient who had not requested a formal hearing but with the following modifications of the Rules:

(a) Rule 4 as to postponement and Rule 16 as to an application being withdrawn or deemed to be withdrawn if the patient ceases to be liable to be detained or subject to guardianship do not apply;

(b) 'notification of the reference' instead of a copy of the application has to be given to the responsible authority under Rule 5;

(c) Rule 27 (3) and (5) as to notification of the decision of a Tribunal and reason therefore to the applicant applies as though the Minister were applicant;

(d) the Minister may if he thinks fit withdraw the reference at any time before it is determined by the Tribunal.

References by Home Secretary (Rule 19)

References by the Home Secretary are to be considered by a Tribunal in whatever informal manner they think appropriate. They may interview the patient and shall do so if he so requests. After considering the references the Tribunal are to give their advice thereon to the Home Secretary.

Proceedings in Private (Rule 20)

In respect of informal determinations on applications and in respect of references by the Minister or the Home Secretary, the proceedings of a Tribunal are to take place in private but the Tribunal may, if they think fit, authorise any person to attend.

(d) Formal Hearings

The following rules apply only when the applicant has requested a formal hearing.[1]

Notice of Hearing (Rule 22)

The Tribunal must give seven days' notice of the date, time and place of the hearing to the applicant, to the responsible authority, to any person who received a notice of the application under Rule 7 and to any other person who, in the opinion of the Tribunal, should have an opportunity of being heard.

[1] Rules 3 (3) and 21.

Decision as to Formal Hearing (Rule 23)

If the patient is the applicant the Tribunal may consider whether a formal hearing would be detrimental to his health, and must do so if the authority's statement includes an opinion by the responsible medical officer that it would be detrimental. Where the Tribunal are of opinion that a formal hearing would be detrimental to the patient's health the application is to be determined informally as though a formal hearing had not been requested.

Privacy of Proceedings (Rule 24)

The Tribunal is to sit in private unless the applicant requests a public hearing and the Tribunal are satisfied that such public hearing would not be detrimental to the interests of the patient and would not for any other reason be undesirable.

When sitting in private the Tribunal may admit to the hearing any person or class of persons on such terms and conditions as they consider appropriate. They may exclude from any hearing (*i.e.*, whether in public or private) any person or class of persons they think fit; and may exclude the patient or any other person while they are hearing evidence if, in their opinion, it would be undesirable in the interests of the patient or for other special reasons for the patient or such other person to be present.

Except so far as the Tribunal may direct, information about proceedings before the Tribunal and the names of any persons concerned shall not be made public. The meaning of this is clear as regards applications heard in private but if the hearing is in public it is not quite so clear. It seems however, that it restricts members of the public attending a public hearing from publishing what they hear. If so all newspaper reports even of public hearings are forbidden unless the Tribunal otherwise directs.

Nothing in the foregoing provisions of Rule 24 is to prevent a member of the Council on Tribunals attending a hearing in his capacity as such.

Procedure (Rule 25)

The Tribunal shall give an opportunity to the applicant to address the Tribunal, to give evidence and call witnesses; and the responsible authority and, with the permission of the Tribunal, any other person, may put questions to the applicant or to any witness called by him or on his behalf.

The Tribunal shall give the responsible authority and any other person notified of the hearing under the provisions of Rule 22 an opportunity to address them, to give evidence and to call witnesses and may permit any other person whom they think fit to do so; and the applicant and the responsible authority, and with the permission of the tribunal any other person, may put questions to any person giving evidence before the Tribunal.

Where the patient is the applicant or is called as a witness, the Tribunal may if they consider it desirable in the interests of the patient's health to do so interview the patient or take his evidence in private or in any manner they think appropriate. Subject to the above, any person who has received notice of the hearing may appear and take such part in the proceedings as the Tribunal think proper.

Adjournment for Further Information (Rule 26)

Where it appears to the Tribunal that it is desirable to obtain further information on any point, the Tribunal may adjourn for the information to be obtained in such manner as they may direct or for the applicant or any other person concerned to produce the information.

Where after any such adjournment the Tribunal consider that a resumed hearing is desirable or where a resumed hearing is requested by the applicant or the responsible authority, not less than seven days' notice thereof (or such shorter notice as all persons concerned may agree) shall be given to the applicant, to the responsible authority and to any other person who was notified of the hearing under the provisions of Rule 22 and who appeared at the previous hearing.

(e) Decisions and Miscellaneous Provisions

Decisions (Rule 27)

Decisions which are to be by a majority of the Tribunal, the president having a second or casting vote, are to be recorded in the form prescribed in the Fourth Schedule[1] and signed by the president.

The decision of the Tribunal shall be communicated in writing within seven days to the applicant, the responsible authority, the patient (where he is not the applicant) and to such other persons as the Tribunal may direct, and the Tribunal shall at the same time inform the applicant and the responsible authority of their right to request reasons for the decision in accordance with Rule 27 (5). If, however, the Tribunal consider that it would not be desirable to communicate their decision in writing to the patient (where he is not the applicant) it shall be communicated to him in such a manner as the Tribunal think appropriate.

The reasons for the Tribunal's decision shall be recorded in the form prescribed in the Fifth Schedule to the Rules and signed by the president.

The applicant and the responsible authority may, within three weeks after receiving notice in writing of the decision, request the Tribunal to give their reasons, and the Tribunal shall comply with any such request except where they consider that it would be undesirable to do so in the interests of the patient or for other special reasons.

Except as stated above, the Tribunal may, where they think it proper to do so, prohibit the publication of the text or a summary of the whole or part of their decision or of their reasons, or direct that the text or summary may be published only to such persons and on such conditions as they may prescribe.

Transfer of Proceedings (Rule 28)

Where an application or reference has not been disposed of by the members of the Tribunal appointed for the purpose and the chairman of the Tribunal is of opinion that it is not practicable or not possible without undue delay for the consideration of the application or reference to be completed by those members, he shall make arrangements for it to be disposed of by other members of the Tribunal.

Where a patient in respect of whom an application or reference is pending moves within the jurisdiction of another Tribunal, the proceedings shall, if the chairman of the Tribunal to whom the application or reference was made so directs, be transferred to the Tribunal with the jurisdiction of which the patient has moved, and that Tribunal shall have power to deal with the application or reference as if it had been made to them.

[1] As replaced by new Fourth Sch. contained in Mental Health Review Tribunal (Amendment) Rules S.I. 1976 No. 447 issued in consequence of the 1975 Amendment Act.

Time (Rule 29)

When because the time prescribed by or under the Rules for doing any act expires on a Sunday or public holiday the act cannot be done on that day, it will be in time if done on the next working day. The time appointed in the Rules for doing any act may be extended by the Tribunal or by the chairman on such terms as he or they think fit and such extension may be granted although the application for extension is not made until after the expiration of the time appointed.

Services of Notices, etc. (Rule 30)

Any application, notice or other document required or authorised by these Rules to be sent or given to any person may be sent by prepaid post or delivered —

(a) in the case of a document directed to the Tribunal or chairman of the Tribunal, to their office;

(b) in any other case, to the last known address of the person to whom the document is directed;

and if sent or given to the authorised representative of any person shall be deemed to be sent or given to that person.

Irregularities (Rule 31)

Any irregularity resulting from failure to comply with these Rules before the Tribunal have reached their decision shall not of itself render the proceedings void, but the Tribunal may, and shall if they consider that any person may have been prejudiced, take such steps as they think fit before reaching their decision to cure the irregularity, whether by the amendment of any document, the giving of any notice, the taking of any step or otherwise.

L. MISCELLANEOUS MATTERS UNDER THE MENTAL HEALTH ACT 1959

Part IX of the Mental Health Act 1959, deals with a number of miscellaneous matters, some of which have already been mentioned.

1. Forgery, etc.

Forgery of applications, medical recommendations and other documents required or authorised for the purposes of the Act and false entries or statements are offences punishable summarily or on indictment under s. 125.

2. Ill-treatment of Patients

Ill-treatment of patients whether in-patients or out-patients is similarly an offence under s. 126.

3. Sexual Intercourse with Patients

Section 128 provides:

(1) Without prejudice to s. 7 of the Sexual Offences Act 1956, it shall be an offence, subject to the exception mentioned in this section —

(a) for a man who is an officer on the staff of or is otherwise employed in, or is one of the managers of, a hospital or mental nursing home to have unlawful sexual intercourse with a woman who is for the time being receiving treatment for mental disorder in that hospital or home, or to have such intercourse on the premises of which the hospital or home forms part with a woman who is for the time being receiving such treatment there as an out-patient;

(b) for a man to have unlawful sexual intercourse with a woman who is a mentally disordered patient and who is subject to his guardianship under this Act or is otherwise in his custody or care under this Act or in pursuance of arrangements under Part III of the National Assistance Act 1948, *National Health Service Act 1977*,[1] or as a resident in a residential home for mentally disordered persons within the meaning of Part III of this Act.[2]

(2) It shall not be an offence under this section for a man to have sexual intercourse with a woman if he does not know and has no reason to suspect her to be a mentally disordered patient.

(3) Any person guilty of an offence under this section shall be liable on conviction on indictment to imprisonment for a term not exceeding two years.

(4) No proceedings shall be instituted for an offence under this section except by or with the consent of the Director of Public Prosecutions.

(5) This section shall be construed as one with the Sexual Offences Act 1956; and s. 47 of that Act (which relates to the proof of exceptions) shall apply to the exception mentioned in this section.

4. Homosexual Relations with a Male Patient

By s. 1 (4) of the Sexual Offences Act 1967 the provisions of s. 128 set out above now apply also to buggery or an act of gross indecency by a member of the staff of a hospital with a male patient or by a guardian with a male patient in his care.

It should also be noted that s. 1 (3) of the Sexual Offences Act 1967 lays down that a man who is suffering from severe subnormality cannot in law give any consent which, by virtue of s. 1 (1), would prevent a homosexual act from being an offence. The defence, however, would be open to the other party of proving that he did not know and had no reason to suspect that the man was suffering from severe subnormality.

Except as so made illegal, other homosexual acts by or with male mental patients are now lawful.[3]

5. Sexual Offences — Amendment of the Sexual Offences Act 1956

Section 7 of the Sexual Offences Act 1956, which made unlawful sexual intercourse with a female known to be an idiot or an imbecile, has been repealed and a new section substituted which makes it an offence for a man to have unlawful sexual intercourse with a woman

[1] Words in italics inserted by that Act.
[2] S. 19, to which this is reference, is not repealed by the Nursing Homes Act 1975.
[3] Unless, of course, still outlawed under the general law, *e.g.* where they are not in private.

who is a defective unless he does not know and has no reason to suspect her to be a defective. Also, s. 45 of the Act of 1956 is amended so that *defective* as used in s. 7 of that Act means a person suffering from severe subnormality within the meaning of the Mental Health Act 1959. Section 8 of the Act of 1956 relating to sexual intercourse with a woman under care and treatment, on licence or under guardianship, being no longer necessary having regard to the wider terms of the new s. 7, is repealed.

An order under s. 38 of the Sexual Offences Act 1956, divesting a man of authority over a girl, on his conviction for incest or attempted incest in respect of her, the girl being a defective within the meaning of that Act, may, so far as it has effect for any of the purposes of the Mental Health Act 1959, be rescinded under that section either before or after the girl has attained the age of 18.[1] The relevance of this is in respect of guardianship and also of the powers of the nearest relative under the Act of 1959.

6. Assisting Patients to Absent Themselves Without Leave, etc.

Section 129 provides:

Any person who induces or knowingly assists any other person —
(a) being liable to be detained in a hospital within the meaning of Part IV of this Act, or being subject to guardianship under the Act, to absent himself without leave; or
(b) being in legal custody by virtue of s. 139 of this Act, to escape from such custody;
shall be guilty of an offence.

(2) Any person who knowingly harbours a patient who is absent without leave or is otherwise at large and liable to be retaken under this Act, or gives him any assistance with intent to prevent, hinder or interfere with his being taken into custody or returned to the hospital or other place where he ought to be, shall be guilty of an offence.

An offence under this section shall be liable —
(a) on summary conviction, to imprisonment for term not exceeding six months or to fine not exceeding £100 or to both;
(b) on conviction on indictment to imprisonment for a term not exceeding two years or to a fine, or to both.

7. Obstruction

Section 130 (1) provides:

Any person who refuses to allow the inspection of any premises, or without reasonable cause refuses to allow the visiting, interviewing or examination of any person by a person authorised in that behalf by or under this Act or to produce for the inspection of any person so authorised any document or record the production of which is duly required by him, or otherwise obstructs any such person in the exercise of his functions, is guilty of an offence.

[4] Section 127. Age 18 substituted by s. 1 (3) of the Family Law Reform Act 1969.

Also any person who insists on being present when requested to withdraw by a person authorised as aforesaid to interview or examine a person in private, is guilty of an offence.[1] Any person guilty of any such offence is liable on summary conviction to imprisonment for a term not exceeding three months or to a fine not exceeding £100, or to both.[2]

8. Prosecutions by Local Social Services and Registration Authorities

Section 131 gives authority to local Social Services Authorities to institute proceedings in respect of offences under Part IX of the Act and to Registration Authorities to institute proceedings in respect of offences under s. 130 in connection with the inspection of any premises, or the visiting, interviewing or examination of any person by a person authorised in that behalf by a Registration Authority. The authority thus given is without prejudice to any provision for requiring the consent of the Director of Public Prosecutions. It is to be observed that so far as local Social Services Authorities and the Registration Authorities are concerned s. 131 is permissive and not mandatory; also that it does not restrict to those Authorities the right of instituting proceedings.

9. Hospitals for Reception of Urgent Cases

Under s. 132 it is the duty of every Regional Health Authority and, in Wales, of every Area Health Authority to give notice to every Local Social Services Authority for an area wholly or partly comprised within the region or area of such Health Authority specifying the hospital or hospitals administered by that Authority in which arrangements are from time to time in force for the reception, in case of special urgency, of patients requiring treatment for mental disorder.

10. Provision of Pocket Money for In-patients

The Secretary of State may pay to persons who are receiving treatment as in-patients (whether liable to be detained or not) in *special hospitals*[3] or other hospitals being hospitals wholly or mainly used for the treatment of persons suffering from mental disorder, such amounts as he thinks fit in respect of their occasional personal expenses where it appears to him that they would otherwise be without resources to meet those expenses.[4] For the purposes of the National Health Service Act 1946 and the National Health Service Reorganisation Act 1973, the

---

[1] Section 130 (2).   [2] Section 130 (3).

[3] *Special hospitals* means institutions provided by the Secretary of State for persons subject to detention under the Act, who in the opinion of the Secretary of State require treatment under conditions of special security on account of their dangerous, violent or criminal propensities.

[4] Section 133 (1).

making of such payments to persons for whom hospital services are provided under those Acts, is to be treated as included among those services.[1]

11. Mentally Disordered Members of Parliament

In s. 137 are set out provisions relating to the vacating of his seat by a member of the House of Commons, authorised to be detained on the ground (however formulated) that he is suffering from mental illness. A member not liable to detention — however serious his mental illness — will not be subject to the provisions of s. 137.

12. Pay, Pensions, etc., of Mentally Disordered Persons

Section 138 provides:

(1) Where a periodic payment falls to be made to any person by way of pay or pension or otherwise in connection with the service or employment of that or any other person, and the payment falls to be made directly out of moneys provided by Parliament or the Consolidated Fund, or other moneys administered by or under the control or supervision of a government department,[2] the authority by whom the sum in question is payable, if satisfied after considering medical evidence that the person to whom it is payable (hereinafter referred to as 'the patient') is incapable by reason of mental disorder of managing and administering his property and affairs, may, instead of paying the sum to the patient, apply it in accordance with the next following subsection.

(2) The authority may pay the sum or such part thereof as they think fit to the institution or person having the care of the patient, to be applied for his benefit, and may pay the remainder (if any) or such part thereof as they think fit —

(a) to or for the benefit of persons who appear to the authority to be members of the patient's family or other persons for whom the patient might be expected to provide if he were not mentally disordered; or

(b) in reimbursement, with or without interest, of money applied by any person either in payment of the patient's debts (whether legally enforceable or not) or for the maintenance or other benefit of the patient or such persons as are mentioned in the foregoing paragraph.

13. Provisions as to Custody, Conveyance and Detention

Section 139 provides:

(1) Any person required or authorised by or by virtue of the Act to be conveyed[3] to any place or to be kept in custody or detained in a place of safety or at any place to which he is taken under s. 66 (5) of this Act[4] shall

---

[1] Section 133 (2).

[2] *Government department* does not include a department of the Government of Northern Ireland. Section 138 (3).

[3] *Convey* includes any other expression denoting removal from one place to another (s. 139 (3)).

[4] *i.e.*, a Part V patient subject to an order restricting discharge, directed by the Home Secretary to be taken to any place in the interests of justice or for the purposes of a public inquiry.

while being so conveyed, detained or kept, as the case may be, to be deemed to be in legal custody.

(2) A constable or any other person required or authorised by or by virtue of this Act to take any person into custody, or to convey[1] or detain any person shall, for the purposes of taking him into custody or conveying or detaining him, have all the powers, authorities, protection and privileges which a constable has within the area for which he acts as constable.

14. Retaking of Patients Escaping from Custody

Section 140 provides:

(1) If any person being in legal custody by virtue of s. 139 of this Ac escapes, he may, subject to the following provisions, be retaken —

(a) in any case, by the person who had his custody immediately before the escape, or by any constable or mental welfare officer;

(b) if at the time of the escape he was liable to be detained in a hospital within the meaning of Part IV of this Act, or subject to guardianship under the Act, by any other person who could take him into custody under s. 40 if he had absented himself without leave.

(2) A person who escapes as aforesaid when liable to be detained or subject to guardianship as mentioned in paragraph (b) of the foregoing subsection (not being a person subject to an order under Part V of the Act restricting his discharge or an order or direction having the like effect as such an order) shall not be retaken under this section after the expiration of the period within which he could be retaken under s. 40 of the Act if he had absented himself without leave on the day of the escape; and s. 40 (3) applies with the necessary modifications accordingly.

(3) A person who escapes while being taken to or detained in a place of safety under s. 135 or s. 136 of this Act shall not be retaken after the expiration of the period of 72 hours beginning with the time when he escapes or the period during which he is liable to be so detained, whichever expires first.

(4) This section, in so far as it relates to the escape of a person liable to be detained in a hospital within the meaning of Part IV of the Act, apply in relation to a person who escapes —

(a) while being taken to or from such a hospital in pursuance of regulations under s. 41 of the Act, or of any order, direction or authorisation under Parts V to VII of this Act; or

(b) while being taken to or detained in a place of safety in pursuance of an order under Part V of this Act pending his admission to such a hospital;

as if he were liable to be detained in that hospital and, if he had not previously been received therein, as if he had been so received.

(5) In computing for the purposes of ss. 63 and 64 of the Act the period of 28 days therein mentioned, no account shall be taken of any time during which the patient is at large and liable to be retaken by virtue of this section.

(6) Section 45 of this Act shall, with any necessary modifications, apply in relation to a patient who is at large and liable to be retaken by virtue of this section as it applies in relation to a patient who is absent without leave within the meaning of s. 40 of the Act, and references therein to s. 40 are to be construed accordingly.

[1] *Convey* includes any other expression denoting removal from one place to another (s. 139 (3)).

u

15. Protection for Acts done in Pursuance of the Act

Section 141 provides:

(1) No person shall be liable, whether on the ground of want of jurisdiction or on any other ground, to any civil or criminal proceedings to which he would have been liable apart from the provisions of this section in respect of any act purporting to be done in pursuance of this Act or any regulations or rules thereunder, or in, or in pursuance of anything done in, the discharge of functions conferred by any other enactment on the authority having jurisdiction under Part VIII of the Act, unless the act was done in bad faith or without reasonable care.

(2) No civil or criminal proceedings shall be brought against any person in any court in respect of any such act without the leave of the High Court,[1] and the High Court shall not give leave under this section unless satisfied that there is substantial ground for the contention that the person to be proceeded against has acted in bad faith or without reasonable care.

(3) This section does not apply to proceedings for an offence under the Act, being proceedings which, under any provision of the Act, can be instituted only by or with the consent of the Director of Public Prosecutions.

This section is widely drafted and it has been held ought to be widely construed.[2] In *Richardson* v. *L.C.C.*[3], Denning, L.J., suggested that the section gave protection to the Authorities even though they misconstrued the Act or had in fact acted without jurisdiction so long as there were no solid grounds for the contention that they had acted in bad faith or without reasonable care. Parker, L.J., in the same case said that the Authorities were allowed to misconstrue statute so long as it could bear that interpretation to the non-legal mind. However in *Buxton* v. *Jayne*,[4] Devlin, L.J., said 'there are limits to which the plaintiffs can be expected to prove a negative'. But in *R.* v. *Runighan* it was held that the section did not apply to informal patients.[5]

In *Pountney* v. *Griffiths*,[6] the House of Lords quashed a conviction for assault by a nurse on a mental patient on the basis that no leave under s. 141 had been sought or obtained. In the Divisional Court in that case[7] it was said that if the nurse used no more than reasonable force to enforce the detention provisions of the Act, no assault would have been committed and he would not have needed the protection of s. 141. If the assault had taken place when the nurse was not on duty or in circumstances in which it could not clearly be justified as an act of control within the terms of the nurse's duty, s. 141 would not apply. The section only applied therefore when more than reasonable force was used when the nurse was carrying out his duties.

---

[1] References to the High Court are to be construed, in relation to Northern Ireland, as references to a judge of the High Court of Northern Ireland (s. 141 (4)).
[2] *Richardson* v. *L.C.C.* [1957] 2 All E.R. 330, 339; *Shackleton* v. *Swift* [1913] 2 K.B. 304.
[3] See previous footnote.　　　[4] [1960] 1 W.L.R. 783.　　　[5] [1977] Crim. L.R. 361.
[6] [1975] 3 W.L.R. 140. *Sub nom. R.* v. *Bracknell Justices ex p. Griffiths.*
[7] [1975] 2 W.L.R. 291.

In neither Court was the extent of these duties discussed and accordingly it would appear that there is still doubt as to *e.g.* whether the section would protect the Authorities for the imposition of treatment even as a result of that detention for treatment.[1] In *Moore* v. *Commissioner of Metropolitan Police*[2] it was held that the application, an interlocutory matter, and that therefore leave was required before an appeal could be made against a judge's order. Finally, it may be mentioned that in *Carter* v. *Commissioner of Metropolitan Police*[3] it was held that the Court is entitled and bound to consider any evidence produced by the proposed defendants.

16. Default Powers of Secretary of State

Section 142 provides:

(1) Where the Minister is of opinion, on complaint or otherwise, that a Local *Social Services*[4] Authority have failed to carry out functions conferred or imposed on the Authority by or under this Act or have in carrying out those functions failed to comply with any regulations relating thereto, he may after such inquiry as he thinks fit make an order declaring the Authority to be in default.

Section 85 (3)–(5) of the National Health Service Act 1977 (which relates to orders declaring, among others, a local authority to be in default under that Act) applies in relation to an order under s. 142 of the Act of 1959.[5]

17. Inquiries

By s. 143 the Secretary of State may cause an inquiry to be held in any case where he thinks it advisable to do so in connection with any matter arising under the Act, and s. 250 of the Local Government Act 1972, applies to any inquiry held under the Act, except that no Local Authority shall be ordered to pay costs in the case of any inquiry unless the Authority is a party thereto[6]. The Tribunals and Inquiries Act 1971 applies to any such inquiry to the extent provided in the Tribunals and Inquiries (Discretionary Inquiries) Order 1975[7].

18. Expenses

Section 144 (1) provides:

There are to be defrayed out of moneys provided by Parliament —
(*a*) any expenses incurred by the Minister[8] or a Secretary of State under the Act;

---

[1] I have discussed the whole question more fully in *The Right of the Mental Patient to his Psychosis* (1975) 39 M.L.R. at p. 17.
[2] [1968] 1 Q.B. 26.   [3] [1975] 1 W.L.R. 507.
[4] Words in italics substituted by Local Government Act 1972.
[5] Section 142 (2) as amended.   [6] Section 143.
[7] S.I. 1975 No. 1379.   [8] Now Secretary of State for Social Services.

(*b*) any sums required for the payment of fees and expenses to medical practitioners acting in relation to a member of the House of Commons under s. 137 of the Act;

   (*c*) any increase attributable to the Act in the sums payable out of moneys provided by Parliament under any other enactment.

19. Application of Act to Scilly Isles

Subsection (4) of s. 130 of the National Health Service Act 1977 (which provides for the extension of that Act to the Isles of Scilly) has effect as if the references to that Act included references to the Mental Health Act 1959.[1]

[1] Section 154 (2).

APPENDIX A

NATIONAL HEALTH SERVICE ACT 1977

PART I

SERVICES AND ADMINISTRATION

Functions of the Secretary of State

1.—1. It is the Secretary of State's duty to continue the promotion in England and Wales of a comprehensive health service designed to secure improvement —

    (*a*) in the physical and mental health of the people of those countries, and

    (*b*) in the prevention, diagnosis and treatment of illness,

and for that purpose to provide or secure the effective provision of services in accordance with this Act.

(2) The services so provided shall be free of charge except in so far as the making and recovery of charges is expressly provided for by or under any enactment, whenever passed.

2. Without prejudice to the Secretary of State's powers apart from this section, he has power —

    (*a*) to provide such services as he considers appropriate for the purpose of discharging any duty imposed on him by this Act; and

    (*b*) to do any other thing whatsoever which is calculated to facilitate, or is conducive or incidental to, the discharge of such a duty.

This section is subject to section 3 (3) below.

3.—(1) It is the Secretary of State's duty to provide throughout England and Wales, to such extent as he considers necessary to meet all reasonable requirements —

    (*a*) hospital accommodation;

    (*b*) other accommodation for the purpose of any service provided under this Act;

    (*c*) medical, dental, nursing and ambulance services;

    (*d*) such other facilities for the care of expectant and nursing mothers and young children as he considers are appropriate as part of the health service;

    (*e*) such facilities for the prevention of illness, the care of persons suffering from illness and the after-care of persons who have suffered from illness as he considers are appropriate as part of the health service;

(*f*) such other services as are required for the diagnosis and treatment of illness.

(2) Where any hospital provided by the Secretary of State in accordance with this Act was a voluntary hospital transferred by virtue of the National Health Service Act 1946, and —

(*a*) the character and associations of that hospital before its transfer were such as to link it with a particular religious denomination, then

(*b*) regard shall be had in the general administration of the hospital to the preservation of that character and those associations.

(3) Nothing in section 2 above or in this section affects the provisions of Part II of this Act (which relates to arrangements with practitioners for the provision of medical, dental, ophthalmic and pharmaceutical services).

4. The duty imposed on the Secretary of State by section 1 above to provide services for the purposes of the health service includes a duty to provide and maintain establishments (in this Act referred to as 'special hospitals') for persons subject to detention under the Mental Health Act 1959 who in his opinion require treatment under conditions of special security on account of their dangerous, violent or criminal propensities.

5.—(1) It is the Secretary of State's duty —

(*a*) to provide for the medical and dental inspection at appropriate intervals of pupils in attendance at schools maintained by local education authorities and for the medical and dental treatment of such pupils (and the additional provisions set out in Schedule 1[1] to this Act have effect in relation to this paragraph);

(*b*) to arrange, to such extent as he considers necessary to meet all reasonable requirements in England and Wales, for the giving of advice on contraception, the medical examination of persons seeking advice on contraception, the treatment of such persons and the supply of contraceptive substances and appliances.

(2) The Secretary of State may —

(*a*) provide invalid carriages for persons appearing to him to be

----

[1] Not here reproduced.

suffering from severe physical defect or disability and, at the request of such a person, may provide for him a vehicle other than an invalid carriage (and the additional provisions set out in Schedule 2[1] to this Act have effect in relation to this paragraph);

(b) arrange to provide accommodation and treatment outside Great Britain for persons suffering from respiratory tuberculosis;

(c) provide a microbiological service, which may include the provision of laboratories, for the control of the spread of infectious diseases (and the Secretary of State may allow persons to use services provided at such laboratories on such terms, including terms as to charges, as he thinks fit);

(d) conduct, or assist by grants or otherwise (without prejudice to the general powers and duties conferred on him under the Ministry of Health Act 1919) any person to conduct, research into any matters relating to the causation, prevention, diagnosis or treatment of illness, and into any such other matters connected with any service provided under this Act as he considers appropriate.

(3) Regulations may provide for the payment by the Secretary of State in such cases as may be prescribed of travelling expenses (including the travelling expenses of a companion) incurred or to be incurred by persons for the purpose of availing themselves of any services provided under this Act.

(4) The Public Health Laboratory Service Board continues in being for the purpose of exercising such functions with respect to the administration of the public health laboratory service (the service referred to in paragraph (c) of subsection (2) above) as the Secretary of State may determine.

(5) The Board shall continue to be constituted in accordance with Part I of Schedule 3 to this Act, and the additional provisions set out in Part II of that Schedule have effect in relation to the Board.

Central Health Services Council and Medical Practices Committee

6.—(1) The Central Health Services Council (in this Act referred to as 'the Central Council') shall have the duty of advising the Secretary of State upon such general matters relating to the services provided under this Act as the Council think fit, and upon any questions relating to those services which he may refer to them.

---

[1] Not here reproduced.

(2) The Central Council shall be constituted in accordance with Schedule 4 to this Act, but the Secretary of State may by order vary that constitution after consultation with the Council; and the supplementary provisions of that Schedule have effect in relation to the Central Council and any standing advisory committee ,constituted under subsection (3) below.

(3) The Secretary of State may, after consultation with the Central Council, by order constitute standing advisory committees for the purpose of advising him and the Council on such of the services provided under this Act as may be specified in the order.

(4) Any committee so constituted shall consist partly of members of the Central Council appointed by the Secretary of State, and partly of persons (whether or not members of the Council) appointed by the Secretary of State after consultation with such representative organisations as he may recognise for the purpose.

(5) It shall be the duty of a committee so constituted to advise the Secretary of State and the Central Council —

(a) upon such matters relating to the services with which the committee are concerned as they think fit, and

(b) upon any questions referred to them by the Secretary of State or the Council relating to those services,

and, if the committee advise the Secretary of State upon any matter, they shall inform the Council, who may express their views on the matter to the Secretary of State.

(6) The Central Council shall make an annual report to the Secretary of State on their proceedings, and on the proceedings of any standing advisory committee constituted under subsection (3) above, and, subject to subsection (7) below, the Secretary of State shall lay that report before Parliament with such comments (if any) as he thinks fit.

(7) If the Secretary of State, after consultation with the Central Council, is satisfied that it would be contrary to the public interest to lay any such report, or a part of any such report before Parliament, he may refrain from so laying that report or that part.

7.—(1) The Medical Practices Committee —

(a) shall consist of a chairman and eight other members appointed by the Secretary of State after consultation with such organisations as he may recognise as representative of the medical profession; and

(b) the chairman and six of the other members shall be medical practitioners, and five at least of those six shall be actively engaged in medical practice.

(2) The Secretary of State may —

    (a) make regulations as to the appointment, tenure of office and vacation of office of the members of the Committee; and

    (b) provide the services of such officers as the Committee may require.

(3) The Committee's proceedings shall not be invalidated by any vacancy in its membership or by any defect in a member's appointment or qualification.

Local administration

8.—(1) It is the Secretary of State's duty to establish by order in accordance with Part I of Schedule 5 to this Act —

    (a) authorities, to be called Regional Health Authorities, for such regions in England as he may by order determine, and

    (b) authorities, to be called either Area Health Authorities or (in accordance with section 9 below) Area Health Authorities (Teaching), for such areas in Wales and those regions as he may by order determine,

and orders determining regions or areas in pursuance of this subsection shall be separate from orders establishing authorities for the regions or areas.

Any reference in the following provisions of this Act to an Area Health Authority includes a reference to an Area Health Authority (Teaching) unless the context otherwise requires.

(2) The Secretary of State may by order vary the region of a Regional Health Authority or the area of an Area Health Authority whether or not the variation entails the determination of a new or the abolition of an existing region or area.

(3) It is the Secretary of State's duty to exercise the powers conferred on him by the preceding provisions of this section so as to secure —

    (a) that the regions determined in pursuance of those provisions together comprise the whole of England, that the areas so determined together comprise the whole of Wales and those regions and that no region includes part only of any area; and

    (b) that the provision of health services in each region can conveniently be associated with a university which has a school of medicine or with two or more such universities.

(4) An order made by virtue of subsection (2) above may (without prejudice to the generality of section 126 (4) below) contain such provisions for the transfer of officers, property, rights and liabilities as the Secretary of State thinks fit.

(5) It is the Secretary of State's duty before he makes an order under subsection (2) to consult with respect to the order —

(*a*) such bodies as he may recognise as representing officers who in his opinion are likely to be transferred or affected by transfers in pursuance of the order; and

(*b*) such other bodies as he considers are concerned with the order.

9.—(1) An order establishing an Authority in pursuance of paragraph (*b*) of section 8(1) above may provide for it to be called an Area Health Authority (Teaching) if and only if the Secretary of State is satisfied that the Authority is to provide for a university or universities substantial facilities for undergraduate or post-graduate clinical teaching.

(2) Where the Secretary of State is satisfied that an Area Health Authority is to provide, or is providing such facilities, he may provide by order for the Authority to be called an Area Health Authority (Teaching), and, where he is satisfied that an Area Health Authority (Teaching) no longer provides such facilities, he may provide by order for the Authority to be called an Area Health Authority.

(3) It is the Secretary of State's duty, before providing that an Authority shall be called or cease to be called an Area Health Authority (Teaching), to consult the university or universities concerned with the facilities in question.

10. It is the duty of each Area Health Authority to establish for its area, in accordance with Part II of Schedule 5 to this Act, a body called a Family Practitioner Committee, and each Family Practitioner Committee has the duty described in section 15 below.

11.—(1) If the Secretary of State considers that a special body should be established for the purpose of performing any functions which he may direct the body to perform on his behalf, or on behalf of an Area Health Authority or a Family Practitioner Committee, he may by order establish a body for that purpose.

(2) The Secretary of State may, subject to the provisions of Part III of Schedule 5 to this Act, make such further provision relating to that body as he thinks fit.

(3) A body established in pursuance of this section shall (without prejudice to the power conferred by subsection (4) below to allocate a particular name to the body) be called a special health authority.

(4) Without prejudice to the generality of the power conferred by this section to make an order (or of section 126(4) below), that order may in particular contain provisions as to —

(*a*) the membership of the body established by the order;

(*b*) the transfer to the body of officers, property, rights and liabilities; and (*c*) the name by which the body is to be known.

(5) It is the Secretary of State's duty before he makes such an order to consult with respect to the order such bodies as he may recognise as representing officers who in his opinion are likely to be transferred or affected by transfers in pursuance of the order.

12. The provisions of Part III of Schedule 5 to this Act have effect, so far as applicable, in relation to —

(*a*) Regional Health Authorities and Area Health Authorities established under section 8 above;

(*b*) Family Practitioner Committees established under section 10 above;

(*c*) any special health authority established under section 11 above.

13.—(1) The Secretary of State may direct a Regional Health Authority, an Area Health Authority of which the area is in Wales or a special health authority to exercise on his behalf such of his functions relating to the health service as are specified in the directions, and (subject to section 14 below) it shall be the duty of the body in question to comply with the directions.

(2) The Secretary of State's functions under subsection (1) above —

(*a*) include any of his functions under enactments relating to mental health and nursing homes, but

(*b*) exclude the duty imposed on him by section 1(1) above to secure the effective provision of the services mentioned in section 15 below.

14.—(1) A Regional Health Authority may direct any Area Health Authority of which the area is included in its region to exercise such of the functions exercisable by the Regional Health Authority by virtue of section 13 above as are specified in the directions, and it is the Area Health Authority's duty to comply with the directions.

(2) If the Secretary of State directs a Regional Health Authority to secure that any of its functions specified in his directions are or are not exercisable by an Area Health Authority it is the Regional Health Authority's duty to comply with his directions.

15.—(1) It is the duty of each Family Practitioner Committee, in accordance with regulations —

(*a*) to administer, on behalf of the Area Health Authority by which the Committee was established, the arrangements made in pursuance of this Act for the provision of general medical services, general dental services, general ophthalmic services and pharmaceutical services for the area of the Authority, and

(b) to perform such other functions relating to those services as may be prescribed.

(2) If it appears to the Secretary of State that, in consequence of regulations made by virtue of the preceding provisions of this section, references to an Area Health Authority in particular provisions of this Act should be construed as references to a Family Practitioner Committee, he may by regulations provide accordingly.

16.—(1) Regulations may provide for functions exercisable by virtue of the provisions of sections 13 to 15 above by a body other than an Area Health Authority, or exercisable by virtue of any provision of this Act by an Area Health Authority, to be exercisable on behalf of the body in question —

(a) by an equivalent body or by another body of which the members consist only of the body and equivalent bodies;

(b) by a committee, sub-committee or officer of the body or an equivalent body or such another body as aforesaid;

(c) in the case of functions exercisable by an Area Health Authority, by a special health authority, an officer of such an authority or a Family Practitioner Committee;

(d) in the case of functions exercisable by a Family Practitioner Committee, by a special health authority, an officer of such an authority or an officer of an Area Health Authority.

(2) For the purposes of subsection (1) above, a Regional or Area Health Authority or a Family Practitioner Committee is equivalent to another body of the same name and a special health authority is equivalent to another such authority.

(3) Nothing in this section shall be construed as precluding any body from acting by an agent where it is entitled so to act apart from this section.

17. The Secretary of State may give directions with respect to the exercise of any functions exercisable by virtue of sections 13 to 16 above, or by an Area Health Authority by virtue of Part II of this Act; and, subject to any directions given by the Secretary of State by virtue of this section —

(a) a Regional Health Authority may give directions with respect to the exercise by an Area Health Authority of which the area is included in its region, of any functions exercisable by the Area Health Authority by virtue of section 14 above.

(b) an Area Health Authority may give directions with respect to the exercise by the Family Practitioner Committee established by it of any functions which are exercisable by the Committee by virtue of section 15 above and are prescribed for the purposes of this paragraph,

and it shall be the duty of the body in question to comply with the directions.

18.—(1) Any directions given by the Secretary of State in pursuance of sections 13 to 17 above shall be given either by regulations or by an instrument in writing, except that —

(*a*) any such directions in pursuance of section 13 above in respect of functions relating to special hospitals, and

(*b*) any such directions in respect of functions conferred on the Secretary of State by section 20(1) or (2) below,

shall only be given by regulations.

(2) Any directions given by an Authority in pursuance of sections 13 to 17 shall be given by an instrument in writing.

(3) Directions given and regulations made under sections 13 to 17 in respect of any function —

(*a*) shall not, except in prescribed cases, preclude a body or person by whom the function is exercisable apart from the directions or regulations from exercising the function, and

(*b*) may in the case of directions given by an instrument in writing be varied or revoked by subsequent directions given in pursuance of those sections and this section (without prejudice to the operation of section 32(3) of the Intepretation Act 1889 in the case of directions given by regulations).

so, however, that an Area Health Authority shall not be entitled to exercise any functions which, by virtue of section 15 above, are exercisable by the Family Practitioner Committee established by the Authority.

Local advisory committees and
Community Health Councils

19.—(1) Where the Secretary of State is satisfied that a committee formed for Wales, or for the region of a Regional Health Authority, is representative of persons of any of the following categories —

(*a*) the medical practitioners, or

(*b*) the dental practitioners, or

(*c*) the nurses and midwives, or

(*d*) the registered pharmacists, or

(*e*) the ophthalmic and dispensing opticians,

of Wales or of the region, then it shall be his duty to recognise the committee.

(2) A committee recognised in pursuance of subsection (1) above shall be called —

 (a) the Welsh Medical, Dental, Nursing and Midwifery, Pharmaceutical or Optical Committee, as the case may be;

 (b) the Regional Medical, Dental, Nursing and Midwifery, Pharmaceutical or Optical Committee, as the case may be, for the region in question.

(3) Where the Secretary of State is satisfied that a committee formed for the area of an Area Health Authority is representative of persons of any of the categories mentioned in paragraphs (a) to (e) in subsection (1) it shall be his duty to recognise the committee.

A committee recognised in pursuance of this subsection shall be called the Area Medical, Dental, Nursing and Midwifery, Pharmaceutical or Optical Committee, as the case may be, for the area in question.

(4) The Secretary of State's duty under subsections (1) and (3) above is subject to paragraph 1 of Schedule 6 to this Act, and that Schedule has effect in relation to a committee recognised in pursuance of this section.

20.—(1) It is the Secretary of State's duty to establish in accordance with this section a council for the area of each Area Health Authority, or separate councils for such separate parts of the areas of those Authorities as he thinks fit, and such a council shall be called a Community Health Council.

(2) The Secretary of State —

 (a) may if he thinks fit discharge this duty by establishing a Community Health Council for a district which includes the areas or parts of the areas of two or more Area Health Authorities, but

 (b) shall be treated as not having discharged that duty unless he secures that there is no part of the area of an Area Health Authority which is not included in some Community Health Council's district.

(3) The additional provisions of Schedule 7 to this Act have effect in relation to Community Health Councils.

Co-operation and assistance

21.—(1) Subject to paragraphs (d) and (e) of section 3(1) above, the services described in Schedule 8 to this Act in relation to —

 (a) care of mothers and young children,

 (b) prevention, care and after-care,

 (c) home help and laundry facilities,

are functions exercisable by local social services authorities, and that Schedule has effect accordingly.

(2) A local social services authority who provide premises, furniture or equipment for any of the purposes of this Act may permit the use of the premises, furniture or equipment —

(a) by any other local social services authority, or

(b) by any of the bodies constituted under this Act, or

(c) by a local education authority.

This permission may be on such terms (including terms with respect to the services of any staff employed by the authority giving permission) as may be agreed.

(3) A local social services authority may provide (or improve or furnish) residential accommodation —

(a) for officers employed by them for the purposes of any of their functions as a local social services authority, or

(b) for officers employed by a voluntary organisation for the purposes of any services provided under this section and Schedule 8.

22.—(1) In exercising their respective functions health authorities and local authorities shall co-operate with one another in order to secure and advance the health and welfare of the people of England and Wales.

(2) There shall be committees, to be called joint consultative committees, who shall advise Area Health Authorities and the authorities in column 2 of the Table below on the performance of their duties under subsection (1) above, and on the planning and operation of services of common concern to those authorities.

(3) Except as provided by an order under the following provisions of this section, each joint consultative committee shall represent one or more Area Health Authorities together with one or more of the authorities in column 2 of the Table above, and an Area Health Authority shall be represented together with each of the authorities associated with that Authority in column 2 of the said Table in one or other of the committees (but not necessarily the same committee).

(4) The Secretary of State shall have power by order to provide for any matter relating to joint consultative committees, and such an order may in particular —

(a) provide for the way in which the provisions of subsections (2) and (3) above are to be carried out, or provide for varying the arrangements set out in those subsections;

(b) provide, where it appears to the Secretary of State appropriate, for an Area Health Authority to be represented on a joint

TABLE

1 Area Health Authority	2 Associated authorities
An Area Health Authority in a metropolitan county in England.	The local authority for each district wholly or partly in the area of the Authority.
An Area Health Authority in a non-metropolitan county in England, or an Area Health Authority in Wales.	The local authority for each county, and also for each district, wholly or partly in the area of the Authority.
An Area Health Authority in Greater London.	The local authority for each London borough wholly or partly in the area of the Authority. Also the Inner London Education Authority, if wholly or partly in the area of the Authority. Also the Common Council of the City of London, if in the area of the Authority.

consultative committee together with a local or other authority whose area is not within the area of the Area Health Authority;

(c) afford a choice to any authorities as to the number of joint consultative committees on which they are to be represented, and provide for the case where the authorities cannot agree on the choice;

(d) authorise or require a joint consultative committee to appoint any sub-committee or to join with another joint consultative committee or other joint consultative committees in appointing a joint sub-committee;

(e) authorise or require the appointment to a joint consultative committee, or to any sub-committee, of persons who are not members of the authorities represented by the joint consultative committee;

(f) require the authorities represented on a joint consultative committee to defray the expenses of the committee, and of any sub-committee, in such shares as may be determined by or under the order, and provide for the way in which any dispute between those authorities concerning the expenses is to be resolved; and

(g) require those authorities to make reports to the Secretary of

State on the work of the joint consultative committee and of any sub-committee.

(5) Before making an order under this section the Secretary of State shall consult with such associations of local authorities as appear to him to be concerned, and with any local authority with whom consultation appears to him to be desirable.

23.—(1) The Secretary of State may, where he considers it appropriate, arrange with any person or body (including a voluntary organisation) for that person or body to provide, or assist in providing, any service under this Act.

In this section 'voluntary organisation' means a body the activities of which are carried on otherwise than for profit, but does not include any public or local authority.

(2) The Secretary of State may make available —

   (a) to any person or body (including a voluntary organisation) carrying out any arrangements under subsection (1) above, or

   (b) to any voluntary organisation eligible for assistance under section 64 or section 65 of the Health Services and Public Health Act 1968 (assistance made available by the Secretary of State or local authorities

any facilities (including goods or materials, or the use of any premises and the use of any vehicle, plant or apparatus) provided by him for any service under this Act; and, where anything is so made available, the services of persons employed by the Secretary of State, or by a health authority in connection with it.

(3) The powers conferred by this section may be exercised on such terms as may be agreed, including terms as to the making of payments by or to the Secretary of State, and any goods or materials may be made available either temporarily or permanently.

(4) The Secretary of State may by order provide that, in relation to a vehicle which is made available by him in pursuance of this section and is used in accordance with the terms on which it is so made available, the Vehicles (Excise) Act 1971 and Part VI of the Road Traffic Act 1972 shall have effect with such modifications as are specified in the order.

(5) Any power to supply goods or materials conferred by this section includes a power to purchase and store them and includes a power to arrange with third parties for the supply of goods or materials by those third parties.

24. Each health authority and the Public Health Laboratory Service Board has power —

(*a*) with the Secretary of State's consent, to enter into and carry out agreements with the relevant Minister under which, at the expense of that Minister, the authority or board acts as the instrument by means of which he furnishes technical assistance in the exercise of the power conferred on him by section 1(1) of the Overseas Aid Act 1966;

(*b*) with the consent of the Secretary of State and the relevant Minister, to enter into and carry out agreements which under the authority or board furnishes, for any purpose specified in that section 1(1), technical assistance (excluding financial assistance) in any country or territory outside the United Kingdom against reimbursement to the authority or board of of the cost of furnishing the assistance.

In this section 'the relevant Minister' means the Minister of the Crown by whom is exercisable the power conferred on the Minister of Overseas Development by that section 1(1) as originally enacted.

25. Where the Secretary of State has acquired —

(*a*) supplies of human blood for the purposes of any service under this Act, or

(*b*) any part of a human body for the purpose of, or in the course of providing, any such service, or

(*c*) supplies of any other substances or preparations not readily obtainable,

he may arrange to make such supplies or that part available (on such terms, including terms as to charges, as he thinks fit) to any person.

This section is subject to section 62 below (restriction of powers under sections 25, 58 and 61).

26.—(1) The Secretary of State may —

(*a*) supply to local authorities, and to such public bodies or classes of public bodies as he may determine, any goods or materials of a kind used in the health service;

(*b*) make available to local authorities, and to those bodies or classes of bodies, any facilities (including the use of any premises and the use of any vehicle, plant or apparatus) provided by him for any service under this Act, and the services of persons employed by the Secretary of State or by a health authority;

(*c*) carry out maintenance work in connection with any land or building for the maintenance of which a local authority is responsible.

In this subsection —

'maintenance work' includes minor renewals, minor improvements and minor extensions; and

'public bodies' includes public bodies in Northern Ireland.

(2) The Secretary of State may supply or make available to persons providing general medical services, general dental services, general ophthalmic services or pharmaceutical services such goods, materials or other facilities as may be prescribed.

(3) The Secretary of State shall make available to local authorities —

(a) any services or other facilities (excluding the services of any person but including goods or materials, the use of any premises and the use of any vehicle, plant or apparatus) provided under this Act,

(b) the services provided as part of the health service by any person employed by the Secretary of State or a health authority, and

(c) the services of any medical practitioner, dental practitioner or nurse employed by the Secretary of State or a health authority otherwise than to provide services which are part of the health service,

so far as is reasonably necessary and practicable to enable local authorities to discharge their functions relating to social services, education and public health.

27.—(1) It is the Secretary of State's duty, before he makes the services of any officer of a health authority available in pursuance of subsection (1)(b) or subsection (3)(b) or (c) of section 26 above, to consult the officer or a body recognised by the Secretary of State as representing the officer about the matter, or to satisfy himself that the health authority has consulted the officer about the matter.

(2) The Secretary of State shall be entitled to disregard the provisions of subsection (1) above in a case where he considers it necessary to make the services of an officer available as mentioned in that subsection for the purpose of dealing temporarily with an emergency, and has previously consulted such a body about the making available of services in an emergency.

(3) For the purposes of subsection (1)(b) or subsection (3)(b) or (c) of section 26 the Secretary of State may give such directions to health authorities to make the services of their officers available as he considers appropriate; and it shall be the health authority's duty to comply with any such directions.

(4) The powers conferred by this section and section 26 may be exercised on such terms as may be agreed, including terms as to the

making of payments to the Secretary of State, and such charges may be made by the Secretary of State in respect of services or facilities provided under subsection (3) of section 26 as may be agreed between the Secretary of State and the local authority or, in default of agreement, as may be determined by arbitration.

(5) The Secretary of State may by order provide that, in relation to a vehicle which is made available by him in pursuance of section 26 and is used in accordance with the terms on which it is so made available the Vehicles (Excise) Act 1971 and Part VI of the Road Traffic Act 1972 shall have effect with such modifications as are specified in the order.

(6) Any power to supply goods or materials conferred by section 26 includes a power to purchase and store them, and a power to arrange with third parties for the supply of goods or materials by those third parties.

28.—(1) In the Local Authorities (Goods and Services) Act 1970 the expression 'public body' includes any health authority and so far as relates to his functions under this Act includes the Secretary of State.

(2) The provisions of subsection (1) above have effect as if made by an order under section 1(5) of that Act of 1970, and accordingly may be varied or revoked by such an order.

(3) Every local authority shall make available to health authorities acting in the area of the local authority the services of persons employed by the local authority for the purposes of the local authority's functions under the Local Authorities Social Services Act 1970 so far as is reasonably necessary and practicable to enable health authorities to discharge their functions under this Act.

(4) Such charges may be made by a local authority for acting under subsection (3) above as may be agreed between the local authority and the Secretary of State or, in default of agreement, as may be determined by arbitration.

Part II

General Medical, General Dental, General Ophthalmic, and Pharmaceutical Services

Since this Part does not directly relate to the National Hospital Service it is not here reproduced.

Part III

Other Powers of the Secretary of State as to the Health Service

Control of maximum prices for medical supplies

57.—(1) The Secretary of State may by order provide for controlling maximum prices to be charged for any medical supplies required for the purposes of this Act.

(2) The Secretary of State may by direction given with respect to any undertaking, or by order made with respect to any class or description of undertakings, being an undertaking or class or description of undertakings concerned with medical supplies required for the purposes of this Act, require persons carrying on the undertaking or undertakings of that class or description —

> (*a*) to keep such books, accounts and records relating to the undertaking as may be prescribed by the direction or, as the case may be, by the order or a notice served under the order;

> (*b*) to furnish at such times, in such manner and in such form as may be so prescribed such estimates, returns or information relating to the undertaking as may be so prescribed.

(3) The additional provisions set out in Schedule 11 to this Act have effect in relation to this section; and

> 'medical supplies' in this section includes surgical, dental and optical materials and equipment; and

> 'undertaking' in this section and that Schedule means any public utility undertaking or any undertaking by way of trade or business.

Additional powers as to services and supplies; and the use of those services and supplies for private patients

58. The Secretary of State may allow persons to make use (on such terms, including terms as to the payment of charges, as he thinks fit) of any accommodation or services provided under this Act and may provide the accommodation or services in question to an extent greater than that necessary apart from this section if he thinks it expedient so to do in order to allow persons to make use of them.

This section is subject to sections 59, 60 and 62 below.

59.—(1) In this section and section 60 below 'the section 58 power' means the Secretary of State's power under section 58 above to afford persons (subject to section 62 below) admission or access to accommodation or services as resident or non-resident private patients at health service hospitals.

(2) The Secretary of State shall not in the exercise of his section 58 power afford a person admission or access to accommodation or services at such a hospital as a private patient unless satisfied that the accommodation or services are required for the purposes of investigation, diagnosis or treatment which —

(*a*) is of a specialised nature or involves the use of specialised equipment or skills; and

(*b*) is not privately available in Great Britain or, if it is so available either —

(i) is not privately available there at a place which is reasonably accessible to the patient; or

(ii) is such that it is in the interests of the health service or of the Scottish health service or of both for it to be carried out on that occasion at that hospital.

In this subsection 'privately available' means available at a satisfactory standard otherwise than at a health service hospital.

(3) The Secretary of State shall not exercise his section 58 power in such a way as to afford persons admission or access to accommodation or services at health service hospitals otherwise than in accordance with the following arrangements.

Those arrangements are such as in his opinion are best suited for securing that all persons admitted or afforded access to accommodation or services at health service hospitals as resident or non-resident patients for the purpose of investigation, diagnosis or treatment of a specialised nature, or involving the use of specialised equipment or skills, are, so far as is practicable, admitted or afforded such access on the basis of medical priority alone, whether they come as private patients or not.

(4) The Secretary of State shall not exercise his section 58 power in such a way as to allow any particular accommodation or facilities at a health service hospital to be reserved or set aside for regular or repeated use in connection with the treatment of persons as private patients.

This subsection is without prejudice to his power to allow such use in connection with the treatment of any particular person afforded admission or access to that accommodation or those facilities.

60.—(1) There shall be made in respect of any exercise of the section 58 power such charges as the Secretary of State may in accordance with subsections (2) and (3) below determine.

(2) Without prejudice to the generality of the Secretary of State's

section 58 power to make and recover charges for any use which he may under that section allow to be made of any accommodation or services provided under this Act, the Secretary of State may in pursuance of subsection (1) above determine different rates or scales of charges —

    (*a*) for different accommodation or services at different health service hospitals or different classes of such hospitals;

    (*b*) for different forms or classes of treatment;

    (*c*) in relation to patients who are, and patients who are not, ordinarily resident in Great Britain;

    (*d*) generally for different accommodation and for different services and in relation to different circumstances.

(3) The charges determined in pursuance of subsection (1) above —

    (*a*) shall be such as will ensure, so far as is practicable, that no increase in the expenses incurred by the Secretary of State under this Act results from any exercise of the section 58 power;

    (*b*) shall include such amounts as appear to the Secretary of State proper and reasonable in respect of costs appearing to him to be properly attributable to capital account; and

    (*c*) in the case of charges for services provided to a private patient at a health service hospital by a whole-time consultant, shall be not less than would be charged by a part-time consultant for providing similar services in similar circumstances to a private patient of his.

(4) Where a health authority receives any sum charged under section 58 for services provided to a private patient by a whole-time consultant

    (*a*) the authority shall retain that sum and use it for the purposes of research and development in medicine or dentistry, but

    (*b*) if the services in question were provided by a consultant employed by a medical or dental school or university, the authority shall, if so directed by the Secretary of State, pay the sum to that school or university to use for those purposes.

(5) Nothing in this section or in section 59 above prevents the Secretary of State from allowing any medical or dental practitioner employed by a health authority to make use of any accommodation or services provided by virtue of this Act to the extent to which the practitioner would be entitled to make such use under the terms of that employment if those terms were as they were or would have been at the passing of the Health Services Act 1976.

(6) In this section —

    'health authority' includes a preserved Board;

    'preserved Board' has the meaning given by section 15(6) of the National Health Service Reorganisation Act 1973;

'whole-time consultant' and 'part-time consultant' mean respectively a consultant employed whole-time or part-time by a health authority, medical or dental school or university.

61.—(1) The Secretary of State may sell or give away, or otherwise dispose of, goods the production or manufacture of which by him is involved in the provision of services under this Act.

(2) He may, in the case of goods referred to in subsection (1) above which are prescribed for the purposes of this section, produce or manufacture them to an extent greater than that necessitated by the provision of such services in order that they may be supplied to persons other than those to whom they are supplied by way of the provision of such services whether or not the first-mentioned persons are engaged in the provision of other services provided under this Act.

(3) This section is subject to section 62 below.

62. The Secretary of State shall exercise the powers conferred on him by the provisions of section 25 above (supplies not readily obtainable) and sections 58 and 61 above only if and to the extent that he is satisfied that anything which he proposes to do or allow under those powers —

(a) will not to a significant extent interfere with the performance by him of any duty imposed on him by this Act to provide accommodation or services of any kind; and

(b) will not to a significant extent operate to the disadvantage of persons seeking or afforded admission or access to accommodation or services at health service hospitals (whether as resident or non-resident patients) otherwise than as private patients.

Further provisions as to payments by patients for health service accommodation and services

63.—(1) The Secretary of State may authorise the accommodation described in this section to be made available, to such extent as he may determine, for patients who give an undertaking (or for whom one is given) to pay such charges for part of the cost as the Secretary of State may determine, and he may recover those charges.

The accommodation mentioned above is —

(a) in single rooms or small wards which is not for the time being needed by any patient on medical grounds;

(b) at any health service hospital or group of hospitals, or a hospital in which patients are treated under arrangements made by virtue of section 23 above, or at the health service hospitals in a particular area or a hospital in which patients are so treated.

(2) The Secretary of State may allow such deductions as he thinks fit from the amount of a charge due by virtue of an undertaking given under this section to be paid for accommodation in respect of any period during which the accommodation is temporarily vacated by the person for whom it is made available.

64. The Secretary of State may require any person —
- (*a*) who is a resident patient for whom the Secretary of State provides services under this Act; and
- (*b*) who is absent during the day for the purpose of engaging in remunerative employment from the hospital where he is a patient,

to pay such part of the cost of his maintenance in the hospital and any incidental cost as may seem reasonable to the Secretary of State having regard to the amount of that person's remuneration, and the Secretary of State may recover the amount so required.

65.—(1) Subject to section 71 below, if the Secretary of State is satisfied, in the case of a health service hospital or group of such hospitals or of the health service hospitals in a particular area, that it is reasonable to do so —
- (a) he may, subject to this section, authorise accommodation and services at the hospital or hospitals in question to be made available to such extent as he may determine; and
- (b) that accommodation and those services shall be available for resident patients who give an undertaking (or for whom one is given) to pay such charges as he may determine in accordance with the following provisions of this section, and the Secretary of State may recover those charges.

(2) The Secretary of State may allow accommodation and services to which an authorisation under subsection (1) above relates to be made available in connection with treatment, in pursuance of arrangements made by a medical practitioner or dental practitioner serving (whether in an honorary or paid capacity) on the staff of a health service hospital of private patients of that practitioner as resident patients.

(3) The Secretary of State, for the purpose of determining charges to be paid under subsection (1) above —
- (*a*) may classify the health service hospitals, and may, in the case of each class, determine in respect of each period of 12 months beginning with 1st April first falling after the date on which the determination is made the charges to be paid under that

subsection in respect of accommodation and services provided during that period at a hospital falling within that class;

(b) in determining such charges in respect of a period the Secretary of State shall have regard, so far as is reasonably practicable, to the total cost (exclusive of costs appearing to him to be properly attributable to capital account) which, by reference to facts known to him at the time of the determination, it is estimated will be incurred during that period in the provision for resident patients of services at hospitals falling within that class; and

(c) may include in any such charges, in such cases as appear to him fit, such amounts as appear to him proper and reasonable to be included by way of contribution to expenditure appearing to him to be properly attributable to capital account.

(4) The Secretary of State may under subsection (3) above determine different charges for different accommodation and for different services and in relation to different circumstances.

(5) The Secretary of State may allow such deduction as he thinks proper from the amount of a charge due by virtue of an undertaking given under this section by or in respect of any patient —

(a) in respect of treatment given to the patient under subsection (2) above; and

(b) in respect of any period during which the accommodation to which the undertaking relates is temporarily vacated by the patient.

(6) Nothing in this section prevents accommodation from being made available for a patient other than one mentioned in subsection (1) above if the use of that accommodation is needed more urgently for him on medical grounds than for a patient so mentioned, and no other suitable accommodation is available.

66.—(1) If the Secretary of State is satisfied, in the case of a health service hospital or group of such hospitals or of the health service hospitals in a particular area, that it is reasonable to do so —

(a) he may, subject to section 71 below, authorise accommodation and services at the hospital or hositals in question to be made available to such extent as he may determine, and

(b) that accommodation and those services shall be available in connection with treatment, in pursuance of arrangements made by a medical practitioner or dental practitioner serving (whether in an honorary or paid capacity) on the staff of any such hospital, of private patients of that practitioner otherwise than as resident patients.

Those patients shall be patients who give an undertaking (or for whom one is given) to pay, in respect of the accommodation and services, such charges as the Secretary of State may determine, and he may recover those charges.

(2) The Secretary of State may under subsection (1) above determine different charges for different accommodation and for different services, and in relation to different circumstances.

(3) No accommodation and no services shall be so made available under subsection (1) above as to prejudice persons availing themselves of services at a hospital otherwise than as private patients.

Withdrawal of health service pay beds and services from private patients

67.—(1) Sections 68 to 71 below have effect for the purpose of —

(a) securing the separation of the facilities available in England and Wales for the prevention, diagnosis and treatment of illness under private arrangements from the facilities available for those purposes at premises vested in the Secretary of State; and

(b) to that end securing the progressive withdrawal of accommodation and services at health service hospitals from use in connection with the treatment of persons at such hospitals as resident or non-resident private patients.

(2) Nothing in this Part of this Act prejudices the operation of paragraph 10(4) of Schedule 5 to this Act (by virtue of which regulations governing the terms of employment of officers employed by an authority within the meaning of sub-paragraph (4) of that paragraph must not contain a requirement that all consultants so employed shall be so employed whole-time).

68.—(1) It continues to be the duty of the Health Services Board to submit to the Secretary of State from time to time in accordance with this section proposals for the progressive revocation of —

(a) the authorisations under section 65(1) above or those granted by virtue of section 71(3) below, and

(b) the authorisations under section 66(1) above or those granted by virtue of section 71(3) below,

and it shall be the Secretary of State's duty to give effect to all proposals so submitted.

(2) The Health Services Board shall in the 6 months beginning with the date on which its first proposals were submitted under section 4(2) of the Health Services Act 1976, and in each successive period of 6 months thereafter, submit further proposals under this section or,

if in all the circumstances it decides that the submission of further proposals in any particular period of 6 months is unnecessary, shall instead prepare and submit to the Secretary of State a report explaining the Board's reasons for that decision.

(3) In formulating proposals under this section the Board shall —
    (a) have regard to the principles set out in section 70 below; and
    (b) consider any representations made to the Board by —
        (i) the Secretary of State;
        (ii) any body which is representative of medical practitioners or dental practitioners or of persons employed in the health service or concerned with the interests of patients at health service hospitals;
        (iii) any other person having a substantial interest in the proposals.

In deciding what advice to give the Board in connection with the formulation of any such proposals the Board's Welsh Committee shall likewise have regard to the principles set out in section 70 and shall consider any representations made to the Committee by any of the persons or bodies above mentioned.

(4) Each set of proposals under this section shall specify —
    (a) the accommodation and services authorisation of which under section 65(1) or section 66(1) should be revoked and
    (b) the date before which the necessary revocations should take effect,

and may specify different dates for different accommodation or services so specified.

69.—(1) Without prejudice to subsection (3) of section 68 above, the Health Services Board, in formulating proposals under that section for the revocation of authorisations given under section 66(1) above in respect of accommodation or services at any particular health service hospital or hospitals, and the Welsh Committee in deciding what advice to give the Board in connection with the formulation of any such proposals —
    (a) shall have regard to the purposes and specialties for which the accommodation or services in quesion are available for use in connection with the treatment of non-resident private patients, and
    (b) shall apply the principles set out in section 70 below separately in respect of different purposes and specialties,

and the Board may formulate separate proposals in respect of different purposes or specialties accordingly.

(2) As regards the revocation of authorisations under section 66(1), any proposals under section 68 relating to —

(a) accommodation available to consultants for the purpose of affording consultations to their private patients, or

(b) accommodation and services available for the following specialties, namely, radiotherapy, diagnostic pathology and diagnostic radiology (including scanning, ultrasonics and methods involving the use of radio-isotopes),

shall be formulated by the Board as separate proposals; and (without prejudice to section 68(1) to (3) above and subsection (1) above) the Board's first proposals under section 4(2) of the Health Services Act 1976 (submitted within 6 months of the passing of that Act or such longer period as the Secretary of State may allow) shall include separate proposals relating to accommodation available to consultants as mentioned in paragraph (a) above.

(3) Without prejudice to section 68 and the preceding provisions of this section, the Health Services Board shall, as regards the revocation of authorisations under section 66(1), submit separate proposals under section 68 relating to —

(a) accommodation and services available for the specialties other than radiotherapy mentioned in subsection (2)(b) above, and

(b) other accommodation and services available for diagnostic purposes,

and shall do so not later than the end of the 12 months following the initial period defined by the Health Services Act 1976 (that is the period of 6 months beginning with the date on which that Act was passed), or, if a period longer than the initial period has been allowed under that Act for the submission of the Board's first proposals under this section, the 12 months following that longer period.

70. The principles referred to in sections 68 and 69 above are —

(a) that accommodation or services at any particular health service hospital or hospitals should remain authorised under section 65(1) or section 66(1) above for use in connection with the treatment of resident or non-resident private patients only while there is a reasonable demand for accommodation and facilities for the private practice of medicine and dentistry in the area or areas served by the hospital or hospitals in question;

(b) that the authorisation of any such accommodation or services under those provisions for use in that connection should be revoked only if sufficient accommodation and facilities for the private practice of medicine and dentistry are otherwise reasonably available (whether privately or at health service hospitals) to meet the reasonable demand for them in the area or areas served by the hospital or hospitals in question;

(c) that the continued authorisation of any such accommodation or services under those provisions for use in that connection should depend on there having been or being taken all reasonable steps to provide, otherwise than at health service hospitals, sufficient reasonable accommodation and facilities for the private practice of medicine and dentistry to meet the reasonable demand for them in the area or areas served by the hospital or hospitals in question;

(d) that failure, in the circumstances mentioned in paragraph (c) above, to take all reasonable steps that could be taken to provide as mentioned in that paragraph would itself be grounds for the Health Services Board, after giving due warning to persons likely to be affected thereby of the likely consequences of such failure, to propose the revocation of the authorisations under those provisions relating to accommodation or services at the hospital or hospitals in question.

71.—(1) No authorisation —

(a) under section 65(1) or section 66(1) above shall be granted, except by virtue of subsection (2) or subsection (4) below; and

(b) shall be, other than one granted on a temporary basis as mentioned in subsection (4), to any extent revoked otherwise than in accordance with proposals submitted to the Secretary of State by the Health Services Board under section 68 above.

(2) The Health Services Board may submit to the Secretary of State proposals for securing that in any case where one or more beds authorised under section 65(1) cease to be available to resident private patients, or any accommodation or services authorised under section 66(1) cease to be available to non-resident private patients, in consequence of the permanent closure of any health service hospital accommodation in England or Wales independently of any proposals submitted by the Board under section 68, the total number of effective beds, or the total amount of effective accommodation or services, as the case may be, so authorised in England or Wales is not thereby reduced below what it would be if —

(a) the closed accommodation had remained in use, but

(b) effect had been given by the Secretary of State to all proposals under section 68 received by him before the submission of the proposals in question under this subsection.

(3) It shall be the Secretary of State's duty to grant such authorisations under section 65(1) or section 66(1), as the case may be, as are needed to give effect to any proposals submitted to him under subsection (2) above.

(4) Where any health service hospital accommodation in England or Wales is temporarily closed (whether at the instance of the Secretary of State or not) for physical or other reasons outside his control, the Secretary of State shall, without the need for any proposals by the Board, grant on a temporary basis such authorisations under section 65(1) or section 66(1) as he would have been able to grant by virtue of subsections (2) and (3) above if —

    (a) the closure had been permanent, and

    (b) the Board had submitted to him any proposals which it could in that case have submitted to him under subsection (2).

(5) Subject to the restrictions imposed by this section, section 65 or, as the case may be, section 66 continue to have effect in relation to any accommodation or services to which an authorisation under section 65(1) or section 66(1) relates.

Use by practitioners of health service facilities for private practice

72.—(1) A person to whom this section applies who wishes to use any relevant health service accommodation or facilities for the purpose of providing medical, dental, pharmaceutical, ophthalmic or chiropody services to non-resident private patients may apply in writing to the Secretary of State for permission under this section.

(2) Any application for permission under this section must specify —

    (a) which of the relevant health service accommodation or facilities the applicant wishes to use for the purpose of providing services to such patients; and

    (b) which of the kinds of services mentioned in subsection (1) above he wishes the permission to cover.

(3) On receiving an application under this section the Secretary of State —

    (a) shall consider whether anything for which permission is sought would interfere with the giving of full and proper attention to persons seeking or afforded access otherwise than as private patients to any services provided under this Act; and

    (b) shall grant the permission applied for unless in his opinion anything for which permission is sought would so interfere.

(4) Any grant of permission under this section shall be on such terms (including terms as to the payment of charges for the use of the relevant health service accommodation or facilities pursuant to the permission) as the Secretary of State may from time to time determine.

(5) The persons to whom this section applies are —

    (a) persons of any of the following descriptions who provide services under Part II of this Act, namely, medical practitioners, dental practitioners, registered pharmacists, and ophthalmic or dispensing opticians; and

(b) other persons who provide pharmaceutical or ophthalmic services under Part II; and

(c) chiropodists who provide services under this Act at premises where services are provided under Part II.

(6) In this section —

(a) 'relevant health service accommodation or facilities', in relation to a person to whom this section applies, means any accommodation or facilities available at premises provided by the Secretary of State by virtue of this Act, being accommodation or facilities which that person is for the time being authorised to use for purposes of Part II; or

(b) in the case of a person to whom this section applies by virtue of paragraph (c) of subsection (5) above, accommodation or facilities which that person is for the time being authorised to use for purposes of this Act at premises where services are provided under Part II.

Information and reports

73. It is the Secretary of State's duty to furnish the Health Services Board with such information as it may reasonably require for the proper discharge of its functions under sections 68 to 71 above.

74. The Secretary of State shall cause every set of proposals submitted to him under sections 68 and 71 above, and every report submitted to him under section 68(2), to be published as soon as practicable after its submission, and shall lay a copy of every such set of proposals or report before each House of Parliament.

75,—(1) There shall be prepared by the Secretary of State on the matters mentioned in subsection (2) below an annual report relating to England and one relating to Wales, and he shall lay a copy of every report under this section before each House of Parliament.

(2) The matters referred to under subsection (1) above are —

(a) the accommodation and services at health service hospitals which in the period covered by the report were available for use in connection with the treatment of private patients by virtue of authorisations under sections 65(1) and 66(1) above;

(b) the extent to which 'the section 58 power' (as defined in section 59(1) above) was exercised in that period;

(c) the extent to which the powers to which section 62 above applies were exercised in that period otherwise than by way of affording persons admission or access to accommodation or services at health service hospitals as resident or non-resident private patients; and

(*d*) the extent to which progress has been made in implementing the common waiting-lists referred to in section 6 of the Health Services Act 1976, and in section 76 below.

76.—(1) The reference in paragraph (*d*) of section 75(2) above to common waiting-lists is to the recommendations made to the Secretary of State by the Health Services Board under section 6(1) of the Health Services Act 1976.

(2) Those recommendations —

(*a*) related to arrangements for affording persons admission or access as resident patients (authorised under section 65 above) or non-resident patients (authorised under section 66 above) to accommodation and services; and

(*b*) were in the Board's opinion the ones best suited for securing that all persons admitted or afforded access to accommodation or services at health service hospitals as resident or non-resident patients are, so far as practicable, admitted or afforded access thereto on the basis of medical priority alone, whether coming as private patients or not.

Regulations as to certain charges

77.—(1) Regulations may provide for the making and recovery in such manner as may be prescribed of such charges as may be prescribed in respect of —

(*a*) the supply under this Act (otherwise than under Part II) of drugs, medicines or appliances (including the replacement and repair of those appliances),

(*b*) such of the pharmaceutical services referred to in Part II as may be prescribed,

and paragraphs (*a*) and (*b*) of this subsection may include the supply of substances and appliances mentioned in paragraph (*b*) of section 5(1) above.

(2) Regulations under subsection (1) above may provide for the grant, on payment of such sums as may be prescribed by those regulations, of certificates conferring on the persons to whom the certificates are granted exemption from charges otherwise exigible under the regulations in respect of drugs, medicines and appliances supplied during such period as may be prescribed, and different sums may be so prescribed in relation to different periods.

(3) The additional provisions of paragraphs 1 and 4 of Schedule 12 to this Act have effect in relation to this section.

78.—(1) Regulations may provide for the making and recovery in such manner as may be prescribed of charges of such amounts as are mentioned in sub-paragraph (1) of paragraph 2 of Schedule 12 to this Act, in respect of the supply under the Act of such dental or optical appliances as are mentioned in that sub-paragraph.

(2) If the Secretary of State, after consultation with the university associated with any hospital providing facilities for clinical dental teaching, is satisfied that it is expedient in the interests of dental training or education that the charges imposed by subsection (1) above should be remitted in the case of dental services provided at that hospital, either generally or subject to limitations or conditions, he may by order provide for that purpose.

Any order made under this subsection may be revoked or varied by a subsequent order made by the Secretary of State after such consultation as is mentioned above.

(3) The additional provisions of paragraphs 2 and 5 of Schedule 12 have effect in relation to this section.

79.—(1) A charge of the amount authorised by this section may be made and recovered, in such manner as may be prescribed, in respect of any services provided as part of the general dental services under Part II of this Act, not being —
  (a) the supply or replacement of appliances mentioned in paragraph 2(1) of Schedule 12 to this Act;
  (b) the repair of appliances other than prescribed appliances;
  (c) the arrest of bleeding; or
  (d) the clinical examination of a patient and any report on that examination.
The additional provisions of paragraphs 3 and 5 of Schedule 12 have effect in relation to this subsection.

(2) Regulations may provide that, in the case of such special dental treatment as may be prescribed, being treatment provided as part of the general dental services, such charges as may be prescribed may be made and recovered by the person providing the services.

80. Regulations may provide for the making and recovery of charges in respect of facilities designated by the regulations as facilities provided in pursuance of paragraph (d) or paragraph (e) of section 3(1) above.

81. Regulations may provide for the making and recovery of such charges as may be prescribed —

(a) by the Secretary of State in respect of the supply by him of any appliance or vehicle which is, at the request of the person supplied, of a more expensive type than the prescribed type, or in respect of the replacement or repair of any such appliance, or the replacement of any such vehicle, or the taking of any such action in relation to the vehicle as is mentioned in paragraph 1 of Schedule 2 to this Act;

(b) by persons providing general dental services or general ophthalmic services in respect of the supply, as part of those services, of any dental or optical appliance which is, at the request of the person supplied, of a more expensive type than the prescribed type or in respect of the replacement or repair of any such appliance.

82. Regulations may provide for the making and recovery of such charges as may be prescribed —

(a) by the Secretary of State in respect of the replacement or repair of any appliance or vehicle supplied by him, or

(b) by persons providing general dental services or general ophthalmic services in respect of the replacement or repair of any dental or optical appliance supplied as part of those services.

if it is determined in the prescribed manner that the replacement or repair is necessitated by an act or omission of the person supplied or (if the act or omission occurred when the person supplied was under 16 years of age) of the person supplied or of the person having charge of him when the act or omission occurred.

83. Regulations made —

(a) under sections 77 to 79 and under sections 81 and 82 above providing for the making and recovery of charges in respect of any services, may provide for the reduction of the sums which would otherwise be payable by a Regional Health Authority, an Area Health Authority or a Family Practitioner Committee to the persons by whom those services are provided by the amount of the charges authorised by the regulations in respect of those services;

(b) for the purposes of section 78(1) in relation to appliances provided as part of the general dental services or the general ophthalmic services under Part II of this Act, may provide for the reduction of the sums which would otherwise be payable by an Area Health Authority or a Family Practitioner Committee to the persons by whom those services are provided by the amount of the charges authorised by section 78(1) in respect of those appliances.

Inquiries, and default and emergency powers

84.—(1) The Secretary of State may cause an inquiry to be held in any case where he deems it advisable to do so in connection with any matter arising under this Act.

(2) For the purpose of any such inquiry (but subject to subsection (3) below) the person appointed to hold the inquiry —

    (*a*) may by summons require any person to attend, at a time and place stated in the summons, to give evidence or to produce any documents in his custody or under his control which relate to any matter in question at the inquiry; and

    (*b*) may take evidence on oath, and for that purpose administer oaths, or may, instead of adminstering an oath, require the person examined to make a solemn affirmation.

(3) Nothing in this section —

    (*a*) requires a person, in obedience to a summons under the section, to attend to give evidence or to produce any documents unless the necessary expenses of his attendance are paid or tendered to him; or

    (*b*) empowers the person holding the inquiry to require the production of the title, or of any instrument relating to the title, of any land not being the property of a local authority.

(4) Any person who refuses or deliberately fails to attend in obedience to a summons under this section, or to give evidence, or who deliberately alters, suppresses, conceals, destroys, or refuses to produce any book or other document which he is required or is liable to be required to produce for the purposes of this section, shall be liable on summary conviction to a fine not exceeding £100 or to imprisonment for a term not exceeding 6 months, or to both.

(5) Where the Secretary of State causes an inquiry to be held under this section —

    (*a*) the costs incurred by him in relation to the inquiry (including such reasonable sum not exceeding £30 a day as he may determine for the services of any officer engaged in the inquiry) shall be paid by such local authority or party to the inquiry as he may direct, and

    (*b*) he may cause the amount of the costs so incurred to be certified, and any amount so certified and directed to be paid by any authority or person shall be recoverable from that authority or person by the Secretary of State summarily as a civil debt.

No local authority shall be ordered to pay costs under this subsection in the case of any inquiry unless it is a party to that inquiry.

(6) Where the Secretary of State causes an inquiry to be held under this section he may make orders —

(a) as to the costs of the parties at the inquiry, and

(b) as to the parties by whom the costs are to be paid,

and every such order may be made a rule of the High Court on the application of any party named in the order.

85.—(1) Where the Secretary of State is of opinion, on complaint or otherwise, that —

(a) any Regional Health Authority;

(b) any Area Health Authority;

(c) any special health authority;

(d) any Family Practitioner Committee;

(e) any local social services authority;

(f) the Medical Practices Committee; or

(g) the Dental Estimates Board;

have failed to carry out any functions conferred or imposed on them by or under this Act, or have in carrying out those functions failed to comply with any regulations or directions relating to those functions, he may after such inquiry as he may think fit make an order declaring them to be in default.

(2) Except where the body in default is a local social services authority, the members of the body shall forthwith vacate their office, and the order —

(a) shall provide for the appointment, in accordance with the provisions of this Act, of new members of the body; and

(b) may contain such provisions as seem to the Secretary of State expedient for authorising any person to act in the place of the body in question pending the appointment of new members.

(3) If the body in default is a local social services authority —

(a) the order shall direct them, for the purpose of remedying the default, to discharge such of their functions, in such manner and within such time or times, as may be specified in the order; and

(b) if the authority fail to comply with any direction given under this subsection within the time so limited, the Secretary of State, instead of enforcing the order by mandamus or otherwise, may make an order transferring to himself such of the functions of the authority as he thinks fit.

(4) Any expenses certified by the Secretary of State to have been incurred by him in discharging functions transferred to him under this

section from a local social services authority shall on demand be paid to him by that authority and shall be recoverable by him from them as a debt due to the Crown; and

(a) the authority or (in the case of a joint board) any constituent local authority thereof shall have the like power of raising the money required as they have of raising money for paying expenses incurred directly by them; and

(b) the payment of any such expenses so incurred by the Secretary of State shall, to such extent as he may sanction, be a purpose for which the authority may borrow money in accordance with the statutory provisions relating to borrowing by that authority.

(5) An order made under this section may contain such supplementary and incidental provisions as appear to the Secretary of State to be necessary or expedient, including —

(a) provision for the transfer to the Secretary of State of property and liabilities of the body in default; and

(b) where any such order is varied or revoked by a subsequent order, provision in the revoking order or a subsequent order for the transfer to the body in default of any property or liabilities acquired or incurred by the Secretary of State in discharging any of the functions transferred to him.

86. If the Secretary of State —

(a) considers that by reason of an emergency it is necessary in order to ensure that a service falling to be provided in pursuance of this Act is provided, to direct that during the period specified by the directions a function conferred on any body or person by virtue of this. Act shall to the exclusion of or concurrently with that body or person be performed by another body or person then

(b) he may give directions accordingly and it shall be the duty of the bodies or persons in question to comply with the directions.

The powers conferred on the Secretary of State by this section are in addition to any other powers exercisable by him.

PART IV

PROPERTY AND FINANCE

Land and other Property

87.—(1) The Secretary of State may acquire —

(a) any land, either by agreement or compulsorily,

(b) any other property,

required by him for the purposes of this Act; and (without prejudice . to the generality of paragraph (*a*) above) land may be so acquired to provide residential accommodation for persons employed for any of those purposes.

(2) The Secretary of State may use for the purposes of any of the functions conferred on him by this Act any property belonging to him by virtue of this Act, and he has power to maintain all such property.

(3) A local social services authority may be authorised to purchase land compulsorily for the purposes of this Act by means of an order made by the authority and confirmed by the Secretary of State.

(4) The Acquisition of Land (Authorisation Procedure) Act 1946 shall apply to the compulsory purchase of land by the Secretary of State under this section, and accordingly shall have effect —

(*a*) as if section 1(1) of that Act (which refers to the compulsory purchase of land by local authorities under public general Acts in force immediately before the commencement of that Act and by the Minister of Transport under certain enactments) included a reference to any compulsory purchase of land by the Secretary of State under this section; and

(*b*) as if this section had been in force immediately before the commencement of that Act.

(5) Section 120(3) of the Local Government Act 1972 (which relates to the application of Part I of the Compulsory Purchase Act 1965 where a council are authorised to acquire land by agreement) applies to the acquisition of land by the Secretary of State under this section in like manner as it applies to such acquisition by a council under that section.

(6) Section 128 of the Town and Country Planning Act 1971 (use and development of consecrated land and burial grounds) applies to consecrated land and land comprised in a burial ground within the meaning of that section which —

(*a*) the Secretary of State holds for any of the purposes of the health service, and

(*b*) has not been acquired by him as mentioned in subsection (1) of that section.

as if that land had been so acquired for those purposes.

88.—(1) All property vested in the Secretary of State in consequence of the transfer of that property under section 6 of the National Health Service Act 1946 (transfer of hospitals) so vests free of any trust existing immediately before that transfer.

(2) The Secretary of State may use any such property for the purpose of any of his functions under this Act, but he shall so far as practicable

secure that the objects for which any such property was used immediately before that transfer are not prejudiced by section 6 of that Act of 1946.

89. Notwithstanding anything contained —
  (*a*) in the constitution or rules of any voluntary organisation formed for the purpose of providing a service of nurses for attendance on the sick in their own homes, or of midwives, or
  (*b*) in any trust deed or other instrument relating to such organisation or service,

any property vested in the organisation or held by any persons on trust for the organisation or service or for any specific purposes connected with the organisation or service may be transferred to the Secretary of State, on such terms as may be agreed between him and the organisation or trustees, with a view to the property being used or held by him for purposes similar to the purposes for which it was previously used or held.

Trusts

90. A health authority has power to accept, hold and administer any property on trust for all or any purposes relating to the health service.

91.—(1) Where —
  (*a*) the terms of a trust instrument authorise or require the trustees, whether immediately or in the future, to apply any part of the capital or income of the trust property for the purposes of any health service hospital, then
  (*b*) the trust instrument shall be construed as authorising or (as the case may be) requiring the trustees to apply the trust property to the like extent, and at the like times, for the purpose of making payments, whether of capital or income, to the appropriate hospital authority.

(2) Any sum so paid to the appropriate hospital authority shall, so far as practicable, be applied by them for the purpose specified in the trust instrument.

(3) In this section 'the appropriate hospital authority' means —
  (*a*) where special trustees are appointed for the hospital, those trustees;
  (*b*) in any other case, the Area Health Authority exercising functions on behalf of the Secretary of State in respect of the hospital.

(4) Nothing in this section applies to a trust for a special hospital, or to property transferred under section 24 of the National Health Service Reorganisation Act 1973.

92.—(1) The Secretary of State may, having regard to any change or proposed change in the arrangements for the administration of a hospital or in the area or functions of any health authority, by order provide for the transfer of any trust property from any health authority or special trustees to any other health authority or special trustees.

(2) If it appears to the Secretary of State at any time that all the functions of any special trustees should be discharged by one or more health authorities then, whether or not there has been any such change as is mentioned in subsection (1) above, he may by order provide for the transfer of all trust property from the special trustees to the health authority, or, in such proportions as he may specify in the order, to those health authorities.

(3) Before so acting the Secretary of State shall consult the health authorities and special trustees concerned.

(4) Where by an order under this section, property is transferred to two or more authorities, it shall be apportioned by them in such proportions as they may agree or as may in default of agreement be determined by the Secretary of State, and the order may provide for the way in which the property is to be apportioned.

(5) Where property is so apportioned, the Secretary of State may by order make any consequential amendments of the trust instrument relating to the property.

93.—(1) This section applies —
  (a) to property transferred under section 23 of the National Health Service Reorganisation Act 1973 (winding-up of hospital endowments funds), and
  (b) to property transferred under section 24 of that Act (transfer of trust property from abolished authorities) which immediately before the day appointed for the purposes of that section was, in accordance with any provision contained in or made under section 7 of the National Health Service Act 1946, applicable for purposes relating to hospital services or relating to some form of research,
and this section continues to apply to the property after any further transfer under section 92 above.

(2) The person holding the property after the transfer or last transfer shall secure, so far as is reasonably practicable, that the objects of any original endowment and the observance of any conditions attached to that endowment, including in particular conditions intended to preserve the memory of any person or class of persons, are not prejudiced by this Part of this Act, or Part II of that Act of 1973.

In this subsection 'original endowment' means a hospital endowment which was transferred under section 7 of that Act of 1946 and from which the property in question is derived.

(3) Subject to subsection (2) above, the property shall be held on trust for such purposes relating to hospital services (including research), or to any other part of the health service associated with any hospital, as the person holding the property thinks fit.

(4) Where the person holding the property is a body of special trustees, the power conferred by subsection (3) above shall be exercised as respects the hospitals for which they are appointed.

94.—(1) Any discretion given by a trust instrument to the trustees of property transferred under —

    (*a*) section 24 of the National Health Service Reorganisation Act 1973 (transfer of trust property from abolished authorities),

    (*b*) section 25 of that Act (transfer of trust property held for health services by local health authorities),

    (*c*) section 92 above,

shall be exercisable by the person to whom the property is so transferred and, subject to section 93 above and the following provisions of this section, the transfer shall not affect the trusts on which the property is held.

(2) Where —

    (*a*) property has been transferred under section 24 of that Act of 1973, and

    (*b*) any discretion is given by a trust instrument to the trustees to apply the property, or income arising from the property, to such hospital services (including research) as the trustees think fit without any restriction on the kinds of hospital services and without any restriction to one or more specified hospitals,

the discretion shall be enlarged so as to allow the application of the property or (as the case may be) of the income arising from the property to such extent as the trustees think fit, for any other part of the health service associated with any hospital.

(3) Subsection (2) above shall apply on any subsequent transfer of the property under section 92 above.

95.—(1) The bodies of trustees (in this Act referred to as special trustees) appointed by the Secretary of State under section 29 of the National Health Service Reorganisation Act 1973 and this section shall (subject to section 92 above) hold and administer the property transferred to them under that Act of 1973.

The special trustees so appointed are bodies of trustees appointed for the hospital or hospitals which, immediately before the day appointed for the purposes of section 29 of that Act of 1973, were controlled and managed by a University Hospital Management Committee or a Board of Governors, but excluding —

(a) a body on whose request an order was made under section 24(2) of that Act of 1973;

(b) a preserved Board within the meaning of section 15(6) of that Act of 1973.

(2) Special trustees have power to accept, hold and administer any property on trust for all or any purposes relating to hospital services (including research), or to any other part of the health service associated with hospitals, being a trust which is wholly or mainly for hospitals for which the special trustees are appointed.

(3) The number of trustees for any hospital or hospitals shall be such as the Secretary of State may from time to time determine after consultation with such persons as he considers appropriate.

(4) The term of office of any special trustee shall be fixed by the Secretary of State but a special trustee may be removed by the Secretary of State at any time during the special trustee's term of office.

96.—(1) Any provision in sections 90 to 95 above for the transfer of any property includes provision for the transfer of any rights and liabilities arising from that property.

(2) Nothing in those sections shall affect any power of Her Majesty, the court (as defined in the Charities Act 1960) or any other person to alter the trusts of any charity.

(3) Nothing in section 12 of the Finance Act 1895 (which requires certain Acts and certain instruments relating to the vesting of property by virtue of an Act to be stamped as conveyances on sale) applies to sections 90 to 95 above or to an order made in pursuance of any of those sections: and stamp duty shall not be payable on such an order.

Finance and Accounts

97.—(1) It is the Secretary of State's duty to pay —

(a) to each Area Health Authority in Wales and each Regional Health Authority the sums needed to defray such expenditure of the Authority as the Secretary of State approves in the prescribed manner;

(b) to each Family Practitioner Committee sums equal to the expenses which the Secretary of State determines are incurred by the Committee for the purpose of performing the functions conferred on the Committee by virtue of this Act; and

(c) to each special health authority sums equal to such of the expenses of the authority as are not defrayed by payments made to the authority in pursuance of subsection (3) below.

(2) It is the duty of each Regional Health Authority to pay to each Area Health Authority of which the area is included in the region of the Regional Health Authority the sums needed to defray such expenses of the Area Health Authority as the Regional Health Authority approves in the prescribed manner.

(3) Where an order establishing a special health authority provides for any expenses of the authority to be defrayed by a Regional or Area Health Authority or by two or more such Authorities in portions determined by or in accordance with the order, it is the duty of each Authority in question to pay to the special health authority sums equal to, or to the appropriate portion of, those expenses.

(4) Sums falling to be paid under this· section shall be payable subject to compliance with such conditions as to records, certificates or otherwise as the Secretary of State may determine.

98.—(1) Accounts, in such form as the Secretary of State may with the approval of the Treasury direct, shall be kept by —

(a) every Regional Health Authority;

(b) every Area Health Authority;

(c) every special health authority;

(d) all special trustees appointed in pursuance of section 29(1) of the National Health Service Reorganisation Act 1973 and section 95(1) above;

(e) the Dental Estimates Board.

Those accounts shall be audited by auditors appointed by the Secretary of State, and the Comptroller and Auditor General may examine all such accounts and any records relating to them, and any report of the auditor on them.

(2) Every such body shall prepare and transmit to the Secretary of State in respect of each financial year annual accounts in such form as the Secretary of State may with the approval of the Treasury direct.

The accounts prepared and transmitted by an Area Health Authority in pursuance of this subsection shall include annual accounts of the Family Practitioner Committees established by the Authority and of any Community Health Council of which the district includes any part of the Authority's area.

(3) The Secretary of State may by regulations provide generally with respect to the audit under subsection (1) above of accounts of bodies to which that subsection applies; and in particular for conferring on the auditor of any of those accounts —

(a) such rights of access to, and production of, books, accounts, vouchers or other documents as may be specified in the regulations; and

(b) such right, in such conditions as may be so specified, to require from any member or officer, or former member or officer, of any such body, such information relating to the affairs of the body as the Secretary of State may think necessary for the proper performance of the auditor's duty under this section.

(4) The Secretary of State shall prepare in respect of each financial year —

(a) in such form as the Treasury may direct, summarised accounts of those Authorities, special authorities and special trustees:

(b) in such form and containing such information as the Treasury may direct, a statement of the accounts of the Dental Estimates Board;

and shall transmit them on or before 30th November in each year to the Comptroller and Auditor General, who shall examine and certify them, and lay copies of them together with his report on them before both Houses of Parliament.

99.—(1) The Secretary of State may by regulations provide, in the case of all or any of the following bodies —

(a) Regional Health Authorities,

(b) Area Health Authorities,

(c) special health authorities,

(d) Family Practitioner Committees,

(e) Community Health Councils, and

(f) the Dental Estimates Board,

for restricting the making of payments by or on behalf of the body otherwise than on such authorisation and subject to such conditions as may be specified in the regulations.

(2) Such provision may be made subject to such exceptions as may be so specified, and those regulations may contain such other provisions as to the making and carrying out by all or any of those bodies of such arrangements with respect to financial matters as the Secretary of State thinks necessary for the purpose of securing that the affairs of such bodies are conducted, so far as reasonably practicable, in such manner as to prevent financial loss and to ensure and maintain efficiency.

(3) The Secretary of State may give directions to any of those bodies as to any matter with respect to which those regulations may be made; and those directions may be specific in character and shall be —

(a) such as appear to him requisite to secure that the affairs of the body are conducted in such a manner as is mentioned in subsection (2) above.

(b) without prejudice to the operation of any such regulations, and shall be compiled with by the body to whom they are given.

100.—(1) There shall be paid out of moneys provided by Parliament such expenses incurred by —

    (a) the Central Council,

    (b) any standing advisory committee constituted under section 6 above,

    (c) the Medical Practices Committee,

    (d) the Tribunal constituted under section 46 above, and

    (e) the Dental Estimates Board,

as may be determined by the Secretary of State with the approval of the Treasury.

(2) Payments made under this section shall be in accordance with regulations made by the Secretary of State and approved by the Treasury, and shall be made at such times and in such manner as the Treasury may direct, and subject to such conditions as to records, certificates, or otherwise as the Secretary of State may with the approval of the Treasury determine.

101. Any sums received by the Secretary of State under this Act shall be paid into the Consolidated Fund, but this section is without prejudice to section 60(4) above.

Miscellaneous provisions as to remuneration,
allowances and superannuation

102.—(1) The Secretary of State may pay such travelling and other allowances, including compensation for loss of remunerative time, as he may, with the approval of the Minister for the Civil Service, determine

    (a) to members of any of the following bodies constituted under this Act —

        (i) the Central Council, any standing advisory committee constituted under section 6 above to advise the Secretary of State and that Council, any committee appointed by that Council under paragraph 4 of Schedule 4 to this Act and any sub-committee appointed by any such standing advisory committee under that paragraph;

        (ii) the Medical Practices Committee;

        (iii) any body on which functions are conferred by regulations under section 32 above;

        (iv) the Dental Estimates Board;

        (v) the Tribunal constituted under section 46 above;

(b) to members of any other body being a body specified in an order made by the Secretary of State as being a body recognised by him to have been formed for the purpose of performing a function connected with the provision of services under this Act.

(2) The Secretary of State may pay to members of any of the following bodies such remuneration as he may, with the approval of the Minister for the Civil Service, determine —

(a) the Medical Practices Committee;

(b) any body on which functions are conferred by regulations under section 32 above;

(c) the Dental Estimates Board;

(d) the Tribunal constituted under section 46 above;

(e) any other body constituted under Part II of this Act, being a body specified in an order made for the purposes of this subsection, with the approval of the Minister for the Civil Service, by the Secretary of State.

(3) Allowances shall not be paid under subsection (1) above except in connection with the exercise or performance of such powers or duties, in such circumstances, as may, with the approval of the Minister for the Civil Service, be determined by the Secretary of State.

(4) Any payments under this section shall be made at such times and in such manner, and subject to such conditions as to records, certificates or otherwise, as the Secretary of State may, with the approval of the Minister for the Civil Service, determine.

103.—(1) If the Secretary of State —

(a) considers it appropriate for remuneration in respect of services provided by any person in pursuance of Part II of this Act to be paid by a particular body, and

(b) apart from this section the functions of the body do not include the function of paying the remuneration,

the Secretary of State may by order confer that function on the body.

(2) Any sums required to enable any body having that function to pay remuneration in respect of such services shall, if apart from this section there is no provision authorising the payment of the sums by the Secretary of State or out of money provided by Parliament, be paid by him.

104.—(1) The Secretary of State may enter into an agreement with the governing body of any hospital to which this section applies —

(a) for admitting officers of the hospital of such classes as may be provided in the agreement to participate, on such terms and conditions as may be so provided, in the superannuation benefits provided under regulations made under section 10 of the Superannuation Act 1972 in like manner as officers of Area Health Authorities; and

(b) those regulations shall apply accordingly in relation to the officers so admitted subject to such modifications as may be provided in the agreement.

(2) The governing body of any hospital to which this section applies shall have all such powers as may be necessary for the purpose of giving effect to any terms and conditions on which their officers are admitted to participate in those superannuation benefits.

(3) This section applies to any hospital (not vested in the Secretary of State) which is used, in pursuance of arrangements made by the governing body of the hospital with the Secretary of State, for the provision of services under this Act.

105.—(1) Where a medical practitioner carries out a medical examination of any person with a view to an application for his admission to hospital for observation or treatment being made under Part IV of the Mental Health Act 1959 the council which is the local authority for the purposes of the Local Authority Social Services Act 1970 for the area where the person examined resides shall, subject to the following provisions of this section, pay to that medical practitioner

(a) reasonable remuneration in respect of that examination and in respect of any recommendation or report made by him with regard to the person examined; and

(b) the amount of any expenses reasonably incurred by him in connection with the examination or the making of any such recommendation or report.

(2) No payment shall be made under this section to a medical practitioner —

(a) in respect of an examination carried out as part of his duty to provide general medical services for the person examined; or

(b) in respect of an examination carried out or any recommendation or report made as part of his duty as an officer of a health authority.

(3) This section shall only apply in a case where it is intended, when the medical examination of the person in question is carried out, that if he is admitted to hospital in pursuance of any such application as mentioned in subsection (1) above, the whole cost of his maintenance and treatment will be defrayed out of moneys provided by Parliament under this Act or the Mental Health Act 1959.

Part V

Health Service Commissioner for England and Health Service Commissioner for Wales

106.—(1) For the purpose of conducting investigations in accordance with this Part of this Act, there shall be appointed —

(*a*) a Commissioner to be known as the Health Service Commissioner for England; and

(*b*) a Commissioner to be known as the Health Service Commissioner for Wales.

(2) Her Majesty may by Letters Patent from time to time appoint a person to be a Commissioner; and a person so appointed shall, subject to subsection (3) below, hold office during good behaviour.

(3) A person appointed to be a Commissioner may be relieved of office by Her Majesty at his own request, or may be removed from office by Her Majesty in consequence of Addresses from both Houses of Parliament, and shall in any case vacate office on completing the year of service in which he attains the age of sixty-five.

(4) A person who is a member of a relevant body (within the meaning of section 109 below) shall not be appointed to be a Commissioner; and a Commissioner shall not become a member of a relevant body.

107.—(1) Subject to subsections (3) and (5) below, there shall be paid to the holder of the office of a Commissioner the same salary as if he were employed in the civil service of the State in such appointment as the House of Commons may by resolution from time to time determine; and any such resolution may take effect from the date on which it is passed, or from such other date as it may specify.

(2) Subject to subsections (6) and (7) below, Schedule 1 to the Parliamentary Commissioner Act 1967 (which relates to pensions and other benefits) has effect with respect to persons who have held office as a Commissioner as it has effect with respect to persons who have held office as the Parliamentary Commissioner for Administration.

(3) The salary payable to a holder of the office of a Commissioner shall be abated by the amount of any pension payable to him in respect of any public office in the United Kingdom or elsewhere to which he has previously been appointed or elected.

(4) In computing the salary of a former holder of the office of Commissioner for the purposes of Schedule 1 to that Act of 1967 there shall be disregarded —

(*a*) any abatement of that salary under subsection (3) above;

(*b*) any temporary abatement of that salary in the national interest; and

(*c*) any voluntary surrender of that salary in whole or in part.

(5) Where —

(*a*) a person holds the office of Parliamentary Commissioner for Administration and one or more of the offices of Health Service Commissioner for Engaland, Health Service Commissioner for Scotland and Health Service Commissioner for Wales he shall, so long as he does so, be entitled only to the salary pertaining to the first-mentioned office; and

(*b*) a person holds two or more of those offices other than that of Parliamentary Commissioner for Administration he shall, so long as he does so, be entitled only to the salary pertaining to such one of those offices as he selects.

(6) A person —

(*a*) shall not be entitled to make simultaneously different elections in pursuance of paragraph 1 of Schedule 1 to that Act of 1967 in respect of different offices mentioned in subsection (5) above, and

(*b*) shall, if he has made or is treated as having made an election in pursuance of that paragraph in respect of such an office, be deemed to have made the same election in respect of all such other offices to which he is, or is subsequently, appointed,

and no account shall be taken for the purposes of that Schedule of a period of service in such an office if salary in respect of the office was not paid for that period.

(7) The Minister for the Civil Service may —

(*a*) by regulations provide that Schedule 1 to that Act of 1967 shall have effect in relation to persons who have held more than one of the offices mentioned in subsection (5) above, and

(*b*) by those regulations modify that Schedule as he considers necessary in consequence of those persons having held more than one of those offices,

and different regulations may be made in pursuance of paragraph 4 of that Schedule in relation to different offices as mentioned.

This subsection is subject to subsection (6) above.

(8) Any salary, pension or other benefit payable by virtue of this section shall be charged on and issued out of the Consolidated Fund.

108.—(1) A Commissioner may appoint such officers as he may determine with the approval of the Minister for the Civil Service as to numbers and conditions of service; and it is the duty of the Health Service Commissioner for Wales to include among his officers such persons having a command of the Welsh language as he considers are needed to enable him to investigate complaints in Welsh.

(2) Any functions of a Commissioner under this Part of this Act may be performed by any officer of the Commissioner authorised by him for that purpose, or by any officer so authorised of another Commissioner mentioned in section 107(5) above.

(3) To assist him in any investigation, a Commissioner may obtain advice from any person who, in his opinion, is qualified to give it, and may pay such fees or allowances to any such person as he may determine with the approval of the Minister for the Civil Service.

(4) The expenses of a Commissioner under this Part of this Act, to such amount as may be sanctioned by the Minister for the Civil Service, shall be defrayed out of money provided by Parliament.

109. In this Part of this Act 'relevant body' means any of the following bodies —

(*a*) Regional Health Authorities;

(*b*) Area Health Authorities;

(*c*) any special health authority established on or before 1st April, 1974;

(*d*) any special health authority established after that 1st April and designated by Order in Council as an authority to which this section applies;

(*e*) Family Practitioner Committee;

(*f*) the Public Health Laboratory Service Board; and

(*g*) the Health Services Board and its Welsh Committee.

Except where the context otherwise requires, any reference in this Part of this Act to a relevant body includes a reference to an officer of the body.

110. The Health Service Commissioner for England shall not conduct an investigation under this Part of this Act in respect of —

(*a*) an Area Health Authority of which the area is in Wales,

(*b*) the Family Practitioner Committee established by such an Authority,

(*c*) a special health authority exercising functions only or mainly in Wales, or

(*d*) the Welsh Committee of the Health Service Board,

and the Health Service Commissioner for Wales shall not conduct such an investigation in respect of a relevant body other than one of those bodies.

111.—(1) A complaint under this Part of this Act may be made by any individual, or by any body of persons whether incorporated or not, not being —

(a) a local authority or other authority or body constituted for purposes of the public service or of local government, or for the purposes of carrying on under national ownership any industry or undertaking or part of an industry or undertaking;

(b) any other authority or body whose members are appointed by Her Majesty or any Minister of the Crown or government department, or whose revenues consist wholly or mainly of money provided by Parliament.

(2) Where the person by whom a complaint might have been made under the preceding provisions of this Part has died, or is for any reason unable to act for himself, the complaint may be made —

(a) by his personal representative, or

(b) by a member of his family, or

(c) by some body or individual suitable to represent him,

but, except as aforesaid and as provided by section 117 below, a complaint shall not be entertained under this Part unless made by the person aggrieved himself.

112. Before proceeding to investigate a complaint —

(a) a Commissioner shall satisfy himself that the complaint has been brought by or on behalf of the person aggrieved to the notice of the relevant body in question, and that that body had been afforded a reasonable opportunity to investigate and reply to the complaint, but

(b) a Commissioner shall disregard the provisions of paragraph (a) in relation to a complaint made by an officer of the relevant body in question on behalf of the person aggrieved if the officer is authorised by virtue of section 111(2) above to make the complaint and the Commissioner is satisfied that in the particular circumstances those provisions ought to be disregarded.

113.—(1) In determining whether to initiate, continue or discontinue an investigation under this Part of this Act, a Commissioner shall, subject to section 110 above and sections 115 and 116 below, act in accordance with his own discretion.

(2) Any question whether a complaint is duly made to a Commissioner under this Part shall be determined by the Commissioner.

114.—(1) A Commissioner —

(a) shall not entertain a complaint under this Part of this Act unless it is made in writing to him by or on behalf of the person aggrieved not later than one year from the day on which the person aggrieved first had notice of the matters alleged in the complaint, but (*b*) may conduct an investigation pursuant to a complaint not made within that period if he considers it reasonable to do so.

(2) The additional provisions contained in Part I of Schedule 13 to this Act, which relate to procedure and other matters have effect for the purposes of this Part.

115. A Commissioner may investigate —
  (*a*) an alleged failure in a service provided by a relevant body, or
  (*b*) an alleged failure of such a body to provide a service which it was a function of the body to provide, or
  (*c*) any other action taken by or on behalf of such a body,
in a case where a complaint is duly made by or on behalf of any person that he has sustained injustice or hardship in consequence of the failure or in consequence of maladministration connected with the other action.

This section is subject to sections 110 and 113 above and section 116 below.

116.—(1) Except as hereafter provided, a Commissioner shall not conduct an investigation under this Part of this Act in respect of any of the following matters —
  (*a*) any action in respect of which the person aggrieved has or had a right of appeal, reference or review to or before a tribunal constituted by or under any enactment or by virtue of Her Majesty's prerogative, or
  (*b*) any action in respect of which the person aggrieved has or had a remedy by way of proceedings in any court of law,
but a Commissioner may conduct an investigation notwithstanding that the person aggrieved has or had such a right or remedy, if satisfied that in the particular circumstances it is not reasonable to expect him to resort or have resorted to it.

(2) Without prejudice to subsection (1) above —
  (*a*) a Commissioner shall not conduct an investigation under this Part in respect of any such action as is described in Part II of Schedule 13 to this Act; and
  (*b*) nothing in sections 110, 113 and 115 above shall be construed as authorising such an investigation in respect of action taken in connection with any general medical services, general dental services, general ophthalmic services or pharmaceutical services by a person providing the services.

(3) Her Majesty may by Order in Council amend Part II of Schedule 13 so as to exclude from it action described in sub-paragraph (3) or (4) of paragraph 19 of that Schedule.

117. Notwithstanding anything in sections 111 and 112 and section 114(1) above, a relevant body —

(*a*) may itself (excluding its officers) refer to a Commissioner a complaint that a person has, in consequence of a failure or maladministration for which the body is responsible, sustained such injustice or hardship as is mentioned in section 115 above if the complaint —

    (i) is made in writing to the relevant body by that person, or by a person authorised by virtue of section 111(2) above to make the complaint to the Commissioner on his behalf, and

    (ii) is so made not later than one year from the day mentioned in section 114(1) above, or within such other period as the Commissioner considers appropriate in any particular case, but

(*b*) shall not be entitled to refer a complaint in pursuance of paragraph (*a*) after the expiry of three months beginning with the day on which the body received the complaint.

A complaint referred to a Commissioner in pursuance of this section shall, subject to section 113 above, be deemed to be duly made to him under this Part of this Act.

118.—(1) Where, at any stage in the course of conducting an investigation under this Part of this Act, the Commissioner conducting the investigation —

(*a*) forms the opinion that the complaint relates partly to a matter which could be the subject of an investigation under Part III of the Local Government Act 1974, then

(*b*) he shall consult about the complaint with the appropriate Local Commissioner within the meaning of Part III of that Act of 1974, and

(*c*) if he considers it necessary, inform the person initiating the complaint under this Part of the steps necessary to initiate a complaint under Part III of that Act of 1974.

(2) Where under subsection (1) above a Commissioner consults with a Local Commissioner in relation to a complaint under this Part of this Act, he may consult that Commissioner about any matter relating to the complaint, including —

(*a*) the conduct of any investigation into the complaint; and

(*b*) the form, content and publication of any report of the results of such an investigation.

(3) Nothing in paragraph 16 of Schedule 13 to this Act applies in relation to the disclosure of information by a Commissioner or his officers in the course of consultations held in accordance with this section.

119.—(1) In any case where a Commissioner conducts an investigation under this Part of this Act, he shall send a report of the results of his investigation —

(a) to the person who made the complaint,

(b) to the relevant body in question,

(c) to any person who is alleged in the complaint to have taken or authorised the action complained of,

(d) if the relevant body in question is not an Area Health Authority for an area in England or a Family Practitioner Committee, to the Secretary of State,

(e) if that body is an Area Health Authority for an area in England, to the Regional Health Authority of which the region includes that area, and

(f) if that body is a Family Practitioner Committee, to the Area Health Authority by which the Committee was established,

but paragraph (d) does not apply in the case of an investigation conducted in respect of the Health Services Board or the Welsh Committee unless the Commissioner thinks fit to publish his report under this subsection.

(2) In any case where a Commissioner decides not to conduct an investigation under this Part, he shall send a statement of his reasons for doing so to the person who made the complaint and to the relevant body in question.

(3) If, after conducting an investigation under this Part, it appears to a Commissioner that the person aggrieved has sustained such injustice or hardship as is mentioned in section 115 above, and that the injustice or hardship has not been and will not be remedied, he may if he thinks fit —

(a) in relation to an investigation conducted in respect of the Health Services Board or the Welsh Committee, lay before each House of Parliament a special report;

(b) in relation to any other investigation, make a special report to the Secretary of State who shall, as soon as is reasonably practicable, lay a copy of the report before each House of Parliament.

(4) Each of the Commissioners shall —

(a) annually lay before each House of Parliament a general report on the performance of his functions under this Part in respect of the Health Services Board and the Welsh Committee, and may from time to time lay before each House of Parliament such other reports with respect to those functions as he thinks fit;

(b) annually make to the Secretary of State a report on the performance of his other functions under this Part, and may from time to time make to the Secretary of State such other reports with respect to those functions as the Commissioner thinks fit, and the Secretary of State shall lay a copy of every such report before each House of Parliament.

(5) For the purposes of the law of defamation, the publication of any matter by a Commissioner in sending or making a report in pursuance of subsection (1), (3) or (4) above, or in sending a statement in pursuance of subsection (2) above, shall be absolutely privileged.

120.—(1) In this Part of this Act and in Schedule 13 to this Act —

'action' includes failure to act, and other expressions connoting action shall be construed accordingly;

'Commissioner' means the Health Service Commissioner for England or the Health Service Commissioner for Wales, and 'Commissioners' means both those persons;

'person aggrieved' means the person who claims or is alleged to have sustained such injustice or hardship as is mentioned in section 115 above; and

'relevant body' has the meaning given by section 109 above, and (except where the context otherwise requires) includes a reference to an officer of the body.

(2) Nothing in this Part of this Act authorises or requires a Commissioner to question the merits of a decision taken without maladministration by a relevant body in the exercise of a discretion vested in that body.

PART VI

MISCELLANEOUS AND SUPPLEMENTARY

General provisions as to charges

121. Regulations may provide for the making and recovery, in such manner as may be prescribed, of such charges —

(a) in respect of such services provided under this Act as may be prescribed, being

(b) services provided in respect of such persons not ordinarily resident in Great Britain as may be prescribed.

Such regulations may provide that the charges are only to be made in such cases as may be determined in accordance with the regulations.

122.—(1) All charges recoverable under this Act by the Secretary of State, a local social services authority, or any body constituted under this Act, may, without prejudice to any other method of recovery, be recovered summarily as a civil debt.

(2) If any person, for the purpose of evading the payment of any charge under this Act, or of reducing the amount of any such charge —

(a) knowingly makes any false statement or false representation, or

(b) produces or furnishes, or causes or knowingly allows to be produced or furnished, any document or information which he knows to be false in a material particular,

the charge, or as the case may be the balance of the charge, may be recovered from him as a simple contract debt by the person by whom the cost of the service in question was defrayed.

Miscellaneous

123.—(1) Where the carrying out of a scheme for the provision by the Secretary of State in pursuance of this Act of hospital accommodation or other facilities will involve the displacement from any premises of persons residing in them, the Secretary of State may make arrangements with one or more of the following bodies —

(a) an authority who are a local authority for the purposes of the Housing Act 1957.

(b) a housing association within the meaning of that Act of 1957,

(c) a housing trust within the meaning of that Act of 1957,

(d) a development corporation established under the New Towns Act 1965, and

(e) the Commission for the New Towns,

for securing, in so far as it appears to him that there is no other residential accommodation suitable for the reasonable requirements of those persons available on reasonable terms, the provision of residential accommodation in advance of the displacement from time to time becoming necessary as the carrying out of the scheme proceeds.

(2) Arrangements under subsection (1) above may include provision for the making by the Secretary of State to the body with whom the arrangements are made of payments of such amounts and for such purposes as may be approved by the Treasury.

124.—(1) The requirements of this section with respect to the notification of births and deaths are in addition to, and not in substitution for, the requirements of any Act relating to the registration of births and deaths.

(2) It is the duty of each registrar of births and deaths to furnish, to the prescribed medical officer of the Area Health Authority of which the area includes the whole or part of the registrar's sub-district, such particulars of each birth and death which occurred in the Authority's area as are entered (on and after 1st April 1974) in a register of births or deaths kept for that sub-district.

(3) Regulations may provide as to the manner in which and the times

at which particulars are to be furnished in pursuance of subsection (2) above.

(4) In the case of every child born, it is the duty —

(*a*) of the child's father, if at the time of the birth he is actually residing on the premises where the birth takes place, and

(*b*) of any person in attendance upon the mother at the time of, or within six hours after, the birth,

to give notice of the birth (as provided in subsection (5) below to the prescribed medical officer of the Area Health Authority for the area in which the birth takes place.

This subsection applies to any child which has issued forth from its mother after the expiry of the twenty-eighth week of pregnancy whether alive or dead.

(5) Notice under subsection (4) above shall be given either —

(*a*) by posting within 36 hours after the birth a prepaid letter or postcard addressed to the prescribed medical officer of the Area Health Authority at his office and containing the required information, or

(*b*) by delivering within that period at that officer's office a written notice containing the required information,

and an Area Health Authority shall, upon application to them, supply without charge to any medical practitioner or midwife residing or practising within their area prepaid addressed envelopes together with the forms of notice.

(6) Any person who fails to give notice of a birth in accordance with subsection (4) above is liable on summary conviction to a fine not exceeding £1, unless he satisfies the court that he believed, and had reasonable grounds for believing, that notice had been duly given by some other person.

Proceedings in respect of this offence shall not, without the Attorney-Generals's written consent, be taken by any person other than a party aggrieved or the Area Health Authority concerned.

(7) A registrar of births and deaths shall, for the purpose of obtaining information concerning births which have occurred in his sub-district, have access at all reasonable times to notices of births received by a medical officer under this section, or to any book in which those notices may be recorded.

125. Section 265 of the Public Health Act 1875 (which relates to the protection of members and officers of certain authorities) has effect as if there were included in the authorities referred to in that section —

(*a*) a Regional Health Authority,

(*b*) an Area Health Authority,

(c) a special health authority, and

(d) a Family Practitioner Committee,

and as if any reference in that section to the Public Health Act 1875 included a reference to this Act.

Supplementary

126.—(1) Any power to make orders or regulations conferred by this Act shall be exercisable by statutory instrument, and a statutory instrument made by virtue of this Act shall be subject to annulment in pursuance of a resolution of either House of Parliament.

This subsection —

(a) is subject to paragraph 15(3) of Schedule 5 to this Act;

(b) does not apply to paragraph 10 of Schedule 11 to this Act.

(2) Any power to make regulations conferred on the Secretary of State by this Act is, if the Treasury so directs, exercisable by the Treasury and the Secretary of State acting jointly, except in the case of —

(a) regulations made under section 32 above;

(b) regulations made under section 77(1) above in respect of charges for the drugs, medicines or appliances referred to in paragraph (a) of that subsection, or under paragraph 1(1) of Schedule 12 to this Act in respect of the remission or repayment of any charge payable under that section in the cases provided for in paragraph 1(1) of that Schedule;

(c) regulations made under paragraph 2(2) of that Schedule;

(d) regulations made under paragraph 2(6) of that Schedule.

(3) Where under any provision of this Act —

(a) power to make an order may be exercisable, or

(b) directions may be given,

that provision includes power to vary or revoke the order or direction, as the case may be, by subsequent order or by subsequent directions.

In relation to directions given by the Secretary of State in pursuance of sections 13 to 17 above this subsection is subject to section 18 above.

(4) Any power conferred by this Act to make orders, regulations, or schemes, and any power conferred by section 18 above to give directions by an instrument in writing, may, unless the contrary intention appears, be exercised —

(a) either in relation to all cases to which the power extends, or in relation to all those cases subject to specified exceptions, or in relation to any specified cases or classes of case, and

(b) so as to make, as respects the cases in relation to which it is exercised —

(i) the full provision to which the power extends or any

      less provision (whether by way of exception or otherwise),
- (ii) the same provision for all cases in relation to which the power is exercised, or different provision for different cases or different classes of case, or different provision as repects the same case or class of case for different purposes of this Act or that section,
- (iii) any such provision either unconditionally, or subject to any specified condition,

and includes power to make such incidental or supplemental provision in the orders, regulations, schemes or directions as the persons making or giving them consider appropriate.

This subsection does not apply to regulations made under section 32 above (but without prejudice to subsection (3) of that section) or to an order made under section 57 above (but without prejudice to paragraph 1(1) of Schedule 11 to this Act).

127. Regulations may provide for all or any of the following matters—
- (*a*) for prescribing the forms and manner of service of notices and other documents;
- (*b*) for prescribing the manner in which documents may be executed or proved;
- (*c*) for prescribing the manner in which resolutions of any bodies (except the Public Health Laboratory Service Board) continued in being by this Act are to be proved;
- (*d*) for exempting judges and justices of the peace from disqualification by their liability to rates.

128.—(1) In this Act, unless the contrary intention appears —

'the Central Council' means the Central Health Services Council referred to in section 6 above;

'certified midwife' means a person who is for the time being certified under the Midwives Act 1951;

'dental practitioner' means a person registered in the dentists register under the Dentists Act 1957;

'dispensing optician' means a person who is registered in the register kept under section 2 of the Opticians Act 1958 of dispensing opticians or a body corporate enrolled in the list kept under section 4 of that Act of such bodies carrying on business as dispensing opticians;

'equipment' includes any machinery, apparatus or appliance, whether fixed or not, and any vehicle;

'functions' includes powers and duties;

'health authority' means a Regional or Area Health Authority or a special health authority;

'the health service' means the health service established in pursuance of section 1(1) above;

'health service hospital' means a hospital vested in the Secretary of State under this Act;

'Health Services Board' means the body established by section 1 of the Health Services Act 1976;

'hospital' means —

(a) any institution for the reception and treatment of persons suffering from illness,

(b) any maternity home, and

(c) any institution for the reception and treatment of persons during convalescence or persons requiring medical rehabilitation, and includes clinics, dispensaries and out-patient departments maintained in connection with any such home or institution, and 'hospital accommodation' shall be construed accordingly;

'illness' includes mental disorder within the meaning of the Mental Health Act 1959 and any injury or disability requiring medical or dental treatment or nursing;

'local authority' means a county council, the Greater London Council, a district council, a London borough council, and the Common Council of the City of London; and includes the King Edward VII Welsh National Memorial Association;

'local education authority' has the same meaning as in the Education Act 1944;

'local social services authority' means the council of a non-metropolitan county, or of a metropolitan district or London borough, or the Common Council of the City of London;

'medical' includes surgical;

'medical practitioner' means a fully registered person within the meaning of the Medical Act 1956;

'medicine' includes such chemical re-agents as are included in a list for the time being approved by the Secretary of State for the purposes of section 41 above;

'modifications' includes additions, omissions and amendments;

'officer' includes servant;

'ophthalmic optician' means a person registered in either of the registers kept under section 2 of the Opticians Act 1958 of ophthalmic opticians or a body corporate enrolled in the list kept under section 4 of that Act of such bodies carrying on business as ophthalmic opticians;

'patient' includes an expectant or nursing mother and a lying-in woman;

'prescribed' means prescribed by regulations made by the Secretary of State under this Act;

'property' includes rights;

'registered nurse' means a nurse registered in the register of nurses established under the Nurses Registration Act 1919 and maintained in pursuance of section 2(1) of the Nurses Act 1957;

'registered pharmacist' means a pharmacist registered in the register of pharmaceutical chemists;

'regulations' means regulations made by the Secretary of State under this Act;

'special hospital' has the meaning given by section 4 above;

'superannuation benefits' means annual superannuation allowances gratuities and periodical payments payable on retirement, death or incapacity, and similar benefits;

'university' includes a university college;

'vuluntary' means not carried on for profit and not provided by a local or public authority;

'Welsh Committee' means the committee constituted under section 1(3) of the Health Services Act 1976.

(2) References in this Act to the purposes of a hospital shall be construed as referring both to the general purposes of the hospital and to any specific purpose of the hospital.

(3) Any reference in this Act to any enactment is a reference to it as amended or applied by or under any other enactment including this Act.

129. Schedule 14 to this Act is hereby given effect, and subject to the transitional provisions and savings contained in that Schedule —

(a) the enactments and the Order specified in Schedule 15 to this Act have effect subject to the amendments (being amendments consequent on this Act) specified in that Schedule, and

(b) the enactments specified in Schedule 16 to this Act (which include enactments which were spent before the passing of this Act) are hereby repealed to the extent specified in the third column of that Schedule,

but nothing in this Act shall be taken as prejudicing the operation of section 38 of the Interpretation Act 1889 (which relates to the operation of repeals).

130.—(1) This Act may be cited as the National Health Service Act 1977.

(2) This Act does not extend to Scotland, except as is mentioned in paragraph 3 of Schedule 11 to this Act.

(3) The following provisions only of this Act apply to Northern Ireland —

(a) this subsection and subsections (1) above and (5) below;

(b) section 57 above and Schedule 11 to this Act;

(c) section 114(2) above and Part I of Schedule 13 to this Act, section 119(5) above, and section 120(1) above so far as it relates to the provisions mentioned in this paragraph;

(d) paragraph 13 of Schedule 14 to this Act so far as it relates to any enactment which extends to Northern Ireland;

(e) paragraph (a) of section 129 above and Schedule 15 to this Act so far as they amend any enactment and order which extends to Northern Ireland;

(f) paragraph (b) of section 129 and Schedule 16 to this Act so far as they repeal any enactment which extends to Northern Ireland.

(4) The Secretary of State may by order provide that this Act shall extend to the Isles of Scilly with such modifications, if any, as are specified in the order, and except as provided in pursuance of this subsection this Act does not extend to the Isles of Scilly.

The Secretary of State may by any such order amend or repeal any provisions contained in the Isles of Scilly Orders 1927 to 1943.

(5) This Act shall come into force on the expiry of the period of one month beginning on the date of its passing.

SCHEDULES

SCHEDULE 1

ADDITIONAL PROVISIONS AS TO THE MEDICAL AND DENTAL INSPECTION AND TREATMENT OF PUPILS

'Not here reproduced'

SCHEDULE 2

ADDITIONAL PROVISIONS AS TO VEHICLES FOR THOSE SUFFERING DISABILITY

'Not here reproduced'

SCHEDULE 3

PUBLIC HEALTH LABORATORY SERVICE BOARD

PART I

CONSTITUTION OF THE PUBLIC HEALTH LABORATORY SERVICE BOARD

1. The Public Health Laboratory Service Board shall be a body corporate.

2. The Board may accept, hold and administer property on trust for any purposes relating to the public health laboratory service or otherwise connected with microbiological research.

3. The Board shall consist of a chairman appointed by the Secretary of State and such other members so appointed as the Secretary of State thinks fit, and the members shall include—

(*a*) not less than two persons appointed after consultation with the Medical Research Council; and

(*b*) not less than two persons with experience as microbiologists, appointed after consultation with such organisations as the Secretary of State thinks appropriate; and

(*c*) not less than two proper officers appointed by a local authority; and

(*d*) not less than one person with experience of service in hospitals; and

(*e*) not less than one medical practitioner engaged in general medical practice, appointed after consultation with such organisations as the Secretary of State may recognise as representative of practitioners so engaged.

4. Subject to paragraph 5 below members shall be appointed for a term of three years.

5. Any member appointed to fill a casual vacancy shall be appointed for the remainder of the term for which his predecessor was appointed.

6. A member may at any time resign his office.

7. A person who is or has been a member of the Board shall be eligible for re-appointment as a member.

8. The Board may elect a deputy chairman and may appoint one or more committees consisting wholly or partly of members of the Board and may delegate to any such committee any of the Board's functions.

9. The proceedings of the Board or any committee appointed by the Board shall not be invalidated by any vacancy in the membership of the Board or committee, or by any defect in the appointment or qualification of any such member.

10. The Board and, subject to any directions of the Board, any committee appointed by them, may regulate their own procedure and fix a quorum for any of their proceedings.

PART II

ADDITIONAL PROVISIONS AS TO THE PUBLIC HEALTH LABORATORY SERVICE BOARD

11. The Board may appoint such officers and servants, on such terms as to remuneration and conditions of service, as the Board may, with the Secretary of State's approval, determine.

12. The Board may pay to its members and to the members of any committee appointed by the Board such travelling and other allowances, including compensation for loss of remunerative time, as the Board may, with the approval of the Secretary of State and the Minister for the Civil Service, determine.

13. The Board shall exercise their functions in accordance with any direction which the Secretary of State may give to them but shall in the exercise of those functions be deemed for all purposes to act as principal.

14. The Secretary of State shall pay to the Board, out of moneys provided by Parliament, such sums as may be necessary to defray the expenditure of the Board incurred with his approval.

15. Any sums received by the Board (otherwise than in exercise of their power under paragraph 2 above, or under paragraph 14 above) shall be paid into the Consolidated Fund.

16. The Board shall keep proper accounts and other records in such form as the Secretary of State may, with the approval of the Treasury determine.

17. The Board shall prepare and transmit to the Secretary of State in respect of each financial year statements of account in such form as the Secretary of State may, with the approval of the Treasury determine.,

18. The Secretary of State shall transmit these statements of accounts on or before 30th November following the financial year to the Comptroller and Auditor General, who shall examine and certify them and lay copies of them together with his report on them before each House of Parliament.

SCHEDULE 4

CENTRAL HEALTH SERVICES COUNCIL AND ADVISORY COMMITTEES

Constitution of Central Council

1.—(1) The number of members of the Central Council shall be not less than forty, and not more than forty-four, of whom—
  (a) thirteen shall be nominated members in accordance with subparagraph (2) below;

(*b*) twenty-seven shall be selected members in accordance with sub-paragraph (5) below; and

(*c*) the remaining members shall be such persons appointed by the Secretary of State as he thinks fit.

(2) The nominated members of the Central Council shall be—

    (*a*) the persons for the time being holding the offices of—

The President of the Royal College of Physicians of London;

The President of the Royal College of Surgeons of England;

The President of the Royal College of Obstetricians and Gynaecologists;

The President of the Royal College of Psychiatrists;

The President of the Royal College of Pathologists;

The President of the Royal College of General Practitioners;

The President of the Royal College of Nursing and National Council of Nurses of the United Kingdom;

The President of the Royal College of Midwives;

The Chairman of the Council of the British Medical Association;

The Chairman of the Council of the British Dental Association;

The President of the Faculty of Community Medicine;

The President of the Pharmaceutical Society of Great Britain; and

    (*b*) one member of the Personal Social Services Council nominated by that body.

(3) Any office-holder specified in paragraph (*a*) of sub-paragraph (2) above may notify the Secretary of State in writing of another member of the body in which he holds office who is to be a member of the Central Council in his place for such period or any part of such period as he holds that office.

(4) The person of whom such notification is given shall be a member of the Central Council—

    (*a*) until he resigns; or

    (*b*) until the office-holder ceases to hold office; or

    (*c*) until the office-holder notifies the Secretary of State in writing that he wishes some other person to be a member in his place or that he wishes to be a member himself.

(5) The selected members of the Central Council, who shall be appointed by the Secretary of State, shall be—

    (*a*) eight medical practitioners;

    (*b*) two dental practitioners;

    (*c*) three registered nurses or certified midwives;

    (*d*) one registered pharmacist;

    (*e*) one registered optician;

    (*f*) seven persons with experience in health service management;

    (*g*) one person with qualifications or experience in social work; and

    (*h*) four persons, who, in the opinion of the Secretary of State, are interested in the health service from the point of view of members of the public.

Before appointing any of the persons specified in paragraphs (*a*) to (*g*) respectively, the Secretary of State shall consult with such organisations as he may recognise as representative of such persons, and before appointing the persons specified in paragraph (*h*) he shall consult with such bodies as appear to him to be appropriate for this purpose.

Supplementary provisions

2. Regulations may make provision with respect to the appointment, tenure

of office and vacation of office of the members of the Central Council, and of any standing advisory committee constituted under section 6 above.

3. The Secretary of State shall appoint a secretary to the Central Council and to each standing advisory committee.

4. The Central Council may appoint such committees, and any standing advisory committee may appoint such sub-committees, as they think fit, and as are approved by the Secretary of State, to consider and report upon questions referred to them by the Central Council or standing advisory committee as the case may be.

Any such committee or sub-committee may include persons who are not members of the Central Council or standing advisory committee as the case may be.

5. The Central Council and any standing advisory committee shall elect one of the members of the Council or committee as the case may be to be chairman of the Council or committee, and shall have power to regulate their own procedure.

6. The proceedings of the Central Council or of any standing advisory committee shall not be invalidated by any vacancy in the membership of the Council or committee, or by any defect in a member's appointment or qualification.

SCHEDULE 5

REGIONAL AND AREA HEALTH AUTHORITIES, FAMILY PRACTITIONER COMMITTEES, AND SPECIAL HEALTH AUTHORITIES

PART I

MEMBERSHIP OF REGIONAL AND AREA HEALTH AUTHORITIES

Regional Health Authorities

1.—(1) A Regional Health Authority shall consist of a chairman appointed by the Secretary of State, and of such number of other members appointed by him as he thinks fit.

(2) Except in prescribed cases, it is the Secretary of State's duty, before he appoints a member of a Regional Health Authority other than the chairman, to consult with respect to the appointment—

(a) such of the following bodies of which the areas or parts of them are within the region of the Authority, namely, county councils, metropolitan district councils, the Greater London Council, London borough councils, and the Common Council of the City of London;

(b) the university or universities with which the provision of health services in that region is, or is to be, associated;

(c) such bodies as the Secretary of State may recognise as being, either in that region or generally, representative respectively of medical practitioners, dental practitioners, nurses, midwives, registered pharmacists and ophthalmic and dispensing opticians, or representative of such other professions as appear to him to be concerned;

(d) any federation of workers' organisations which appear to the Secretary of State to be concerned, and any voluntary organisation within the meaning of section 23 above and any other body which appear to him to be concerned; and (*e*) in the case of an appointment of a member falling to be made after the establishment of the Regional Health Authority in question, that Authority.

Area Health Authorities

2.—(1) Subject to paragraph 4 below, an Area Health Authority for an area in England shall consist of the following members—

(*a*) a chairman appointed by the Secretary of State;

(*b*) the specified number of members appointed by the relevant Regional Authority after consultation (except in prescribed cases) with the bodies mentioned in sub-paragraph (2) below;

(*c*) the specified number of members appointed by the relevant Regional Authority on the nomination of the university or universities specified as being associated with the provision of health services in that Authority's region; and

(*d*) the specified number (not less than four) of members appointed by the specified local authority or local authorities.

(2) The bodies referred to in sub-paragraph (1)(*b*) above are—

(*a*) such bodies as the relevant Regional Authority may recognise as being, either in its region or in the area of the Area Health Authority or generally, representative respectively of medical practitioners, dental practitioners, nurses, midwives, registered pharmacists and ophthalmic and dispensing opticians, or representative of such other professions as appear to the relevant Regional Authority to be concerned;

(*b*) such other bodies (including any federation of workers' organisations) as appear to the relevant Regional Authority to be concerned, excluding any university which has nominated, or is entitled to nominate, a member, and any local authority which has appointed, or is entitled to appoint, a member; and

(*c*) in the case of an appointment of a member falling to be made after the establishment of the Area Health Authority in question, that Authority.

3. Paragraph 2 above applies to an Area Health Authority for an area in Wales as if, for any reference to the relevant Regional Authority, there were substituted a reference to the Secretary of State, and for any reference to England or the region of that Authority there were substituted a reference to Wales.

4. The members of an Area Health Authority (Teaching) shall, in addition to the members appointed in pursuance of paragraph 2 above, include the specified number of members appointed—

(*a*) in the case of such an Authority the area of which is in England, by the relevant Regional Authority from among persons appearing to that Authority to have knowledge of and experience in, the administration of a hospital providing substantial facilities for under-graduate or post-graduate clinical teaching; and

(*b*) in the case of such an Authority the area of which is in Wales, by the Secretary of State from among persons appearing to him to have such knowledge and experience.

Supplemental

5.—(1) For the purposes of paragraphs 2 to 4 above—

(*a*) 'local authority' means the council of a non-metropolitan county, a metropolitan district and a London borough, the Inner London Education Authority, and the Common Council of the City of London;

(b) 'the relevant Regional Authority' means the Regional Health Authority of which the region includes the area of the Area Health Authority in question; and

(c) 'specified' means specified in the order establishing the Area Health Authority in question, or, where another order provides for it to be called an Area Health Authority (Teaching), in that other order.

(2) Where—

(a) an order establishing an Area Health Authority, or another order providing for it to be called an Area Health Authority or an Area Health Authority (Teaching), specifies more than one university in pursuance of paragraph 2(1)(c) above, the order may contain provision as to which of the universities shall (either severally or jointly) nominate all or any of the members falling to be nominated in pursuance of that provision;

(b) such an order specifies more than one local authority in pursuance of paragraph 2(1)(d) above, the order may provide for each of the local authorities to appoint in pursuance of paragraph 2(1)(d) the number of members specified in the order in relation to that local authority.

PART II

MEMBERSHIP OF FAMILY PRACTITIONER COMMITTEES

6.—(1) Subject to paragraph 7 below, a Family Practitioner Committee shall consist of thirty members, of whom—

(a) eleven shall be appointed by the Area Health Authority responsible for establishing the Committee, and at least one of them must be, but not every one of them shall be, a member of the Authority;

(b) four shall be appointed by the local authority entitled in pursuance of paragraph 2(1)(d) above to appoint members of that Authority or, where two or more local authorities are so entitled, by those authorities acting jointly;

(c) eight shall be appointed by the Local Medical Committee for the area of that Authority, and one of them must be, but not more than one of them shall be, a medical practitioner having the qualifications prescribed in pursuance of section 38 above (ophthalmic services);

(d) three shall be appointed by the Local Dental Committee for that area;

(e) two shall be appointed by the Local Pharmaceutical Committee for that area;

(f) one shall be an ophthalmic optician appointed by such members of the Local Optical Committee for that area as are ophthalmic opticians;

(g) one shall be a dispensing optician appointed by such members of that Local Optical Committee as are dispensing opticians.

The members of a Family Practitioner Committee shall from time to time, in accordance with such procedure as may be prescribed, select one of their members to be the chairman of the Committee.

(2) If any appointment falling to be made in pursuance of sub-paragraph (1) above by, or by certain members of, a Local Committee is not made before

such date as the Area Health Authority in question may determine for that appointment, the appointment shall be made by that Authority, to the exclusion of the Committee or members in question.

(3) A Local Committee—

(a) the members of which are mentioned in paragraphs (*f*) and (*g*) of sub-paragraph (1) may, if they think fit, appoint, in addition to the member of the Family Practitioner Committee appointed by them, an ophthalmic or, as the case may be, a dispensing optician to be the deputy of the member so appointed; and

(b) by which such a practitioner as is mentioned in paragraph (*c*) of that sub-paragraph is appointed in pursuance of that paragraph as a member of a Family Practitioner Committee may if it thinks fit appoint another practitioner to be his deputy.

A deputy appointed in pursuance of this sub-paragraph may, while the member for whom he is deputy is absent from any meeting of the relevant Family Practitioner Committee, act as a member of that Committee in the place of the absent member.

7.—(1) If it appears to the Secretary of State that, by reason of special circumstances affecting the area of an Area Health Authority, it is appropriate that the Family Practitioner Committee established by the Authority should not be in accordance with paragraph 6 above, he may by order provide that that paragraph shall apply in relation to the Committee with such modifications as are specified in the order.

(2) It is the Secretary of State's duty—

(a) before he makes an order under sub-paragraph (1) above in respect of any Family Practitioner Committee, to consult that Committee with respect to the order; and

(b) in making any such order, to have regard to the desirability of maintaining, so far as practicable, the same numerical proportion as between members falling to be appointed by different bodies in pursuance of paragraph 6 apart from any modification.

PART III

SUPPLEMENTARY PROVISIONS

Corporate Status

8. Each Regional Health Authority, Area Health Authority, special health authority and Family Practitioner Committee (herinafter in this Schedule referred to severally as 'an authority') shall be a body corporate.

Pay and allowances

9.—(1) The Secretary of State may pay to the chairman of an authority other than a Family Practitioner Committee such remuneration as he may determine with the approval of the Minister for the Civil Service.

(2) The Secretary of State may provide as he may determine with the approval of the Minister for the Civil Service for the payment of a pension, allowance or gratuity to or in respect of the chairman of an authority other than such a Committee.

(3) Where a person ceases to be chairman of an authority other than such a Committee, and it appears to the Secretary of State that there are special cir-

cumstances which make it right for that person to receive compensation, the Secretary of State may make to him a payment of such amount as the Secretary of State may determine with the approval of the Minister for the Civil Service.

(4) The Secretary of State may pay to a member of an authority, or of a committee or sub-committee of an authority, such travelling and other allowances (including attendance allowance or compensation for the loss of remunerative time) as he may determine with the approval of the Minister for the Civil Service.

(5) Allowances shall not be paid in pursuance of sub-paragraph (4) above except in connection with the exercise, in such circumstances as the Secretary of State may determine with the approval of the Minister for the Civil Service, of such functions as he may so determine.

(6) Payments under this paragraph shall be made at such times, and in such manner and subject to such conditions, as the Secretary of State may determine with the approval of the Minister for the Civil Service.

Staff

10.—(1) An authority other than a Family Practitioner Committee may employ, on such terms as it may determine in accordance with regulations and such directions as may be given by the Secretary of State, such officers as it may so determine; and regulations made for the purposes of this sub-paragraph may contain provision—

(a) with respect to the qualifications of persons who may be employed as officers of an authority;

(b) requiring an authority to employ, for the purpose of performing prescribed functions of the authority or any other body, officers having prescribed qualifications or experience; and

(c) as to the manner in which any officers of an authority are to be appointed.

(2) Regulations may provide for the transfer of officers from one authority to another which is not a Family Practitioner Committee, and for arrangements under which the services of an officer of an authority are placed at the disposal of another authority or a local authority.

(3) Directions may be given—

(a) by the Secretary of State to an authority to place services of any of its officers at the disposal of another authority,

(b) subject to any directions given by the Secretary of State in pursuance of this sub-paragraph, by a Regional Health Authority to an Area Health Authority of which the area is included in its region to place services of any of its officers at the disposal of another such Area Health Authority,

(c) by the Secretary of State to any authority other than a Family Practitioner Committee to employ as an officer of the authority any person who is or was employed by another authority and is specified in the direction,

(d) by a Regional Health Authority to an Area Health Authority of which the area is included in its region to employ as an officer of the Area Health Authority any person who is or was employed by an authority other than the Area Health Authority and is specified in the direction, and it shall be the duty of an authority to which directions are given in pursuance of this sub-paragraph to comply with the directions.

(4) Regulations made in pursuance of this paragraph shall not require that all consultants employed by an authority are to be so employed whole-time.

11.—(1) It shall be the duty of the Secretary of State, before he makes regulations in pursuance of paragraph 10 above, to consult such bodies as he may recognise as representing persons who, in his opinion, are likely to be affected by the regulations.

(2) Subject to sub-paragraph (3) below, it is the Secretary of State's duty, or, as the case may be, a Regional Health Authority's, before he or the Authority gives directions to an authority in pursuance of sub-paragraph (3) of paragraph 10 above in respect of any officer of an authority—

(a) to consult the officer about the directions; or

(b) to satisfy himself or itself that the authority of which he is an officer has consulted the officer about the placing or employment in question; or

(c) to consult, except in the case of a direction in pursuance of paragraph (c) or paragraph (d) of paragraph 10(3), with respect to the directions such body as he or the Authority may recognise as representing the officer.

(3) If the Secretary of State or Regional Health Authority—

(a) considers it necessary to give directions in pursuance of paragraph (a) or paragraph (b) of paragraph 10(3) for the purpose of dealing temporarily with an emergency, and

(b) has previously consulted bodies recognised by him or the Authority as representing the relevant officers about the giving of directions for that purpose,

the Secretary of State or the Authority shall be entitled to disregard sub-paragraph (2) above in relation to the directions.

Miscellaneous

12. Provision may be made by regulations as to—

(a) the appointment and tenure of office of the chairman and members of an authority;

(b) the appointment of, and the exercise of functions by, committees and sub-committees of an authority (including joint committees and joint sub-committees of two or more authorities, and committees and sub-committees consisting wholly or partly of persons who are not members of the authority in question); and

(c) the procedure of an authority, and of such committees and sub-committees as are mentioned in sub-paragraph (b) above.

13. An authority may pay subscriptions, of such amounts as the Secretary of State may approve, to the funds of such bodies as he may approve.

14. The proceedings of an authority shall not be invalidated by any vacancy in its membership, or by any defect in a member's appointment.

15.—(1) An authority shall, notwithstanding that it is exercising any function on behalf of the Secretary of State or another authority, be entitled to enforce any rights acquired in the exercise of that function, and be liable in respect of any liabilities incurred (including liabilities in tort) in the exercise of that function, in all respects as if it were acting as a principal.

Proceedings for the enforcement of such rights and liabilities shall be brought, and brought only, by or, as the case may be, against the authority in question in its own name.

(2) An authority shall not be entitled to claim in any proceedings any privilege of the Crown in respect of the discovery or production of documents.

This sub-paragraph shall not prejudice any right of the Crown to withhold or procure the withholding from production of any document on the ground that its disclosure would be contrary to the public interest.

(3) The Secretary of State may by order provide—

(a) that any right which a Regional Hospital Board, a Board of Governors or a Hospital Management Committee was entitled to enforce by virtue of section 13 of the National Health Service Act 1946 immediately before 1st April 1974, and

(b) that any liability in respect of which such a board or committee was liable by virtue of that section immediately before that day,

shall, on and after that day, be enforceable by or, as the case may be, against a health authority specified in the order as if the health authority so specified were concerned as a principal with the matter in question and did not exercise functions on behalf of the Secretary of State.

A statutory instrument containing only an order made by virtue of this sub-paragraph shall be laid before Parliament after being made.

16. Provision may be made by regulations with respect to the recording of information by an authority, and the furnishing of information by an authority to the Secretary of State or another authority.

SCHEDULE 6

ADDITIONAL PROVISIONS AS TO LOCAL ADVISORY COMMITTEES

1.—(1) Where the Secretary of State is satisfied that a committee formed for Wales, or for the region of a Regional Health Authority, or the area of an Area Health Authority, is representative of—

(a) any category of persons (other than a category mentioned in section 19(1) above) who provides services forming part of the health service, or

(b) two or more of any of the categories mentioned in that sub-section and paragraph (a) above,

and that it is in the interests of the health service to recognise the committee, it shall be his duty to recognise it in pursuance of this sub-paragraph, and to determine that it shall be known by a name specified in the determination.

(2) Where a committee recognised in pursuance of sub-paragraph (1) above appears to the Secretary of State to represent categories of persons which include a category mentioned in section 19(1), he shall not be required by virtue of that subsection to recognise a committee representing persons of that category.

2. The Secretary of State may, by notice in writing served on any member of a duly recognised committee, withdraw his recognition of the committee if he considers it expedient to do so—

(a) where the committee is recognised in pursuance of section 19(1) or (3) above or paragraph 1(1)(a) above, with a view to recognising in pursuance of paragraph 1(1)(b) another committee representing categories of persons which include the category represented by the recognised committee; or

(b) where the committee is recognised in pursuance of paragraph 1(1)(b), with a view to recognising in pursuance of any of the provisions of section 19 and paragraph 1 other committees which together are representative of the categories in question.

3. It is the duty of any duly recognised committee for Wales—
    (a) to advise the Secretary of State on the provision by him of services of a kind provided by the categories of persons of whom the committee is representative, and
    (b) to perform such other functions as may be prescribed.

4. It is the duty of a committee duly recognised by reference to the region of a Regional Health Authority or the area of an Area Health Authority—
    (a) to advise the Authority on the Authority's provision of services of a kind provided by the categories of persons of whom the committee is representative, and
    (b) to perform such other functions as may be prescribed,
and it shall be the duty of the Authority to consult the committee with respect to such matters, and on such occasions, as may be prescribed.

5. An Authority may defray such expenses incurred by a committee in performing the duty imposed on the committee by paragraphs 3 or 4 above as the Authority considers reasonable, and those expenses may include travelling and other allowances and compensation for loss of remunerative time at such rates as the Secretary of State may determine with the approval of the Minister for the Civil Service.
In this paragraph 'an Authority' means—
    (a) in relation to any duly recognised committee for Wales, the Secretary of State;
    (b) in relation to the region of a Regional Health Authority, that Regional Health Authority;
    (c) in relation to the area of an Area Health Authority, that Area Health Authority.

SCHEDULE 7

ADDITIONAL PROVISIONS AS TO COMMUNITY HEALTH COUNCILS

1. It is the duty of a Community Health Council (in this Schedule referred to as a 'Council')—
    (a) to represent the interests in the health service of the public in its district; and
    (b) to perform such other functions as may be conferred on it by virtue of paragraph 2 below.

2. Regulations may provide as to—
    (a) the membership of Councils (including the election by members of a Council of a chairman of the Council);
    (b) the proceedings of Councils;
    (c) the staff, premises and expenses of Councils;
    (d) the consultation of Councils by Area Health Authorities with respect to such matters, and on such occasions, as may be prescribed;
    (e) the furnishing of information to Councils by Area Health Authorities, and the rights of members of Councils to enter and inspect premises controlled by Area Health Authorities;
    (f) the consideration by Councils of matters relating to the operation of

the health service within their districts, and the giving of advice by Councils to Area Health Authorities on such matters;

(g) the preparation and publication of reports by Councils on such matters, and the furnishing and publication by Area Health Authorities of comments on the reports; and

(h) the functions to be exercised by Councils in addition to the functions exercisable by them by virtue of paragraph 1(a) above and the preceding provisions of this paragraph.

3. It is the Secretary of State's duty to exercise his power to make regulations in pursuance of paragraph 2(a) above so as to secure as respects each Council that—

(a) at least one member of the Council is appointed by each local authority of which the area or part of it is included in the Council's district, and at least half of the members of the Council consist of persons appointed by those local authorities;

(b) at least one third of the members are appointed in a prescribed manner by bodies (other than public or local authorities) of which the activities are carried on otherwise than for profit;

(c) the other members of the Council are appointed by such bodies, and in such manner and after such consultations as may be prescribed; and

(d) no member of the Council is also a member of a Regional Health Authority or Area Health Authority.

4. Nothing in paragraph 3 above affects the validity of anything done by or in relation to a Council during any period during which, by reason of a vacancy in the membership of the Council or a defect in the appointment of a member of it, a requirement included in regulations in pursuance of that paragraph is not satisfied.

5. The Secretary of State may by regulations—

(a) provide for the establishment of a body—

(i) to advise Councils with respect to the performance of their functions, and to assist Councils in the performance of their functions; and

(ii) to perform such other functions as may be prescribed; and

(b) provide for the membership, proceedings, staff, premises and expenses of that body.

6. The Secretary of State may pay to members of Councils and any body established under paragraph 5 above such travelling and other allowances (including compensation for loss of remunerative time) as he may determine with the consent of the Minister for the Civil Service.

7. In this Schedule—

'local authority' means the council of a London borough, or of a county or district as defined in relation to England in section 270(1) of the Local Government Act 1972, or of a county or district mentioned in section 20(3) of that Act (which relates to Wales) or the Common Council of the City of London, and

'district', in relation to a Council, means the locality for which it is established, whether that locality consists of the area or part of the area of an Area Health Authority, or such an area or part together with the areas or parts of the areas of other Area Health Authorities,

and the district of a Council must be such that no part of it is separated from the rest of it by territory not included in the district.

SCHEDULE 8

LOCAL SOCIAL SERVICES AUTHORITIES

Care of mothers and young children

1.—(1) A local social services authority may, with the Secretary of State's approval, and to such extent as he may direct shall, make arrangements for the care of expectant and nursing mothers and of children who have not attained the age of 5 years and are not attending primary schools maintained by a local education authority.

(2) A local social services authority may make and recover from persons availing themselves of the services provided under this paragraph such charges (if any) in respect of residential accommodation, day nurseries, child-minders, food or articles provided as the authority consider reasonable, having regard to the means of those persons.

Prevention, care and after-care

2.—(1) A local social services authority may, with the Secretary of State's approval, and to such extent as he may direct shall, make arrangements for the purpose of the prevention of illness and for the care of persons suffering from illness and for the after-care of persons who have been so suffering and in particular for—

(*a*) the provision, equipment and maintenance of residential accommodation for the care of persons with a view to preventing them from becoming ill, the care of persons suffering from illness and the after-care of persons who have been so suffering;

(*b*) the provision, for persons whose care is undertaken with a view to preventing them from becoming ill, persons suffering from illness and persons who have been so suffering, of centres or other facilities for training them or keeping them suitably occupied and the equipment and maintentance of such centres;

(*c*) the provision, for the benefit of such persons as are mentioned in paragraph (*b*) above, of ancillary or supplemental services; and

(*d*) as regards persons suffering from mental disorder within the meaning of the Mental Health Act 1959, the appointment of officers to act as mental welfare officers under that Act and, in the case of such persons so suffering as are received into guardianship under Part IV of that Act (whether the guardianship of the local social services authority or of other persons), the exercise of the functions of the authority in respect of them.

Such an authority shall neither have the power nor be subject to a duty to make under this paragraph arrangements to provide facilities for any of the purposes mentioned in section 15(1) of the Disabled Persons (Employment) Act 1944.

(2) No arrangements under this paragraph shall provide for the payment of money to persons for whose benefit they are made except—

(*a*) in so far as they may provide for the remuneration of such persons engaged in suitable work in accordance with the arrangements; or

(*b*) to persons who—

(i) are, or have been, suffering from mental disorder within the meaning of the Mental Health Act 1959,

    (ii) are under the age of 16 years, and

    (iii) are resident in accommodation provided under the arrangements, of such amounts as the local social services authority think fit in respect of their occasional personal expenses where it appears to that authority that no such payment would otherwise be made.

(3) The Secretary of State may make regulations as to the conduct of premises in which, in pursuance of arrangements made under this paragraph, are provided for persons whose care is undertaken with a view to preventing them from becoming sufferers from mental disorder within the meaning of that Act of 1959 or who are, or have been, so suffering, residential accommodation or facilities for training them or keeping them suitably occupied.

(4) Any such regulations may in particular confer on the Secretary of State's officers so authorised such powers of inspection as may be prescibed by the regulations.

(5) A local social services authority may recover from persons availing themselves of services provided in pursuance of arrangements under this paragraph such charges (if any) as the authority consider reasonable, having regard to the means of those persons.

Home help and laundry facilities

3.—(1) It is the duty of every local social services authority to provide on such a scale as is adequate for the needs of their area, or to arrange for the provision on such a scale as is so adequate, of home help for households where such help is required owing to the presence of—

    (a) a person who is suffering from illness, lying-in, an expectant mother, aged, handicapped as a result of having suffered from illness or by congenital deformity, or

    (b) a child who has not attained the age which, for the purposes of the Education Act 1944 is, in his case, the upper limit of the compulsory school age,

and every such authority has power to provide or arrange for the provision of laundry facilities for households for which home help is being, or can be, provided under this sub-paragraph.

(2) A local social services authority may recover from persons availing themselves of help or facilities provided under this paragraph such charges (if any) as the authority consider reasonable, having regard to the means of those persons.

SCHEDULE 9

Tribunal for Purposes of Section 46

'*Not here reproduced*'

SCHEDULE 10

Additional Provisions as to Prohibition of Sale of Medical Practices

'*Not here reproduced*'.

SCHEDULE 11

ADDITIONAL PROVISIONS AS TO THE CONTROL OF MAXIMUM PRICES FOR MEDICAL SUPPLIES

Orders and directions

1.—(1) Any power of making orders under section 57 above includes power to provide for any incidental and supplementary provisions which the Secretary of State thinks it expedient for the purposes of the order to provide.

(2) An order under section 57 may make such provisions (including provision for requiring any person to furnish information) as the Secretary of State thinks necessary or expedient for facilitating the introduction or operation of a scheme of control for which provision has been made, or for which, in his opinion, it will or may be found necessary or expedient that provision should be made, under that section.

(3) An order under section 57 may prohibit the doing of anything regulated by the order except under the authority of a licence granted by such authority or person as may be specified in the order, and may be made so as to apply either to persons or undertakings generally or to any particular person or undertaking or class of persons or undertakings, and so as to have effect either generally or in any particular area.

(4) The Interpretation Act 1889 shall apply to the interpretation of any order made under section 57 as it applies to the intrepretation of an Act of Parliament and for the purposes of section 38 of that Act any such order shall be deemed to be an Act of Parliament.

Notices, authorisations and proof of documents

2.—(1) A notice to be served on any person for the purposes of section 57 above, or of any order or direction made or given under that section, shall be deemed to have been duly served on the person to whom it is directed if—
  (*a*) it is delivered to him personally; or
  (*b*) it is sent by registered post or the recorded delivery service addressed to him at his last or usual place of abode or place of business.

(2) Where under section 57 and this Schedule a person has power to authorise other persons to act thereunder, the power may be exercised so as to confer the authority either on particular persons or on a specified class of persons.

(3) Any permit, licence, permission or authorisation granted for the purposes of section 57 may be revoked at any time by the authority or person empowered to grant it.

(4) Every document purporting to be an instrument made or issued by the Secretary of State or other authority or person in pursuance of section 57 and this Schedule or any provisions so having effect and to be signed by or on behalf of the Secretary of State, or that authority or person, shall be received in evidence and shall until the contrary is proved, be deemed to be an instrument made or issued by the Secretary of State, or that authority or person.

(5) Prima facie evidence of any such instrument as is described in subparagraph (4) above may in any legal proceedings (including arbitrations) be given by the production of a document purporting to be certified to be a true copy of the instrument by or on behalf of the Secretary of State or other authority or person having power to make or issue the instrument.

Territorial extent

3. So far as any provisions contained in or having effect under section 57 above and this Schedule impose prohibitions, restrictions or obligations on persons, those provisions apply to all persons in the United Kingdom and all persons on board any British ship or aircraft, not being an excepted ship or aircraft, and to all other persons, wherever they may be, who are ordinarily resident in the United Kingdom and who are citizens of the United Kingdom and Colonies or British protected persons.

In this paragraph—
'British aircraft' means an aircraft registered in—
   (*a*) any part of Her Majesty's dominions;
   (*b*) any country outside Her Majesty's dominions in which for the time being Her Majesty has jurisdiction;
   (*c*) any country consisting partly of one or more colonies and partly of one or more such countries as are mentioned in paragraph (*b*) above;
'British protected person' means the same as in the British Nationality Acts 1948 to 1965;
'excepted ship or aircraft' means a ship or aircraft registered in any country for the time being listed in section 1(3) of the British Nationality Act 1948 or in any territory administered by the government of any such country, not being a ship or aircraft for the time being placed at the disposal of, or chartered by or on behalf of, Her Majesty's Government in the United Kingdom.

False documents and false statements

4.—(1) A person shall not, with intent to deceive—
   (*a*) use any document issued for the purposes of section 57 above and this Schedule or of any order made under that section;
   (*b*) have in his possession any document so closely resembling such a document as is described in paragraph (*a*) above as to be calculated to deceive;
   (*c*) produce, furnish, send or otherwise make use of for purposes connected with that section and this Schedule or any order or direction made or given under that section, any book, account, estimate, return, declaration or other document which is false in a material particular.

(2) A person shall not, in furnishing any information for the purposes of section 57 and this Schedule or of any order made under that section, make a statement which he knows to be false in a material particular or recklessly make a statement which is false in a material particular.

Restrictions on disclosing information

5. No person who obtains any information by virtue of section 57 above and this Schedule shall, otherwise than in connection with the execution of that section and this Schedule or of an order made under that section, disclose that information except for the purposes of any criminal proceedings, or of a report of any criminal proceedings, or with permission granted by or on behalf of a Minister of the Crown.

Offences by corporations

6. Where an offence under this Schedule committed by a body corporate is proved to have been committed with the consent or connivance of, or to be attributable to any neglect on the part of, any director, manager, secretary or

other similar officer of the body corporate or any person who was purporting to act in any such capacity, he, as well as the body corporate, shall be guilty of that offence and shall be liable to be proceeded against and punished accordingly.

In this paragraph, the expression 'director', in relation to a body corporate established by or under any enactment for the purpose of carrying on under national ownership any industry or part of an industry or undertaking, being a body corporate whose affairs are managed by its members, means a member of that body corporate.

Penalties

7.—(1) If any person contravenes or fails to comply with any order made under section 57 above, or any direction given or requirement imposed under that section, or contravenes or fails to comply with this Schedule (except for paragraph 8(3) or paragraph 9(4) below) he is, save as otherwise expressly provided, guilty of an offence.

(2) Subject to any special provisions contained in this Schedule, a person guilty of such an offence shall—

    (a) on summary conviction, be liable to imprisonment for a term not exceeding three months or to a fine not exceeding £100, or to both; or

    (b) on conviction on indictment, be liable to imprisonment for a term not exceeding two years or to a fine not exceeding £500, or to both.

(3) Where a person convicted on indictment of such an offence is a body corporate, no provision limiting the amount of the fine which may be imposed shall apply, and the body corporate shall be liable to a fine of such amount as the court thinks just.

Production of documents

8.—(1) For the purposes—

    (a) of securing compliance with any order made or direction given under section 57 above by or on behalf of the Secretary of State, or

    (b) of verifying any estimates, returns or information furnished to the Secretary of State in connection with section 57 or any order made or direction given under that section,

an officer of the Secretary of State duly authorised in that behalf has power, on producing (if required to do so) evidence of his authority, to require any person carrying on an undertaking or employed in connection with an undertaking to produce to that officer forthwith any documents relating to the undertaking which that officer may reasonably require for the purpose set out above.

(2) The power conferred by this paragraph to require any person to produce documents includes power—

    (a) if the documents are produced, to take copies of them or extracts from them and to require that person, or where that person is a body corporate, any other person who is a present or past officer of, or is employed by, the body corporate, to provide an explanation of any of them;

    (b) if the documents are not produced, to require the person who was required to produce them to state, to the best of his knowledge and belief, where they are.

(3) If any requirement to produce documents or provide an explanation or make a statement which is imposed by virtue of this paragraph is not complied

with, the person on whom the requirement was so imposed is guilty of an offence and liable on summary conviction to imprisonment for a term not exceeding three months or to a fine not exceeding £100, or to both.

Where a person is charged with such an offence in respect of a requirement to produce any document, it shall be a defence to prove that they were not in his possession or under his control and that it was not reasonably practicable for him to comply with the requirements.

9.—(1) If a justice of the peace is satisfied, on information on oath laid on the Secretary of State's behalf, that there are any reasonable grounds for suspecting that there are on any premises any documents of which production has been required by virtue of paragraph 8 above and which have not been produced in compliance with that requirement, he may issue a warrant under this paragraph.

A warrant so issued may authorise any constable, together with any other persons named in the warrant and any other constables—

(*a*) to enter the premises specified in the information (using such force as is reasonably necessary for the purpose); and

(*b*) to search the premises and take possession of any documents appearing to be such documents as are mentioned above, or to take in relation to any documents so appearing any other steps which may appear necessary for preserving them and preventing interference with them.

(2) Every warrant issued under this paragraph shall continue in force until the end of the period of one month after the date on which it is issued.

(3) Any documents of which possession is taken under this paragraph may be retained for a period of three months or, if within that period there are commenced any proceedings for an offence under section 57 above and this Schedule to which they are relevant, until the conclusion of those proceedings.

(4) Any person who obstructs the exercise of any right of entry or search conferred by virtue of a warrant under this paragraph, or who obstructs the exercise of any rights so conferred to take possession of any documents, is guilty of an offence and liable on summary conviction to imprisonment for a term not exceeding three months or to a fine not exceeding £50, or to both.

Northern Ireland

10.—(1) So far as the Secretary of State's power under section 57 above and this Schedule is exercisable in relation to Northern Ireland—

(*a*) he may, to such extent and subject to such restrictions as he thinks proper, by order delegate that power either to a Northern Ireland department or departments specified in that order or to the appropriate Northern Ireland department or departments; and

(*b*) where any power is so delegated to the appropriate Northern Ireland department or departments, that power shall be exercised by such Northern Ireland department or departments as the Secretary of State may by order specify.

(2) The power of the Secretary of State to make an order under subparagraph (1)(*b*) above shall be exercisable by statutory instrument; and where a power to make orders has been delegated in pursuance of subparagraph (1)—

(*a*) any order made in pursuance of that power shall be made by statutory instrument; and (*b*) the Statutory Instruments Act 1946 shall apply in like manner as if the order had been made by the Secretary of State.

(3) The references in section 57(1) and (2) above to this Act include any corresponding enactments of the Parliament of Northern Ireland or the Northern Ireland Assembly.

SCHEDULE 12

ADDITIONAL PROVISIONS AS TO REGULATIONS FOR THE MAKING AND RECOVERY OF CHARGES

Regulations under section 77—charges for drugs, medicines or appliances, or pharmaceutical services

1.—(1) No charge shall be made under section 77(1) above in relation to the supply of drugs, medicines and appliances referred to in paragraph (*a*) of that subsection in respect of—

   (*a*) the supply of any drug, medicine or appliance for a patient who is for the time being resident in hospital, or

   (*b*) the supply of any drug or medicine for the treatment of venereal disease, or

   (*c*) the supply of any appliance (otherwise than in pursuance of paragraph (*b*) of section 5(1) above) for a person who is under 16 years of age or is undergoing full-time education in a school, or

   (*d*) the replacement or repair of any appliance in consequence of a defect in the appliance as supplied,

and regulations may provide for the remission or repayment of any charge payable under paragraph (*a*) of section 77(1) in such other cases as may be prescribed.

(2) Regulations made under section 77(1) above in relation to the pharmaceutical services referred to in paragraph (*b*) of that subsection may provide for the remission or repayment of the charges made by those regulations in the case of such persons as may be prescribed.

Regulations under section 78—charges for dental or optical appliances

2.—(1) The dental and optical appliances mentioned in the first column below, and the charges mentioned in the second column, are the appliances and charges referred to in section 78(1) above.

Appliance	*Charge*
The dentures described in regulations made under section 78(1) and this paragraph.	The amount or the maximum amount prescribed by regulations made under section 78(1) and this paragraph.
Glasses other than children's glasses— The lenses described in regulations made under section 78(1) and this paragraph.	The amount or the maximum amount prescribed by regulations made under section 78(1) and this paragraph.
Frames.	The current specified cost.

In this sub-paragraph—

'children's glasses' means glasses for which a standard type of children's frame as described in the Statement referred to below is used and which are supplied for a person who was, at the time of the examination or testing of sight leading to the supply of the glasses or of the first such examination or testing, under 16 years of age or receiving full-time education in a school, and

'current specified cost', in relation to frames supplied under Part II of this Act, means the sum specified in the Statement as the sum payable for frames of that description by the person to whom they are supplied, and in relation to frames supplied under this Act otherwise than under Part II means a sum equal to the sum so specified, or in the case of frames of a description for which no sum is so specified, such sum as may be determined by or in accordance with directions given by the Secretary of State,

and for the purposes of this provision 'the Statement' means the Statement published by the Secretary of State pursuant to the provisions of regulation 10 of the National Health Service (General Ophthalmic Services) Regulations 1974 or any corresponding regulation for the time being in force.

(2) Regulations may—

    (a) vary the amount or maximum amount of any charge authorised by section 78(1) for any dental or optical appliance, and this power includes power to direct that the charge shall not be payable; or

    (b) vary the descriptions of appliances for which any such charge is authorised;

and regulations made for the purposes of section 78(1) may be made so as to take effect—

    (i) in the case of appliances supplied under this Act otherwise than under Part II, where the examination or testing of sight (otherwise than under that Part) leading to the supply of those appliances, or the first such examination or testing, takes place on or after the date on which the regulations come into force;

    (ii) in the case of dental appliances supplied under Part II, where the contract or arrangement between the person by whom and the person to whom the appliances are supplied is made on or after that date;

    (iii) in the case of optical appliances supplied under Part II, where the testing of sight leading to the supply of those appliances, or the first such testing, takes place on or after that date.

(3) No charge shall be made under section 78(1) in respect of any appliance supplied otherwise than under Part II to a patient for the time being resident in a hospital.

(4) No charge shall be made under section 78(1) in respect of the supply of a dental appliance if at the relevant time the person for whom that appliance was supplied—

    (a) was under 16 years of age or was receiving full-time education in a school; or

    (b) was an expectant mother or had borne a child within the previous twelve months.

(5) No charge shall be made under section 78(1) for the supply under this Act of lenses for any glasses if—

    (a) the person for whom the glasses are supplied was at the relevant time of the age of 10 or more and either under the age of 16 or receiving full-time education in a school; and

    (b) the frames of the glasses are of any description specified in the Statement referred to in sub-paragraph (1) above, or any corresponding regulation for the time being in force.

(6) Regulations made with respect to any exemption under sub-paragraph (4) or sub-paragraph (5) above may provide that it shall be a condition of the exemption that such declaration is made in such form and manner, or such certificate or other evidence is supplied in such form and manner, as may be prescribed.

(7) In sub-paragraphs (4) and (5), 'the relevant time' means—

    (a) in relation to a dental appliance supplied otherwise than under Part II, or to an optical appliance supplied under this Act, the time of the examination or testing of sight leading to the supply of the appliance, or the first such examination or testing;

    (b) in relation to a dental appliance supplied under Part II, the time of the making of the contract or arrangement in pursuance of which the appliance is supplied.

(8) References in section 78 and in this paragraph to the supply of appliances shall be construed as including references to their replacement, but no charge shall be made under those provisions in respect of the replacement of dentures or lenses if the replacement is required in consequence of loss or damage.

Regulations under section 79—charges for dental treatment

3.—(1) The amount of the charge payable under section 79(1) above in respect of services provided in pursuance of any contract or arrangement shall be (subject to sub-paragraph (3) below) the current authorised fee for all services so provided in respect of which a charge is payable under that section or a prescribed sum, whichever is the less.

In this sub-paragraph 'current authorised fee', in relation to any services, means the fee authorised in accordance with regulations for the time being in force under this Act as the fee payable to the practitioner in respect of those services, but does not include—

    (a) any fee so authorised in respect of a visit to a patient by a practitioner or

    (b) any fee or part of a fee payable by the patient in pursuance of regulations under—

        (i) section 79(2) above;

        (ii) section 81 above, in relation to paragraph (b) of that section;

        (iii) section 82 above, in relation to paragraph (b) of that section.

(2) Regulations may vary the amount or the maximum amount of any charge (including power to direct that the charge shall not be payable) authorised by section 79(1); and no charge shall be made under that section for any services provided in pursuance of a contract or arrangement under which the first examination took place before 29th May 1952.

(3) Where any services in respect of which a charge is payable under section 78 above are provided in pursuance of a contract or arrangement, the charges payable under that section and section 79(1) in respect of all services provided in pursuance of the contract or arrangement shall not exceed a prescribed sum in the aggregate.

(4) No charge shall be made under section 79(1) in respect of services pro-

vided for any person who, on the date of the contract or arrangement for the services—

    (*a*) was under 21 years of age (other than for services in respect of the relining of a denture or the addition of teeth, bands or wires to a denture),

    (*b*) was under 16 years of age or was receiving full-time education in a school,

    (*c*) was an expectant mother or had borne a child within the previous 12 months,

if (in any such case) a declaration to that effect is made by or on behalf of that person in such form and manner as may be prescribed.

    (5) Regulations under section 79(1), in relation to—

    (*a*) the persons described in paragraphs (*b*) and (*c*) of sub-paragraph (4) above, and

    (*b*) any exemption in respect of the relining of a denture or the addition of teeth, bands or wires to a denture,

may provide that it shall be a condition of the exemption that such declaration is made in such form and manner, or such certificate or other evidence supplied in such form and manner, as may be prescribed.

Miscellaneous Provisions

4. For the purposes of paragraph (*a*) of section 5(1) above and paragraph 1(*a*) of Schedule 1 to this Act (which provide for the Secretary of State to arrange for the free medical treatment of certain pupils) any charge made in pursuance of regulations under this Act in respect of the supply of drugs, medicines or appliances shall be disregarded.

5. Regulations may provide for the remission or repayment of any charges which, in pursuance of section 78(1) above or section 79(1) above, are payable apart from this paragraph by a person whose income as calculated in accordance with regulations is at less that the prescribed rate, in respect of the supply or replacement of dental or optical appliances or in respect of services provided as part of the general dental services.

6. For the purposes of sections 77 and 78 above and of this Schedule, a bridge, whether fixed or removable, which takes the place of any teeth shall be deemed to be a denture having that number of teeth; and the reference in paragraph (*a*) of section 79(1) to appliances described in paragraph 2(1) of this Schedule shall be construed accordingly.

7. References in this Schedule to full-time education in a school mean full-time instruction in a school within the meaning of the Education Act 1944 or the Education (Scotland) Act 1962.

SCHEDULE 13

ADDITIONAL PROVISIONS AS TO THE HEALTH SERVICE COMMISSIONER FOR ENGLAND AND THE HEALTH SERVICE COMMISSIONER FOR WALES

PART I

PROCEDURAL AND OTHER PROVISIONS

Procedure in respect of investigations

1. Where the Commissioner proposes to conduct an investigation pursuant to a complaint under Part V of this Act, he shall afford to the relevant body

concerned, and to any other person who is alleged in the complaint to have taken or authorised the action complained of, an opportunity to comment on any allegations contained in the complaint.

2. Every such investigation shall be conducted in private, but except for that the procedure for conducting an investigation shall be such as the Commissioner considers appropriate in the circumstances of the case.

3. Without prejudice to the generality of paragraph 2 above, the Commissioner may obtain information from such persons and in such manner, and make such enquiries, as he thinks fit, and may determine whether any person may be represented, by counsel or solicitor or otherwise, in the investigation.

4. The Commissioner may, if he thinks fit, pay to the person by whom the complaint was made and to any other person who attends or furnishes information for the purposes of an investigation under Part V of this Act—

(a) sums in respect of expenses properly incurred by them,

(b) allowances by way of compensation for the loss of their time,

in accordance with such scales and subject to such conditions as may be determined by the Minister for the Civil Service.

5. The conduct of an investigation under Part V of this Act shall not affect any action taken by the relevant body concerned, or any power or duty of that body to take further action with respect to any matters subject to the investigation.

6. Where the person aggrieved has been removed from the United Kingdom under any Order in force under the Immigration Act 1971 he shall, if the Commissioner so directs, be permitted to re-enter and remain in the United Kingdom, subject to such conditions as the Secretary of State may direct, for the purposes of the investigation.

Evidence

7. For the purposes of an investigation under Part V of this Act the Commissioner may require any employee, officer or member of the relevant body concerned or any other person who in his opinion is able to furnish information or produce documents relevant to the investigation to furnish any such information or produce any such document.

8. For the purposes of any such investigation the Commissioner shall have the same powers as the Court (which in this Schedule means, in relation to England and Wales, the High Court, in relation to Scotland, the Court of Session, and in relation to Northern Ireland, the High Court of Northern Ireland) in respect of the attendance and examination of witnesses (including the administration of oaths or affirmations and the examination of witnesses abroad) and in respect of the production of documents.

9. No obligation to maintain secrecy or other restriction upon the disclosure of information obtained by or furnished to persons in Her Majesty's service, whether imposed by any enactment or by any rule of law, shall apply to the disclosure of information for the purposes of an investigation under Part V of this Act.

The Crown shall not be entitled in relation to any such investigation to any such privilege in respect of the production of documents or the giving of evidence as is allowed by law in legal proceedings.

10. No person shall be required or authorised by Part V of this Act and this Schedule to furnish any information or answer any question relating to pro-

ceedings of the Cabinet or of any committee of the Cabinet or to produce so much of any document as relates to such proceedings.

For the purposes of this paragraph a certificate issued by the Secretary of the Cabinet with the approval of the Prime Minister and certifying that any information, question, document, or part of a document so relates shall be conclusive.

11. Subject to paragraph 9 above, no person shall be compelled for the purposes of an investigation under Part V of this Act to give any evidence or produce any document which he could not be compelled to give or produce in civil proceedings before the Court.

Obstruction and contempt

12. If any person without lawful excuse obstructs the Commissioner or any officer of the Commissioner in the performance of his functions under Part V of this Act and this Schedule, or is guilty of any act or omission in relation to an investigation under that Part which, if that investigation were a proceeding in the Court, would constitute contempt of court, the Commissioner may certify the offence to the Court.

13. Where an offence is certified under paragraph 12 above, the Court may inquire into the matter and, after hearing any witnesses who may be produced against or on behalf of the person charged with the offence, and after hearing any statement that may be offered in defence, deal with him in any manner in which the Court could deal with him if he had committed the like offence in relation to the Court.

14. Nothing in paragraphs 12 and 13 above shall be construed as applying to the taking of any such action as is mentioned in paragraphs 5 and 6 above.

Secrecy of information

15. The Commissioner and his officers hold office under Her Majesty within the meaning of the Official Secrets Act 1911.

16. Information obtained by the Commissioner or his officers in the course of or for the purposes of an investigation under Part V of this Act shall not be disclosed except—

(a) for the purposes of the investigation and of any report to be made in respect of the investigation under that Part,

(b) for the purposes of any proceedings for an offence under the Official Secrets Acts 1911 to 1939 alleged to have been committed in respect of information obtained by the Commissioner or any of his officers by virtue of that Part or for an offence of perjury alleged to have been committed in the course of an investigation under that Part or for the purposes of an inquiry with a view to the taking of such proceedings, or

(c) for the purposes of any proceedings under paragraphs 12 and 13 above,

and the Commissioner and his officers shall not be called upon to give evidence in any proceedings (other than those mentioned in this paragraph) of matters coming to his or their knowledge in the course of an investigation under that Part.

17. A Minister of the Crown may give notice in writing to the Commissioner, with respect to any document or information specified in the notice, or any class of documents or information so specified, that in the Minister's

opinion the disclosure of that document or information, or of documents or information of that class, would be prejudicial to the safety of the State or otherwise contrary to the public interest.

18. Where a notice under paragraph 17 above is given nothing in this Schedule shall be construed as authorising or requiring the Commissioner or any officer of the Commissioner to communicate to any person or for any purpose any document or information specified in the notice, or any document or information of a class so specified.

PART II

Matters not subject to investigation by the Health Service Commissioner for England or the Health Service Commissioner for Wales

19. The following matters are not subject to investigation by the Health Service Commissioner for England or the Health Service Commissioner for Wales —

(1) Action taken in connection with the diagnosis of illness or the care or treatment of a patient, being action which, in the opinion of the Commissioner in question, was taken solely in consequence of the exercise of clinical judgment, whether formed by the person taking the action or any other person.

(2) Action taken by a Family Practitioner Committee in the exercise of its functions under the National Health Service (Service Committees and Tribunal) Regulations 1974, or any instrument amending or replacing those regulations.

(3) Action taken in respect of appointments or removals, pay, discipline, superannuation or other personnel matters in relation to service under this Act.

(4) Action taken in matters relating to contractual or other commercial transactions, other than in matters arising from arrangements between a relevant body and another body which is not a relevant body for the provision of services for patients by that other body; and in determining what matters arise from such arrangements there shall be disregarded any arrangements for the provision of services at an establishment maintained by a Minister of the Crown for patients who are mainly members of the armed forces of the Crown.

(5) Action which has been, or is, the subject of an inquiry under section 84 above.

SCHEDULE 14

TRANSITIONAL PROVISIONS AND SAVINGS

General

1.—(1) In so far as —
    (a) any agreement, appointment, apportionment, authorisation, determination, instrument, order or regulation made by virtue of an enactment repealed by this Act, or
    (b) any approval, consent, direction, or notice given by virtue of such an enactment, or
    (c) any complaint made or investigation begun by virtue of such an enactment, or

(d) any other proceedings begun by virtue of such an enactment, or

(e) anything done or having effect as if done,

could, if a corresponding enactment in this Act were in force at the relevant time, have been made, given, begun or done by virtue of the corresponding enactment, it shall, if effective immediately before the corresponding enactment comes into force, continue to have effect thereafter as if made, given, begun or done by virtue of that corresponding enactment.

(2) Where —

    (a) there is any reference in this Act (whether express or implied) to a thing done or required or authorised to be done, or to a thing omitted, or to an event which has occurred, under or for the purposes of or by reference to or in contravention of any provisions of this Act, then

    (b) that reference shall be construed (subject to its context) as including a reference to the corresponding thing done or required or authorised to be done, or omitted, or to the corresponding event which occurred, as the case may be, under or for the purposes of or by reference to or in contravention of any of the corresponding provisions of the repealed enactments.

2. Where any instrument or document refers either expressly or by implication to an enactment repealed by this Act the reference shall (subject to its context) be construed as or as including a reference to the corresponding provision of this Act.

3. Where any period of time specified in an enactment repealed by this Act is current at the commencement of this Act, this Act has effect as if its corresponding provision had been in force when that period began to run.

Medical schools in London

4. Notwithstanding the repeal by this Act of section 15 of the National Health Service Act 1946 —

    (a) where a scheme was prepared and submitted under subsection (1) and approved under subsection (2) of that section, that scheme may be amended by a new scheme in accordance with subsection (3) of that section; and

    (b) any scheme prepared, submitted and approved under that section, or as amended under paragraph (a) above, shall continue to have effect, or have effect, as if that section had not been repealed.

Section 36 of the National Health Service Act 1946

5. Notwithstanding the repeal by this Act of section 36 of the National Health Service Act 1946 (compensation for loss of right to sell a medical practice) that section shall continue to have such effect as may be necessary for the purposes of sections 1 to 7 of the National Health Service (Amendment) Act 1949.

The saving made by this paragraph applies to section 51 of the National Health Service Reorganisation Act 1973 (which amended section 36 of the National Health Service Act 1946), and to any regulations made under that section 36 which were in force immediately before the coming into force of this Act.

Local Acts and charters

6.—(1) Where at the passing of the National Health Service Act 1946 —

    (a) there was in force a local or private Act or charter containing provisions which appear to the Secretary of State either to be inconsistent with any of the provisions of that Act of 1946 as reproduced in this Act, or to have been made redundant in consequence of the passing of that Act of 1946, then

(b) the Secretary of State may by order make such alterations, whether by amendment or by repeal, in the local or private Act or charter as appear to him to be necessary for the purpose of bringing its provisions into conformity with the provisions of that Act of 1946 as so reproduced, or for the purpose of removing redundant provisions, as the case may be.

(2) Any provision of a charter defining or restricting —

(a) the objects of any hospital to which section 6 of that Act of 1946 applied, or

(b) the purposes for which any property transferred to the Secretary of State or the Board of Governors of a teaching hospital by virtue of that Act of 1946 may be used,

shall cease to have effect.

Persons authorised to provide pharmaceutical services

7.—(1) A person who for three years immediately before 16th December 1911 acted as a dispenser to a medical practitioner or a public institution is in the same position in relation to the undertaking referred to in section 43(2) above regarding the dispensing of medicines as a registered pharmacist.

(2) Nothing in the provisions of the National Health Service Act 1946 as those provisions are reproduced in this Act affects the rights and privileges conferred by the Apothecaries Act 1815 upon any person qualified under that Act to act as an assistant to any apothecary in compounding and dispensing medicines.

Disqualification of practitioners

8. Where by virtue of section 42(8) of the National Health Service Act 1946 a person's name was, immediately before the coming into force of this Act, disqualified for inclusion in any list referred to in section 42(1) of that Act, that person's name is disqualified for inclusion in any list referred to in section 46(1) above, until such time as the Tribunal or the Secretary of State directs to the contrary.

Regulations made under section 49 above shall have effect for the purposes of this paragraph.

Definition of 'local authority'

9. The definition of 'local authority' in section 128(1) above includes any joint board constituted under the Public Health Act 1936 or under the Public Health (London) Act 1936 or any enactment repealed by those Acts, or any port health authority constituted under those Acts or under any Act passed before those Acts.

Sections 3 and 4 of the Health Services and Public Health Act 1968

10.—(1) Notwithstanding the repeal by this Act of section 3 of the Health Services and Public Health Act 1968 (transitional provisions relating to accommodation and treatment of private patients), sub-section (2) of that section continues to have the same effect in relation to an undertaking given before 31st March 1969 under section 5 of the National Health Service Act 1946 (accommodation for private patients) as it had immediately before the coming into force of this Act.

(2) An undertaking given before the coming into force of section 4(1) of the Health Services and Public Health Act 1968 in respect of payment under section 4 of the National Health Service Act 1946 (accommodation available on part payment) continues to have the same effect as it had immediately before the coming into force of this Act.

Vehicles under section 33 of the Health Services and Public Health Act 1968

11. The provision of vehicles as mentioned in section 33 of the Health Services and Public Health Act 1968, and the taking of any such action as is mentioned in subsection (2) of that section, shall for the purposes of the National Health Service Act 1946 be treated as having been included among hospital and specialist services provided under Part II of that Act of 1946 as from its commencement.

Prevention, care and after-care

12. Any arrangements made under section 28(1) of the National Health Service Act 1946 by a local health authority which were in force immediately before 9th September 1968 shall—

    (a) so far as they could be made under paragraph 2(1) of Schedule 8 to this Act, continue to have effect as if so made;

    (b) so far as they relate to any matters falling within section 3(1) of the Disabled Persons (Employment) Act 1958, continue to have effect as if made under that section.

Saving of amendments

13.—(1) Notwithstanding the repeal by this Act of section 76 and Part I of Schedule 10 to the National Health Service Act 1946, and section 57(1) and Schedule 4 to the National Health Service Reorganisation Act 1973—

    (a) the amendments made by Part I of Schedule 10 to that Act of 1946 to the Voluntary Hospitals (Paying Patients) Act 1936 and to the Public Health Act 1936, and

    (b) the amendments made by paragraphs 2 to 4, 6 to 9, 40, 44, 45, 48 and 49, 56 and 57, 61, 63 and 64, 68 to 71, 73 to 78, 80 to 83, 86 to 91, 93, 95 and 96, 99, 102, 106 to 109, 111, 122 and 123, 124(1) to (4), 125 to 128, 130 to 134, 136 and 151 and 152 of Schedule 4 to that Act of 1973,

shall continue to have the same effect as they had immediately before the coming into force of this Act, subject to any amendments made by this Act.

(2) Nothing in this Act affects the Secretary of State's power under section 58 of the National Health Service Reorganisation Act 1973 to bring into force paragraph 131 of Schedule 4 to that Act.

Transfers of property by voluntary organisations

14. Notwithstanding the repeal by this Act of section 23(2) of the National Health Service (Amendment) Act 1949, section 23(1) of that Act shall be deemed to have had effect as from 5th July 1948.

Mental Health Act 1959

15.—(1) Any regulations under section 7 of the Mental Health Act 1959 in force immediately before 9th September 1968, shall, so far as they could be made under paragraph 2 of Schedule 8 to this Act, have effect as if so made.

(2) Any institution provided under section 97 of the Mental Health Act 1959, or deemed to be so provided when that section came into force, shall be deemed to be provided in pursuance of section 4 above.

The National Health Service Reorganisation Act 1973

16.—(1) Nothing in this Act affects any remaining duty of the Secretary of State in connection with the arrangements for the reorganisation of the health service in accordance with section 1 of the National Health Service Reorganisation Act 1973.

(2) The repeal by this Act of section 57(1) of and Schedule 4 to the National Health Service Reorganisation Act 1973 does not affect any exercise of the Secretary of State's powers in relation to that Schedule conferred on him by section 15(3) of that Act.

Complaints in respect of preserved Boards or bodies abolished under section 14 of the National Health Service Reorganisation Act 1973

17.—(1) Regulations may provide that where a relevant body within the meaning of section 34 of the National Health Service Reorganisation Act 1973 is abolished by virtue of section 14 of that Act, any prescribed provisions of Part V of this Act and Schedule 13 to this Act shall apply, with or without prescribed modifications, in relation to a complaint which —

(a) was duly made to a Commissioner under Part V before the date of the abolition, or

(b) was made in accordance with the regulations within the period of one year beginning with that date.

(2) For so long as a Board of Governors of a teaching hospital is a preserved Board within the meaning of section 15(6) of the National Health Service Reorganisation Act 1973, that Board of Governors shall be treated as if it were a relevant body for the purposes of Part V of this Act by virtue of section 109 above.

Permission deemed to have been granted under section 9(5) of the Health Services Act 1976

18. Where under any arrangements terminated by virtue of section 9(5) of the Health Services Act 1976—

(a) a person was deemed to have been granted under that section permission to use accommodation and facilities to the same extent and for the same purposes as were covered by those arrangements, then

(b) that person shall be deemed to have been granted under section 72 above the like permission (and the provisions of that section shall apply accordingly).

SCHEDULE 15

'Not here reproduced'.

SCHEDULE 16

'Not here reproduced'.

APPENDIX B

OTHER STATUTES

The Health Services and Public Health Act 1968

Much of the Act was amended by the 1973 *Reorganisation Act and consolidated into the National Health Service Act* 1977. *Some sections are still in force. Only those sections (or parts of sections) which remain and which affect the National Hospital Service are reproduced here.*

PART III

NOTIFIABLE DISEASES AND FOOD POISONING

Cases of notifiable disease and food poisoning to be reported to local authority

48.—(1) If a duly qualified medical practitioner becomes aware, or suspects, that a patient whom he is attending within the district of a local authority is suffering from a notifiable disease[1] or from food poisoning, he shall unless he believes, and has reasonable grounds for believing, that some other such practitioner has complied with this subsection with respect to the patient, forthwith send to the medical officer of health of that district a certificate stating —

    (*a*) the name, age and sex of the patient and the address of the premises where the patient is;

    (*b*) the disease or, as the case may be, particulars of the poisoning from which the patient is, or is suspected to be, suffering and the date, or approximate date, of its onset; and

    (*c*) if the premises aforesaid are a hospital, the day on which the patient was admitted thereto, the address of the premises from whence he came there and whether or not, in the opinion of the person giving the certificate, the disease or poisoning from which the patient is, or is suspected to be, suffering was contracted in the hospital.

(2) *The officer who receives the certificate aforesaid shall, on the day of its receipt (if possible) and in any case within forty-eight hours after its receipt, send a copy of the certificate—*

    (a) *to the Area Health Authority within whose area are situate the premises whose address is specified in the certificate by*

[1] For definition of '*notifiable disease*' see s. 343 of the Public Health Act 1936 as amended by s. 47 of this Act; see also ss. 56 and 57 of this Act. For further information see pp. 465–467

virtue of paragraph (a) *of the foregoing subsection; and* (b) *if the certificate is given with respect to a patient in a hospital who came there from premises outside the district of the local authority within whose district the hospital is situate and the certificate states that the patient did not contract the disease or the poisoning in the hospital—*

(i) *to the proper officer for the district within which the premises from which the patient came are situate, and*

(ii) *to the Area Health Authority for the area in which those premises are situate if that Authority is not responsible for the administration of the hospital, and*

(iii) *to the proper officer of the relevant port health authority constituted in pursuance of section 2 of the Public Health Act 1936 if those premises were a ship or hovercraft situate within the port health district for which that authority is constituted.*[1]

(3) *Repealed by* 1973 *Act Schedule* 4 *paragraph* 122 (2) *and Schedule* 5.

(5) In this section, 'hospital' means any institution for the reception and treatment of persons suffering from illness, any maternity home and any institution for the reception and treatment of persons during convalescence or persons requiring medical rehabilitation, and 'illness' includes mental disorder within the meaning of the Mental Health Act 1959 and any injury or disability requiring medical, surgical or dental treatment or nursing.

Fees for certificates under section 48

50.—(3) For the avoidance of doubt it is hereby declared that the fact that a medical practitioner who gives a certificate under section 48 of this Act holds the office to whose holder the certificate is required to be sent does not disentitle him to payment of the fee (if any) payable for the certificate.

PART IV

MISCELLANEOUS MATTERS

Provisions applicable to England and Wales and Scotland

Provisions of instruction for officers of hospital authorities and other persons employed, or contemplating employment, in certain activities connected with health or welfare.

63.—(1) The Minister of Health may, either directly or by entering into arrangements with others,—

(*a*) provide, for persons employed or having it in contemplation

---

[1] New subsection in italics substituted by 1973 Act Sch. 4 para. 122 (1).

to be employed as officers or servants of a *Regional Health Authority, Area Health Authority or a special health authority*[1] such instruction as appears to him conducive to securing their efficiency as such officers or servants; . . .

(3) The Minister of Health may allow instruction provided under this section to be given to persons other than persons described in subsection (1) above, and he may under this section provide instruction to an extent greater than that necessitated by the requirements of persons so described if he thinks it expedient so to do in order to allow such other persons to receive such instruction.

(5) Instruction under this section may be provided on such terms, including terms as to payment of charges, as the Minister of Health thinks fit.

(6) The Minister of Health may, with the approval of the Treasury,—

   (a) make grants and pay fees to persons or bodies with whom arrangements under subsection (1) above are made for the provision of instruction under this section; and

   (b) pay travelling and other allowances to persons availing themselves of such instruction.

Financial assistance by the Minister of Health and the Secretary of State to certain voluntary organisations.

64.—(1) The Minister of Health may, upon such terms and subject to such conditions as he may, with the approval of the Treasury, determine, give to a voluntary organisation to which this section applies assistance by way of grant or by way of loan, or partly in the one way and partly in the other.

(2) This section applies to a voluntary organisation whose activities consist in, or include, the provision of a service similar to a relevant service, the promotion of the provision of a relevant service or a similar one, the publicising of a relevant service or a similar one or the giving of advice with respect to the manner in which a relevant service or a similar one can best be provided.

(3) In this section[2]—

   (a) *'the relevant enactments' means —*

      (i) *Parts III and IV of the Children and Young Persons Act* 1933

      (ii) Repealed

      (iii) *Part III of the National Assistance Act* 1948

      (iv) *the Children Act* 1948

      (v) *the Adoption Act* 1958

[1] Words in italics substituted by 1973 Act Sch. 4 para. 124 (1).
[2] New definition in italics substituted by Children Act 1975 Sch. 3 para. 46 as amended by 1977 Act Sch. 15 para. 46.

(vi) *the Children Act 1958*

(vii) *Section 9 of the Mental Health Act 1959*

(viii) *Section 10 of the Mental Health Act 1959, so far as it relates to cases mentioned in paragraph* (a) *of that section*

(ix) *Section 2* (1) (f) *of the Matrimonial Proceeding (Magistrates' Courts) Act 1960*

(x) *the Children and Young Persons Act 1963, except Part II and section 56*

(xi) *this Act*

(xii) *the Adoption Act 1968*

(xiii) *Section 7* (4) *of the Family Law Reform Act 1969*

(xiv) *The Children and Young Persons Act 1969, except so far as it relates to any voluntary home designated as mentioned in section 39* (1) *of that Act as a controlled or assisted community home*

(xv) *Section 43 of the Matrimonial Causes Act 1973*

(xvi) Repealed

(xvii) *the Children Act 1975*

(xviii) *the National Health Service Act 1977.*[1]

(b) 'relevant service' means a service which must or may, by virtue of the relevant enactments, be provided or the provision of which must or may, by virtue of those enactments, be secured by the Minister of Health or the Council of a *non-metropolitan county, metropolitan district*[2] or London borough or the Common Council of the City of London or a service for the provision of which an *Area Health Authority*[2] is, by virtue of Part IV of the National Health Service Act 1946, under a duty to make arrangements; and

(c) 'voluntary organisation' means a body the activities of which are carried on otherwise than for profit, but does not include any public or local authority. . . .

Payments in respect of travelling expenses of visitors to patients in special hospitals . . .

66.—(1) The Minister of Health may, in accordance with arrangements made by him with the approval of the Treasury, make payments, at such rates as may be determined under those arrangements, to persons of such class or description as may be so determined in respect of travelling expenses necessarily incurred by them in making visits to patients for the time being detained under the Mental Health Act 1959 in special hospitals. . . .

[1] New definition in italics substituted by Children Act 1975 Sch. 3 para. 46 as amended by 1977 Act Sch. 15 para. 46.

[2] Words in italics substituted by 1973 Act Sch. 4 para 125 (2).

PART V

GENERAL

THE NATIONAL HEALTH SERVICE REORGANISATION ACT 1973

The greater part of this Act has been taken into the 1977 Consolidation. Some sections are re-enacted but are also not repealed. Most of these relate to trust instruments existing in 1977 affecting the preserved Boards of Governors under section 15 of the 1973 Act. It is possible that had these sections been repealed even if they had been re-enacted the trusts might have been affected.

Other sections relating mainly to transitional arrangements consequent on the Re-organisation remain untouched by the 1977 Act. They have a real but limited life ahead of them. It is understood that both types will be repealed by some future Statute Laws Repeal Act.

In this work it is not necessary to produce these sections. The reader who requires more is referred to the full Queen's Printer's edition of the Act.

PART II

ABOLITION OF CERTAIN AUTHORITIES AND TRANSFER OF PROPERTY, STAFF AND ENDOWMENTS ETC.

Abolition of certain authorities

14.—(1) All Regional Hospital Boards, Hospital Management Committees and Executive Councils, the Joint Pricing Committee for England, the Welsh Joint Pricing Committee and, except as provided by the following section, all Boards of Governors shall cease to exist on the appointed day; and on that day any authority which is a local health authority by virtue of section 19 of the principal Act[1] shall cease to be a local health authority and all joint boards constituted in pursuance of that section shall cease to exist.

(2) The Secretary of State may by order make such provision as he considers appropriate in anticipation or in consequence of the abolition by the preceding subsection of any body or in connection with the winding up of the body's affairs; and if a body abolished by that subsection has, as respects a period before the appointed day, not performed a duty imposed on the body by *subsection* (1) *or* (2) *of section* 98 *of the National Health Service Act* 1977[2] (which relate to accounts), then—

---

[1] I.e. the 1946 Act.   [2] Words in italics substituted by 1977 Act Sch. 15 para 58.

z

(*a*) it shall be the duty of the Secretary of State to secure that the duty so imposed is performed by a Regional or Area Health Authority or special health authority determined by him; and

(*b*) that section shall have effect in relation to the body and period in question as if for references to each financial year in sub-sections (3) and (4) there were substituted references to that period and as if the word 'annual' in subsection (3) were omitted.

15.—(1) The Secretary of State may by order provide that the preceding section shall, while the order is in force, not apply to any body specified in the order which is the Board of Governors of a teaching hospital mentioned in Schedule 2 to this Act[1].

(2) An order made by virtue of the preceding subsection—

(*a*) must be made before the appointed day except in a case falling within paragraph (*c*) of this subsection;

(*b*) shall provide for the order to cease to have effect, unless it is previously revoked, on the expiration of a period specified in the order (which shall not be longer than five years beginning with the date on which the order is made);

(*c*) may be made after the appointed day in respect of a preserved Board for the purpose of securing that the Board continues to be a preserved Board for a further period; and

(*d*) may at any time be revoked by order by the Secretary of State; and it shall be the duty of the Secretary of State, before he makes an order in pursuance of the preceding subsection or paragraph (*d*) of this subsection, to consult the University of London and the Board of Governors in question about the order.

(3) The Secretary of State may by order provide that, in relation to a preserved Board and any person, thing, right, liability or other matter whatsoever connected with the Board,—

(*a*) any provision of this Act which repeals or amends any enact-ment and is specified in the order shall not apply;

(*b*) any enactment which, apart from any provision made by virtue of the preceding paragraph, is repealed or amended by this Act shall have effect with such modifications as are specified in the order; and

(*c*) such provisions of this Act and any instrument in force by virtue of this Act as are specified in the order shall have effect with such modifications as are so specified;

but nothing in this Act, and in particular nothing in any provision of this Act amending section 55 of the principal Act (which relates to

---

[1] The Schedule is not reproduced here but the hospitals concerned are named on p. 23.

accounts) shall affect the application of that section to a preserved Board.

(4) The Secretary of State may by order—

    (*a*) provide that a preserved Board shall cease to exercise functions with respect to the administration of any hospital specified in the order;

    (*b*) confer on a preserved Board such functions as are specified in the order with respect to the administration of a hospital so specified (whether or not apart from the order the Board has functions with respect to the administration of that hospital); and

    (*c*) provide that this Act and any instrument in force by virtue of this Act shall, in relation to any person, thing, right, liability or other matter whatsoever connected with the hospital in question, have effect with such modifications as are specified in the order.

(5) Where a Board of Governors ceases to be a preserved Board this Act and any instrument in force by virtue of this Act shall, in relation to the Board and any person, thing, right, liability and other matter whatsoever connected with the Board, have effect with the substitution of a reference to the date of the cesser for the first reference in subsection (1) of the preceding section and the reference in subsection (2) of that section to the appointed day and with such further modifications as the Secretary of State may by order specify.

(5a) So far as may be necessary for the purposes of subsections (3) to (5) above, any reference in those subsections to this Act, or to any instrument in force by virtue of this Act, shall (as the case may be) include a reference to—

    (a) any provision of this Act which has been repealed and re-enacted by the National Health Service Act 1977;

    (b) any instrument in force by virtue of a provision of this Act which has been repealed and re-enacted by that Act of 1977.[1]

(6) In this Act 'preserved Board' means a Board of Governors to which by virtue of this section the preceding section does not for the time being apply; and any question whether a person, thing, right, liability or other matter whatsoever is for the purposes of this section connected with a Board of Governors or a hospital shall be determined by the Secretary of State.

Sections 16 and 17 deal with the transfer of property used for health purposes from local authorities and Executive Councils consequent on the reorganisation.

Sections 18 and 19 deal with the transfer of staff employed on health

---

[1] New subsection added by 1977 Act Sch. 15 para. 59.

functions, consequent on the reorganisation. As regards the individual the principal effect of these provisions is to change his employer but on terms which are, taken as a whole, not less favourable than under his previous contract. Section 20 establishes Health Service Staff Commissions whose task it is to oversee the transfer of staff and inter alia 'to keep under review the arrangements made by relevant bodies for recruiting and engaging employees'.

The main effect of sections 18-20 is now spent but the sections are still live in the sense that employees may still have recourse to these provisions as regards some individual items of their contracts of employment. Despite this the sections are not here reproduced. They are not repealed by the 1977 Act.

THE NURSING HOMES ACT 1975

Meaning of 'nursing home' and 'mental nursing home'

1.—(1) In this Act 'nursing home' means, subject to subsection (2) below, any premises used, or intended to be used, for the reception of, and the providing of nursing for, persons suffering from any sickness, injury or infirmity.

(2) In this Act 'nursing home' includes a maternity home (that is to say, any premises used, or intended to be used, for the reception of pregnant women, or of women immediately after childbirth), but does not include—

(*a*) any hospital or other premises maintained or controlled by a Government department, a local authority as defined in subsection (3) below, or any other authority or body constituted by special Act of Parliament or incorporated by Royal Charter: or

(*b*) any mental nursing home as defined in section 2 below.

(3) In subsection (2) (*a*) above 'local authority' means a county council, the council of a district or London borough, the Common Council of the City of London, the Sub-Treasurer of the Inner Temple, and the Under Treasurer of the Middle Temple.

2.—(1) In this Act 'mental nursing home' means, subject to subsection (2) below, any premises used, or intended to be used, for the reception of, and the provision of nursing or other medical treatment (including care and training under medical supervision) for, one or more mentally disordered patients (meaning persons suffering, or appearing to be suffering, from mental disorder), whether exclusively or in common with other persons.

(2) In this Act 'mental nursing home' does not include any hospital as defined in subsection (3) below, or any other premises managed by a Government department or provided by a local authority.

(3) In subsection (2) above 'hospital' means—

    (a) any hospital vested in the Secretary of State by virtue of the *National Health Service Act 1977*;[1]

    (b) any accommodation provided by a local authority, and used as a hospital by or on behalf of the Secretary of State under *the National Health Service Act 1977*[1]; and

    (c) any special hospital within the meaning of *section 4 of the National Health Service Act 1977.*[1]

Registration and conduct of nursing homes and mental nursing homes

3.—(1) Any person who carries on a nursing home or a mental nursing home without being registered under this Act in respect of that home shall be guilty of an offence.

(2) An application for registration under this Act—

    (a) shall be made to the Secretary of State;

    (b) shall be accompanied by a fee of such amount as the Secretary of State may by regulations prescribe;

    (c) in the case of a mental nursing home, shall specify whether or not it is proposed to receive in the home patients who are liable to be detained under the provisions of the Mental Health Act 1959.

(3) Subject to section 4 below, the Secretary of State shall, on receiving an application under subsection (2) above, register the applicant in respect of the home named in the application, and shall issue to the applicant a certificate of registration.

(4) Where a person is registered in pursuance of an application stating that it is proposed to receive in the home such patients as are described in subsection (2) (c) above—

    (a) that fact shall be specified in the certificate of registration; and

    (b) the particulars of the registration shall be entered by the Secretary of State in a separate part of the register.

(5) The certificate of registration issued under this Act in respect of any nursing home or mental nursing home shall be kept affixed in a conspicuous place in the home, and if default is made in complying with this subsection the person carrying on the home shall be guilty of an offence.

[1] Words in italics substituted by 1977 Act.

4. The Secretary of State may refuse to register an applicant in respect of a nursing home or a mental nursing home if he is satisfied—

    (*a*) that the applicant, or any person employed or proposed to be employed by the applicant at the home, is not a fit person (whether by reason of age or otherwise) to carry on or be employed at a home of such a description as that named in the application; or

    (*b*) that, for reasons connected with situation, construction, state of repair, accommodation, staffing or equipment, the home is not, or any premises used in connection therewith are not, fit to be used for such a home; or

    (*c*) that the home is, or any premises used in connection therewith are, used, or proposed to be used, for purposes which are in any way improper or undesirable in the case of such a home; or

    (*d*) in the case of a home other than a maternity home—

        (i) that the home is not, or will not be, under the charge of a person who is either a registered medical practitioner or a qualified nurse, and is or will be resident in the home; or

        (ii) that there is not, or will not be, a proper proportion of qualified nurses among the persons having the superintendence of, or employed in the nursing of the patients in, the home; or

    (*e*) in the case of a maternity home—

        (i) that the person who has, or will have, the superintendence of the nursing of the patients in the home is not either a qualified nurse or a certified midwife; or

        (ii) that any person employed, or proposed to be employed, in attending any woman in the home in childbirth, or in nursing any patient in the home, is not either a registered medical practitioner, a certified midwife, a pupil midwife, or a qualified nurse.

5.—(1) The Secretary of State may make regulations as to the conduct of nursing homes and mental nursing homes, and such regulations may in particular—

    (*a*) make provision as to the facilities and services to be provided in such homes;

    (*b*) provide that a contravention of or failure to comply with any specified provision of the regulations shall be an offence against the regulations.

(2) In the case of nursing homes, regulations made under subsection (1) above may empower the Secretary of State to limit the number of persons, or persons of any description, who may be received into any

such home, and enable registration of any such home to be made subject to the condition that persons shall not be received into the home in excess of the number fixed for the home in accordance with the regulations.

6.—The Secretary of State may make regulations—

(*a*) with respect to the registration of persons under this Act in respect of nursing homes and mental nursing homes, and in particular with respect to—

   (i) the making of applications for registration;

   (ii) the refusal and cancellation of registration; and

   (iii) appeals to magistrates' courts against refusals and cancellations of registration;

(*b*) with respect to the keeping of records relating to nursing homes and mental nursing homes and with respect to the notification of events occurring in such homes:

(*c*) with respect to entry into and the inspection of premises used or reasonably believed to be used as a nursing home;

(*d*) providing that a contravention of or failure to comply with any specified provision of the regulations shall be an offence against the regulations.

7. The Secretary of State may at any time cancel the registration of a person in respect of a nursing home or a mental nursing home—

(*a*) on any ground which would entitle him to refuse an application for the registration of that person in respect of that home;

(*b*) on the ground that that person has been convicted of an offence against the provisions of this Act relating to nursing homes or mental nursing homes, or on the ground that any other person has been convicted of such an offence in respect of that home;

(*c*) on the ground that any condition imposed by section 8 (1) and (2) below has not been complied with;

(*d*) on the ground that that person has been convicted of an offence against regulations made under section 5 or section 6 above.

8.—(1) It shall be a condition of the registration of any person in respect of a mental nursing home that the number of persons kept at any one time in the home (excluding persons carrying on, or employed in, the home, together with their families) does not exceed such number as may be specified in the certificate of registration.

(2) Without prejudice to subsection (1) above, any such registration may be effected subject to such conditions (to be specified in the certificate of registration) as the Secretary of State may consider

appropriate for regulating the age, sex or other category of persons who may be received in the home in question.

(3) If any condition imposed by or under subsection (1) or (2) above is not complied with, the person carrying on the home shall be guilty of an offence.

9.—(1) Subject to the provisions of this section, any person authorised in that behalf by the Secretary of State may at any time, after producing, if asked to do so, some duly authenticated document showing that he is so authorised, enter and inspect any premises which are used, or which that person has reasonable cause to believe to be used, for the purposes of a mental nursing home, and may inspect any records kept in pursuance of section (6) (*b*) above.

(2) A person authorised under subsection (1) above to inspect a mental nursing home may visit and interview in private any patient residing in the home who is, or appears to be, suffering from mental disorder—

    (*a*) for the purpose of investigating any complaint as to his treatment made by or on behalf of the patient; or

    (*b*) in any case where the person so authosised has reasonable cause to believe that the patient is not receiving proper care;

and where the person so authorised is a medical practitioner, he may examine the patient in private, and may require the production of, and inspect, any medical records relating to the patient's treatment in that home.

(3) Regulations made under section 5 above may make provision with respect to the exercise on behalf of the Secretary of State of the powers conferred by this section, and may in particular provide—

    (*a*) for imposing conditions or restrictions with respect to the exercise of those powers in relation to mental nursing homes which, immediately before 1st November 1960, were registered hospitals as defined in sub-section (4) below, and

    (*b*) subject as aforesaid, for requiring the inspection of mental nursing homes under subsection (1) above to be carried out on such occasions, or at such intervals, as the regulations may prescribe.

(4) In subsection (3) (*a*) above, 'registered hospital' means a hospital registered as mentioned in section 231 (9) of the Lunacy Act 1890.

(5) Any person who refuses to allow the inspection of any premises, or without reasonable cause refuses to allow the visiting, interviewing or examination of any person by a person authorised in that behalf under this section or to produce for the inspection of any person so authorised any document or record the production of which is duly

required by him, or otherwise obstructs any such person in the exercise of his functions, shall be guilty of an offence.

(6) Without prejudice to the generality of subsection (5) above, any person who insists on being present when requested to withdraw by a person authorised as aforesaid to interview or examine a person in private, shall be guilty of an offence.

10.—(1) This section applies to any mental nursing home the particulars of the registration of which are entered in the separate part of the register referred to in paragraph (*b*) of section 3 (4) above, and in subsections (2) and (3) below 'patient' means a person suffering or appearing to be suffering from mental disorder.

(2) If the registration of any such home is cancelled under section 7 above at a time when any patient is liable to be detained in the home under the provisions of the Mental Health Act 1959, the registration shall, notwithstanding the cancellation, continue in force until the expiry of the period of two months beginning with the date of the cancellation, or until every such patient has ceased to be so liable, whichever first occurs.

(3) If the person registered in respect of any such home (not being one of two or more persons so registered) dies at a time when any patient is liable to be so detained, the registration shall continue in force until the expiry of the period of two months beginning with the death, or until every such patient has ceased to be so liable, or until a person other than the deceased has been registered in respect of the home, whichever first occurs.

(4) A registration continued in force by virtue of subsection (3) above shall continue in force—

(*a*) as from the grant of representation to the estate of the deceased, for the benefit of the personal representative of the deceased; and

(*b*) pending the grant of such representation, for the benefit of any person approved for the purpose by the Secretary of State.

(5) For the purposes of this Act, a person for whose benefit the registration continues in force by virtue of subsection (3) above shall be treated as registered in respect of the home.

Offences

11.—(1) Proceedings in respect of an offence under section 3 (1) or (5) above relating to a nursing home shall not, without the written consent of the Attorney General, be taken by any person other than a party aggrieved or the Secretary of State.

(2) A local social services authority may institute proceedings for any offence under section 9 (5) or (6) above.

12. A person guilty of an offence under section 3 (1) above shall be liable on summary conviction to a fine not exceeding £50 or, in the case of a second or subsequent offence, to imprisonment for a term not exceeding three months, or to a fine not exceeding £50, or to both such imprisonment and fine.

13.—(1) A person guilty of an offence under section 3 (5) above shall be liable on summary conviction—

    (*a*) to a fine not exceeding £5; and,

    (*b*) subject to subsection (2) below, to a further fine not exceeding £2 for each day on which the offence continues after conviction.

(2) The court by which a person is convicted of an original offence under subsection (1) above may fix a reasonable period from the date of conviction for compliance with any directions given by the court; and where the court has fixed such a period, the daily penalty prescribed by that subsection shall not be recoverable in respect of any day before the expiry of that period.

14. A person guilty of an offence against regulations made under section 5 or section 6 above shall be liable on summary conviction to a fine not exceeding £20.

15. A person guilty of an offence referred to in section 8 (3) above shall be liable on summary conviction to a fine not exceeding £20.

16. A person guilty of an offence under section 9 (5) or (6) above shall be liable on summary conviction to imprisonment for a term not exceeding three months or to a fine not exceeding £100, or to both such imprisonment and fine.

17.—(1) Subsection (2) below applies to—

    (*a*) an offence under section 3 (1) or (5) above;

    (*b*) an offence against regulations made under section 5 above so far as that section relates to nursing homes;

    (*c*) an offence against regulations made under section 6 above.

(2) Where an offence referred to in subsection (1) above which has been committed by a body corporate is proved to have been committed with the consent or connivance of, or to be attributable to any neglect on the part of, any director, manager, secretary or other similar officer of the body corporate, or any person purporting to act in any such capacity, he as well as the body corporate shall be deemed to be guilty of that offence, and shall be liable to be proceeded against and punished accordingly.

Miscellaneous and supplemental

18.—(1) The Secretary of State may grant exemption from the operation of the provisions of this Act in respect of any nursing home or mental nursing home as respects which he is satisfied that it is being, or will be, carried on in accordance with the practice and principles of the body known as the Church of Christ Scientist.

(2) It shall be a condition of any exemption granted under this section that the home in question shall adopt and use the name of Christian Science house.

(3) An exemption granted under this section may at any time be withdrawn by the Secretary of State if it appears to him that the home in question is no longer being carried on in accordance with the said practice and principles.

19.—(1) Any regulations under this Act shall be made by statutory instrument which shall be subject to annulment in pursuance of a resolution of either House of Parliament.

(2) The power to make regulations conferred on the Secretary of State by section 6 above shall, if the Treasury so directs, be exercisable by the Treasury and the Secretary of State acting jointly.

(3) Any power conferred by this Act to make regulations under section 5 above so far as the power in that section relates to nursing homes, or under section 6 above, may, unless the contrary intention appears, be exercised—

(*a*) either in relation to all cases to which the power extends, or in relation to all those cases subject to specified exceptions, or in relation to any specified cases or classes of case; and

(*b*) so as to make, as respects the cases in relation to which it is exercised—

   (i) the full provision to which the power extends or any less provision (whether by way of exception or otherwise):

   (ii) the same provision for all cases in relation to which the power is exercised, or different provision for different cases or different classes of case, or different provision as respects the same case or class of case for different purposes of those sections;

   (iii) any such provision either unconditionally or subject to any specified condition;

and includes power to make such incidental or supplemental provision in the regulations as the persons making them consider appropriate.

20.—(1) Except where the contrary intention appears, in this Act—

'local social services authority' means a council which is a local authority for the purpose of the Local Authority Social Services Act 1970;

'maternity home' has the meaning given by section 1(2) above;

'mental disorder' has the meaning given by section 4 of the Mental Health Act 1959 (definition and classification of mental disorder), and 'mentally disordered' shall be construed accordingly;

'mental nursing home' has the meaning given by section 2 above;

'nursing home' has the meaning given by section 1 above;

'pupil midwife' means a person who is undergoing training with a view to becoming a certified midwife, and for that purpose attending women in childbirth, as part of a course of practical instruction in midwifery recognised by the Central Midwives Board;

'qualified nurse' means subject to subsection (2) below, a person registered in the general part of the register of nurses required to be kept under the Nurses Act 1957, or a person who had before 1st July 1928 completed a three years course of training in a hospital which was during the period of her training, or subsequently became, a training school approved by the General Nursing Council for England and Wales, or the General Nursing Council for Scotland, or the General Nursing Council for Northern Ireland, for the purpose of admission to the general part of that register.

(2) In relation to any premises used or intended to be used solely for the reception of, and the provision of nursing for, a class of patients in whose case the requisite nursing can be suitably and adequately provided by nurses of a class whose names are contained in some part of the register of nurses required to be kept under the Nurses Act 1957, other than the general part of that register, references in the definition of 'qualified nurse' in subsection (1) above to the general part of the register shall be construed as including references to that other part of the register.

(3) References in this Act to any enactment shall, except in so far as the context otherwise requires, be construed as references to that enactment as amended or applied by or under any other enactment including this Act.

21. So far as section 125 (forgery, false statements, etc.), section 141 (protection for acts done) or section 143 (inquiries) of the Mental Health Act 1959 immediately before the commencement of this Act in relation to any provision re-enacted by this Act, those sections shall apply in relation to the corresponding provision of this Act.

22.—(1) – (3) which give effect to the Schedules are not reproduced.

(4) Nothing in this Act shall be taken as prejudicing the operation of section 38 of the Interpretation Act 1889 (which relates to the operation of repeals).

23.—(1) This Act does not extend to Scotland or Northern Ireland.

(2) The Secretary of State may by order direct that the provisions of this Act relating to mental nursing homes shall, subject to such exceptions, adaptations and modifications as may be specified in the order, extend to the Isles of Scilly, but except as so applied this Act shall not extend to the said Isles.

(3) Any order made by the Secretary of State under subsection (2) above may be varied or revoked by a subsequent order of the Secretary of State made in like manner and subject to the like conditions as the original order.

24.—(1) This Act may be cited as the Nursing Homes Act 1975.

(2) *The Act was brought into force by the Commencement Order S.I. 1975, No. 1781.*

HEALTH SERVICES ACT 1976

PART I

THE HEALTH SERVICES BOARD AND ITS COMMITTEES

1.—(1) There shall be a body, to be called the Health Services Board (in this Act referred to as 'the Board'), which shall have the functions assigned to it by this Act.

(2) The Board shall consist of five members appointed by the Secretary of State in accordance with Part I of Schedule 1 to this Act.

(3) Without prejudice to the power of the Board to set up any other committees, there shall be constituted in accordance with Part II of the said Schedule 1—

(a) a Scottish Committee of the Board ('the Scottish Committee') having the general duty of advising the Board on the performance of its functions in relation to matters affecting Scotland; and

(b) a Welsh Committee of the Board ('the Welsh Committee') having the General duty of advising the Board on the performance of its functions in relation to matters affecting Wales.

(4) At any meeting of the Board or of the Scottish or Welsh Committee for the purpose of considering or dealing with any application

for an authorisation under section 12 below or any proposed alteration of the terms of any such authorisation, the Board or Committee shall be assisted by four assessors selected in accordance with Part III of the said Schedule 1.

(5) In deciding how to perform any of its functions in relation to any matter affecting Scotland or Wales the Board shall obtain and consider the advice of the Scottish Committee or the Welsh Committee, as the case may be.

(6) The supplementary provisions contained in Parts IV to VI of the said Schedule 1 shall have effect with respect to the Board and its committees and assessors.

PART II

USE OF NATIONAL HEALTH SERVICE FACILITIES BY PRIVATE PATIENTS, ETC.

Sections 2 – 11 are either repealed by the 1977 Act or their effect is largely spent and they are not reproduced here.

PART III

CONTROL OF HOSPITAL BUILDING OUTSIDE NATIONAL HEALTH SERVICE, ETC.

12.—(1) Subject to subsection (3) below, no person shall execute any controlled works unless—

   (*a*) he is authorised in writing by the Board to do so and the works are in accordance with the terms of the authorisation; or

   (*b*) the works are executed in accordance with planning permission in force in pursuance of the Town and Country Planning Act 1971 or the Town and Country Planning (Scotland) Act 1972 and granted (otherwise than by a development order within the meaning of that Act) either before the passing of this Act or in consequence of an application for such permission which was made before 12th April 1976.

(2) In this part of this Act—

   'controlled works' means—

      (*a*) works for the construction of controlled premises or of a controlled extension of controlled premises; or

      (*b*) works for converting any premises into controlled premises;

   'controlled premises' means premises at which there are or are to be facilities for the provision of all or any of the following services, namely—

(*a*) the carrying out of surgical procedures under general anaesthesia;

(*b*) obstetrics;

(*c*) radiotherapy;

(*d*) renal dialysis;

(*e*) radiology or diagnostic pathology.

being premises which, if situated or to be situated in Greater London, provide or will provide one hundred or more beds for the reception of patients or, if situated or to be situated elsewhere, provide or will provide seventy-five or more beds for the reception of patients;

'controlled extension', in relation to any controlled premises, means works designed—

(*a*) to extend, adapt or be used in conjunction with the controlled premises; or

(*b*) to extend or adapt works used in conjunction with the controlled premises.

(3) Subsection (1) above—

(*a*) does not apply in the case of works that are to be executed by or on behalf of the Crown or for the purposes of a visiting force; but

(*b*) in the case of works that are to be executed otherwise than as aforesaid, shall apply notwithstanding any interest of the Crown in the land on which, or in any premises in connection with which, the works are to be executed.

13.—(1) Every application for an authorisation shall be made to the Board, and on receipt of any such application the Board shall send a copy of it to the Secretary of State.

(2) On receiving an application for an authorisation the Board shall consider whether, having regard to the matters mentioned in subsection (3) below, the execution of the works in question—

(*a*) would to a significant extent interfere with the performance by the Secretary of State of any duty imposed on him by the *National Health Service Act 1777*[1] to provide accommodation or services of any kind; or

(*b*) would to a significant extent operate to the disadvantage of persons seeking or afforded admission or access to any accommodation or services provided by the Secretary of State under that Act[2] (whether as resident or non-resident patients) otherwise than as private patients.

and shall grant the authorisation unless, having regard to those matters,

----

[1] Words in italics substituted by 1977 Act.   [2] Words substituted by 1977 Act.

it is satisfied that the execution of the works would do either or both of the things mentioned in paragraphs (a) and (b) above.

(3) The matters referred to in subsection (2) above are, in relation to the works in question—

(a) how much accommodation or additional accommodation the works would provide;

(b) what facilities or additional facilities the works would enable to be provided;

(c) what staffing requirements or additional staffing requirements the works would give rise to.

(4) An authorisation may contain such terms as the Board thinks appropriate, including in particular, without prejudice to the generality of the preceding provisions of this subsection, terms as to the duration of the authorisation and the place at which or area within which the works may be executed: and the Board may, with the consent of the person to whom an authorisation was issued, alter any of its terms at any time.

14.—(1) Any person who proposes to make, after the coming into force of this Part of this Act, an application for planning permission for any notifiable works must, before making the application, notify the Board of the proposed application by giving to it a notice in the prescribed form.

(2) A notice under this section must contain the prescribed information about—

(a) the notifiable works for which planning permission is to be applied for; and

(b) the purposes for which any hospital premises that will result from or be directly affected by the execution of those works are to be used.

(3) On receipt of a notice under this section which is in the prescribed form and contains the information required by subsection (2) above the Board shall issue to the person by whom the notice was given a written acknowledgment—

(a) identifying the notice and stating the date on which it was received by the Board; and

(b) acknowledging that it complies with the requirements of this section.

(4) In any proceedings for an offence under section 18(2)(a) below, an acknowledgement under subsection (3) above shall be conclusive evidence of the matters which it states or acknowledges.

(5) It shall be the duty of the Board to furnish the Secretary of State with such of the information contained in any notice received by the

Board under this section as he may reasonably require for the proper discharge of his functions under the *National Health Service Act* 1977[1] and Part II of this Act.

(6) Subsection (3) of section 12 above shall apply in relation to subsection (1) above as it applies in relation to subsection (1) of that section.

(7) In this Part of this Act—

'notifiable works' means—

    (*a*) works for the construction of hospital premises or of an extension of hospital premises; or

    (*b*) works for converting any premises into hospital premises. not being in either case, works for which an authorisation is required:

'hospital premises' means premises of any prescribed class, being premises used or to be used for the prevention, diagnosis or treatment of illness or for the reception of patients;

'extension', in relation to any hospital premises, means works designed—

    (*a*) to extend, adapt or be used in conjunction with the hospital premises; or

    (*b*) to extend or adapt works used in conjunction with the hospital premises.

15.—(1) This section applies to works that consist of, or include, controlled works.

(2) An application made after the coming into force of this Part of this Act for planning permission for works to which this section applies shall be of no effect unless it is accompanied by a copy of an authorisation in force for all of those works in the planning area or district concerned for which an authorisation is required.

(3) Where at the time when this Part of this Act comes into force—

    (*a*) an application for planning permission made on or after 12th April 1976 is pending, or any appeal to the Secretary of State connected with such an application is pending, or the time within which such an appeal may be begun has not expired; and

    (*b*) if the application had been made after the coming into force of this Part of this Act it would have been of no effect by virtue of subsection (2) above.

the application shall be of no effect, or as the case may be the appeal shall be stayed or sisted or not begun, until the authority to which the application was made is furnished with the document which would

---

[1] Words in italics substituted by 1977 Act.

under subsection (2) above have been required to accompany the application if it had been made after the coming into force of this Part of this Act.

(4) Where by virtue of the preceding subsection a prohibition imposed by that subsection on the beginning of an appeal ceases to be so imposed, the appeal may be begun during a period which begins with the cessar and is equal to so much of the time within which the appeal could have been begun apart from the prohibition as was unexpired when the prohibition was so imposed.

(5) In this section—

'local planning authority' has the same meaning as in the Town and Country Planning Act 1971;

'planning authority' has the same meaning as in the Town and Country Planning (Scotland) Act 1972;

'planning permission' has the same meaning as in the said Act of 1971 or 1972, as the case may be;

'the planning area or district concerned' means, in England and Wales, the area of the local planning authority or, in Scotland, the district of the planning authority, as the case may be.

(6) Subsection (3) of section 12 above shall apply in relation to subsection (2) above as it applies in relation to subsection (1) of that section.

16.—(1) The Secretary of State may by regulations make provision—

(a) as to the manner and form in which any application for an authorisation is to be made to the Board;

(b) as to the manner in which any notice under section 14 above is to be given to the Board, and as to the form in which any acknowledgment under subsection (3) of that section is to be issued by the Board;

(c) for requiring such reasonable fees as may, with the consent of the Treasury, be prescribed to be paid in connection with any application for an authorisation;

(d) as to the quorum and procedure of the Board in relation to applications for authorisations;

(e) as to the circumstances in which the Board may or must afford the applicant for an authorisation a hearing by the Board or, in such cases as may be prescribed, the Scottish or Welsh Committee, and for determining the locality of, and entitling persons other than the applicant to appear and be heard at, such a hearing;

(f) as to the time to be allowed on any such application for the production of evidence or the taking of any prescribed steps for the purposes of such a hearing;

(g) for requiring persons to attend and give evidence or produce documents at such hearings, and for authorising the administration of oaths to persons so attending;

(h) for enabling any person entitled to appear otherwise than as a witness at any such hearing to be represented by another person, whether professionally qualified or not;

(i) for prescribing anything which under this Part of this Act is required or authorised to be prescribed.

(2) Without prejudice to the generality of paragraph (e) of subsection (1) above, provision shall be made by regulations under that subsection for requiring the Board not to refuse an application for an authorisation unless the applicant has been afforded a hearing such as is mentioned in that paragraph.

(3) Regulations under subsection (1) above may, for the purpose of securing compliance with requirements imposed by virtue of any provisions included in the regulations by virtue of paragraph (g) of that subsection, provide that a person who without reasonable excuse fails to comply with such a requirement shall be liable on summary conviction to a fine not exceeding such amount not greater than £100 as may be prescribed.

(4) The Secretary of State may by regulations provide for the appointment by him of inspectors to act, under the direction of the Board, for the purposes of this Part of this Act, except so far as it relates to notifiable works, and for conferring on such inspectors such powers (including powers of entry and inspection) as the Secretary of State considers necessary for those purposes.

(5) Any powers conferred on inspectors by regulations made in pursuance of subsection (4) above shall, to the extent that the regulations so provide, be exercisable in relation to—

(a) premises or land owned by, but not occupied by or for the purposes of, the Crown; and

(b) works on such land which have been or are being executed otherwise than by or on behalf of the Crown or for the purposes of a visiting force.

17.—(1) When an application for an authorisation is refused or granted by the Board and the decision to refuse or grant it, as the case may be, involves a question of law, then—

(a) if the application is refused, the applicant or, if the applicant was afforded a hearing by the Board, the applicant or any other person who appeared (in person or not) and was heard at the hearing may on that question appeal from the Board's decision to the court; or

(b) if the application is granted in a case in which the applicant was afforded a hearing by the Board, any other person who so appeared and was heard may on that question appeal as aforesaid.

(2) In the preceding subsection "the court" means—
(a) In England and Wales, the High Court;
(b) in Scotland, the Court of Session.

(3) An appeal under this section must be brought before the end of the three months beginning with the date on which the applicant is notified of the Board's decision on his application.

(4) The Board and the Secretary of State and (if he would not be so entitled apart from this subsection) the applicant shall each be entitled to appear and be heard on any appeal under this section.

(5) Rules of court relating to appeals under this section may provide for excluding so much of section 63(1) of the Supreme Court of Judicature (Consolidation) Act 1925 as requires appeals to the High Court to be heard and determined by a Divisional Court; but no appeal to the Court of Appeal shall be brought by virtue of this section except with the leave of the High Court or the Court of Appeal.

(6) In relation to proceedings in the High Court or the Court of Appeal or the Court of Session brought by virtue of this section the power to make rules of court shall include power to make rules prescribing the powers of the court with respect to—
(a) the giving of any decision which might have been given by the Board on the application;
(b) the remitting of the application, with the court's decision on any question of law decided by it on appeal, for re-hearing and determination by the Board;
(c) the giving of directions to the Board.

(7) On any appeal brought under or by virtue of this section the court may, if the decision is in favour of the appellant, order the Board (whether or not it appears on the appeal) to pay the costs or, in Scotland, the expenses of the appellant or any other person.

(8) An appeal shall lie, with the leave of the Court of Session or the House of Lords, from any decision of the Court of Session under this section, and such leave may be given on such terms as to costs or otherwise as the Court of Session or the House of Lords may determine.

18.—(1) Any person who contravenes section 12(1) of this Act shall be guilty of an offence and liable on summary conviction to a fine not exceeding £400 or on conviction on indictment to a fine.

(2) Any person who—

    (*a*) without reasonable excuse fails to comply with the requirements of section 14(1) and (2) above in relation to an application for planning permission for any notifiable works; or

    (*b*) knowingly or recklessly furnishes a notice which is false in a material particular in purported compliance with section 14(1) above,

shall be guilty of an offence and liable on summary conviction to a fine not exceeding £400.

(3) Any person who—

    (*a*) intentionally obstructs an inspector appointed by virtue of regulations made in pursuance of section 16(4) above in the exercise of any power of entry or inspection conferred on him by regulations so made; or

    (*b*) without reasonable excuse fails to comply with any requirement imposed by such an inspector by virtue of regulations so made,

shall be guilty of an offence and liable on summary conviction to a fine not exceeding £400.

(4) Where an offence under any of the preceding provisions of this section has been committed by a body corporate and is proved to have been committed with the consent or connivance of, or to be attributable to any neglect on the part of, a director, manager, secretary or other similar officer of the body corporate or any person who was purporting to act in any such capacity, he as well as the body corporate shall be guilty of that offence and shall be liable to be proceeded against and punished accordingly.

(5) Where the affairs of a body corporate are managed by its members, subsection (4) above shall apply in relation to the acts and defaults of a member in connection with his functions of management as if he were a director of the body corporate.

19.—(1) The paragraph set out in subsection (2) below shall be inserted—

    (*a*) after paragraph (*c*) of section 4 of the Nursing Homes Act 1975, as paragraph (*cc*); and

    (*b*) after paragraph (*b*) of the proviso in section 1(3) of the Nursing Homes Registration (Scotland) Act 1938, as paragraph (*bb*),

so as to afford, in each case, an additional ground for refusing to register, or cancelling the registration of, a person in respect of a nursing home or mental nursing home.

(2) The said paragraph is—

    '( ) that the home or any premises to be used in connection

therewith consists of or include works executed in contravention of section 12(1) of the Health Services Act 1976;'.

(3) In section 16(1) of the Mental Health (Scotland) Act 1960 (prerequisites of registration of private hospital) the following paragraph shall be inserted after paragraph (b)—

'(bb) that neither the hospital nor any premises to be used in connection therewith consists of or include works executed in contravention of section 12(1) of the Health Services Act 1976;'

(4) In each of the following provisions (penalites for carrying on a nursing home, mental nursing home or private hospital without registration) namely—

(a) section 12 of the Nursing Homes Act 1975;

(b) section 1(1) of the Nursing Homes Registration (Scotland) Act 1938;

(c) section 22(1) of the Mental Health (Scotland) Act 1960;

for the words from 'shall be liable' onwards there shall be substituted the words 'shall be liable on summary conviction to a fine not exceeding £400 or on conviction on indictment to a fine'.

20. In this Part of this Act—

'authorisation' means an authorisation required by section 12(1) above;

'controlled works' has the meaning given by section 12(2) above;

'hospital premises' has the meaning given by section 14(7) above;

'notifiable works' has the meaning given by section 14(7) above;

'prescribed' means prescribed by regulations made by the Secretary of State;

'visiting force' means any such body, contingent or detachment of the forces of any country as is a visiting force for the purposes of any of the provisions of the Visiting Forces Act 1952.

Part IV

Supplementary and General

S.21 Not here reproduced

22.—(1) Any power conferred by this Act to make regulations—

(a) may be exercised so as to make different provision for different areas or in relation to different cases or different circumstances to which the power is applicable, and to make any provision to which the power extends subject to such exceptions, limitations and conditions (if any) as the Secretary of State considers necessary or expedient;

(b) includes power to make such incidental or supplemental provision in the regulations as the Secretary of State considers appropriate; and

(c) shall be exercisable by statutory instrument, which shall be subject to annulment in pursuance of a resolution of either House of Parliament.

(2) Before making any regulations under paragraph 10 of Schedule 1 to this Act or under any provision of Part III of this Act, the Secretary of State shall consult with—

   (a) the Board;

   (b) such bodies as he may recognise as being representative of medical practitioners or dental practitioners; and

   (c) such other bodies as appear to him to be representative of interests likely to be substantially affected by the regulations.

23.—(1) In this Act—

   'the 1947 Act' means the National Health Service (Scotland) Act 1947;

   'the national health services' means the health services established in England and Wales and in Scotland respectively in pursuance of section 1 of the principal Act;

   'NHS hospital' means a hospital vested in the Secretary of State;

   'the principal Act' means, for England and Wales, the National Health Service Act 1946 or, for Scotland, the National Health Service Scotland) Act 1947;

and, unless the context otherwise requires, any expression to which a meaning is assigned by the principal Act for the purposes of that Act has that meaning also for the purposes of this Act.

(2) Except so far as the context otherwise requires, any reference in this Act to an enactment is a reference to it as amended by or under any other entactment, including this Act.

S.23(6) Not here reproduced.

S.24 Not here reproduced.

SCHEDULES

SCHEDULE 1

THE HEALTH SERVICES BOARD AND ITS COMMITTEES

PART I

THE BOARD

1.—(1) The Board shall comprise—

(a) a chairman appointed after consultation with the bodies mentioned in paragraphs (a) and (b) of sub-paragraph (2) below;

(b) two medical practitioners appointed after consultation with the bodies mentioned in paragraph (a) of that sub-paragraph; and

(c) two other persons appointed after consultation with the bodies mentioned in paragraph(b) of that sub-paragraph.

(2) Those bodies are—

(a) such bodies as the Secretary of State may recognise as being representative of medical practitioners or dental practitioners;

(b) such bodies not falling within paragraph (a) above as the Secretary of State may recognise as being representative of persons employed in one or other of the national health services or concerned with the interests of patients at NHS hospitals.

PART II

THE SCOTTISH AND WELSH COMMITTEES

2.—(1) The Scottish Committee and the Welsh Committee shall each be constituted in accordance with the following provisions of this paragraph; and in those provisions 'the Committee' means the Scottish Committee or the Welsh Committee, as the case may be.

(2) The Board shall designate, with the consent of the Secretary of State, a member of the Board as a member of the Committee ('the designated member').

(3) The Committee shall comprise—

(a) a chairman who, if the designated member is the chairman of the Board, shall be the designated member, but who shall otherwise be a person appointed by the Secretary of State after consultation with the bodies mentioned in paragraphs (a) and (b) of paragraph 1(2) above;

(b) two medical practitioners appointed by the Secretary of State after consultation with the bodies mentioned in paragraph

(a) of paragraph 1(2) above or, if the designated member is a member of the Board appointed under paragraph 1(1)(b) above, one medical practitioner so appointed by the Secretary of State; and

(c) two other persons appointed by the Secretary of State after consultation with the bodies mentioned in paragraph (b) of paragraph 1(2) above or, if the designated member is a member of the Board appointed under paragraph 1(1) (c) above, one other person so appointed by the Secretary of State.

PART III

ASSESSORS

3. Of the four assessors required by section 1(4) above for any such meeting of the Board or of the Scottish or Welsh Committee as is there mentioned, one shall be selected by the Board or that Committee, as the case may be, from each of the lists maintained by the Board under the following paragraph.

4.—(1) The Board shall prepare and maintain four lists of persons to act as assessors in accordance with section 1(4) above.

(2) Of those lists—

(a) one shall comprise medical or dental practitioners having special knowledge and experience of one or more of the services mentioned in the definition of 'controlled premises' in section 12(2) above;

(b) one shall comprise persons having special knowledge and experience of nursing;

(c) one shall comprise persons having special knowledge and experience of hospital administration;

(d) one shall comprise persons having special knowledge and experience of the design and construction of hospitals.

(3) Before placing a person on any of the lists the Board shall consult with the Secretary of State and the bodies mentioned in paragraphs (a) and (b) of paragraph 1(2) above.

PART IV

SUPPLEMENTARY PROVISIONS RELATING TO THE BOARD AND ITS COMMITTEES AND ASSESSORS

Incorporation and status

5. The Board shall be a body corporate.

6. The Board shall not be regarded as the servant or agent of the Crown, or as enjoying any status, immunity or privilege of the Crown.

Tenure of office, etc.

7.—(1) Subject to paragraphs 8 and 9 below, a person shall hold and vacate office as chairman or a member of the Board in accordance with the terms of the instrument appointing him to that office.

(2) Every appointment as chairman or a member of the Board shall be for a period of not less than three years.

8. A person may at any time resign his office as chairman or a member of the Board by giving the Secretary of State a notice in writing signed by that person and stating that he resigns that office.

9.—(1) If the Secretary of State is satisfied that a member of the Board—

    (*a*) has been absent from meetings of the Board for a period longer than six consecutive months without the permission of the Board; or

    (*b*) has become bankrupt or made an arrangement with his creditors; or

    (*c*) is incapacitated by physical or mental illness; or

    (*d*) is otherwise unable or unfit to discharge the functions of a member,

the Secretary of State may declare his office as a memger to be vacant and shall notify the declaration in such manner as the Secretary of State thinks fit; and thereupon the office shall become vacant.

(2) In the application of the preceding sub-paragraph to Scotland, for the references in paragraph (*b*) to a member's having become bankrupt and to a member's having made an arrangement with his creditors there shall be substituted respectively references to sequestration of a member's estate having been awarded and to a member's having made a trust deed for behoof of his creditors or a composition contract.

10.—(1) The Secretary of State shall by regulations provide for the appointment by him, after the appropriate consultation, of—

    (*a*) a deputy chairman to act in place of the chairman of the Board and, for each other member of the Board, a deputy member to act in his place;

    (*b*) a deputy chairman to act in place of the chairman of the Scottish Committee and, for each other member of that Committee, a deputy member to act in his place;

    (*c*) a deputy chairman to act in place of the chairman of the Welsh Committee and, for each other member of that Committee, a deputy member to act in his place;

and in this sub-paragraph 'appropriate consultation' means consultation with the bodies with whom consultation was required by paragraph 1 or 2 above prior to the appointment of the person in whose place the deputy is to act.

(2) Regulations under this paragraph shall provide that a deputy, while he is acting in place of a member of the Board or of the Scottish or Welsh Committee (but not otherwise), shall be deemed to be a member of the Board or of that Committee, as the case may be, but that paragraphs 12 and 13 below shall not apply to him.

11. The Board shall pay to its members, and to the members of the Scottish Committee and the Welsh Committee, and to persons acting as assessors in accordance with section 1(4) above, such remuneraation and allowances as the Secretary of State may with the approval of the Minister for the Civil Service determine.

12. Where—
    (a) a person ceases to be a member of the Board; or
    (b) a person (not being a member of the Board) ceases to be a member of the Scottish Committee or the Welsh Committee,
in circumstances which, in the opinion of the Secretary of State, make it right that he should receive compensation, the Secretary of State shall, with the approval of the Minister for the Civil Service, direct the Board to make to that person a payment of such amount as the Secretary of State may with the approval of that Minister determine.

13. The Board shall, as regards any member of the Board or any member of the Scottish Committee or the Welsh Committee (not being a member of the Board) in whose case the Secretary of State may with the approval of the Minister for the Civil Service, so determine, pay such pension, allowance or gratuity to or in respect of him or make such payments towards the provisions of such pension, allowance or gratuity, as the Secretary of State may, with the approval of that Minister, determine.

Staff

14. The Board may, with the approval of the Secretary of State given with the consent of the Minister for the Civil Service as to numbers and as to remuneration and other terms and conditions of service, appoint such officers as it may think fit.

15. Employment with the Board shall be included among the kinds of employment to which a superannuation scheme under section 1 of the Superannuation Act 1972 can apply, and accordingly in Schedule 1 to that Act (in which those kinds of employment are listed) the words 'Health Services Board' shall be inserted after the words 'Gaming Board for Great Britain.'

Proceedings and instruments

16. Subject to section 1(4) above and any regulations made under section 16(1) above, the quorum of the Board and the arrangements relating to its procedure and business shall be such as the Board may determine.

17. The validity of any proceedings of the Board shall not be affected by any vacancy among the members of the Board or by any defect in the appointment of a member or of an assessor.

18.—(1) A document purporting to be duly executed under the common seal of the Board shall be received in evidence and shall be deemed to be so executed unless the contarry is proved.

(2) A document purpoting to be signed on behalf of the Board shall be received in evidence and shall be deemed to be so signed unless the contrary is proved.

19. Paragraphs 16, 17 and 18(2) above shall apply to the Scottish Committee and the Welsh Committee as they apply to the Board.

Finance

20. The Secretary of State shall pay to the Board expenses incurred or to be incurred by it under paragraphs 11 to 14 above and, with the approval of the Minister for the Civil Service given with the consent of the Treasury, shall pay to the Board such sums as the Secretary of State thinks fit for enabling the Board to meet other expenses.

21.—(1) The accounting year of the Board shall be the twelve months ending on 31st March.

(2) It shall be the duty of the Board—

    (a) to keep proper accounts and proper records in relation to the accounts;

    (b) to prepare in respect of each accounting year a statement of accounts in such form as the Secretary of State may direct with the approval of the Treasury; and

    (c) to submit to the Secretary of State before the end of the month of September next following the accounting year to which the statement relates.

(3) The Secretary of State shall transmit each statement of accounts received by him in pursuance of this paragraph to the Comptroller and Auditor General before the end of the month of November next following the accounting year to which the statement relates, and the Comptroller and Auditor General shall examine, certify and report on the statement and lay copies of it and of his report before each House of Parliament.

Annual report

22.—(1) As soon as practicable after the end of each calendar year the Board shall make to the Secretary of State a report on the performance of its functions during that year.

(2) The Secretary of State shall lay a copy of every report under this paragraph before each House of Parliament.

Supervision by Council on Tribunals

23.—(1) The Tribunals and Inquiries Act 1971 shall be amended in accordance with the following provisions of this paragraph (being provisions for bringing the functions of the Board and the Scottish and Welsh Committees under Part III of this Act under the supervision of the Council on Tribunals).

(2) In section 8(2), as amended by section 3(*a*) of the Consumer Credit Act 1974, after '5A' insert '7A', and after '35' insert '37A'.

(3) In Schedule 1, after paragraph 7 insert—

'Hospital building
7A. The Health Services Board and its Welsh Committee, in respect of their functions under Part III of the Health Services Act 1976.'

(4) In Schedule 1, after paragraph 37 insert—

'Hospital building
37A. The Scottish Committee of the Health Services Board, in respect of the Committee's functions under Part III of the Health Act 1976.'

House of Commons Disqualification Act 1975

24. In Part II of Schedule 1 to the House of Commons Disqualification Act 1975 (bodies of which all members are disqualified under that Act) there shall (at the appropriate places in alphabetical order) be inserted the following entries:—

'The Health Services Board.
The Scottish Committee of the Health Services Board.
The Welsh Committee of the Health Services Board.'

Part V repealed by 1977 Act.

PART VI

LIABILITY OF SCOTTISH COMMITTEE TO INVESTIGATION BY HEALTH SERVICE COMMISSIONER FOR SCOTLAND

29. Part VII of the National Health Service (Scotland) Act 1972 (the Health Service Commissioner for Scotland) shall have effect subject to the following provisions of this Part of this Schedule.

30.—(1) In section 45(1) of the said Act of 1972 (definition of 'body subject to investigation'), after paragraph (e) add—

'(f) the Scottish Committee of the Health Services Board.'

(2) In section 48 of that Act (reports by Commissioner), after subsection (5) add—

'(6) In the case of the Scottish Committee of the Health Services Board, the preceding provisions of this section have effect subject to paragraphs 31 and 32 of Schedule 1 to the Health Services Act 1976'.

31. Section 48 (reports by Commissioner) of the said Act of 1972 shall have effect subject to the following modifications, that is to say—

    (a) in relation to an investigation conducted under the said Part VII in repect of the Scottish Committee—

        (i) paragraph (d) of subsection (1) (report to be sent to Secretary of State) shall not apply, but the Health Commissioner for Scotland may, if he thinks fit, publish his report under that subsection; and

        (ii) subsection (3) (special report) shall have effect with the substitution for the words from 'make a special report to the Secretary of State' to the end of the subsection of the words 'lay before each House of Parliament a special report';

APPENDIX C

SELECTED STATUTORY INSTRUMENTS

In this appendix, I have not reproduced the dates of making, laying or coming into operation or the recital of the powers under which the instruments are made or the signatories of the Secretaries of State who made the various orders quoted. I have reproduced the footnotes and the 'explanatory notes' which appear at the end of each instrument in the Stationary Office edition.

Schedule 14 of the 1977 Act preserves the instruments and ensures that references in them to sections repealed and re-enacted by that Act are now to be taken as references to the corresponding provisions of the 1977 Act. I have noted, as footnotes, the corresponding provisions of the 1977 National Health Service Act. Such notes are indicated by the letters '(J.J.)'.

The National Health Service (Expenses in attending Hospitals) Regulations 1950 S.I. 1950 No. 1222

1.—(1) These regulations may be cited as the National Health Service (Expenses in attending Hospitals) Regulations 1950, and shall come into operation on the first day of September, 1950.

(2) The Interpretation Act 1889, applies to the interpretation of these regulations as it applies to the interpretation of an Act of Parliament.

2. The National Health Service (Expenses in attending Hospitals) Regulations 1948, are hereby revoked.

3. The Minister shall pay the travelling expenses necessarily incurred or to be incurred by a person (including the travelling expenses of a companion) in attending a hospital or clinic for the purpose of availing himself of hospital and specialist services if it is determined under such arrangements as may from time to time be made by the Minister that, in the circumstances of the case, the payment of such expenses by the patient would involve hardship:

Provided that—

(a) If it is determined under such arrangements as aforesaid that the patient may reasonably be required to bear a part of such expenses the balance only shall be payable by the Minister; and

(b) The travelling expenses of a companion shall not be payable by the Minister if it is determined under such arrangements as aforesaid that, having regard to the age or health of the patient or other relevant circumstances, it was necessary for the patient to be accompanied.

The National Health Service Functions (Directions to Authorities) Regulations 1974 S.I. 1974 No. 24

PART I

GENERAL

Citation and commencement

1. These regulations may be cited as the National Health Service Functions (Directions to Authorities) Regulations 1974 and shall come into operation: in the case of regulations 1, 2, 3(3)(i), 3(3)(j) and regulations 5 and 7, so far as they relate to regulation 3(3)(j), 8th February 1974; and in the case of the remainder of the regulations, 1st April 1974.

Interpretation

2.—(1) In these regulations, unless the context otherwise requires:—
'the Act of 1946' means the National Health Service Act 1946(a);
'the Act of 1968' means the Health Services and Public Health Act 1968(b);
'the Act of 1973' means the National Service Reorganisation Act 1973;
'Area Authority' means an Area Health Authority;
'health authority' means a Regional Authority, an Area Authority or a special health authority;
'Regional Authority' means a Regional Health Authority;
'regulation' means a regulation of these regulations;
'relevant Regional Authority' means the Regional Health Authority of which the region includes the area of the Area Authority in question.

(2) References in these regulations to any enactment or regulations shall include references to such enactment or regulations as amended by any subsequent enactment, order or regulations.

(3) The rules for the construction of an Act of Parliament contained in the Interpretation Act 1889(c) shall apply for the purposes of the interpretation of this instrument as they apply for the purposes of the interpretation of an Act of Parliament and in relation to any revocation effected thereby as if the instrument and the regulations revoked by it and any regulations revoked by the regulations so revoked were Acts of Parliament and if each revocation were a repeal.

(a) 1946 c. 81.　　　(b) 1968 c. 46.　　　(c) 1889 c. 63.

PART II

REGIONAL AUTHORITIES

Functions exercisable by Regional Authorities

3. Subject to the provisions of regulation 4 and to such limitations as the Secretary of State may direct with respect to the exercise of any function and in accordance with any directions he may give, a Regional Authority shall exercise on behalf of the Secretary of State, as respects its region and anywhere outside its region that the Secretary of State may direct, his functions relating to the health service under—

(1) The following provisions of the Act of 1946 and of any regulations made thereunder, namely—

(*a*) section 3(2)[1] with respect to the making and recovering of charges for the supply, replacement or repair of appliances;

(*b*) section 3(3)[2] with respect to the payment of travelling expenses;

(*c*) section 4[3] with respect to authorising hospital accommodation to be made available on payment of part of the cost thereof;

(*d*) section 4[3] with respect to the making available of such accommodation on part payment and recovery of charges;

(*e*) section 16(1)[4] with respect to conducting, or assisting any person to conduct, research; and

(*f*) section 58(1)[5] with respect to the acquisition of land; and

(2) The following provisions of the Act of 1968 and of any regulations made thereunder, namely—

(*a*) section 1(1)[6] and 2[7] with respect to authorising hospital accommodation and services to be made available for private patients as resident patients or otherwise than as resident patients;

(*b*) section 1(2)[8] with respect to allowing accommodation and services, authorised to be made available under the said section 1(1),[9] to be made available in connection with the treatment, in pursuance of arrangements may be medical or dental practitioners, of their private patients as resident patients;

(*c*) section 1(1),[9] 1(2),[8] 1(5)[10] and 2[11] with respect to making available hospital accommodation and services for private patients as resident patients or otherwise than as resident patients; to the recovery of charges for such accommodation and services; to determining such charges in the case of a patient, not being a

---

[1] Now 1977 Act ss. 81 and 82 (J.J.)
[2] Now 1977 Act s. 5 (3) (J.J.)
[3] Now 1977 Act s. 63 (J.J.)
[4] Now 1977 Act s. 5 (2) (J.J.)
[5] Now 1977 Act s. 87 (1) (J.J.)
[6] Now 1977 Act s. 65 (1) (J.J.)
[7] Now 1977 Act s. 66 (J.J.)
[8] Now 1977 Act s. 65 (2) (J.J.)
[9] Now 1977 Act s. 65 (1) (J.J.)
[10] Now 1977 Act s. 65 (5) (J.J.)
[11] Now 1977 Act s. 66 (J.J.)

resident patient, where no such determination has been made by the Secretary of State;

(*d*) section 31[1] with respect to allowing persons to make use of any services provided under the Health Service Acts, deciding on what terms such services may be so used and the provision of such services to an extent greater than otherwise necessary;

(*e*) section 32[2] with respect to the disposal of goods and the production and manufacture of them otherwise than for national health service purposes;

(*f*) section 63(1), 63(3), 63(5) and 63(6), with respect to provision for the instruction of officers of health authorities and other persons employed or contemplating employment by health authorities or in activities connected with health or welfare; and

(*g*) section 64 with respect to giving financial assistance to voluntary organisations; and

(3) The following provisions of the Act of 1973 and of any regulations made thereunder, namely—

(*a*) section 2(1)[3] with respect to the provisions of services considered appropriate for the purposes of discharging any duty imposed on the Secretary of State by the Health Service Acts and the doing of any other thing calculated to facilitate the discharge of such duty;

(*b*) section 2(2)(*a*)[4] and 2(2)(*b*)[5] with respect to the provision of hospital accommodation and other accommodation for the purposes of any service provided under the Health Service Acts;

(*c*) section 2(2)(*c*)[6] with respect to the provision of medical, dental, nursing and ambulance services;

(*d*) section 2(2)(*d*)[7] with respect to the provision of facilities for the care of nursing expectant mothers and young children and the making and recovery of charges in respect of facilities designated as being facilities so provided;

(*e*) section 2(2)(*e*)[8] with respect to the provision of facilities for the prevention of illness, the care of persons suffering from illness and the after care of persons who have suffered from illness and the making and recovery of charges for facilities designated as being facilities so provided;

(*f*) section 2(2)(*f*)[9] with respect to the provision of such other services as are required for the diagnosis and treatment of illness;

[1] Now 1977 Act s. 58 (J.J.)
[2] Now 1977 Act s. 61 (J.J.)
[3] Now 1977 Qct s. 2 (J.J.)
[4] Now 1977 Act s. 3 (1) (*a*) J.J.)
[5] Now 1977 Act s. 3 (1) (*b*) (J.J)
[6] Now 1977 Act s. 3(1) (*c*) (J.J.)
[7] Now 1977 Act ss. 3 (1) (*d*) and 80 (J.J.)
[8] Now 1977 Act ss. 3 (1) (*e*) and 80 (J.J.)
[9] Now 1977 Act s. 3 (1) (*f*) (J.J.)

(g) section 3(1) and 3(2)[1] with respect to the provision for the medical and dental inspection and treatment of pupils;

(h) section 4[2] with respect to making arrangements for the giving of advice on contraception, for the medical examination of persons seeking such advice, for the treatment of such persons and for the supply of contraceptive substances and appliances;

(i) section 8(1), 8(2), and 8(3)[3] with respect to the recognition of regional advisory committees;

(j) section 8(7)[4] with respect to the recognition of area advisory committees;

(k) section 11(1)[5] with respect to the supply of goods, services, and other facilities to local authorities and other public bodies, and carrying out maintenance work in connection with any land or buildings held by a local authority;

(l) section 11(2)[6] with respect to the supply of prescribed goods, materials or other facilities to persons providing general medical services, general dental services, general ophthalmic services or pharmaceutical services;

(m) section 11(3)[7] with respect to making available any services or other facilities and the services of persons to enable local authorities to discharge their functions relating to social services, education and public health;

(n) section 11(4)[8] with respect to consultation before the services of any officer of a health authority are made available;

(o) section 11(6)[9] with respect to the agreement of terms and the making of charges in respect of services or facilities provided;

(p) section 12(3)[10] wth respect to the agreement of charges to be made by a local authority for the services of persons employed by the local authority made available to enable health authorities to discharge their functions under the Health Service Acts;

(q) section 13(1)[11] with respect to arranging with any person or body (including a voluntary organisation) for such person or body to provide or assist in providing any service under the Health Service Acts;

(r) section 13(2)[12] with respect to making available to certan persons and bodies (including voluntary organisations) facilities and services of persons employed in connection with such facilities;

(s) section 13(3)[13] wth respect to the agreement of terms and the making of payments in respect of facilities or services provided;

[1] Now 1977 Act s. 5 (1) and Sch. 1 (J.J.)
[2] Now 1977 Act ss. 5 (1) and 77 (J.J.)
[3] Now 1977 Act s. 19 and Sch. 6 (J.J.)
[4] Now 1977 Act s. 20 and Sch. 6 (J.J.)
[5] Now 1977 Act s. 26 (1) (J.J.)
[6] Now 1977 Act s. 26 (2) (J.J.)
[7] Now 1977 Act s. 26 (3) (J.J.)
[8] Now 1977 Act s. 27 (1) and (2) (J.J.)
[9] Now 1977 Act s. 27 (4) (J.J.)
[10] Now 1977 Act s. 28 (4) (J.J.)
[11] Now 1977 Act s. 23 (1) (J.J.)
[12] Now 1977 Act s. 23 (2) (J.J.)
[13] Now 1977 Act ss. 23 (3) and (4) (J.J.)

(*t*) section 41(1) and 41(2)[1] with respect to the supervision of nursing homes and mental nursing homes;

(*u*) section 43(1)[2] with respect to making available accommodation provided under the Health Service Acts for use in connection with the provision of general medical services, general dental services, general ophthalmic services or pharmaceutical services;

(*v*) section 43(2)[3] with respect to making available facilities at accommodation provided under the Health Service Acts to a medical or dental practitioner, a registered pharmacist, an ophthalmic or dispensing optician or any other person, as may be determined, who provides services under the Health Service Acts, for use for private practice;

(*w*) section 43(4)[4] with respect to making available, in premises provided under the Health Service Acts, such facilities as are required for clinical teaching and for research connected with clinical medicine or clinical dentistry; and

(*x*) section 53(1)[5] and 53(3)[6] with respect to the acquisition of property, other than land, required for the purposes of the Health Service Acts and the use and maintenance of any property belonging to the Secretary of State by virtue of any of those Acts; and

(4) The provisions of section 28(2) of the Mental Health Act 1959(**a**) with respect to the approval of medical practitioners as having special experience in the diagnosis or treatment of mental disorder; and

(5) The provisions of section 17(1) of the Chronically Sick and Disabled Persons Act 1970(**b**) with respect to securing, so far as practicable, that hospital in-patients, who are not themselves elderly but are suffering from a condition of chronic illness or disability, are not cared for in any part of the hospital normally used wholly or partly for the care of elderly persons.

Restriction on exercise of certain functions by Regional Authorities

4.—(1) The exercise of any function by a Regional Authority in accordance with directions given in the last foregoing regulation shall be subject to the following provisions of this regulation in so far as they relate to the exercise of such function.

(2) Nothing in these regulations shall be taken as giving directions for

---

(**a**) 1959 c. 72.   (**b**) 1970 c. 44.
[1] Now 1975 Nursing Homes Act ss. 3–10 (J.J.)
[2] Now 1977 Act s. 52 (J.J.)
[3] Now repealed by Health Services Act 1976 (J.J.)
[4] Now unnecessary under the consolidation (J.J.)
[5] Now 1977 Act s. 87 (1) (J.J.)
[6] Now 1977 Act s. 87 (2) and (4) (J.J.)

the exercise of any function, conferred upon or vested in the Secretary of State, with respect to the making of any order or regulations.

(3) Accommodation shall only be made available under section 4[1] of the Act of 1946 to such extent as the Secretary of State may from time to time approve.

(4) Nothing in these regulations shall enable a Regional Authority to exercise the function of the Secretary of State under section 58(1) of the Act of 1946[2] with respect to the compulsory acquisition of land.

(5) Accommodation and services shall be made available at any hospital under either section 1[3] or section 2[4] of the Act of 1968 only to such extent as the Secretary of State may from time to time approve.

(6) The power of the Secretary of State under section 2(1) of the Act of 1973[5] shall be exercisable by a Regional Authority to such extent only as is necessary for the proper exercise, in relation to the region of that authority or anywhere outside that region in relation to which the Secretary of State has directed, of one or more other functions which the Secretary of State has directed the Regional Authority to exercise on his behalf.

(7) In exercising the duty under section 2(2)(c) of the Act of 1973[6] to provide ambulance services, each Regional Authority, in the region of which is included any of the areas set out in Part I of the Schedule[7] to these regulations, shall make arrangements for the function of providing an ambulance service for all such areas to be exercised on its behalf by such one of the four Regional Authorities, in the regions of which any such areas are included, as may be agreed between those four authorities and the arrangements made for the provision of such service, which shall be known as the London Ambulance Service, shall be such as have been approved by the Secretary of State and have been agreed between those four authorities;

Provided that the arrangements made may be varied at any time subject to such approval and agreement as aforesaid.

(8) Where arrangements are made with medical practitioners for the vaccination or immunisation of persons against disease, every medical practitioner providing general medical services shall so far as reasonably practicable, be given an opportunity to participate in those arrangements.

(9) The use of facilities for the purpose of private practice at accommodation provided by virtue of the Health Service Acts shall be permitted under section 43(2) of the Act of 1973[8] only to such an extent as,

[1] Now 1977 Act s. 63 (J.J.)
[2] Now 1977 Act s. 87 (1) (J.J.)
[3] Now 1977 Act s. 65 (J.J.)
[4] Now 1977 Act s. 66 (J.J.)
[5] Now 1977 Act s. 2 (J.J.)
[6] Now 1977 Act s. 3 (1) (e) (J.J.)
[7] Not here reproduced.
[8] Repealed by Health Services Act 1976 (J.J.)

and on such terms and conditions as, the Secretary of State may, from time to time, approve.

(10) Approval of a medical practitioner for the purposes of section 28(2) of the Mental Health Act 1959 as having special experience in the diagnosis or treatment of mental disorder shall only be given after having carried out such consultations and after having obtained such advice and for such period as the Secretary of State shall direct.

PART III

AREA AUTHORITIES IN ENGLAND

Functions to be made exercisable by Area Authorities in England

5.—(1) Subject to the provisions of paragraphs (2) and (3) of this regulation and of regulation 6 and to such limitations as the Secretary of State may direct with respect to the exercise of any function and in accordance with any directions he may give, every Regional Authority shall secure, by direction given by an instrument in writing, that each of the Area Authorities of which the area is included in its region shall subject as aforesaid and in accordance with any direction which may be given by the Secretary of State or, subject to any such directions, by the relevant Regional Authority exercise, as respects its area, such other parts of the region of the relevant Regional Authority as the relevant Regional Authority may direct, and anywhere outside its area that the Secretary of State may direct, such of the Secretary of State's functions relating to the health service as are specified in regulation 3.

(2) Each Regional Authority shall secure that no directions are given to any Area Authority, of which the area is included in its region, directing any such Area Authority to exercise any function under any provision specified in regulation 3(1)(*c*), 3(2)(*a*) or 3(3)(*i*).

(3) Each Regional Authority shall secure that no directions to exercise the function of providing ambulance services under the provision specified in regulation 3(3)(*c*) are given to any Area Authority, of which the area is included in its region, unless such Area Authority is one set out in Part II of the Schedule[1] to these regulations.

Restriction on exercise of functions by Area Authorities in England

6.—(1) The exercise of any function by an Area Authority in accordance with directions given by the relevant Regional Authority shall be subject to the provisions of regulation 4(2), 4(3), 4(5), 4(8), 4(9), and 4(10) in so far as they relate to the exercise of such function.

[1] Not here reproduced

(2) The power of the Secretary of State under section 2(1) of the Act of 1973[1] shall be exercisable by an Area Authority, to which directions for the exercise of such power have been given by the relevant Regional Authority, to such extent only as is necessary for the proper exercise, in relation to the area of that Area Authority or anywhere outside that area in relation to which the Secretary of State or the relevant Regional Authority has directed, of one or more other functions which the relevant Regional Authority has directed to be exercisable by the Area Authority.

PART IV

AREA AUTHORITIES IN WALES

Functions exercisable by Area Authorities in Wales

7. Subject to the provisions of regulation 8 and to such limitations as the Secretary of State may direct with respect to the exercise of any function and in accordance with any directions he may give, an Area Authority in Wales shall exercise on behalf of the Secretary of State, as respects its area and anywhere outside its area that the Secretary of State may direct, his functions relating to the health service under any provision specified in regulation 3 except such provisions as are specified in regulations 3(1)(*c*), 3(2)(*a*) and 3(3)(*i*).

Restrictions on exercise of certain functions by Area Authorities in Wales

8.—(1) The exercise of any function by an Area Authority in Wales in accordance with directions given in regulation 7 shall be subject to the provisions of regulation 4(2), 4(3), 4(5), 4(8), 4(9) and 4(10) in so far as they relate to the exercise of such function.

(2) Nothing in these regulations shall enable an Area Authority in Wales to exercise the functions of the Secretary of State under section 58(1) of the Act of 1946[2] with respect to the compulsory acquisition of land.

(3) The power of the Secretary of State under section 2(1) of the Act of 1973[3] shall be exercisable by an Area Authority in Wales to such extent only as is necessary for the proper exercise, in relation to the area of that Authority or anywhere outside that area in relation to which the Secretary of State has directed, of one or more other functions which the Secretary of State has directed the Area Authority to exercise on his behalf.

[1] Now 1977 Act s. 2 (J.J.)
[2] Now 1977 Act s. 87 (1) (J.J.)
[3] Now 1977 Act s.3. (J.J.)

PART V

REVOCATIONS

Revocation of regulations under Mental Health Act 1959

9. Regulations 3 and 5 of the Mental Health (Hospital and Guardianship) Regulations 1960(a) are hereby revoked.

EXPLANATORY NOTE

(This Note is not part of the Regulations.)

Directions are given in these Regulations by the Secretary of State to Regional Health Authorities and to Area Health Authorities in Wales to exercise, on his behalf, certain of his functions relating to the national health service and directions are given as to which of those functions Regional Health Authorities must, or must not, direct should be exercisable by Area Health Authorities in England.

The National Health Service (Venereal Disease) Regulations 1974 S.I. 1974 No. 29

Citation, commencement and interpretation

1.—(1) These regulations may be cited as the National Health Service (Venereal Diseases) Regulations 1974 and shall come into operation on 1st April 1974.

(2) The rules for the construction of Acts of Parliament contained in the Interpretation Act 1889(b) shall apply for the purposes of the interpretation of these regulations as they apply for the purposes of the interpretation of an Act of Parliament.

Confidentiality of information

2. Every Regional Health Authority and every Area Health Authority shall take all necessary steps to secure that any information capable of identifying an individual obtained by officers of the Authority with respect to persons examined or treated for any sexually transmitted disease shall not be disclosed except—

    (*a*) for the purpose of communicating that information to a medical practitioner, or to a person employed under the direction of a medical practitioner in connection with the treat-

(a) S.I. 1960/1241 (1960 II, p. 1903).   (b) 1889 c. 63.

ment of persons suffering from such disease or the prevention of the spread thereof, and

(b) for the purpose of such treatment or prevention.

EXPLANATORY NOTE

(This Note is not part of the Regulations).

The National Health Service (Venereal Diseases) Regulations 1968 (S.I. 1968/1624) imposed on hospital authorities an obligation to secure that information about venereal diseases obtained by their officers should be treated as confidential. These Regulations replace the 1968 Regulations which lapse on the repeal of section 12 of the National Health Service Act 1946 (c. 81), and impose similar obligations on health authorities. They also extend the scope of the obligation so as to include all sexually transmitted diseases and not only those commonly known as venereal diseases.

The National Health Service Functions (Administration Arrangements) Regulations 1974 S.I. 1974 No. 36

Citation and commencement

1. These regulations may be cited as the National Health Service Functions (Administration Arrangements) Regulations 1974 and shall come into operation on 14th February 1974.

Interpretation

2.—(1) In these regulations, unless the context otherwise requires:—
'the Act of 1946' means the National Health Service Act 1946(a);
'the Act of 1973' means the National Health Service Reorganisation Act 1973;
'Area Authority' means an Area Health Authority;
'Committee' means a Family Practitioner Committee;
'Regional Authority' means a Regional Health Authority;
'relevant Regional Authority' in relation to any Area Authority means the Regional Authority of which the region includes the area of the Area Authority in question;
and any other expression to which a meaning is assigned by the Act of 1946 has that meaning in these regulations.

(2) For the purposes of these regulations a Regional Authority is equivalent to another Regional Authority, an Area Authority is equivalent to another Area Authority and a Committee is equivalent to

(a) 1946 c. 81.

another Committee; but nothing in these regulations shall be construed as precluding a Regional Authority, an Area Authority or a Committee from acting by an agent where it is entitled so to act apart from these regulations.

(3) References in these regulations to any enactment shall include references to such enactment as amended by any subsequent enactment, order or regulations.

(4) The rules for the construction of an Act of Parliament contained in the Interpretation Act 1889(a) shall apply for the purposes of the interpretation of these regulations as they apply for the purposes of the interpretation of an Act of Parliament.

Arrangements by Regional Authorities for exercise of functions

3. Subject to any directions which may be given by the Secretary of State as to the exercise of any function exercisable by a Regional Authority by virtue of any direction given under section 7 of the Act of 1973,[1] any Regional Authority so directed to exercise any function may arrange with an equivalent body, a committee or sub-committee of such equivalent body, with another body of which the members consist only of the Regional Authority and equivalent bodies, or with an officer of an equivalent body or such other body as aforesaid, for the exercise of such function on its behalf.

Arrangements by Area Authorities for exercise of functions

4.—(1) Subject to the following paragraph of this regulation, to any directions which may be given by the Secretary of State, and, in the case of an Area Authority in England, to any directions given by the relevant Regional Authority with respect to the exercise of any function exercisable by virtue of a direction given under section 7(2) of the Act of 1973,[2] an Area Authority by which any function is exercisable by virtue of any provision of the Health Service Acts may arrange with an equivalent body, a committee or sub-committee of such equivalent body, with another body of which the members consist only of the Area Authority and equivalent bodies, or with an officer of an equivalent body or such other body as aforesaid, for the exercise of such function on its behalf.

(2) The duty of an Area Authority to make arrangements for the provision of general medical services, general dental services, general ophthalmic services and pharmaceutical services, in so far as such duty relates to—

    (*a*) the referral to the Medical Practices Committee of applications

---

(a) 1889 c. 63.

[1] Now 1977 Act ss. 13 to 18 (J.J.)   [2] Now 1977 Act s. 14 (J.J.)

for inclusion in a list of medical practitioners who undertake to provide general medical services;

(*b*) acceptance of applications for inclusion in a list of dental practitioners undertaking to provide general dental services or of persons undertaking to provide general ophthalmic services or pharmaceutical services; and

(*c*) any rights and liabilities arising in connection with any such applications or by virtue of inclusion in any such list as aforesaid;

shall be a function exercisable on behalf of the Area Authority, in accordance with regulations and any directions given by the Secretary of State, by the Committee established for the area of that Authority.

Arrangements by Family Practitioner Committees for exercise of functions

5.—(1) Subject to the following paragraph of this regulation and to any directions given by the Secretary of State, a Committee may arrange with an equivalent body, or another body of which the members consist only of the Committee and equivalent bodies, a sub-committee appointed by such equivalent body or an officer of any Area Authority which has established such equivalent body, for the exercise on its behalf of any function exercisable by the Committee.

(2) The functions of a Committee under section $7(3)(a)^1$ of the Act of 1973 in regard to the examination, checking and pricing of prescriptions for drugs, medicines and appliances supplied under arrangements made by an Area Authority for the provision of pharmaceutical services, shall be exercisable on behalf of a Committee established in England by the Prescription Pricing Authority**(a)** and on behalf of a Committee established in Wales by the Welsh Health Technical Services Organisation**(b)** and arrangements shall be made by Committees in accordance with directions given by the Secretary of State with respect to the exercise of such functions.

EXPLANATORY NOTE

(This Note is not part of the Regulations.)

These regulations make provision for functions relating to the National Health Service to be exercisable on each others behalf by bodies established under the National Health Service Reorganisation Act 1973.

(a) S.I. 1974/9.   **(b)** S.I. 1973/1624 (1973 III, p. 5070)
[1]Now 1977 Act s. 15

The National Health Service (Amendment of Trust Instruments) Order 1974 S.I. 1974 No. 63

Citation, commencement and interpretation

1.—(1) This order may be cited as the National Health Service (Amendment of Trust Instruments) Order 1974 and shall come into operation on 15th February 1974.

(2) In this order a reference to the holder of an office is a reference to the person who from time to time is the holder of that office, a reference to 'the Act' is a reference to the National Health Service Reorganisation Act 1973, and the expressions 'a charity', 'charity trustees' and 'trusts' have the same meaning as in the Charities Act 1960 (a).

(3) The rules for the construction of Acts of Parliament contained in the Interpretation Act 1889(b) shall apply for the purposes of the interpretation of this order as they apply for the purposes of the interpretation of an Act of Parliament.

Appointment of New Trustees

2. Where under the trusts of any charity connected with hospital purposes, not being a charity incorporated under the Companies Acts 1948 to 1967 or by charter, the charity trustees immediately before 1st April 1974 include the holder of an office connected with a Regional Hospital Board, a Hospital Management Committee (including a University Hospital Management Committee) or a Board of Governors which is not a preserved Board, those trustees shall instead include by virtue of this order the holder of such office as may be designated—

(*a*) where a charity trustee is the holder of an office connected with a Regional Hospital Board in England, by the Regional Health Authority the region of which includes all or most of the region of the Regional Hospital Board;

(*b*) where a charity trustee is the holder of an office connected with a Board of Governors which is not a preserved Board or a University Hospital Management Committee and the charity is wholly or mainly associated with a Teaching Hospital or University Hospital for which Special Trustees are appointed under section 29 of the Act[1] by the Area Health Authority which will be wholly or mainly responsible for that hospital, on the nomination of those Special Trustees.

(*c*) where a charity trustee is—

(i) the holder of an office connected with a Hospital Man-

(a) 1960 c. 58.   (b) 1889 c. 63.
[1] Now also 1977 Act s. 95 (J.J.)

agement Committee which is not a University Hospital Management Committee; or

(ii) the holder of an office connected with the Board of Governors of a Teaching Hospital or University Hospital Management Committee of a University Hospital for which Special Trustees have not been appointed.

and the hospital or hospitals with the purposes of which the charity is connected and which are controlled and managed by that Board or that Committee will be administered by more that one Area Health Authority after 1st April 1974, by those Area Health Authorities either jointly or severally, as they may agree;

(d) in any other case, by the Area Health Authority which will administer the hospital or hospitals with the purposes of which the charity is connected.

Vesting of Trust Property

3. Where immediately before 1st April 1974 any property belonging to a charity connected with hospital purposes is held as sole trustee or sole trustees by the holder or holders of an office or offices to which article 2 of these regulations applies, that property shall by virtue of this order vest (on the same trusts) on 1st April 1974 or on the date of designation, whichever is the later, in the holder or holders of the office designated under the provisions of article 2 of this order.

Exercise of Powers

4.—(1) Where immediately before 1st April 1974 any power (including a power to appoint trustees but not including any power by virtue of being a charity trustee thereof) with respect to a charity connected with hospital purposes, not being a charity incorporated under the Companies Acts 1948 to 1967 or by charter, is under the trusts of the charity vested in, or in the holder of an office connected with, a Regional Hospital Board, a Board of Governors which is not a preserved Board or a Hospital Management Committee (including a University Hospital Management Committee) that power shall, subject to paragraph (2) below, on 1st April 1974 vest—

(a) where the power is vested in, or in the holder of an office connected with, a Regional Hospital Board, in the Regional Health Authority the region of which includes all or most of the region of the Regional Hospital Board or, as the case may be, in the holder of an office connected with and designated by that Authority;

(b) subject to sub-paragraph (c) below where the power is vested in, or in the holder of an office connected with, a Hospital Management Committee (including a University Hospital

Management Committee) or a Board of Governors of a teaching hospital which is not a preserved Board—

    (i) where the power relates to a hospital or hospitals which will be administered by one Area Health Authority, in that Area Health Authority or, as the case may be, the holder of an office connected with and designated by that Authority;

    (ii) where the power relates to a hospital or hospitals which will be administered by more than one Area Health Authority, in those Area Health Authorities acting jointly or, as the case may be, the holder of an office connected with one of those Area Health Authorities designated jointly by those Authorities;

  (c) where the charity to which the power relates is wholly or mainly associated with a Teaching Hospital or University Hospital for which Special Trustees are appointed, a designation under sub-paragraph (b) above shall be made by the Authority or Authorities concerned, on the nomination of those Special Trustees.

(2) Where a designation of an officer is made after 1st April 1974, the vesting in that designated officer of the power referred to in paragraph (1) of this article shall take effect on the later date.

Designations

5. Any designations under this order shall be by instrument in writing.

Choice of Trustees, etc.

6. In making designations under this order a Regional Health Authority and an Area Health Authority, and in making nominations Special Trustees, shall secure that so far as is practicable the offices of the new trustees designated under this order or the offices of persons to whom powers are transferred by this order, shall correspond as closely as possible to the offices of the trustees, or of those persons, as they exist immediately before 1st April 1974.

EXPLANATORY NOTE

(This Note is not part of the Order).

Various trust instruments contain references to Hospital Authorities which are to be abolished under the National Health Service Reorganisation Act 1973 or to offices connected with them. This Order makes provision for those references to be replaced by references to Health Authorities and offices connected with them but does not alter any trust.

The National Health Service (Preservation of Boards of Governors) Order 1974 S.I. 1974 No. 281

Citation, duration and interpretation

1.—(1) This order may be cited as The National Health Service (Preservation of Boards of Governors) Order 1974 and shall come into operation on 31st March 1974.

(2) Unless previously revoked this order shall cease to have effect on the expiration of 5 years beginning with the date on which it is made.

(3) In this order 'the Act' means the National Health Service Re-organisation Act 1973.

(4) The rules for the construction of Acts of Parliament contained in the Interpretation Act 1889**(a)** shall apply for the purposes of the interpretation of this order as they apply for the purposes of the interpretation of an Act of Parliament.

Preservation of certain Boards of Governors of teaching hospitals

2. Section 14 (Abolition of Authorities) of the Act shall, while this order is in force, not apply to any Board of Governors of a teaching hospital mentioned in Schedule 1 to this order.

Scope of Order

3. The following provisions have effect in relation to a preserved Board and any person, thing, right, liability or other matter whatsoever connected with a preserved Board.

Repeals and amendments not to apply

4. So much of section 57(1) and (2) of, and schedules 4 and 5 to, the Act as repeals or amends enactments specified in Schedule 2 to this order shall not apply.

Modification of enactments otherwise repealed or amended

5. The enactments set out in column 1 in Schedule 3 to this order which are repealed or amended by the Act shall have effect with such modifications as are specified in column 2 of that schedule.

Provisions of Act to have effect with modifications

6. The enactments specified in column 1 of Schedule 4 to this order shall have effect with such modifications as are specified in column 2 of that schedule.

(a) 1889 c. 63.

Article 2

SCHEDULE 1

TEACHING HOSPITALS OF WHICH THE BOARDS OF GOVERNORS ARE PRESERVED

The Hospitals for Sick Children
The National Hospitals for Nervous Diseases
The Royal National Throat, Nose and Ear Hospital
The Moorfields Eye Hospital
The Bethlem Royal Hospital and the Maudsley Hospital
St. John's Hospital for Diseases of the Skin
The Royal National Orthopaedic Hospitals
The National Heart and Chest Hospitals
St. Peter's Hospitals
The Royal Marsden Hospital
Queen Charlotte's Hospital for Women
The Eastmen Dental Hospital

Article 4

SCHEDULE 2

REPEALS AND AMENDMENTS NOT TO APPLY.

THE PUBLIC HEALTH ACT 1936**(a)**

Section 169(1)	Removal to Hospital of Person suffering from Notifiable Disease
Section 244	Removal to Hospital of Person in Common Lodging House suffering from Notifiable Disease

THE NATIONAL HEALTH SERVICE ACT 1946**(b)**

Section 3(1)	Provisions of Hospital and specialist services
Section 7(1), (2), (3), (7), (8)(a), (9), (10) and (11)(a)	Endowments of Voluntary Hospitals vesting in Boards of Governors
Section 11(8) and (10)	Designation of teaching hospitals
Section 12(3)	Duties of Boards of Governors
Section 13	Legal Status of Boards of Governors
Section 14, as amended by section 9(1) of the Health Services and Public Health Act 1968**(c)**	Employment of Officers
Section 16(2)	Research
Section 54(1)(b)	Payments to Boards of Governors
Section 55(2), as amended by section 28(3) of the Health Services and Public Health Act 1968, and (4)	Accounts

(a) 1936 c. 49.   **(b)** 1946 c. 81.   **(c)** 1968 c. 46.

Section 60	Power of Trustees to make payments to Boards of Governors
Section 62	Provisions of Special Schools
Section 66, as amended by section 12 of the National Health Service (Amendment) Act 1949**(a)**	Qualifications and terms of service of officers
Section 72	Protection of members and officers
Schedule 3 Part IV, as amended by section 29 of, and Schedule 1 to, the National Health Service (Amendment) Act 1949 and section 78(2) of, and Schedule 4 to, the Health Services and Public Health Act 1968	Supplementary provisions relating to Boards of Governors

THE NATIONAL HEALTH SERVICE (AMENDMENT) ACT 1949

| Section 18(4) | Superannuation of officers |
| Section 25(2), as substituted by Schedule 7 to the Mental Health Act 1959**(b)** | Payment to officers of Boards of Governors |

THE NATIONAL HEALTH SERVICE ACT 1952**(c)**

| Section 7(6) | Reduction of sums otherwise payable by Boards of Governors to persons who may recover charges |

THE LANDLORD AND TENANT ACT 1954**(d)**

| Section 57(6) | Protection of Government Departments and Local Authorities applied to hospitals |

THE NURSES ACT 1957**(e)**

Section 13(1)	Expenditure for the purposes of training nurses
Section 14	Exclusions of right to receive contributions towards training of nurses
Section 33(1)	Definition of Boards of Governors and teaching hospital

THE MENTAL HEALTH ACT 1959

| Section 59(1)(*a*) | Definition of 'the Managers' |

THE RADIO-ACTIVE SUBSTANCES ACT 1960**(f)**

| Section 14(1) | Application of Acts to the Crown |

THE REDUNDANCY PAYMENTS ACT 1965**(g)**

| Schedule 3 Paragraph 2 | Reference to Board of Governors of a teaching hospital |

(a) 1949 c. 93.   **(b)** 1959 c. 72.   **(c)** 1952 c. 25   **(d)** 1954 c. 56
(e) 1957 c. 15   **(f)** 1960 c. 34.   **(g)** 1965 c. 62

THE BUILDING CONTROL ACT 1966(a)

Section 5(1)	Reference to body corporate constituted under section 11 of the National Health Service Act 1946

THE PARLIAMENTARY COMMISSIONER ACT 1967(b)

Schedule 3 Paragraph 8	Action on behalf of Secretary of State by Board of Governors of a teaching hospital not subject to investigation

THE LEASEHOLD REFORM ACT 1967(c)

Section 28(5)(d) and (6)(c)	Application to Boards of Governors

THE HEALTH SERVICES AND PUBLIC HEALTH ACT 1968

Section 6	Power of Board of Governors to administer services outside hospital
Section 29(1)	Regulation of financial arrangements
Section 34	Superannuation of officers of private hospitals used by the Board of Governors
Section 36(1)(a)(ii)	Payment of travelling and other allowances
Section 63(1)(a), (4) and so much of paragraph (8) as provides that 'Board of Governors of a teaching hospital' has the same meaning as in the National Health Service Act 1946	Instruction of officers

THE POST OFFICE ACT 1969(d)

Section 86(1)	So much of paragraph (a) of the definition of national health service authority as refers to the Board of Governors of a teaching hospital

THE ROAD TRAFFIC ACT 1972(e)

Section 156(1)(b), (2)(a) and (3)	Payments for treatment

Article 5

SCHEDULE 3

MODIFICATION OF ENACTMENTS OTHERWISE REPEALED OR AMENDED

THE NATIONAL HEALTH SERVICE ACT 1946 Section 57(1), amended by paragraph 32 of Schedule 4 to the Act	The amended provision shall have effect as if references to a Regional Health Authority included references to a preserved Board

(a) 1966 c. 27   (b) 1967 c. 13   (c) 1967 c. 88.   (d) 1969 c. 48.   (e) 1972 c. 20.

Schedule 3 Part III, repealed by Schedule 5 to the Act	The provision shall not be repealed but shall have effect as if for the words 'Regional Hospital Board for the area' there were substituted the words 'Regional Health Authority for the region'

THE NATIONAL ASSISTANCE ACT 1948(a)

Section 21(7)(c), amended by paragraph 44 of Schedule 4 to the Act	The amended provision shall have effect as if it included a reference to a Board of Governors of a teaching hospital

THE NURSES ACT 1957

Section 11(2)(c)(ii), amended by paragraph 71(2) of Schedule 4 to the Act	The amended provision shall have effect as if for sub-section 2(c)(ii) there were substituted the words '(2)(c)(ii) Boards of Governors of teaching hospitals situated in the region'
Section 16 amended by paragraph 75 of Schedule 4 to the Act	The provision as amended shall have effect as if it included a reference to a Board of Governors of a teaching hospital situated in the region
Section 33(2), repealed by Schedule 5 to the Act	The provision shall not be repealed but shall have effect as if for the word 'areas' there was substituted the word 'regions'
Schedule 2, paragraph 1(b) (Appointments by Boards of Governors), amended by paragraph 78(2) of Schedule 4 to the Act	The provision as amended shall have effect as if it included a reference to persons appointed by Boards of Governors of teaching hospitals situated in the region

THE PUBLIC RECORDS ACT 1958(b)

Schedule 1 as amended by paragraph 82 of Schedule 4 to the Act	The amended provision shall have effect as if references to Regional Health Authorities included references to preserved Boards

THE LOCAL GOVERNMENT ACT 1972(c)

Section 113(1A) (placing officers at the disposal of other authorities) added by paragraph 151(1) of Schedule 4 to the Act	The provision as added shall have effect as if references to a Regional Health Authority included references to a Board of Governors of a teaching hospital

(a) 1948 c. 29.   (b) 1958 c. 51.   (c) 1972 c. 70.

Article 6

SCHEDULE 4

PROVISIONS OF ACT TO HAVE EFFECT WITH MODIFICATIONS

PROVISIONS OF THE ACT	MODIFICATION;
Section 11[1] (Supply of goods and services by the Secretary of State)	
Section 12[2] (Supply of goods and services by Local Authorities)	References to a Health Authority shall include references to a preserved Board
Section 13[3] (Facilities for Voluntary Organisations and other bodies)	
Section 26(1)[4] (Power to make transfers of trust property)	
Section 29(2)[5] (Power of Special Trustees to hold trust property)	References to Special Trustees shall include references to preserved Boards
Section 45[6] (Overseas Aid)	The reference to an Area Health Authority shall include a reference to a preserved Board

EXPLANATORY NOTE

(This Note is not part of the Order.)

This Order preserves from abolition under section 14 of the National Health Service Reorganisation Act 1973 the Boards of Governors of the Teaching Hospitals specified in Schedule 1 (Article 2 of the Order) and applies in relation to these preserved Boards various statutory provisions with or without modification (Articles 4 to 6 and Schedules 2, 3 and 4).

The National Health Service (Remuneration and Conditions of Service) Regulations 1974 S.I. 1974 No. 296

1. These regulations may be cited as the National Health Service (Remuneration and Conditions of Service) Regulations 1974 and shall come into operation on 1st April 1974.

2.—(1) In these regulations, unless the context otherwise requires:—
'the Act' means the National Health Service Reorganisation Act 1973;

[1] Now 1977 Act s. 26 (J.J.)
[2] Now 1977 Act s. 28 (J.J.)
[3] Now 1977 Act s. 23 (J.J.)
[4] Now see also 1977 Act s. 92 (1) (J.J.)
[5] Now see also 1977 Act s. 95 (2) (J.J.)
[6] Now 1977 Act s 24 (J.J.)

'authority' means a Regional or Area Health Authority or a special health authority;

'officer' means an officer of an authority;

'negotiating body' means any body accepted by the Secretary of State as a proper body for negotiating remuneration and other conditions of service for officers or any class of officers.

(2) The rules for the construction of Acts of Parliament contained in the Interpretation Act 1889**(a)** shall apply for the purpose of the interpretation of these regulations as they apply for the purpose of the interpretation of an Act of Parliament.

3.—(1) Subject to paragraph (3) of this regulation, the remuneration of any officer who belongs to a class of officers whose remuneration has been the subject of negotiations by a negotiating body and has been approved by the Secretary of State after considering the result of those negotiations shall be neither more nor less than the remuneration so approved whether or not it is paid out of moneys provided by Parliament.

(2) Subject as aforesaid, where conditions of service, other than conditions with respect to remuneration, of any class of officers have been the subject of negotiations by a negotiating body and have been approved by the Secretary of State after considering the result of those negotiations, the conditions of service of any officer belonging to that class shall include the conditions so approved.

(3) The remuneration or other conditions of service approved under paragraphs (1) and (2) of this regulation may in the case of an individual officer or of officers of a particular description be varied by an authority only as may be provided for by directions given by the Secretary of State.

EXPLANATORY NOTE

(This Note is not part of the Regulations.)

These regulations provide for the determination of the remuneration or other conditions of service of officers employed by certain authorities in the National Health Service.

The National Health Service (Appointment of Consultants) Regulations 1974 S.I. 1974 No. 361

Citation and commencement

1. These regulations may be cited as the National Health Service (Appointment of Consultants) Regulations 1974 and shall come into operation on 1st April 1974.

(a) 1889 c. 63.

Interpretation

2.—(1) In these regulations, unless the context otherwise requires:—

'appropriate body' means any of the following bodies, namely, the Royal College of Physicians of London, the Royal College of Surgeons of England or its associated Faculties of Anaesthetists or Dental Surgery, the Royal College of Obstetricians and Gynaecologists, the Royal College of Pathologists, the Royal College of Psychiatrists or the Faculty of Radiologists whichever in the opinion of the Authority concerned is the most appropriate body having regard to the proposed appointment;

'Area Authority (Teaching)' means an Area Health Authority (Teaching);

'Authority' means a Regional Health Authority or Area Health Authority (Teaching) and includes Authorities acting jointly in accordance with regulation 6;

'Committee' means an Advisory Appointments Committee constituted in accordance with these regulations;

'consultant in the specialty' means a consultant specialising or who has recently specialised in the branch of medicine or dentistry with which the proposed appointment is concerned;

'lay member' means a person who is not a registered dental or medical practitioner or an officer of an Authority;

'member of the hospital staff' means, in relation to a medical appointment, a member of consultant status of the medical staff of a hospital in which an applicant will, if appointed to a post, be employed and, in relation to a dental appointment, a member of consultant status of a dental staff of such a hospital, or, if there is no dental staff, a member of consultant status of the medical staff of such a hospital;

'professional member' means, where a medical appointment is to be made a registered medical practitioner and, where a dental appointment is to be made, a registered dental practitioner;

'Regional Authority' means a Regional Health Authority;

'relevant Area Authority' means the Area Health Authority administering any hospital or hospitals in which an applicant will, if appointed to a post, be employed.

(2) Unless the context otherwise requires, any reference in these regulations to a numbered regulation is a reference to the regulation bearing that number in these regulations, and any reference in a regulation to a numbered paragraph is a reference to the paragraph bearing that number in that regulation.

(3) The rules for the construction of Acts of Parliament contained

in the Interpretation Act 1889(a) shall apply for the purposes of the interpretation of these regulations as they apply for the purposes of the interpretation of an Act of Parliament.

Appointments to which the regulations apply

3.—(1) The provisions of these regulations shall apply with respect to the appointment of any medical or dental officer to the post of consultant on the staff of any hospital in England providing hospital accommodation other than the appointment of any person in any of the classes specified in regulation 4.

(2) For the purposes of this regulation 'appointment' includes any appointment to a post, whether existing or new, and whether whole-time or part-time.

Exempted appointments.

4.—(1) The classes referred to in regulation 3 to which these regulations do not apply are:—

(a) professors, readers or other members of a medical or dental professorial unit of a University who will receive no remuneration (other than any distinction award) from the Authority for their hospital appointments;

(b) consultants who have reached the age of 65, or in the case of mental health officers as defined in the National Health Service (Superannuation) Regulations 1961(b) as amended(c), the age of 60, and who will receive no remuneration for the hospital appointments;

(c) clinical teachers who are already officers of any Area Authority (Teaching) and whose appointment is to be made by a Regional Authority primarily to enable them to give clinical instruction to students in a non-teaching hospital;

(d) persons who are primarily engaged in research which necessitates their appointment to the staff of a hospital and who will receive no remuneration (other than any distinction award) for that appointment from the Authority;

(e) persons to be appointed to posts which are, with the approval of the Secretary of State, expressly limited in duration;

(f) redundant officers whose employment, or whose last employment by an Authority (including a Regional Health Authority in Scotland or an Area Health Authority in Wales) is, or was, in a post as consultant;

(g) consultants employed in posts by an Authority who are transferred to the employment of another Authority with the

(a) 1889 c. 63.   (b) S.I. 1961/1441 (1961 II, p. 2824).
(c) The amending regulations are not relevant to the subject matter of these regulations.

approval of the Secretary of State as part of a local reorganisation to fill posts the duties of which are substantially the same as the posts in which they were employed by the Authority which originally employed them;

(*h*) persons employed by Universities or officers of the Medical Research Council or the Public Health Laboratory Board who are engaged in providing services for the National Health Service in posts equivalent to posts of consultant status, who are transferred to the employment of an Authority with the approval of the Secretary of State, to fill posts the duties of which are substantially the same as the posts in which they were employed immediately before the date of such transfer.

(2) In this regulation 'redundant officers' means persons whose employment has been terminated owing to redundancy or other local change of organisation and whose names have at the direction of the Secretary of State for Social Services, the Secretary of State for Scotland or the Secretary of State for Wales been notified to one or more Authorities as officers to whom this regulation applies; and 'employment' includes part-time employment, whether or not the officer is also employed by another Authority, but does not include employment in a post where the appointment was expressly limited in duration.

Advertisement of vacancy

5.—(1) Where an Authority proposes to make an appointment to a vacancy in any office to which these regulations apply, the Authority shall place an advertisement, specifying the exact nature of the appointment and the closing date for receipt of applications, in not less than two publications circulating throughout England and Wales which are commonly used for similar advertisements relating to the profession concerned:

Provided that where such advertisement is not reasonably practicable the Authority shall advertise the vacancy in such other publications as it considers appropriate.

(2) Any advertisement shall state the effect of paragraph 8 of Schedule 4 to these regulations.

(3) The Secretary of State may if he thinks fit authorise an Authority to dispense with the requirements of regulation 5 (1) in relation to an appointment to any post or class of post.

Constitution and procedure of Advisory Appointments Committees

6.—(1) For the purpose of filling each vacancy in any office to which these regulations apply an Advisory Appointments Committee shall be constituted—

(*a*) where the appointment is to be made by a Regional Authority in accordance with Schedule 1 to these regulations;

(*b*) where the appointment is to be made by an Area Authority (Teaching) in accordance with Schedule 2 to these regulations;

(*c*) where a Regional Authority or an Area Authority (Teaching) propose to appoint the same person to fill posts in hospitals in respect of which they respectively exercise functions, and agree not to constitute separate Committees but to act jointly, in accordance with Schedule 3 to these regulations.

(2) Where two or more Regional Authorities or two or more Area Authorities (Teaching) agree jointly to appoint the same person to two or more posts in hospitals in respect of which they respectively exercise functions as aforesaid they shall, instead of constituting separate committees, act jointly in all respects for the constitution of a single committee under Schedules 1, 2 or 3 hereto as the case may be.

(3) The provisions of Schedules 1, 2 and 3 hereto shall have effect subject to the general provisions as to Committees contained in Schedule 4 to these regulations.

Selection by Advisory Appointments Committees

7.—(1) The Authority shall refer to the Committee all applications received by the Authority on or before the closing date specified in the said advertisement and may also refer an application received after that date if the Authority is satisfied that there is a reasonable explanation for the failure to make such an application by such date.

(2) The Committee shall consider all applications so referred to them and they shall select from the applications the person or persons the Committee shall consider suitable for the appointment and submit the appropriate name or names to the Authority together with any comments they may wish to make.

(3) If in the opinion of the Committee none of the applicants is suitable for the appointment they shall so inform the Authority.

Appointment by Authority

8. An Authority shall not make an appointment to a vacancy to which these regulations apply except from persons selected by a Committee under regulation 7.

Travelling and subsistence expenses

9. Members of the Committee shall be entitled to receive from the Authority or, where Authorities are acting jointly, from the Authority to which nominations are required to be sent by paragraph 3 of Schedule

4 hereto, such payments in respect of travelling and subsistence expenses as are payable to members of the Authority performing an approved duty.

Revocation of regulations

10. The National Health Service (Appointment of Consultants) Regulations 1969(a) are hereby revoked.

Regulation 6(1)

SCHEDULE 1

APPOINTMENTS BY REGIONAL HEALTH AUTHORITIES

1. The Authority shall constitute a Committee of seven members.

2. Five members shall be nominated by the Authority and of those five—
   (a) one shall be a lay member and
   (b) four shall be professional members and of those four—
   (i) one shall be nominated after consultation with the University or Universities associated with the provision of hospital services in the region of the Regional Authority, and
   (ii) one shall be a consultant in the relevant speciality, not being employed within the region of the Regional Authority, nominated after consultation with the appropriate body.

3. Two members shall be nominated by the relevant Area Authority, and of those two one shall be a lay member and the other a member of the hospital staff.

Regulation 6 (1)

SCHEDULE 2

APPOINTMENTS BY AREA AUTHORITIES (TEACHING)

1. The Authority shall constitute a Committee of seven members.

2. All the members shall be nominated by the Authority and of those members—
   (a) two shall be lay members, one of whom shall be nominated after consultation with the University associated with the provision of hospital services in the area of the Authority, and
   (b) two shall be consultants in the relevant speciality who are not members of the hospital staff and of those two—
   (i) one shall be nominated after consultation with the Regional Authority of the region, and
   (ii) one, not being employed within the region of the Regional Authority, shall be nominated after consultation with the appropriate body;
   (c) one shall be a professional member of the hospital staff;

(a) S.I. 1969/163 (1969 I, p. 419)

(d) two shall be professional members nominated after consultation with the University associated with the provision of hospital services in the area of the Authority.

Regulation 6(1)

SCHEDULE 3

APPOINTMENTS BY REGIONAL AUTHORITIES OR AREA AUTHORITIES (TEACHING) ACTING JOINTLY

1. The Authorities acting jointly shall constitute a Committee.

2. Five members shall be nominated by the Authorities acting jointly and of those five—
   (a) two shall be lay members, one of whom shall be nominated after consultation with the University associated with the provision of hospital services in the area of the Authority, and
   (b) three shall be professional members and of those three—
       (i) one shall be a consultant in the relevant speciality, not being employed within the region of the Regional Authority, nominated after consultation with the appropriate body, and
       (ii) two shall be nominated after consultation with the University associated with the provision of hospital services in the area of the Authority.

3. Two professional members shall be nominated by each Authority at least one of whom shall be a member of the hospital staff.

Regulation 6(3)

SCHEDULE 4

GENERAL PROVISIONS APPLYING IN ALL CASES

1. Where the Authority or Authorities acting jointly are satisfied that one or more local Authorities have an interest in the appointment to be considered they may, after consultation with them, nominate to the Committee an additional member or members up to a maximum of five.

2. Where under paragraph 3 of Schedule 1 or paragraph 3 (b) of Schedule 3 members of a Committee are required to be nominated by the relevant Area Authority and more than one Area Authority is a relevant Authority each such Area Authority shall nominate a member of the hospital staff and the Committee shall be enlarged accordingly.

3. Nominations shall be sent to the Administrator of the Regional Authority or Area Authority (Teaching) or, where Authorities are acting jointly, to the Administrator or such Authority as they may agree. If the same person is nominated by more than one body, only the first of the nominations to reach the Administrator shall be valid and he shall forthwith inform the other body concerned accordingly, and that body shall then make a fresh nomination.

4. The Administrator shall provide the Committee with such clerical and other assistance as the chairman of the Committee may require.

5. The Chairman shall be one of the lay members of the Committee appointed by the Authority who shall be so designated by the Authority. The Chairman shall convene any meeting of the Committee and if present at any such meeting shall preside. If the Chairman is not present at any meeting of the Committee such member of the Committee as the members present choose shall preside.

6. The Committee shall meet to consider their selection and may adjourn as necessary: subject to the provisions of this Schedule the procedure of the Committee shall be such as they think fit.

7. The Committee may require any applicant to attend before them for the purpose of an interview.

8. The Committee shall disqualify any candidates who have canvassed any member of the Committee, the Regional Authority, Area Authority (Teaching) or any relevant Area Authority.

9. In the event of an equality of votes the chairman shall not have a second or casting vote.

10. The selection made by the Committee shall not be invalidated by any vacancy or failure to nominate or by any defect in the nomination or qualification of any member of the Committee.

11. No selection shall be made if more than one of the lay members nominated under Schedules 1, 2 or 3 or of the members nominated by any body under those Schedules is absent, or if more than two members in all are absent.

12. When in the opinion of an Authority or Authorities acting jointly more than one appropriate body is appropriate in relation to the appointment to be considered, the Authority or Authorities acting jointly may after consultation with the appropriate bodies nominate to a Committee a further consultant in a relevant speciality:

Provided that no more than one additional member shall be nominated in respect of each appropriate body.

EXPLANATORY NOTE

(*This Note is not part of the Regulations.*)

These Regulations make provision for the constitution by Regional Health Authorities and Area Health Authorities (Teaching) of Advisory Appointments Committees in relation to the appointment by them of consultants in hospitals.

The National Health Service (Appointment of Consultants) (Wales) Regulations 1974 S.I. 1974 No. 477

Citation and commencement

1. These regulations may be cited as the National Health Service (Appointment of Consultants) (Wales) Regulations 1974 and shall come into operation on 1st April 1974.

Interpretation

2.—(1) In these regulations, unless the context otherwise requires—

'appropriate body' means any of the following bodies, namely, the Royal College of Physicians of London, the Royal College of Surgeons of England or its associated Faculties of Anaesthetists or Dental Surgery, the Royal College of Obstetricians and Gynaecologists, the Royal College of Pathologists, the Royal College of Psychiatrists or the Faculty of Radiologists which, in the opinion of the Authority concerned, is the most appropriate body having regard to the proposed appointment:

'Authority' means an Area Health Authority for an area in Wales and includes Authorities acting jointly in accordance with regulation 6;

'Committee' means an Advisory Appointments Committee constituted in accordance with these regulations;

'consultant in the specialty' means a consultant specialising or who has recently specialised in the branch of medicine or dentistry with which the proposed appointment is concerned;

'lay member' means a person who is not a registered medical or dental practitioner or an officer of an Authority;

'professional member' means, where a medical appointment is to be made, a registered medical practitioner, and, where a dental appointment is to be made, a registered dental practitioner.

'Welsh Medical Committee' means the Committee recognised by the Secretary of State under section 8 of the National Health Service Reorganisation Act 1973[1] as being representative of the medical practitioners of Wales.

(2) Any reference in these regulations to a numbered regulation or schedule is a reference to the regulation or schedule bearing that number in these regulations.

(3) The Interpretation Act 1889(a) shall apply to the interpretation of these regulations as it applies to the interpretation of an Act of Parliament.

Appointments to which the regulations apply

3.—(1) The provisions of these regulations shall apply with respect to the appointment of any medical or dental officer to the post of consultant on the staff of any hospital in Wales providing hospital accommodation other than the appointment of any person in any of the classes specified in regulation 4.

(2) For the purposes of this regulation 'appointment' includes any

(a) 1889 c. 63.   [1] s. 19 of the 1977 Act (J.3.)

appointment to a post, whether existing or new, and whether whole-time or part-time.

Exempted appointments

4.—(1) The classes referred to in regulation 3 to which these regulations do not apply are:—

(*a*) professors, readers or other members of a medical or dental professorial unit of a University who will receive no remuneration (other than any distinction award) from the Authority for their hospital appointments;

(*b*) consultants who have reached the age of 65, or in the case of mental health officers as defined in the National Health Service (Superannuation) Regulations 1961(b) as amended(c), the age of 60, and who will receive no remuneration for their hospital appointments;

(*c*) persons employed by Universities or who are officers of the Medical Research Council or the Public Health Laboratory Board engaged in providing services for the National Health Service in posts equivalent to posts of consultant status, and who are transferred to the employment of an Authority with the approval of the Secretary of State, to fill posts the duties of which are substantially the same as the posts in which they were employed immediately before the date of such transfer.

(*d*) persons who are primarily engaged in research which necessitates their appointment to the staff of a hospital and who will receive no remuneration (other than any distinction award) for that appointment from the Authority;

(*e*) persons to be appointed to posts which are, with the approval of the Secretary of State, expressly limited in duration;

(*f*) redundant officers whose employment, or whose last employment by an Authority (or by a Regional Health Authority or an Area Health Authority outside Wales) is, or was, in a post as consultant; and

(*g*) consultants employed in posts by an Authority who are transferred to the employment of another Authority with the approval of the Secretary of State as part of a local reorganisation to fill posts the duties of which are substantially the same as the posts in which they were employed by the Authority which originally employed them.

(2) In this regulation 'redundant officers' means persons whose employment has been terminated owing to redundancy or other local change of organisation, and whose names have at the direction of the

(a) S.I. 1961/1441 (1961 II, p. 2824).
(b) The amending regulations are not relevant to the subject matter of the regulations.

Secretary of State for Social Services, the Secretary of State for Wales or the Secretary of State for Scotland been notified to one or more Authorities as officers to whom this regulation applies; and 'employment' includes part-time employment, whether or not the officer is also employed by another Authority, but does not include employment in a post where the appointment was expressly limited in duration.

Advertisement of vacancy

5.—(1) Where an Authority propose to make an appointment to a vacancy in any office to which these regulations apply, the Authority shall place an advertisement, specifying the exact nature of the appointment and the closing date for receipt of applications, in not less than two publications circulating throughout England and Wales, which are commonly used for similar advertisements relating to the profession concerned; provided that where such advertisements is not reasonably practicable the Authority shall advertise the vacancy in such other publications as they consider appropriate.

(2) Any advertisement shall state the effect of paragraph 7 of Schedule 3.

Constitution and procedure of Advisory Appointments Committees

6.—(1) For the purpose of filling each vacancy in any office to which these regulations apply, an Advisory Appointments Committee shall be constituted:—

(*a*) where the appointment is to be made by an Area Health Authority, in accordance with Schedule 1; or

(*b*) where the appointment is to be made by an Area Health Authority (Teaching), in accordance with Schedule 2.

(2) Where two or more Authorities agree to appoint the same person to fill posts in hospitals in respect of which they respectively exercise functions, they shall, instead of constituting separate Committees, act jointly in all respects for the constitution of a single Committee under Schedule 1 or 2 as the case may be.

(3) The provisions of Schedules 1 and 2 shall have effect subject to the general provisions as to Committees contained in Schedule 3.

Selection by Advisory Appointments Committees

7.—(1) The Authority shall refer to the Committee all applications received by the Authority on or before the closing date specified in the said advertisement and may also refer an application received after that date if the Authority are satisfied that there is a reasonable explanation for the failure to make such an application by such date.

(2) The Committee shall consider all applications so referred to them and they shall select from the applications the person or persons considered by them to be suitable for the appointment or appointments and submit the appropriate name or names to the Authority together with any comments they may wish to make.

(3) If in the opinion of the Committee none of the applicants is suitable for the appointment they shall so inform the Authority.

Appointment by Authority

8. An Authority shall not make an appointment to a vacancy to which these regulations apply except from persons selected by a Committee under regulation 7.

Travelling and subsistence expenses

9. Members of a Committee shall be entitled to receive from the Authority or, where Authorities are acting jointly, from the Authority to which nominations are required to be sent by paragraph 1 of Schedule 3, such payments in respect of travelling and subsistence expenses as are payable to members of the Authority performing an approved duty.

Employment by a single Authority of a consultant appointed jointly

10. Where two or more Authorities agree to appoint the same person to fill posts in hospitals in respect of which they respectively exercise functions, those Authorities shall make arrangements for the person appointed to be employed by such one of those Authorities as may be agreed, or failing agreement as the Secretary of State may direct and for the services of the person appointed to be made available to the other Authority or Authorities so as to enable all the posts to which he was appointed to be filled.

Regulation 6(1)

SCHEDULE 1

APPOINTMENTS BY AREA HEALTH AUTHORITIES

1. The Authority shall constitute a Committee of seven members.

2. Three members shall be nominated by the Authority and of these three, one shall be a lay member of the Authority, one shall be a lay member of another Authority, and one shall be a consultant employed within the area of the Authority.

3. One member shall be a consultant in the speciality not being employed in Wales nominated by the appropriate body.

4. One member shall be a professional member nominated by the Welsh National School of Medicine.

5. Two members shall be professional members employed within the area of another Authority in Wales nominated by the Welsh Medical Committee.

6. Where two or more Authorities (not including an Area Health Authority (Teaching)) decide jointly to constitute a single committee, in addition to persons nominated to that committee under paragraphs 3, 4 and 5 of this Schedule, each Authority shall nominate a lay member of the Authority and a consultant employed within the area of the Authority, and the Authorities shall jointly nominate a lay member of an Authority not included among them and the Committee shall be enlarged accordingly.

Regulation 6(1)

SCHEDULE 2

APPOINTMENTS BY AREA HEALTH AUTHORITIES (TEACHING)

1. The Authority shall constitute a Committee of nine members.

2. Three members shall be nominated by the Authority and of those three, one shall be a lay member of the Authority and two shall be consultants employed within the area of the Authority.

3. One member shall be a consultant in the speciality not being employed in Wales nominated by the appropriate body.

4. One member shall be a lay member nominated by the Welsh National School of Medicine.

5. Three members shall be professional members nominated by the Welsh National School of Medicine.

6. One member shall be a professional member employed within the area of another Authority nominated by the Welsh Medical Committee.

7. Where an Area Health Authority (Teaching) and one or more other Area Health Authorities decide jointly to constitute a single committee, in addition to persons nominated to that committee under paragraphs 3, 4, 5 and 6 of this Schedule, each Authority shall nominate a lay member of the Authority and a consultant employed within the area of the Authority and the Committee shall be enlarged accordingly.

Regulation 6(3)

SCHEDULE 3

GENERAL PROVISIONS APPLYING IN ALL CASES

1. Nominations shall be sent to the Administrator to the Authority, or where Authorities are acting jointly, to the Administrator to such Authority as they may agree; and, where the same person is nominated by more than one body, only the first of the nominations to reach the Administrator shall be valid and he shall forthwith inform the other body concerned accordingly, and that body shall then make a fresh nomination.

2B

2. The Chairman of the Committee shall be one of the lay members of the Committee nominated by the Authority who shall be so designated by the Authority. Where a Committee is constituted by two or more Authorities acting jointly, the Chairman shall be nominated by the Authority by which the person appointed will be employed under regulation 10.

3. The Chairman shall convene any meeting of the Committee and if present at any such meeting shall preside. If the Chairman is not present at any meeting of the Committee such member of the Committee as the members present choose shall preside.

4. The said Administrator shall provide the Committee with such clerical and other assistance as the Chairman may require.

5. The Committee shall meet to consider their selection and may adjourn as necessary; subject to the provisions of this Schedule the procedure of the Committee shall be such as they think fit.

6. The Committee may require any applicant to attend before them for the purpose of an interview.

7. The Committee shall disqualify any candidate who has canvassed any member of the Committee or of the Authority or Authorities concerned.

8. In the event of an equality of votes the Chairman shall not have a second or casting vote.

9. The selection made by the Committee shall not be invalidated by any vacancy or failure to nominate or by any defect in the nomination or qualification of any member of the Committee.

10. No selection shall be made, if more than one of the lay members nominated under Schedules 1 or 2 is absent, or if more than two members in all are absent.

11. Where in the opinion of the Authority more than one appropriate body is appropriate in relation to the appointment to be considered, the Authority may, after consultation with the appropriate bodies, nominate to a Committee a further consultant in the speciality: Provided that no more than one additional member shall be nominated in respect of each appropriate body.

EXPLANATORY NOTE

(*This Note is not part of the Regulations.*)

These Regulations make provision for the constitution by Area Health Authorities in Wales of Advisory Appointments Committees in relation to the appointment by them of consultants in hospitals.

The National Health Service (Professions Supplementary to Medicine) Regulations 1974 S.I. 1974 No. 494

Citation and Commencement

1. These Regulations may be cited as the National Health Service (Professions Supplementary to Medicine) Regulations 1974, and shall come into operation on the 1st April 1974.

Interpretation

2.—(1) In these Regulations, the expression 'local authority' has the meaning assigned to it in section 33 (1) of the National Assistance Act 1948**(a)**.

(2) For the purposes of these Regulations a person is registered in respect of a profession if his name is on the register maintained under the Professions Supplementary to Medicine Act 1960**(b)** by the Board for that profession.

(3) The rules for the construction of Acts of Parliament contained in the Interpretation Act 1889**(c)** shall apply for the purposes of the interpretation of these Regulations as they apply for the purposes of the interpretation of an Act of Parliament.

Employment of officers

3.—(1) No person shall be employed as an officer of an authority to which this regulation applies, in the capacity of chiropodist, dietician, medical laboratory technician, occupational therapist, orthoptist, physiotherapist, radiographer or remedial gymnast, unless:—

    (*a*) he is registeted in respect of the profession appropriate to the work for which he is employed; or

    (*b*) immediately before the 1st April 1974, he was an officer employed in the capacity of chiropodist, dietitian, medical laboratory technician, occupational therapist, orthoptist, physiotherapist, radiographer or remedial gymnast, within the meaning of regulation 2 of the National Health Service (Professions Supplementary to Medicine) Regulations 1964**(d)**, as amended**(e)** or was employed in such a capacity for the purposes of Part III of the National Assistance Act 1948 by a local authority or by a voluntary organisation acting on behalf of such an authority.

(2) The authorities to which this regulation applies are:—

    (*a*) Regional Health Authorities;

    (*b*) Area Health Authorities;

    (*c*) special health authorities.

EXPLANATORY NOTE

(This Note is not part of the Regulations.)

These Regulations prohibit the employment for the purposes of providing services under the national health service, as reorganised by

(a) 1948 c. 29.   (b) 1960 c. 66.   (c) 1889 c. 63.
(d) 1964/940 (1964 II, p. 2100).   (e) S.I. 1968/270 (1968 I, p. 806).

the National Health Service Reorganisation Act 1973, of chiropodists, dietitians, medical laboratory technicians, occupational therapists, orthoptists, physiotherapists, radiographers or remedial gymnasts unless they are registered under the Professions Supplementary to Medicine Act 1960 or were employed in such capacity immediately before 1st April 1974 in the national health service or local authority welfare services.

**The National Health Service (Speech Therapists)
Regulations 1974 S.I. 1974 No. 495**

Citation and commencement

1. These Regulations may be cited as the National Health Service (Speech Therapists) Regulations 1974, and shall come into operation on 1st April 1974.

Interpretation

2.—(1) In these Regulations, subject to the provisions of paragraph (2) of this regulation, expressions to which a meaning is assigned by the National Health Service Act 1946(a), as amended by the National Health Service Reorganisation Act 1973, have that meaning.

(2) In relation to Scotland, the expressions 'Regional Hospital Board', 'local health authority' and 'education authority' have the same meaning as in the National Health Service (Scotland) Act 1947(b).

(3) The rules for the construction of Acts of Parliament contained in the Interpretation Act(c) shall apply for the purposes of the interpretation of these Regulations as they apply for the purposes of the interpretation of an Act of Parliament.

Employment of Officers

3. No person shall be employed as an officer of an authority to which this regulation applies, in the capacity of a speech therapist, unless he satisfies one of the following conditions:—

(1) He holds a certificate issued by the College of Speech Therapists (hereinafter in this regulation referred to as 'the College').
  (*a*) certifying that he has attended a course of training, and passed an examination, approved by the Secretary of State; or
  (*b*) certifying that the College are satisfied that he has, in a country or territory outside the United Kingdom, attended a course of training and passed an examination recognised by the College and approved by the Secretary of State.

(a) 1946 c. 81.   (b) 1947 c. 27.   (c) 1889 c. 63.

(2) His name is included in a list, kept by the Secretary of State for Social Services or the Secretary of State for Wales, of persons not qualified in accordance with the foregoing provisions of this Regulation, who have satisfied the Secretary of State that their training and experience are adequate for employment as speech therapists.

(3) His name is included in a list of persons suitable for employment as speech therapists kept by the Secretary of State for Scotland or the Secretary of State for Northern Ireland.

(4) He was immediately before 1st April 1974 employed as a speech therapist:—
    (*a*) by a Regional Hospital Board or the Welsh Hospital Board; or
    (*b*) by a Board of Governors of a teaching hospital; or
    (*c*) by a local health authority or a local education authority; or
    (*d*) by a Regional Hospital Board, local health authority or education authority in Scotland; or
    (*e*) in the Northern Ireland health service.

4. The authorities to which the foregoing Regulation applies are:—
    (*a*) Regional Health Authorities;
    (*b*) Area Health Authorities;
    (*c*) special health authorities.

EXPLANATORY NOTE

(This Note is not part of the Regulations.)

These Regulations prescribe the conditions under which a speech therapist may be employed for the purposes of providing services under the national health service as reorganised by the National Health Service Reorganisation Act 1973.

The National Health Service Financial (No. 2) Regulations 1974 S.I. 1974 No. 541

Citation and commencement

1. These regulations may be cited as the National Health Service Financial (No. 2) Regulations 1974 and shall come into operation on 1st April 1974.

Interpretation

2.—(1) In these regulations, unless the context otherwise requires—
'the Act' means the National Health Service Act 1946;

'the Reorganisation Act' means the National Health Service Reorganisation Act 1973;

'auditor' means an auditor appointed by the Secretary of State under section 55(2)[1] of the Act;

'enactment' includes a provision in a Statutory Instrument;

'Health Authority' means a Regional or Area Health Authority;

"Prescription Pricing Authority' means the special health authority constituted by the Prescription Pricing Authority (Establishment and Constitution) Order 1974(a);

'Welsh Health Technical Services Organisation' means the special health authority constituted by the Welsh Health Technical Services Organisation (Establishment and Constitution) Order 1973(b);

(2) Unless the context otherwise requires, references in these regulations to an enactment shall be construed as references to that enactment as amended by any subsequent enactment.

(3) Unless the context otherwise requires, any reference in these regulations to a numbered regulation is a reference to the regulation bearing that number in these regulations, and any reference in a regulation to a numbered paragraph is a reference to the paragraph bearing that number in that regulation.

(4) References in any other regulations to the regulations revoked by these regulations or to any provision thereof shall be construed as references to these regulations or to the corresponding provision hereof, as the case may be.

(5) The rules for the construction of Acts of Parliament contained in the Interpretation Act 1889(c) shall apply for the purposes of the interpretation of these regulations as they apply for the purposes of the interpretation of an Act of Parliament.

Estimates

3.—(1) Subject to paragraph (5), each Regional Health Authority shall submit to the Secretary of State such estimates of such expenditure, income and capital receipts in such form, by such dates, for such financial years and accompanied by such relevant information as he may specify.

(2) The Secretary of State may approve any such estimates with or without modification and subject to such conditions as he thinks fit and may at any time vary such approval or conditions.

(3) Subject to paragraph (5), each Area Health Authority in England shall submit to the Regional Health Authority in whose region it is

(a) S.I. 1974/9 (1974 I, p. 14).   (b) S.I. 1973/1624 (1973 III, p. 5070).
(c) 1889 c. 63.

[1] Now 1977 Act s. 98 (1) (J.J.)

included, and each Area Health Authority in Wales shall submit to the Secretary of State, such estimates of such expenditure, income and capital receipts in such form, by such dates, for such financial years and accompanied by such relevant information as the Regional Health Authority or the Secretary of State may specify.

(4) Subject to regulation 4, the Regional Health Authority or the Secretary of State may approve any such estimates with or without modification and subject to such conditions as the Regional Health Authority or the Secretary of State thinks fit and may at any time vary such approval or conditions.

(5) A Regional Health Authority shall not be required to submit to the Secretary of State, an Area Health Authority in England shall not be required to submit to a Regional Health Authority, and in Wales shall not be required to submit to the Secretary of State, estimates of payments to be made by a Family Practitioner Committee to persons for the provision of services under Part IV of the Act or estimates of any sums which may be due from such persons in respect of that provision.

Community Health Councils

4. Modification under regulation 3(4) by a Regional Health Authority or the Secretary of State of the estimates of an Area Health Authority may include modification by the incorporation in or addition to those estimates of the approved estimates of such Community Health Council as they may respectively specify; and may incorporate arrangements with that Area Health Authority for the payment of sums equal to such expenses of that Community Health Council as are included in such approved estimates.

Standing Financial Instructions

5.—(1) Each Health Authority shall make and may from time to time vary Standing Financial Instructions for the regulation of the conduct of its members and officers in relation to all financial matters with which it is concerned including those relating to the provision of services to a Family Practitioner Committee.

(2) Each Health Authority shall incorporate in such Standing Financial Instructions such requirements as the Secretary of State may direct and may not vary such requirements otherwise than as such directions may provide.

Annual Accounts

6.—(1) Each Health Authority and body of Special Trustees shall transmit its annual accounts (including in the case of a Health Authority account in respect of any property held on trust, and in the case of an

Area Health Authority the annual accounts of any Family Practitioner Committee which it has established and the annual accounts of any Community Health Council whose approved estimates were the subject of a modification under regulation 4 of the estimates of that Area Health Authority) to the Secretary of State by such date after the end of each financial year and in such form as he, with the approval of the Treasury, may direct and each Area Health Authority and each body of Special Trustees in England shall send a copy of such accounts to the Regional Health Authority in whose region it is included.

(2) Each Health Authority and body of Special Trustees shall maintain such records relating to its accounts and shall comply with such conditions as to certificates relating to such accounts as the Secretary of State may direct.

Audit of Accounts

7.—(1) Each Health Authority and body of Special Trustees shall make available to an auditor at all reasonable times such books, accounts, vouchers and other documents of the Health Authority or body and their officers as the auditor may require on giving reasonable notice thereof in writing to the Health Authority or body.

(2) Each Health Authority shall require such member or officer (including an officer whose services are placed at the disposal of a Family Practitioner Committee or Community Health Council), each body of Special Trustees shall require such Special Trustee, and each Family Practitioner Committee shall require such member to attend before the auditor to give such information relating to the affairs of such Authority, body or Committee for the purpose of an audit as he may require on giving reasonable notice thereof in writing to such Authority, body or Committee.

Losses and damages

8. Where a loss occurs or a claim for damages or compensation is made against a Health Authority that Authority shall follow such procedures, maintain such records and make such reports in relation thereto as the Secretary of State may require.

Treasurer

9.—(1) Each Regional Health Authority shall appoint an officer as Regional Treasurer and each Area Health Authority shall appoint an officer as Area Treasurer.

(2) Without prejudice to the generality of the functions of officers of Health Authorities, the duties of the Regional Treasurer and the Area Treasurer shall include the provision of financial advice to the Health

Authority and its officers, supervision of the implementation of the Health Authority's financial policies, the design, implementation and supervision of systems of financial control and the preparation and maintenance of such accounts, certificates, estimates, records and reports as the Health Authority may require for the purpose of carrying out its duties under these regulations, and in the case of an Area Treasurer the like provision to the Family Practitioner Committee established by the Health Authority of which he is the Area Treasurer.

Dental Estimates Board

10.—(1) The Dental Estimates Board shall appoint as Financial Officer such person as may be approved by the Secretary of State.

(2) Without prejudice to the generality of the functions of officers of the Dental Estimates Board, the duties of the Finance Officer shall include the provision of financial advice to the Dental Estimates Board or any of its committees, the design, implementation and supervision of systems of financial control, and the preparation and maintenance of such accounts, certificates, estimates, records and reports as the Board may require for the purpose of carrying out its duties under these regulations.

(3) Regulations 3, 5, 6, 7 and 8 shall apply to the Dental Estimates Board as if it were a Regional Health Authority.

Prescription Pricing Authority

11. Regulation 10 shall apply to the Prescription Pricing Authority with the substitution of the words 'Prescription Pricing Authority' for the words 'Dental Estimates Board'.

Welsh Health Technical Services Organisation

12.—(1) The Welsh Health Technical Services Organisation shall appoint its Chief Administrator as its Chief Financial Officer.

(2) Regulation 9(2) shall apply to the Chief Financial Officer as if he were the Area Treasurer of an Area Health Authority in Wales.

(3) Regulations 3, 5, 6, 7 and 8 shall apply to the Welsh Health Technical Services Organisation as they apply to an Area Health Authority in Wales.

Revocation

13. Part III of the National Health Service (Executive Councils and Dental Estimates Board) Financial Regulations 1969(a) and the National Health Service Financial Regulations 1974(b) are hereby revoked.

(a) S.I. 1969/1581 1969 III, p. 5047).   (b) S.I. 1974/282.

EXPLANATORY NOTE

(This Note is not part of the Regulations.)

These regulations supersede with corrections the National Health Service Financial Regulations 1974 which have not yet come into operation. They provide for the preparation, the submission for approval and the approval of estimates of income and expenditure by Area Health Authorities and Regional Health Authorities. They also provide for any approvals to be subject to conditions and modifications; require annual accounts to be kept and audited and standing financial instructions to be prepared to govern the conduct of members and staff of those authorities. Provision is also made to apply the regulations as appropriate to Special Trustees, the Prescription Pricing Authority and the Welsh Health Technical Services Organisation as well as to the Dental Estimates Board. The Health Authorities are also required to appoint a Treasurer whose duties are set out and to keep such accounts of losses or claims for damages as they may be required to do.

APPENDIX D

SUNDRY DEPARTMENTAL CIRCULARS

In this Appendix, I have left those circulars I have quoted virtually unannotated, i.e. I have left them in the form in which they were originally published. Of course the guidance and instructions contained therein must be read in the light of the re-organisation with the change from hospital management committees to Area Health Authorities etc., and in the light of the now existing provisions in statutes and statutory instruments. So far as I am able to trace they are all still operative at the date of writing.[1]

CLAIMS AND LEGAL PROCEEDINGS

(*Text of circulars R.H.B.* (49) 128 *and H.M.* (54) 32)

1. It was stated in H.M.C.(48)51, B.G.(48)55 that a further Memorandum would be sent to Boards and Committees in regard to actions in respect of rights or liabilities accrued or incurred *after* the appointed day. This Memorandum primarily deals with this class of case.

2. The rights and liabilities arising in connection with the control and management of a hospital obviously cover a wide range of matters and where legal advice becomes necessary the authority should place the matter in the hands of solicitors. The procedure to be followed in this respect is discussed in paragraph 4 of this Memorandum.

3. Attention is particularly drawn to section 13 of the National Health Service Act 1946, under which Boards, notwithstanding that they are exercising functions on behalf of the Minister, and Committees, notwithstanding that they may be exercising functions on behalf of the Regional Hospital Board, are entitled to enforce any rights acquired, and are liable in respect of any liabilities incurred (including liabilities in tort), in the exercise of those functions, in all respects as if the Board or Committee were acting as a principal, and all proceedings for the enforcement of such rights and liabilities, shall be brought by or against the Board or Committee in their own name. The functions of the Boards and Committees are, of course, regulated by the National Health Service (Functions of Regional Hospital Boards, etc.) Regulations 1948. The Minister is advised that, having regard to the provisions

[1] September 1977

of section 13, proceedings should in regard to the matters falling within that section, be brought by or against Boards or Committees, and that the Ministry should not be made a party to the proceedings. In cases, therefore, where legal proceedings are threatened it is desirable that the claimant's solicitor should be informed, if an opportunity occurs, of the view taken as to the correct defendant, and the plaintiff would seem to be under no disadvantage if he sues the Board or Committee and not the Minister. In cases, however, where, through ignorance of the correct procedure or otherwise, the Ministry is sued instead of the Board or Committee, the matter should, unless the plaintiffs' solicitor is prepared to amend the proceedings, be brought at once to the notice of the Ministry, as it will probably be necessary, in a High Court case, to issue a summons under Order XVI[1] of the Rules of the Supreme Court for striking out the Ministry from the proceedings and substituting the appropriate Board or Committee.

4. In the case of non-teaching hospitals, it is difficult to be precise as to the steps to be taken to secure legal representation, but the Minister visualises that claims against authorities will generally be made against the Hospital Management Committee and that the Committee will instruct solicitors to deal with the matter. The case may, however, have been dealt with in its early stages by the Regional Board's solicitor and it may, therefore, be more convenient for him to deal with the matter to its conclusion, although the proceedings may be instituted against the Committee. Again if the Board have the services of a full-time salaried solicitor, the appropriate course may well be for that solicitor to deal with the case and for the matter to be referred to him when the intervention of a solicitor becomes necessary. The arrangements to be made will be largely a matter of agreement between the authorities, with due regard to considerations of expense. The Minister would, generally speaking, regard it as undesirable that in an action against one authority the point should be taken that the function was being exercised by another authority. Similarly, as regards claims by an authority, while, if the matter clearly arises out of a function of the Committee, the action will normally be brought in the name of the Committee and conducted by the Committee's solicitor, there may well be cases where the matter is best handled by the Board's solicitor
In the case of teaching hospitals these complications do not arise.

As indicated later in this Memorandum, there may be exceptional cases involving matters of importance where it will be appropriate for the Solicitor to the Ministry of Health to act in the matter although the proceedings are in the form by or against a Board or Committee.

5. It is indicated in para. 6 of R.H.B.(49)127; H.M.C.(49)107;

[1] Now Order 15, r. 6.

B.G.(49)112 that the authority there given to effect settlement of claims where the sum involved does not exceed £500, is subject to the provisions of this Memorandum. The authority there given must be read in the light of the following observations because it is not intended that in all cases, however important, the authority's legal advisers shall be at liberty to carry through the procceedings without reference to the Ministry merely because a settlement out of court is not proposed. Without attempting to give an exhaustive list of cases on which the Ministry should be consulted, it is clear that reference should be made to the Minister in regard to the following matters:

(a) Cases involving the construction of the Act and the Regulations thereunder. In such cases it will be appreciated that the Ministry are likely to have views as to the proper construction and may indeed have acted on a view contrary to that taken by the authority's legal advisers.

(b) Cases where an application is being threatened for leave to apply for a writ[1] of mandamus, prohibition or certiorari against the authority.

(c) Cases involving legal questions of first-class importance although not falling within (a) or (b). A case falling under this category would be one involving the respective liabilities of the hospital authority and a medical practitioner in respect of an injury suffered by a patient, which it was proposed to treat as a test case and might be suitable to take to the Court of Appeal or even the House of Lords.

In cases of the above category the Ministry should be consulted, particularly as to Counsel to be employed, and there may be cases where it is thought desirable for the Solicitor to the Ministry of Health to deal with the case in order that a Law Officer of the Crown can be briefed to argue the case.

The Ministry should be advised immediately of any case where damages are awarded against a Board or Committee by a Court, together with any recommendations of the Board or Committee, in order that the question of an appeal may be considered.

6. An important class of case with which the authority will be concerned are claims by a patient in respect of alleged negligence by a member of the nursing staff or by the doctor or doctors who attended to the case. Ordinarily where the claim is based on negligent treatment by a nurse, it is to be expected that the authority will be sued as her employer and that the nurse will not be made a separate defendant. If,

---

[1] *Sic*; should read 'an order' since orders were substituted for the old prerogative writs (except *habeas corpus*) by the Administration of Justice (Miscellaneous Provisions) Act 1938.

however, the nurse is joined in the proceedings the authority are authorised to see to her defence, if she so desires, and in such cases the solicitor acting for the authority would normally act for the defendant nurse as well. There may, of course, be cases where the nurse has acted quite outside the scope of her authority or for other reasons ought to be left to conduct her own defence. If such a position appears to arise. the case should be referred to the Ministry for consideration.

The position as regards a doctor, whether he is a resident medical officer or a visiting specialist practitioner, is somewhat different. In these cases, in view of the somewhat conflicting authorities as to the liability of a hospital for negligent treatment by medical practitioners, it is likely that the doctor will be sued as well as the authority, even though the doctor may be a resident medical officer employed at a salary. In these cases the doctor will normally be represented by solicitors instructed by his defence organisation.

Generally speaking, whatever the form of the proceedings, authorities are not authorised to undertake the defence of hospital doctors who may be sued in respect of alleged negligence and in the normal case, should, if it is sought to make them liable for negligent acts of a doctor, take such steps as are open to them under the Law Reform (Married Women and Tortfeasors) Act 1935, to obtain a contribution from him in respect of damages that may be recovered.[1]

7. Section 21 of the Limitation Act 1939, which provides that action shall not be brought against public authorities except where commenced within one year of the event complained of, should not be relied on except with the approval of the Ministry.

(Section 21 of the Limitation Act 1939, has been repealed as from June 4th, 1954, by the Law Reform (Limitation of Actions, etc.) Act, 1954, and the Minister has instructed hospital authorities to plead statutory limitation automatically without reference to him. Where the time for bringing proceedings in respect of a cause of action expired before June 4th, 1954, the Minister has indicated that any proceedings commenced on or after that date should be dealt with as follows:

(a) *proceedings commenced before the end of 1954 should be dealt with in accordance with paragraph 7* (supra).

(b) *in proceedings commenced after the end of 1954 which would be time-barred if the new periods of limitation were applicable, the limitation should be pleaded automatically without reference to the Ministry.*

(c) *in proceedings commenced after the end of 1954 which would not be time-barred if the new periods were applicable, the limitation*

---

[1] But see now Ministry Circular H.M. (54) 32 which indicates that medical practitioners who belong to a defence organisation should not ordinarily be brought in as third parties for the purpose.

should not be pleaded without the approval of the Ministry.[1])

8. Authorities will from time to time have to initiate proceedings. In such circumstances, they should take action as indicated in paragraph 4.

9. In respect of road accident cases treated in hospitals, the special statutory rights to recover

(a) from vehicle drivers, the cost of emergency treatment, and

(b) from insurance companies, the cost of subsequent in-patient and out-patient treatment to the amounts provided for in section 36 (3) of the Road Traffic Act 1930, as enacted in section 33 of the Road and Rail Traffic Act 1933,

are, since the appointed day, exercisable by Boards of Governors and Hospital Management Committees: see the amendment of the Road Traffic Acts 1930 and 1934, made by the Tenth Schedule to the National Health Service Act 1946, and paragraph 5 (9) of the National Health Service (Functions of Regional Hospital Boards, etc.) Regulations 1948. The amendment of section 36 (2) of the Road Traffic Act 1930, by section 33 of the Road and Rail Traffic Act, 1933, and the right to obtain information from the police under section 17 (1) of the Road Traffic Act, 1934, will be noted.

11.[2] Except in cases being dealt with by insurers, authorities will be handling the payment of workmen's compensation to former employees of pre-1948 authorities. They should take the action which is necessary from time to time in relation to such payments (*e.g.*, enquiries as to employment, medical examinations) and should, as may be necessary, place the cases in the hands of solicitors. In the consideration of any proposals for lump sum settlements, enquiry should be directed to (a) the use which is proposed to be made by the workman of the lump sum, (b) his position apart from the compensation, and any provisional settlement should be referred to the Ministry for consideration.

September 15*th*, 1949

LEGAL PROCEEDINGS

(Text of circular H.M. (54) 32)

Summary: The present policy of taking legal action to secure contributions from doctors in respect of whose negligence successful claims may be brought against hospitals authorities is to be modified. In future, where any doctor who may be liable is a member of a Defence Society and that body accepts responsibility for him, any payment made to the plaintiff is to be apportioned between the doctor(s) and the hospital authority as agreed privately between them or, in default of agreement, in equal shares.

---

[1] Ministry Circular H.M. (54) 73. The reader should also refer to pp. 266–273.
[2] *Sic.* no para. 10

1. As Boards and Committees are aware, it has been the Minister's policy (see paragraph 6 of R.H.B. (49) 128) that where proceedings are brought against a hospital authority and/or a doctor employed by them for alleged negligence by the doctor the authority should not undertake the defence of the doctor and that if it is sought to make them liable for negligent acts of a doctor employed by them, they should normally take such steps as are open to them under the Lew Reform (Married Women and Tortfeasors) Act, 1935, to obtain a contribution from him in respect of damages which may be recovered. It has been represented to the Minister that this policy may tend to prejudice that successful conduct of the defence which is in the interest of doctor and hospital authority alike. The Minister has therefore reviewed the position in consultation with representatives of the profession and the Defence Societies and has agreed with them the revised procedure set out in this memorandum.

2. Actions may be brought against the hospital authority alone, or against one or more members of their medical staff alone, or against the hospital authority and a member or members of the medical staff jointly. The arrangements set out in the two succeeding paragraphs will apply to all three classes of action so far as regards medical practitioners who are to be defended by the Medical Defence Union or the Medical Protection Society or the Medical and Dental Defence Union of Scotland. As regards medical practitioners not so defended the arrangements hitherto in force should continue even in actions in which the new arrangements are being applied to other parties defended as above.

3. Where both the hospital authority and one or more hospital doctors are cited by the plaintiff as defendants, the following arrangements will apply:

    (1) Any defendant may, on notifying the other(s), decide to settle the case out of court at any stage in the proceedings, but if he does so, he must accept sole liability for payment of the whole sum for which the case is settled; but each defendant shall pay his own costs.

    (2) If the defendants decide to explore the possibility of settlement out of court (and a settlement is ultimately effected), the payment made to the plaintiff shall be borne between the defendants agreed to be liable in such proportion as they may agree between themselves or, in default of agreement on the proportions in equal shares.

    (3) If the defendants agree to defend the action in court the procedure should be as follows:

        (a) the defendants should try to agree before the action comes to court on the proportion in which any dam-

ages and costs which may be awarded to the plaintiff
shall be borne between them;

(b) if this proves impossible, the defendants should try to
reach such agreement after the trial of the action;

(c) failing agreement under (a) or (b) the damages and costs
awarded to the plaintiff shall be borne in equal shares
between such defendants as are held liable.

(4) In exceptional circumstances where some important legal or
professional principle is involved, any defendant may give
notice to the other before delivery of defence by either party
that sub-paragraphs (1)–(3) above shall not apply; and the
normal legal processes will then be open to all defendants.

4. Where either the hospital authority alone or a hospital doctor
alone is cited as defendant in the action, the defendant will have
complete discretion whether to fight the action or to attempt to settle
it out of court. The hospital or the doctor soley cited shall not take
legal action to obtain a contribution from the other, nor cite the other
unless requested so to do when the request shall be conceded forthwith
The Defence Societies recognise, however, that there will be cases
where, although one of their members has not been cited, they might
properly be asked to make a contribution towards any payment made
by the hospital authority to the plaintiff, because the action or inaction
of the practitioner in question was a material factor in the negligence
complained of. Conversely, in actions in which a hospital doctor alone
is cited, there may be circumstances in which the Defence Society asks
the hospital authority to make a similar contribution. In either case
the procedure should follow the principles set out in paragraph 3 (2)
and (3) above, as if the party not cited were a defendant.

5. The success of the new arrangements set out above clearly depends
on mutual confidence between the defendants and a fully co-operative
attitude on the part of both parties from the beginning, and hospital
authorities are urged to bear this in mind. There should be full consultation at the request of either party in the formulation of the defence.
In any case where, in accordance with paragraph 4, there is a possibility
of a contribution being requested from a hospital authority or a doctor
who has not been cited, full information about the incident and the
possibility of such a request should be exchanged at the earliest opportunity, which normally should be as soon as the Statement of
Claim has been delivered, and in event not later than delivery of
Defence.

6. The principles of paragraph 5 of R.H.B. (49) 128 (which require
hospital authorities to obtain the Minister's prior authority to settling
any case out of court for a sum exceeding £500 plus costs and also to

consult the Minister on cases raising certain major legal issues) continue to apply. Where, however, in a case to be settled out of court, the sum to be paid is apportioned between a hospital authority and one or more members of its medical staff, the Minister's authority need be obtained only where the sum apportioned to the hospital authority (not the total sum) exceeds £500.

7. It has been the normal practice of the Defence Societies to claim the protection of section 21 of the Limitation Act 1939, where action is not commenced within one year of the occurrence of the cause of action. Hospital authorities should, as hitherto, not plead this section except with the Minister's prior approval. No liability under paragraphs 3 or 4 for any damages or costs, other than his own costs, should be regarded as falling on any doctor where the hospital authority or the Minister is satisfied that exemption from liability could be successfully claimed under section 21.

8. The provisions of this circular should be applied to all proceedings, which are commenced on or after the 1st day of April, 1954, and also if it is agreed by, or on behalf of, the hospital authority and the doctor or doctors concerned, to any proceedings which are pending on that date and in which judgment has not been given.

March 29th, 1954.

N.B.—By a subsequent circular, H.M. (54) 43, the Minister has extended the arrangements to dentists belonging to Defence Societies.

PSYCHIATRIC HOSPITAL SERVICES

(Text of circular H.M. (61) 110)

Supply of Information about Psychiatric Patients engaged in Legal Proceedings

1. Hospitals will sometimes be asked to disclose the statutory documents authorising the detention in hospital of a patient suffering from mental disorder. Advice on the procedure which should be used in dealing with such requests is contained in paragraph 3 of H.M. (59) 88 and in paragraphs 263–6 of the memorandum on Parts I, IV to VII and IX of the Mental Health Act 1959, which was enclosed with H.M. (60) 69.

2. Requests for the supply of other information about psychiatric patients should be dealt with on the lines indicated in H.M. (59) 88, which applies to hospital patients generally. The following additional considerations arise, however, in connection with mentally disordered patients:

(*a*) Where the consent of the patient is needed to the disclosure of information the doctor in charge of the patient's treatment should be consulted first, even though the patient may, in fact, be prepared to give his consent; if the doctor considers that the patient's mental condition is such as to cast doubt on his ability to manage his own affairs, the hospital should also consult the patient's solicitors or his nearest relative before disclosing any information. In any event, where solicitors are known to be acting for the patient, the patient should be advised to consult them before giving his personal consent to disclosure by the hospital. If the patient's affairs are subject to control by the Court of Protection the Receiver's advice should be obtained; if some financial matter is at stake, and although there is doubt as to the patient's ability to manage his own affairs, no Receiver has been appointed, the Court of Protection should be consulted.

(b) Paragraph 4 of H.M. (54) 88 recommends that where medical matters are involved the medical staff should be consulted before information is disclosed. In the case of mentally disordered patients information such as the facts and dates of admission or discharge may also have clinical significance, and if such information is requested the doctor in charge of the patient's treatment should be consulted.

3. Paragraph 8 of H.M. (59) 88 is cancelled.

REPATRIATION OF MENTALLY DISORDERED ALIENS

4. Paragraphs 277 and 278 of the Memorandum on Parts I, IV to VII and IX of the Mental Health Act 1959 (H.M. (60) 69) give guidance on the procedure to be adopted for the repatriation in certain circumstances of aliens receiving in-patient treatment for mental illness.

5. Difficulty has arisen in some cases because hospital authorities have made firm arrangements for the removal of patients without first providing the Home Office with sufficient information to enable the Secretary of State to make an order for removal under section 90 of the Mental Health Act.

6. Application to the Home Office is unnecessary if the patient (whether or not accompanied by an escort) is able and willing to travel, powers of detention are not required, and suitable arrangements for the journey have been made. In every other case, however, proposals for the removal of an alien should be made in writing to the Home Office (Aliens' Department, D.M. Group). Hospitals should confirm that the alien is receiving treatment for mental illness as an in-patient; indicate whether it is in the patient's interest to remove him and, if so, why;

and say what arrangements have been, or could be, made for the patient's care and treatment abroad and also what approach has been made to the Consulate for passports, visas, etc. It will be helpful to tell the Home Office what travel arrangements are proposed and whether any necessary escort can be provided; but travel reservations should not be confirmed until the Home Office has decided, in consultation as necessary with the Ministry of Health, whether an authority under section 90 should be issued or whether the patient should be repatriated under other powers.

7. The Home Office do not wish to be informed of the admission or, except in the above circumstances, of the subsequent movements of alien psychiatric patients (Board of Control Circular No. 1017 was cancelled by H.M. (60) 69).

INSPECTION BY H.M. INSPECTORS OF FACTORIES OF WORKSHOPS IN PSYCHIATRIC AND OTHER HOSPITALS

8. The statutory powers of H.M. Inspectors of Factories to inspect workshops in psychiatric hospitals where patients only are engaged in manual labour (the only hospital staff being those having care of patients) lapsed on November 1st, 1960, with the dissolution of the Board of Control. In future Factory Inspectors will visit only on request.

9. Hospitals should make use of the services of Inspectors to ensure that a high standard of safety, health and welfare is maintained in those workshops previously subject to inspection. The circumstances in which it might be appropriate to seek their assistance include:

    (*a*) The setting up of a new workshop.

    (*b*) The introduction of moving machinery or of a potentially dangerous process into an existing workshop.

    (*c*) The occurrence of an accident resulting in serious personal injury, where the advice of a factory inspector might be of value.

10. Requests for visits should be addressed to the appropriate District Inspector of Factories, who will make any written report direct to the Hospital Authority requesting the visit.

11. Similar arrangements with the Inspectors of Factories should be made for other types of hospitals in which patients are engaged in manual labour under comparable conditions.

12. The Inspectors of Factories' statutory powers to enter and inspect hospital laundries, electrical stations and places where hospital staffs are engaged in manual work are unaffected.

INDIAN AND PAKISTANI NATIONALS

13. Though the arrangements whereby the Board of Control was notified of the admission to hospital of mentally disordered nationals of India and Pakistan are no longer in force, the Minister is confident that hospitals will give every assistance if approached direct by the Medical Adviser to the High Commissioner for India or by the High Commissioner for Pakistan about individual Indian or Pakistani patients. The High Commissioner for India is particularly concerned with the welfare of students and, in this connection, his medical adviser would be glad to be informed (at India House, Aldwych, London, W.C.2) of any Indian student whose stay in hospital as a psychiatric patient (whether informally or under compulsory powers) is longer than a few weeks.

November 22nd, 1961

CUSTODY OF UNOFFICIAL FUNDS AND PATIENTS' MONIES

(Text of circular H.M. (62) 2)

Unofficial Funds

1. It often happens that unofficial funds, for example, money collected by a League of Friends or a chaplain, or subscriptions to a sports club, are left in a hospital safe or other place of security on hospital premises. There is no objection of principle to this, and where it is simply a matter of the occasional use of the safe for overnight security the arrangement can be informal, provided it is made clear that the Exchequer is not to be held liable for any loss whatever the cause.

2. Where, however, unofficial funds are deposited as a regular arrangement or for any length of time, certain more formal safeguards are necessary to protect the Exchequer against, for example, claims for reimbursement of unofficial funds stolen while in the hospital safe. The details of the safeguards are a matter for individual authorities to settle, but the Minister thinks it right to set out the main points to be covered. The following list of precautions has been drawn up with this in mind and the Minister asks authorities to ensure that their arrangements give at least this degree of protection.

    (i) A written agreement absolving the Board or Committee from responsibility for any loss should be obtained from the individual or organisation concerned. The appendix to this memorandum sets out a form of agreement which might be modified to suit individual circumstances.

(ii) The name of the organisation and of its financially responsible officer should be recorded in the minutes of the Board or Committee.

(iii) Boards and Committees should see that the amounts of unofficial cash in their care do not become too large, *e.g.*, by fixing an upper limit for each organisation in relation to its function and to the banking facilities conveniently available.

(iv) Boards and Committees should endeavour, as far as practicable, to ensure that members of their staff responsible for the handling of official cash do not at the same time hold an office of financial responsibility in any organisation whose funds are deposited within the hospital.

(v) Persons responsible for unofficial cash should be required, before handing it over for safe keeping, to secure it, *e.g.*, in a locked box or sealed packet, in such a way that it can readily be identified as their property and so as to guard against unauthorised interference.

3. There is no objection to National Savings stamps or cash for stamp schemes being kept in hospital safes, provided the consent of the hospital secretary or other responsible officer is obtained, and he is kept informed of the amounts deposited. Such lodgments are regarded by the National Savings Committees as their representative's personal responsibility to them, and it is to the representative, and not to the Savings Committee, that the hospital authority should look for any necessary indemnity.

Patient's Monies

4. This memorandum supersedes R.H.B. (49) 28/H.M.C. (49) 20/B.G. (49) 22 which dealt with the custody of patients' monies, and R.H.B. (50) 28/H.M.C. (50) 27 which dealt with the safe custody of money belonging to mentally subnormal patients. The following arrangements for safe custody are intended to apply to money belonging to all patients.

5. Patients should be warned that the Board or Committee cannot accept responsibility for cash or valuables not deposited for safe custody.

6. Cash accepted for safe custody should, except as indicated in paragraph 7 below, be paid to the Exchequer Bank Account and treated for funding purposes as Exchequer Cash and for accounting purposes as 'Other Creditors'. The liability to the patient is the exact amount accepted for safe custody.

7. If a patient hands over or accumulates more than £100 and maintains such a balance for three months, an appropriate amount should be reserved for the patient's immediate needs and the rest should be

deposited in a Trustee or Post Office Savings Bank or a Bank Deposit Account subject to the following conditions:

(a) if the patient is capable of understanding the transactions involved, he should be encouraged to open an account in his own name and be given any necessary help in opening and operating it. Savings Bank books or other documents relating to patients' accounts must be kept in a safe place;

(b) if the patient is incapable of understanding the transactions or is unwilling to open an account even with assistance, his money should be paid into a Patients' Savings Account, opened in the name of the hospital authority and operated by nominated officers. Interest on the account should be divided among all the participating patients, having regard to the sum deposited by each. The Minister is advised that it is illegal for interest on a bulk account for patients to be appropriated to the non-Exchequer funds of the hospital for the benefit of patients generally. If the hospital authority, in operating such an account, wishes to go beyond the limits imposed by the Savings Bank authority on sums deposited, it should apply for approval to the National Debt Commissioners.

8. Paragraph 7 is not applicable when action has been or needs to be taken to protect the patient's estate under Part VIII of the Mental Health Act 1959. H.M. (60) 80 gives advice on this part of the Mental Health Act and on the circumstances in which the management of a mentally disordered patient's affairs should be referred to the Court of Protection.

9. Repayments to a patient of sums accepted under paragraph 6 should be made from the Chief Financial Officer's Imprest Acccount, or from a patient's money Imprest Account reimbursed solely by duly authorised payments from the main account of the Board or Committee. All cash received from or on behalf of patients should be banked and any disbursements to them or on their behalf should be made as above and not from cash received from patients.

A proper discharge should be secured for all payments; if there is any possibility that the suitability of a patient's signature as a discharge might be questioned , the payment should be certified by an independent witness. All transactions should be subject to the supervision and overall responsibility of the Chief Financial Officer. The advice given in paragraph 8 of the Appendix to H.M. (56) 85 should also be considered.

10. Every patient who has handed over money to the hospital and who is capable of understanding the transactions involved should be informed, at least annually, of the total amount held for him. If he requests a detailed account he should be given it. Patients' Savings Books

should be submitted annually to the Post Office Savings Bank for the addition of accrued interest.

January 5th, 1962.

APPENDIX TO H.M. (62) 2

FORMS OF AGREEMENT RELATING TO DEPOSIT OF MONIES OR OTHER PROPERTY

1. Deposit by an individual

To the...(Board) (Committee)

In consideration of the consent given by you to the deposit by me in your custody from time to time, without benefit or reward to you, of such monies, chattels and other property as you may at your discretion permit to be so deposited,

I, (*name*)..of (*address*)......................

....hereby undertake and agree

    (1) not to make any claim against you in respect of any loss, damage or expense arising in any circumstances whatsoever from or in connection with any such deposit;

       and

    (2) to keep you indemnified from and against all actions, claims, costs and expenses arising as aforesaid which may be brought or made against you or incurred by you.

            Dated the....................day of..........................19......

Signed in the presence of

Name ....

Address ....

....

Occupation ....

                         Depositor's Signature
        Note: The depositor should sign over
              a sixpenny postage stamp.[1]

2. Deposit by an organisation

To the...(Board) (Committee)

The (*name of organisation*)...

(hereinafter called 'the Society'), by (*name of authorised officer*)..................

.... of (*address*) ....

duly authorised in that behalf, in consideration of the consent given by you to the deposit by the Society in your custody from time to time, without benefit or reward to you, of such monies, chattels and other property as you may at your discretion permit to be so deposited, hereby undertake and agree

    (1) not to make any claim against you in respect of any loss, damage or expense arising in any circumstances whatsoever from or in connection with any such deposit;

       and

---

[1] A sixpenny stamp is no longer necessary, the fixed stamp duty on agreements under hand having been abolished.

(2) to keep you indemnified from and against all actions, claims, costs and expenses arising as aforesaid which may be brought or made against you or incurred by you.

Dated the.....................day of........................19.........

Signed in the presence of

Name ....

Address ....

....

Occupation ....

Signature of Society's authorised agent.

Note: The Society's authorised agent should sign over a sixpenny postage stamp.[1]

SCOTTISH HOSPITAL SERVICE

LEGAL DOCUMENTS OF PATIENTS: HOSPITAL STAFF RESPONSIBILITIES

S.H.M. 58/80 (*being text of circular issued by the Department of Health for Scotland, now the Scottish Home and Health Department*).

1. Hospital medical and nursing staff are from time to time asked to sign as witnesses documents which have been signed by patients, *e.g.*, patients' wills, etc. It has become clear that current practice varies as between hospitals and that in many cases hospital staff are in doubt as to whether or not they should act as witnesses. The purpose of this memorandum is to give guidance on this topic.

2. Generally it is accepted as a duty of all citizens to assist the course of law by witnessing signatures to documents when required. Hospital staff should accordingly be encouraged to help patients in every reasonable way in the execution of a will or other legal document, particularly in cases where the patient is seriously ill. Similarly, hospital authorities should allow facilities for the signing of such documents at any time, even if not in visiting hours.

3. Where arrangements are being made for a deed to be signed by a patient and the medical officer concerned with his treatment is of the view that the patient does not realise or is incapable of realising the nature of the act of signing and of its consequences the medical officer or hospital staff should decline to witness, and the Solicitor or other persons presenting the will or other document for signature should be informed of the reason for so doing: in addition the medical officer should make a notation in the case records giving the reasons for his views and, if possible, obtain confirmation of such opinion from another medical officer.

---

[1] A sixpenny stamp is no longer necessary, the fixed stamp duty on agreements under hand having been abolished.

4. Where a patient reaches hospital and is in possession of a will this should under no circumstances be given to any relative of the patient. The patient's consent should be obtained to the sending of the will to his/her banker or lawyer. If this cannot be done then the will should be retained in safe custody by the hospital authorities.

5. Should any member of the hospital staff have doubts regarding the execution of a will or other legal document, advice can be obtained from —[1]

6. Boards should ensure that hospital staff are aware of their responsibilities in these matters.

Department of Health for Scotland,
Edinburgh, 1. *November 28th*, 1958.

STAFF: CONDITIONS OF SERVICE

Machinery for dealing with Disciplinary Cases
(*Text of circular R.H.B.* (51) 80)

The attached memorandum on the procedure for dealing with disciplinary cases in the National Health Service is forwarded for the attention of Regional Hospital Boards, Hospital Management Committees and Boards of Governors, Pending the conclusion of a Whitley agreement on the subject, Boards and Committees are asked to take steps to ensure that their practice in this matter is governed by the principles and procedure set out in the memorandum.

August 8th, 1951.

MEMORANDUM

1. This memorandum is concerned with procedure for dealing with disciplinary cases involving members of the staffs of Regional Hospital Boards, Boards of Governors, Hospital Management Committees, Executive Councils and other employing authorities consitituted under the National Health Service Act, 1946 (apart from the machinery for the termination of the appointment of a consultant, which is set out in paragraph 16 of the Terms and Conditions of Service of Hospital Medical and Dental Staff). This subject has been considered by the General Whitley Council but up to the present no agreement has been reached and there is no generally agreed procedure for dealing with cases that arise.

2. In these circumstances the Minister thinks that some general interim guidance would be appropriate, and this memorandum sets out lines of procedure which in his opinion should govern the practice of employing authorities in this matter. The procedure suggested should,

---

[1] Here I have omitted address of Scottish legal officer concerned.

of course, be regarded as provisional, pending agreement on the Whitley Council, and is subject to review in the light of Whitley agreement. Employing authorities are accordingly asked to review their own procedure for dealing with cases of discipline and see whether it can be improved on the lines indicated in the following paragraphs.

3. The procedure is intended for cases where the more serious forms of disciplinary action are involved, and not for minor matters where for instance all that is needed is a word from the officer's immediate superior. It provides machinery for appeal to the employing authority for officers who are aggrieved, or opportunities for personal hearing, if so desired, before a final decision is reached. But it is perhaps unnecessary to say that, although satisfactory appeal machinery is very important, what is more important is a sound practice for dealing with cases at an early stage.

4. All procedure should provide for proper warning, wherever possible, of serious matters likely to involve disciplinary action, and for a right of appeal to the employing authority, or opportunity for personal hearing, before a final decision is reached. It is important to ensure, not only that justice is done and injustice avoided, but also that justice is seen to be done. The existence of a regular procedure is a valuable safeguard of this.

In reviewing their own procedure employing authorities are asked to bear these principles in mind and to follow them in making any adaptation of their own practice that may be necessary in the light of this memorandum.

5. There are broadly two types of case and different provision needs to be made for each.

(i) Employees whose employment can be terminated by an individual officer of the authority or by a committee or sub-committee of the employing authority under delegated powers;

(ii) Employees whose employment can be terminated only by a decision of the full employing authority.

6. *Employees whose employment can be terminated by an individual officer or by a committee or sub-committee of the employing authority under delegated powers.*

An employee of a Regional Hospital Board, Hospital Management Committee, or Board of Governors, an Executive Council, the Dental Estimates Board, or a Joint Pricing Committee, who is aggrieved by disciplinary action, including dismissal, should have the right of appeal to his employing authority. The authority should from amongst its own members set up an appeals committee to hear the appeal and the employee should have the right of appearing personally before the committee, either alone, or with a representative of his professional organisation or trade union, or with a friend not appearing in a professional capacity. This appeal committee should not include any members directly involved in the circumstances leading to the disciplinary action or, where disciplinary action taken by a committee or sub-committee of the authority is the subject of appeal, members of that committee or sub-committee. The report of the committee should be submitted to the full employing authority who should thereupon reach a decision on the case.

It is important that appeals should be made and disposed of quickly and time limits would be appropriate. It is suggested that any appeal should be lodged within three weeks of the receipt by the employee of notice of the disciplinary action, and the hearing should take place within five weeks of the receipt of the appeal.

7. *Employees whose employment can be terminated only by a decision of the full employing authority.*

This should be taken to include the authority's more senior grades, *e.g.*, senior professional (including nursing), administrative, or technical staff, whether or not the employing authority has developed powers of dismissal or disciplinary action to a committee or sub-committee. (In the case of such staff the Minister considers that the authority should never have devolved power of dismissal to a particular officer, and they should review any decision they have taken as regards devolution of the power to a committee or sub-committee so as to assure themselves that such devolution is appropriate. It should in any case not be a function of a House Committee in a hospital.)

If circumstances arise which might lead to disciplinary action, including dismissal, no decision in regard to the matter should be taken by the employing authority without affording the employee an opportunity of being heard. The employee should have the right of appearing personally at the hearing, either alone, or with a representative of his professional organisation or trade union, or with a friend not appearing in a professional capacity. At the hearing no member of the authority who is directly involved in the circumstances that appear to indicate the need for disciplinary action should have a part in the decision which the employing authority must thereupon make.

8. These arrangements do not prejudice the right of the employing authority to take immediate action (whether by suspension from duty or by dismissal) where this is required in cases of a very serious nature.

9. The appeal procedure which has been suggested is for appeal to the employing authority. In this paragraph, and throughout the memorandum, the term 'employing authority' is used to mean the authority whose function it is to appoint and dismiss employees of the grade in question. The procedure does not provide any *right* of appeal to any

other authority beyond the employing authority. If an aggrieved employee after having exhausted the appeal procedure within his employing authority seeks to appeal to some authority beyond the immediate employing authority and applies, for instance, to the Minister or, in the case of Hospital Management Committee staffs, to the Regional Hospital Board, it is for the Minister, or the Board, at their discretion to decide what they shall do in regard to the application. Further consideration would depend upon the circumstances as they were found in the particular case: it would be for the Minister, or the Board, to decide, and their intervention could not be claimed as a matter of right by the individual employee. In exercising discretion in such circumstances a Board should bear in mind that it is desirable that appeals be heard by persons who have not taken a direct part in the original decision against which the appeal is made.

MEDICAL AND DENTAL STAFF

DISCIPLINARY PROCEEDINGS IN CASES RELATING TO HOSPITAL MEDICAL AND DENTAL STAFF

(Text of circular H.M. (61) 112)

Summary—Guidance is given on the procedure to be followed in serious disciplinary cases involving hospital doctors or dentists.

General

1. This memorandum sets out lines of procedure which, in the Minister's opinion, should govern the practice of hospital employing authorities in handling serious disciplinary charges, for example, where the outcome of disciplinary action could be the dismissal of the medical or dental officer concerned, and for cases of this kind applies the guidance contained in R.H.B. (51) 80 but replaces that contained in H.M. (56) 98. The lines of procedure proposed are designed to ensure that justice is done and injustice avoided both to the practitioner and to the public.

2. The arrangements described below do not prejudice the right of the authority to take immediate action (*e.g.*, suspension from duty) where this is required in cases of a very serious nature.

3. There are broadly three types of case which may involve medical or dental staff:

    (*a*) Cases involving personal conduct;

    (*b*) Cases involving professional conduct;

    (*c*) Cases involving professional competence.

It is for the authority to decide into which category the case falls.

Cases involving personal conduct

4. In cases involving personal conduct, the position of a doctor or

dentist is no different from that of other hospital staff. Accordingly the provisions from time to time applicable to hospital staff generally apply in such cases. These are at present those set out in the memorandum attached to R.H.B. (51) 80, of which a copy is reproduced as an appendix.[1] These provisions are, however, currently under review.

Cases involving Professional Conduct and Professional Competence

(i) *Preliminary Investigation — Establishment of prima facie case*

5. The first step when an incident occurs or a complaint is made involving the professional conduct or competence of a medical or dental officer should be for the Chairman of the Board or Hospital Management Committee (whichever is the appointing authority) to decide whether there is a prima facie case, which, if well founded, could result in serious disciplinary action such as dismissal. Such preliminary enquiries, if any, as are necessary before this decision is reached should be in the hands of the Senior Administrative Medical Officer on behalf of a Regional Hospital Board or of the Secretary on behalf of a Board of Governors or Hospital Management Committee, whichever is the appointing authority. In appropriate cases the legal adviser or solicitor to the Board should be called in to assist. Where the matter arises from an incident for which an accident report has been made in accordance with H.M. (55) 66, the Chairman before reaching his decision should have regard to the accident report but normally no subsequent use should be made of the report in the proceedings except insofar as it is used by the appointing authority's solicitors in preparing the case to be presented to the investigating panel (see paragraph 8 below).

6. Unless the Chairman decides forthwith that there is no prima facie case the doctor or dentist should be warned in writing immediately of the nature of the incident which has been alleged or of the complaint which has been made, and that the question of an enquiry which might lead to serious disciplinary action is under consideration. Copies of all relevant correspondence should be sent to the practitioner and he should be informed that any comments made by him will be placed before the Chairman and any investigating panel which may be appointed. The practitioner should be given reasonable time to make representations and to seek advice, if he so wishes, before any final decision is taken on whether an enquiry is necessary.

7. If, on considering the allegation or the complaint made and the practitioner's comments, if any, in reply to the written warning given in accordance with paragraph 6, the Chairman decides that a prima facie case exists and that there is a dispute as to the facts, the Board or Committee should proceed to an enquiry as in paragraphs 8–15. If the Chair-

---

[1] For text of memorandum see R.H.B. (51) 80 on pp. 736–739

man decides that a prima facie case exists, but there is no substantial dispute as to the facts, any subsequent disciplinary action which the Board or Committee may take should comply with the guidance contained in the memorandum attached to R.H.B. (51) 80 (see appendix).[1] An enquiry on the lines laid down in paragraphs 8–15 below will normally be unnecessary also where, in a matter affecting the practitioner's professional conduct or competence, the facts in question have been the subject of a criminal charge on which he has been found guilty in a court of law.

(ii) *Enquiry*

8. An investigating panel, the composition of which should differ with the type of enquiry, should be set up by the authority responsible for appointing the practitioner. No member of the panel should be associated with the hospital in question. In all cases the panel should be small, normally of three persons including a legally qualified chairman, not being either an officer of the Ministry of Health or a member or officer of the Board or Committee concerned, who will be nominated in each case which arises by the Minister from a panel appointed by the Lord Chancellor. Payment should be made by the Board to the chairman at the rate of . . . .[2] for each day on which the investigating panel sits. This fee covers any preparatory work required and any time spent on preparation of reports. Travelling and subsistence expenses of both the chairman and members of the panel shall be payable in accordance with the National Health Service (Travelling Allowances, etc.) (No. 2) Regulations, 1961 (S. I. 1961 No. 1792). In cases involving professional conduct, the members other than the chairman should contain an equal proportion of professional and lay persons, unless the charges relate only to relationships between a doctor or a dentist and his professional colleagues, when it would clearly be appropriate to have a panel wholly or predominantly of professional members apart frôm the chairman. In cases involving solely professional competence, all the other members should be professionally qualified and it will probably be appropriate that at least one of their number should be in the same speciality as the practitioner whose professional competence has been called in question, and it may sometimes be appropriate that one of them should be a practitioner from another hospital in the same grade. Before the professional members are chosen there should be consultation with the Joint Consultants Committee. In the case of a dental officer the appointment of the professional members should be made after consultation with the Hospitals Group of the British Dental Association.

9. The terms of reference of the panel should include the nature of the incident or complaint against the practitioner who should be informed

[1] For H.M. (51) 80, see pp. 736–739. [2] Amount here omitted as subject to alteration.

of the setting up of the panel and its terms of reference and given not less than twenty-one days notice in order to prepare his case. He should be provided as soon as possible with copies of any correspondence or written statements made. A copy of the list of witnesses referred to in paragraph 10 and the main points on which they can give evidence should be furnished to the practitioner as long as possible before the hearing if he so requests unless for any exceptional reason the chairman of the panel gives authority for the names of witnesses not to be provided in advance of the hearing.

10. It is important that the enquiry should elicit all the relevant facts of the case. A list of witnesses should be drawn up with the main points on which they can give evidence; in the case of a Regional Hospital Board this task might with advantage be undertaken by the Legal Adviser or Solicitor to the Board, assisted by the Senior Administrative Medical Officer. Subsequently at the hearing the case should be presented by the Legal Adviser or Solicitor who should conduct an examination of the witnesses before the investigating panel. In the case of a Board of Governors or a Hospital Management Committee, these tasks would no doubt be undertaken by the Board's or Committee's Solicitor acting on the instructions of the Board which will normally be given through their Secretary.

11. The practitioner should have the right to appear personally before the investigating panel and to be represented (legally or otherwise) and to hear all the evidence presented to the panel. He should have the right to cross-examine all witnesses and to produce his own witnesses, and they and he may also be subjected to cross-examination. The question of what is to happen upon any application for adjournment in the event of the illness or unavoidable absence of the practitioner or any witness should be a matter for the Chairman to decide in accordance with the normal procedure for similar enquiries.

12. The procedure and rules as regards the admission of evidence before the investigating panel should be determined by the chairman who may, if he wishes, hold a preliminary meeting with the parties (or their representatives) for the purpose.

13. The report of the investigating panel should be divided into two parts. The first part should set out the Committee's findings on all the relevant facts of the case but contain no recommendations as to action. The second part should contain a view as to whether the practitioner is at fault and may, at the request of the authority appointing the panel, contain recommendations as to disciplinary action. In no circumstances should the investigating panel itself be given disciplinary powers.

14. The panel should send the practitioner a copy of the first part of their report and should allow a period of fourteen days for the sub-

mission to them of any proposals for corrections of fact or for setting out in greater detail the facts on any particular matter which has arisen. It would be for the panel to decide whether to accept any proposed amendments and whether any further hearing was necessary to enable them thus to decide. Subject to this procedure, the facts as set out in the panel's report should be accepted as established in any subsequent consideration of the matter.

15. The Board or Committee should then receive the report of the investigating panel and decide what action to take. In the event of the investigating panel finding that the practitioner is at fault, the substance of their views on the case and recommendations in the second part of their report should be made available to him in good time before the meeting of the Board or Committee and he should be given the opportunity to put to them any plea which he may wish to make in mitigation before they reach any conclusion as to action.

16. **Rights of certain officers under Section 16 of the Terms and Conditions of Service of Hospital Medical and Dental Staff.**

This memorandum is without prejudice to the provisions of Section 16 of the Terms and Conditions of Service of Hospital Medical and Dental Staff, relating to a consultant or senior hospital medical or dental officer who considers that his appointment is being unfairly terminated.

REPORTING OF ACCIDENTS IN HOSPITALS

(*Text of Ministry circular H.M.* (55) 66)

1. From time to time accidents or other untoward occurrences arise at hospitals which may give rise to complaints followed by claims for compensation or legal proceedings, and which may also call for immediate enquiry and action to prevent a repetition. Though comparatively few in number, such occurrences cover a very wide range: cases where the treatment of a patient is unsuccessful through some mishap, cases such as a patient's being given wrong medicine or burnt with a hot water bottle, and accidents to patients, visitors or staff such as a fall on hospital premises.

2. Unless statements about any occurrences of this kind are obtained at the time, and a report based on the statements drawn up at once, it is often difficult to find out the facts, secure evidence of how the incident occurred, or determine responsibility for it; and this gives rise to particular difficulty for hospital solicitors when complaints or claims are made, or legal proceedings commenced without previous warning. Similarly without a contemporaneous report it may not be possible to take action urgently needed to prevent the occurrence of the same mishap again.

2C

3. It is therefore most desirable — as is already the practice of many hospitals — that a brief report should be prepared by the Secretary of the Board of Governors or Hospital Management Committee as soon as possible after any occurrence of the kind in question, giving the name of any person injured, the names of all witnesses, details of the injuries and the full facts of the occurrence and of the action taken at the time. This report should have attached to it a statement from each of the persons present in the form attached to this memorandum. It should be regarded as the responsibility of the senior hospital officer present at any such occurrence to make a statement in this form immediately to the Secretary, and the responsibility of the Secretary to obtain a similar statement from all others present at the occurrence who have evidence to contribute. In mental and mental deficiency hospitals where arrangements already exist for reporting accidents involving patients (and for reports to the Board of Control in certain instances) this procedure should not be regarded as replacing the existing one but rather as supplementing it in such manner as may be neccesary to meet the special requirements of this memorandum.

4. If these reports and statements are to be of full value to the hospital's solicitor it is essential that they should be confidential and privileged documents. In order that professional privilege may be claimed for them they must be regarded as, in essence, communications between the hospital's solicitor and his client.

5. Since, however, it may be necessary for the hospital authority — Regional Board, Management Committee or Board of Governors — to be informed of the circumstances to enable immediate action to be taken, and since the authority may be sued jointly with an officer alleged to be responsible for the occurrence and it will be the hospital authority who are instructing their solicitor if they are sued, there is no reason why the report should not be put before the authority for consideration. But it should in no circumstances be given any general circulation to the hospital's staff. It must also be borne in mind that privilege cannot be claimed for any correspondence or other documents relating to action in connection with the occurrence (including the minutes of the hospital authority's meetings), other than the report itself or documents made in connection with its preparation.

6. No report or copy of it should be given to any member of the staff concerned in the occurrence. If this were done, professional privilege could no longer be claimed for it. If any member of the staff, having made a report, desires a copy of it, whether for his professional organisation or otherwise, the proper procedure to protect the privilege is for the officer's solicitor (which in an appropriate case will include the solicitor of a professional organisation) to obtain it by a request

addressed to the hospital's solicitor, which request should be met. (The Minister is, however, advised that the report would not be regarded as coming into the possession of the officer if he were a member of the hospital authority and received it solely in that capacity.)

7. As a matter of procedure, it is desirable for the establishment of privilege that a general request should be made to each hospital authority by their solicitor that a report should be prepared for his use in the event of any claim arising from an occurrence at the hospital. There is, however, no reason why the report on any particular occurrence should be sent to the solicitor unless and until a claim is actually made or proceedings commenced, and it may well be felt more convenient that it should be kept in the office of the Secretary of the Board or Committee until that time.

8. The solicitor to each Regional Board should ask all Hospital Management Committees in his region for a report to be prepared for his use on any occurrence where the Board may possibly be sued for any action or negligence on the part of hospital staff employed directly by the Board and — where he acts also as solicitor to the Hospital Management Committee — on any occurrence where the Committee themselves may be sued. Boards of Governors, and Hospital Management Committees who are advised by solicitors other than the solicitor to the Regional Board, should discuss the whole matter with their own solicitors with a view to being given a general request on the same lines. (In the case of non-teaching hospitals the report will often have to be regarded as being prepared both for the Regional Board's solicitor and for the Management Committee's solicitor.)

9. This procedure has been evolved in consultation with representatives of the medical and dental professions and the defence societies.

July 7th, 1955

CONFIDENTIAL

.... HOSPITAL/CLINIC

Report of Accidents or other untoward occurrences to Patients, Staff, or any other Persons on the Premises

Name in full ....   Case No.....................................
                                               (where appropriate)

Home address.............................
                                     Date of Birth.............................

              ....   Sex ....

Particulars of Occurrences

Nature and extent of injuries...

....

How caused...

Where occurrence took place ....

Date and time of occurrence ....

In the case of hospital staff, was the injured person on or off duty at the
     time ....

Names and addresses   ....

     of any witnesses   ....

                       ....

Description of apparatus or equipment involved................................

Has it been retained for inspection..

Further details and remarks (e.g. action or treatment in progress, action taken
     after occurrence)...

....

....

                              (Signed) ....

                              Description   ....

Date ....

NOTE.

This form with attached Reports is to be treated as confidential and is prepared for the use of the Solicitors to the R.H.B. and H.M.C. or B.G. in the event of a complaint arising or legal proceedings being brought.

It should be completed as soon as possible after the occurrence and forwarded to the Secretary of the Board of Governors or Hospital Management Committee.

SUPPLY OF INFORMATION ABOUT HOSPITAL PATIENTS ENGAGED IN LEGAL PROCEEDINGS

(Text of circular H.M. (59) 88)

1. Hospital authorities are frequently asked by solicitors and others, for information about patients who have been, or are being, treated there. It is desirable that such requests should be addressed to and handled by the Secretary of the Board or Committee (as is no doubt the normal practice) who will, of course, in the great majority of cases, have to consult and be guided in his reply by the medical or dental staff concerned. Legal advice may also be needed.

2. There are two main types of case in which hospital authorities are likely to be asked for information: that where the patient or his representative is taking or contemplating proceeds (or making a claim) against the Board or Committee or a member of their staff or both; and that where the patient is, or may be, engaged in litigation with a third party (the proceedings being taken either by or against the patient), and neither the hospital authority nor their staff are directly involved.

3. Where a request for records or reports is made on what are manifestly insubstantial grounds, the hospital cannot be expected to grant it, but where information is being sought in pursuance of a claim of *prima facie* substance against the Board or Committee or a member of their staff or both, the decision is more difficult and each request must be examined on its own merits, in the light of legal advice, and of course in consultation with any member of their medical or dental staff directly concerned in the outcome of the claim (in this connection see H.M. (54) 32). The production of case notes and similar documents is not obligatory before the stage of discovery in the actual proceedings is reached, but the Minister does not feel that Boards and Committees, especially as they are public authorities, would either wish or be well advised to maintain their strict rights in this connection except for some good reason bearing on the defence to the particular claim or on the ground that the request is made without substantial justification.

4. Where the information is required in a matter which has nothing to do with the hospital or any member of its staff, *e.g.*, in litigation between the patient and a third party, hospital authorities should be prepared to help by providing, as far as possible, the information asked for subject always to the consent of the patient. Sometimes the information sought may be entirely unrelated to medical matters — *e.g.*, the date of the patient's admission or discharge; whether he was a private patient and signed the appropriate form of undertaking; and if so, the amount paid by way of hospital charges. Such information may properly be given by the Secretary of the Board or Committee, without reference

to the medical staff. But in all cases — and they will undoubtedly be the majority — where medical matters are in any way involved (*e.g.*, where information is wanted about the diagnosis made on admission, details of treatment, conditions on discharge, or prognosis) the doctor or dentist who was in charge of the patient's treatment at the hospital, or his successor, should be consulted. It is self-evident that this must be done when a medical or dental report is being asked for. But the principle is equally important when the request is only for extracts from the case notes, since it is necessary for the doctor or dentist to ensure that any extracts which are made are not misleading, and also that their disclosure to the patient cannot in any way be harmful medically to him — it would, no doubt, often be undesirable to let the patient himself have so detailed a report or such full extracts from the medical records as it would be proper to give to his general practitioner. This decision is one which can be made only by a professionally qualified person. At the same time it is imperative that no material information which can in any way be relevant to the matter should be withheld in such a way as to convey a wrong picture. Reports about accidents prepared in accordance with H.M. (55) 66 are privileged documents, and therefore are not affected by this memorandum.

5. Where the request for information comes, not from the patient himself or his representative, but from some other party or the representative of some other party who is engaged in legal proceedings with him, no information of any kind should be supplied until written consent of the patient or his representative has been obtained, unless, of course, a witness or document has been subjected to subpoena or discovery by the courts. The only other exception made to this rule should be where information is sought on behalf of another hospital Board or Committee (or a member of their staff), against whom the patient is bringing proceedings. In all appropriate cases the doctor in charge of the patient, or his successor, should be consulted as in paragraph 4.

6. The question of the circumstances in which a member of the medical or dental staff of the hospital may charge a fee for supplying information has given rise to some doubt. The position is governed by paragraph 14 of the Terms and Conditions of Service. Where the patient about whom information is required is at the time under observation or treatment at the hospital, the doctor or dentist is not entitled to make a charge (*i.e.*, the work is in category I) unless it it necessary for him to make a special examination of the patient to enable him to furnish the information. Where the patient is not under observation or treatment at the hospital, or where a special examination is necessary, preparation of a report comes under category II and a doctor or dentist is entitled to make a charge. Some difficulty may arise

where the patient or his representative asks not for a medical report but for extracts from the case notes. In such cases the doctor or dentist, though not called upon to prepare a report, will often have to examine the case notes in detail in order to make the relevant extracts to provide information which will neither be misleading nor prejudicial medically to the patient. Where an appreciable amount of work is involved in doing this it could, in the Minister's view, reasonably be regarded as equivalent to the preparation of a report, so that the doctor or dentist would be entitled to charge a suitable fee. The amount and quality of the work will, however, vary so much that it seems undesirable to suggest any standard fee or scale of fees.

7. No hospital charge should be made for the supply of information in the circumstances described in this memorandum, unless significant additional expenditure has to be incurred specifically for the purpose of providing it.

8. Cancelled H.M. (61) 110.

9. The principles in this memorandum are also intended to apply to records of patients treated under section 5 of the National Health Service Act 1946, in so far as they concern the activities of hospitals. But since these records mainly arise from the private work of consultants, any request for information which involves possible claims against the hospital or the consultant must be decided upon by agreement between them.

September 23rd, 1959

PRESERVATION AND DESTRUCTION OF HOSPITAL RECORDS

(*Text of circular H.M.* (61) 73)

1. The statutory arrangements for the disposal of public records have, as from 1st January, 1959, been changed by the Public Records Act 1958, which replaces the Public Record Office Acts 1838–1898. The effect of the new Act is that Government Departments and other authorities responsible for public records have now a duty to make proper arrangements for selecting under the guidance of the Public Record Office those of their records which should be permanently preserved and for disposing of the rest. The authority of a Parliamentary destruction schedule is no longer required. There are also provisions for records destined for permanent preservation to be transferred to suitable places of deposit and in due course made available for public inspection. Records of National Health Service hospitals are defined as public records for the purposes of the Act with the following exceptions:

(1) Records of endowments passing to Boards of Governors under section seven of the National Health Service Act 1946.

(2) Records relating to funds held by Hospital Boards and Committees under sections fifty-nine and sixty of the said Act.

(3) Records of private patients admitted under section five of the said Act.

Selection and disposal of records

2. The Schedule transmitted with H.M. (56) 103, authorising the destruction of various types of hospital records, is superseded. In its place, the lists contained in Appendices A and B below, drawn up in consultation with the Public Record Office, should be observed as the guide for selection and disposal of hospital records. Appendix A lists classes which should not be destroyed at all. Appendix B lists those which may be destroyed. In any case where a hospital wishes to destroy documents but there is doubt whether Appendix B gives authority for this to be done the Ministry or the Keeper of Public Records, Public Record Office, Chancery Lane, London, W.C.2, should be consulted before any action is taken. The decision to destroy should also be subject to the special reservations set out in paragraphs 4 to 7 below.

No documents should be destroyed which is or might be relevant to legal proceedings which have begun or to a pending claim or other matter which could result in legal proceedings.

3. The Act places a positive duty on an organisation subject to it to segregate and take proper care of documents which ought to be permanently preserved. Documents rejected as not required for permanent preservation should be destroyed as soon as, after the expiry of the specified retention periods, they cease to have usefulness for the purposes of the hospital. Disposal of rejected documents in a way other than by destruction (*e.g.*, by presentation) has to be approved by the Lord Chancellor (the Minister responsible for the supervision of public records), and application for such approval should be made through the Keeper of Public Records.

4. The actual period of retention of medical records (*i.e.*, part IV in Appendix B) should be determined by medical considerations with particular reference to clinical and research requirements. A joint committee of the Royal College of Physicians and the Royal College of Surgeons has considered the question of what proportion of these records it would be desirable to preserve permanently for research purposes and has made recommendations, of which account has been taken in compiling the list of classes in Appendix A and also in special arrangements which it is proposed to make with particular hospitals for the preservation of a suitable sample of selected classes of these records.

5. Hospitals which for special reasons consider it desirable and practicable not to destroy any or certain of their clinical records should treat such records as designated for permanent preservation and

regard the contents of paragraphs 9 to 17 below as applicable to them.

6. Paragraph 4 of H.M. (56) 103 requested that, if any former E.M.S. medical records were found to be still in the possession of a hospital, the hospital concerned should inform the Ministry of Pensions and National Insurance, Norcross, Blackpool, Lancs. (to whom they should have gone after the end of the war), so that their transfer to that Ministry could be arranged. In the event of any further records of this kind coming to light, the same action should be taken.

7. One of the main objects of the Act is to ensure the preservation of any documents which are, or may in future become, of historical interest. It prohibits in any case the disposal of any documents of earlier date than 1660. Hospitals should consider very carefully before disposing of documents of any great age, even though they may fall under the head of one of the classes in Appendix B; any created before 1858 (in which year the Medical Act was passed) should always be selected for preservation; and caution should be exercised over the rejection of any more than, say, fifty years old. Similarly any more recent document in such a class should be preserved if there is any reason for supposing that it may be of historical interest.

8. Paragraphs 12 and 13 of H.M. (54) 47 referred to the microfilming of medical records (regarding hospital records in general). The Note to the former Schedule indicated that any document of which the Schedule authorising the eventual destruction might be microfilmed after two years, the original then being destroyed and the microfilm retained for at least the remainder of the authorised retention period. The finding of the Committee on Departmental Records (Cmd. 9163), after careful investigation of the use of microphotography for archival purposes, was that the high overall cost of reproduction of records on microfilm would be much more than the cost of providing storage accommodation for the original documents. In view of this conclusion, and of other disadvantages mentioned in the Committee's report, microfilming is not now recommended as a method of reducing the bulk of documents held. If documents have been selected for permanent preservation, the original documents must be preserved; it is not permissible to preserve microfilm copies in their place.

Transfer of records

9. The Act directs the transfer of all records selected for preservation not later than thirty years after their creation either to the Public Record Office or to another place of deposit appointed by the Lord Chancellor; provided that they may be retained after that time if the person responsible for them considers that they ought to be retained for administrative purposes or any other special reason and the Lord Chancellor has been informed of the facts and given his approval.

10. Hospitals having records thirty years and more old intended for permanent preservation which they consider should be retained in their own keeping are requested to inform the Keeper of Public Records (at the address given in paragraph 2 above), with a view to obtaining the Lord Chancellor's approval. Retention until the time when records become fifty years old will normally have the Lord Chancellor's concurrence. But it is the intention of the Act (see paragraph 15 below) that records should become available for public inspection when they are fifty[1] years old, unless there is good reason for access being withheld or made subject to special conditions or restrictions. Hospitals are therefore asked to give careful consideration to the need to retain old records for administrative purposes beyond the age specified in the Act; bearing in mind that they can always recall them, should they need to refer to them from the place of deposit (see paragraph 14 below).

11. If hospitals wish for any reason to retain records which are to be permanently preserved and have ceased to be of administrative value they should consult the Keeper of Public Records.

Place of deposit

12. The Public Record Office is the normal place of deposit for public records which are to be permanently preserved. The Act however provides for particular classes of public records to be deposited in some other place if the Lord Chancellor considers that it affords suitable facilities for their safe keeping and inspection by the public and if the authority responsible for the place agrees. Hospital records are regarded by the Lord Chancellor as a category of documents which will most appropriately be deposited in a local record repository or, in the case of records of a medical nature, in the library of a medical institution.

13. Hospitals having records available for transfer are asked, if they propose to transmit them to a particular place, to inform the Keeper of Public Records, having previously ascertained that the authority responsible is prepared to accept them.

14. The Act provides that records in the Public Record Office or other appointed place of deposit shall be temporarily returned, if asked for, to the office from which they were transferred.

Access to records

15. The Act provides that public records transferred to the Public Record Office or other appointed place of deposit shall be available for public inspection; but not until they have been in existence for fifty[1] years or such other period, longer or shorter, as the Lord Chancellor may prescribe with the approval or at the request of the Minister or other authority concerned. It also provides that access to transferred

---

[1] Now *thirty* under the Public Records Act 1967.

records can be withheld or made subject to special conditions if the authority previously responsible for them considers that on grounds of confidentiality this is desirable, and if the Lord Chancellor concurs.

16. In view of the confidential character of medical records and other records containing information about individual patients, the Lord Chancellor intends at the request of the Minister of Health to direct that such records should not be made available for public inspection in the place of deposit until they are a hundred years old. Other types of hospital records will become available for public inspection when they are fifty[1] years old, unless in a particular case the Lord Chancellor has at the request of the Minister or the hospital authority concerned pre-scribed a different period. In all cases where a record covers a number of years the period, whatever its length, will be reckoned from the date of the last paper or entry.

17. The Act provides that documents closed to the public in general may nevertheless be made available to the holder of special permission to see them obtained from the department or body concerned. Hospital authori-ties should exercise the greatest discretion in granting such permission in the case of medical records and other documents containing informa-tion about patients. It is advised that they should require from persons seeking such permission a signed undertaking not to identify any in-dividual patient's case by name in any work resulting from such research.

18. In all matters of doubt as to the application of the new procedure in particular cases or treatment of documents or groups of documents where the question of proper disposal is in doubt the Ministry or the Keeper of Public Records should be consulted.

Psychiatric patients

19. When a patient is transferred to another hospital or to guardian-ship, the originals of the documents relating to his detention will, in future, be transferred to the receiving hospital or local health authority, who will be able to destroy them at the times specified in Appendix B. When transfers occurred before 1st November, 1960, however, the trans-ferring hospital may find itself holding originals of documents author-ising detention under the Lunacy and Mental Treatment, etc. Acts and, because the patient is no longer in their care, they will not know when is an appropriate time to destroy the documents. These should therefore be forwarded, at some convenient opportunity, to the receiving hospital (or other receiving authority) which should pass them on again if the patient has been further transferred or, if he has not, may destroy them at the times specified in the Appendix B.

20. It will sometimes happen that a patient who has been discharged from one hospital will within seven years of his discharge be compul-

[1] Now thirty years, under s. 1 of the Public Records Act 1967.

sorily admitted to another hospital for psychiatric treatment. If the first hospital does not know of this, the original documents in its possession will be regarded as liable to destruction seven years after discharge; but if it does know and there is no prospect of the patient being transferred back to that hospital, the documents relating to the patient's detention should be sent to the hospital where he is. They should be kept with the similar later documents and should be regarded as forming part of them for the purpose of deciding when they may be destroyed.

21. Where copies of documents have been retained on the transfer of a patient after 1st November, 1960, in accordance with paragraph 115 of the memorandum on Parts I, IV to VII and IX of the Mental Health Act, 1959, enclosed with H.M. (60) 69, the date of which they may be destroyed is at the discretion of the Board or Committee. From the point of view of giving the hospital full protection in the event of legal proceedings, the ideal arrangement would be to keep them for the same period as the originals. This might be secured by asking the hospital to which the patient had been transferred to send a notification when he was discharged or died. Otherwise the copies should be retained for such a period (which may well be lengthy) as the Committee thinks will substantially achieve the same result.

22. The position of records relating to psychiatric patients, other than documents relating to the detention of an individual, is to be further reviewed when the Minister receives the report of his Working Party on the methods of record keeping and standardisation of forms for psychiatric patients (H.M. (60) 2) and further advice may be issued. In the meantime, all such records should continue to be retained.

23. Memorandum H.M. (56) 103 is hereby cancelled.

July 26th, 1961.

APPENDIX A

Classes of Documents which are Not to be Destroyed

1. Minute books, including minute books of governing bodies (and their sub-committees).

2. Title deeds and correspondence relating to the transfer of hospital property to the Minister; to the apportionment and vesting in the Minister of interests in premises used partly for hospital and partly for other purposes; to the purchase, disposal and leasing of property; to the grant of leases, easements, licences and other rights over property by or to the Minister; and to the transfer and discharge of mortages.

3. Correspondence and other documents relating to town and country planning matters and having a permanent value.

4. Accounts and statements prepared in pursuance of regulations 19 and 20 of the National Health Service (Hospital Accounts and Financial Provisions) Regulations 1948 (S.1. 1948 No. 1414).

5. One set of annual reports of each hospital authority, including annual reports of governing bodies of former voluntary hospitals.

6. Documents relating to building and engineering works:
   (i) Contract documents, drawings, bills of quantities and other documents of permanent value (i.e. excluding those covered by Item 15 of Appendix B).
   (ii) Site plans, surveys, record drawings, etc., having a permanent value.
   (iii) Record documents relating to major projects which have been abandoned or deferred.

7. Central inventories of:
   (i) Permanent or fixed equipment.
   (ii) Furniture and surgical, diagnostic and therapeutic equipment, not held on store charge, having a minimum life of five years.

8. Documents of permanent value relating to benefactions, special donations and memorials of any sort covered by sections 7 (7), 59 and 60 of the National Health Service Act 1946, including all trusts created since 5th July, 1948.

9. Post-mortem books.

10. Summaries of clinical notes taken (Front Sheets, Registrars' books, etc.).

11. Discharge Books containing corrected diagnoses.

12.* In psychiatric hospitals, the following documents, most of which were prescribed in the Lunacy and Mental Treatment Acts 1890 to 1930, the Mental Deficiency Acts 1913 to 1938, the Mental Treatment Rules 1948, and the Mental Deficiency Regulations 1948.
Visitors' Books.
General Registers.
Post-mortem Records.
Medical Records or patients' records (including cards for General Register Office and nursing record (non-statutory)).
Hospital Cards (non-statutory).
Patients' Books.
Alphabetical Register.
Register of mechanical restraint and seclusion.
Casualty Books.
Day and night nursing report books.
and any similar document relating to psychiatric patients which is used after 1st November, 1960, in psychiatric *or other hospitals*, for similar purposes.

13. All documents of earlier date than 1858.

14. Superannuation records: Duplicate forms S.D.55A, B, C, and D and their successors for subsequent septennia.

APPENDIX B

CLASSES OF DOCUMENTS WHICH MAY BE DESTROYED

Number and Class of Documents	Period after which Documents may be destroyed
Part I—Financial	
1. Estimates: including supporting calculations and statistics.	Three years after the end of the financial year to which they relate.

* To be preserved provisionally: see paragraph 22 of this memorandum.

Number and Class of Documents	Period after which Documents may be destroyed
Part I—Financial—*cont.*	
2. Audit reports	The same.
3. Principal Ledger Records: including such documents as cash book, ledgers, income and expenditure journals, etc.	Six years after the end of the financial year to which they relate.
4. Minor Accounting Records:	
(*a*) Pass-books, bank statements of accounts, paying-in slips, cheque counterfoils and cancelled and discharged cheques other than cheques bearing printed receipts; accounts of petty cash expenditure; travelling and subsistence accounts; minor vouchers, including duplicate receipt books; income records; laundry lists and receipts; forms A.P.1, 2, 3 and 4 (used in connection with the supply of surgical appliances), etc.	Two years after the end of the financial year to which they relate.
(*b*) Debtors' records	Two years after the end of the financial year in which the accounts are paid or are written off.
5. Cost accounts prepared in accordance with regulation 21 of the National Health Service (Hospital Accounts and Financial Provisions) Regulations 1948, or any similar or amending regulations.	Three years after the end of the financial year to which they relate.
6. Bills and receipts: including cheques bearing printed receipts.	Six years after the end of the financial year to which they relate.
7. Documents, other than those referred to in Item 8 of Appendix A, relating to benefactions, special donations and memorials of any sort covered by Sections 7 (7), 59 and 60 of the National Health Service Act 1946, and to trusts created since 5th July, 1948.	Six years after the end of the financial year in which the trust moneys became finally spent, or the gift in kind was accepted.
8. Salaries and Wages Records (i.e. employees' pay cards and personal pay records).	Eleven years after the end of the financial year to which they relate.
9. Pay Sheets and Records of unpaid salaries and wages.	Six years after the end of the financial year to which they relate.

Number and Class of Documents	Period after which Documents may be destroyed
Part II—Stores, Equipment and Buildings	
10. Major Stores Records: stores ledgers and equivalents.	Six years after the end of the financial year to which they relate.
11. Minor Stores Records: requisitions, issues notes, transfer vouchers, goods received books, etc.	Two years after the end of the financial year to which they relate.
12. Agreements and simple contracts (and documents subsidiary to these) which are only of temporary or minor importance, i.e., short-term agreements and minor contracts; papers preliminary or subsidiary to contracts; documents relating to contracts for the supply of goods.	Six years after the end of the financial year in which the agreement or contract expires.
13. Engineers' inspection reports on boilers, lifts, etc.	When the plant to which they relate goes finally out of use.
14. Minor Supplies Records: including invitations to tender and unaccepted tenders, routine papers relating to catering and demands for furniture, equipment, stationery and other supplies.	Two years after the end of the financial year to which they relate.
15. Records (other than those referred to in Item 6 of Appendix A) relating to capital and other building works or improvements: including plans and specifications prepared for temporary purposes and papers relating to them.	Two years after they have ceased to be effective.
16. Inventories not in current use of utensils, instruments, bedding, etc., not held on store charge, having a life of less than five years.	Two years after the end of the financial year in which the inventories were in use.
Part III—Establishment and Statistics	
17. Major Establishment Records: including personal files, letters of appointment, contracts, references and related correspondence and records of sick leave.	Six years after the officer leaves the service of the hospital or on the date on which the officer would reach the age of 70, whichever is the later, provided that if an adequate summary of the personal and health record is kept for this period the main records may be destroyed six years after the officer leaves the service of the hospital.

Number and Class of Documents	Period after which Documents may be destroyed
Part III—Establishment and Statistics—*cont.*	
18. Minor Establishment Records: including attendance books, annual leave records, time sheets, duty rosters, clock cards and other documents of ephemeral importance.	Two years after the end of the year to which they relate.
19. Documents relating to unsuccessful applications for posts.	One year after the vacancy was filled.
20. Superannuation Records: (*a*) Original forms S.D.56	Two years after the end of the financial year in which the officer left the service of the employing authority.
(*b*) Original forms Prem. (P) 5A	The same.
21. Statistical and other returns which were required for ephemeral purposes only and have ceased to be effective.	One year after the end of the period to which they relate.
22. Annual statistical returns required by the Ministry of Health.	Six years after the end of the period to which they relate.
Part IV—Medical	
23. Mass miniature radiography records, including microfilms.	Five years after the date on which the film was taken.
24. Blood Transfusion Service: laboratory records relating to donors.	One year after the resignation or death of the donor.
25. Medical records and allied documents in hospitals: (*a*) *Medical records including: Clinical notes (which includes reports from pathological, radiological and other special departments, X-rays, electrocardiographic and electroencephalographic records). (*b*) Blood Transfusion Records .. (*c*) Consent forms of all types .. (*d*) Four-hourly temperature charts	Six years after conclusion of treatment of,[1] where the patient dies in hospital, three years after death.

---

* See also Items 9 to 13 of Appendix A.   [1] Presumably 'of' should read 'or'.

Number and Class of Documents	Period after which Documents may be destroyed
Part IV—Medical—*cont.*	
26. Records of all types of special departments (including almoners' records).	Six years from date of last entry.
27. Operation books	The same.
28. Casualty notes	The same.
29. Day and night nursing report books ..	Six years from date of last entry.
30. Ancillary records, including prescriptions, department registers, appointment sheets, attendance registers, etc.	The same.
31. Appliance Order Forms Nos. 1, 2 and 3 ..	The same.
32. Records relating to dangerous drugs and poisons: (*a*) Registers, records books, prescriptions and other documents kept, issued or made under the Dangerous Drugs Regulations 1953: (i) Registers, books or records ..	Two years from date of last entry.
(ii) Other documents	Two years from date on which issued or made.
(*b*) Non-statutory records relating to dangerous drugs.	Two years from date on which issued or made.
(*c*) Records of medicines included in the First Schedule to the Poisons Rules, 1960 (and Rules repealed by those rules), and supplied to out-patients.	Two years from the date of the last entry relating to the supply of such a medicine.
33. Documents prescribed in the Lunacy and Mental Treatment Acts 1890 to 1930, the Mental Deficiency Acts 1913 to 1938, the Mental Treatment Rules 1948, and the Mental Deficiency Regulations 1948: (*a*) Dispensary book or medicine card or sheet.	Two years after the last entry.
(*b*) Register of dysentry and diarrhoea ..	Two years after the last entry
(*c*) Caution cards	Two years after patient's discharge, removal or death.
(*d*) List of patients in wards	One year after the last entry.
(*e*) Diary for Visiting Medical Officers ..	Two years after the last entry.

Number and Class of Documents	Period after which Documents may be destroyed
Part IV—Medical—*cont.*	
34. Undertakings signed by patients admitted to beds designated under Section 4 or Section 5 of the National Health Service Act, 1946.	Six years.
Part V—Miscellaneous	
35. Any documents relating to legal actions or to complaints, including accident record sheets.	Six years after the end of the financial year in which the incident occurred; or, where an action has been commenced, when legally advised.
36. Documents relating to contractual arrangements with hospitals, etc., outside the National Health Service:	
(*a*) Documents relating to the contractual arrangements.	Six years from the termination of the arrangement.
(*b*) Documents relating to periodical financial settlements made under the contract.	Six years after the end of the financial year to which they relate.
37. Records of patients' property handed in for safe custody.	Six years after the end of the financial year in which the property was disposed of.
38. Correspondence and other papers of minor or ephemeral importance, not covered by the foregoing classes: including — advertising matter; covering letters; reminders and letters making appointments; anonymous or unintelligible letters; drafts; duplicates of documents known to be preserved elsewhere (unless they have important minutes on them); indexes and registers compiled for temporary purposes; routine reports; punched cards; and other documents which have ceased to be of value on settlement of the matter involved.	Forthwith.

Number and Class of Documents	Period after which, Documents may be destroyed
Part V—Miscellaneous—*cont*.	
39. Documents relating to the detention of an individual mentally disordered patient (including documents prescribed in the Mental Health (Hospital and Guardianship) Regulations, 1960, required under the Mental Health Act, 1959, documents described in or required by earlier, superseded, legislation and documents relating to detention which are not statutorily prescribed or required):	
(*a*) Patients who have been *finally* discharged from hospital care (including out-patient care), whether the care was compulsory or had become informal by the date of discharge.	Seven years from the date of discharge or from reaching the age of 21, whichever is the later.
(*b*) Patients who have died	Three years from the date of death.

ROAD SAFETY ACT 1967

(Text of circular H.M. (67) 64)

Summary—This memorandum draws the attention of hospital authorities to the provisions in Part I of the Safety Act enabling the police to require a driver, who following a road accident is at a hospital as a patient, to provide specimens for the purpose of the Act.

1. Part I of the Road Safety Act 1967 coming into operation on 9th October 1967 makes it an offence to drive with a proportion of alcohol in the blood exceeding the prescribed limit and enables the police in certain circumstances to require drivers to provide specimens of breath for breath tests and of blood or urine for laboratory tests. When following a road accident a driver is at a hospital as a patient the Act enables the police to require him to provide specimens for these tests while he is at the hospital, provided the doctor in immediate charge of the case does not object on the grounds that this would be prejudicial to the proper care or treatment of the patient. It is not intended that the police should seek to invoke these provisions of the Act in every case of a driver suspected of having been drinking who is at a hospital as a patient after an accident, for example a patient who is seriously injured or ill; on the other hand, a driver who has an accident after he has been drinking should not necessarily escape the provisions of the Act simply because he is at a hospital.

2. The procedure, so far as it may affect a driver who is at a hospital as a patient, whether an in-patient or an out-patient, following an accident, is given in greater detail in the following paragraphs. Apart from the need for the hospital doctor in immediate charge of the patient to be notified of the proposal to require provision of a specimen and his power to object, hospital staff will not be involved in the taking of the specimens or their evaluation for the purposes of the Act. Specimens of breath and urine will be taken by a police constable and specimens of blood by a police doctor and the laboratory tests will be carried out in forensic science laboratories. The necessary equipment for breath tests and for the taking of specimens of blood and urine will be provided by the police. There is no provision in the Act for the taking of urine specimens by catheter.

Breath Test

3. Section 2 (2) (*b*) of the Act provides that where a driver is at a hospital as a patient following a road accident a constable in uniform may require him to take a breath test at the hospital, but the requirement is not to be made if the doctor in immediate charge of the case is not first notified of the proposal to make the requirement or if he objects on the grounds that the provision of a specimen of breath or the requirement to provide it would be prejudicial to the proper care or treatment of the patient. Tests may not be made on a patient without his consent, nor on an unconscious patient.

4. The notification by the constable and any objection by the doctor would both normally be given orally.

5. The doctor in immediate charge of the case would be the doctor attending the patient. If he is in any doubt whether or not to object he can consult his senior. The grounds on which he can object are wide enough to enable him to object on the grounds that the test would interfere with the examination, diagnosis or treatment of the patient as well as that it would be likely to be detrimental to the patient's health.

6. The doctor may object on the above grounds at the beginning or at a later stage, having first not objected; if he objects at any stage before the specimen has been provided, the constable may not proceed. The breath test will be taken at the hospital and a person at a hospital as a patient may not be required to go elsewhere to take the test, nor under the provisions of Section 2 (4) or 2 (5) of this Act will he be subject to arrest without warrant, unless and until he is no longer at hospital as a patient.

Laboratory Tests

7. Section 3 (2) provides that a person at a hospital as a patient may be required by a constable to provide a specimen for a labroratory test if

he has been required to take a breath test after an accident, whether at the hospital or elsewhere, and either the test is positive or he fails or refuses to take it and the constable has reasonable cause to suspect him of having alcohol in his body. On making the requirement the constable must, in accordance with Section 3 (10), warn the person that failure to provide a specimen may make him liable to a penalty.

8. As in the case of a breath test, the constable must first notify the doctor in immediate charge of the case of the proposal to require a person to provide a specimen and the doctor has the same power to object on the same grounds as in the case of a breath test, and also on the grounds that the warning would be prejudicial to the proper care or treatment of the patient.

9. If the doctor offers no objection to the taking of specimens for a laboratory test the procedure will be as follows:

   (i) The person will first be requested to provide a specimen of blood. This may be taken only with his consent and by a police doctor, and will be a very small quantity of capillary blood;

  (ii) if he refuses to provide a specimen of blood he will be asked to provide two specimens of urine within an hour;

 (iii) if he refuses or fails to provide two specimens of urine within an hour he will be offered another chance to provide a specimen of blood.

10. What is said in paragraphs 4, 5 and 6 above applies also to laboratory tests. Specimens may not be taken from a patient without his consent nor from an unconscious patient.

General

11. The Home Office will be advising Chief Police Officers that they may consider it useful to discuss the arrangements generally with the hospital authorities in their areas in advance of the Act coming into force, approaching Regional Hospital Boards and Boards of Governors in the first instance. Detailed discussions will be needed between the police and individual hospitals. Hospital authorities are asked to co-operate in these discussions and to bring into them such administrative, medical and nursing staff as may be appropriate.

12. The following points should be made known to all medical staff concerned:

   (i) Under the Act a patient at a hospital is not liable to arrest without warrant, nor can he be required to go elsewhere to give the specimens of breath, blood or urine.

  (ii) Specimens may not be taken from a patient without his consent, and a specimen may not be taken from an unconscious patient or by catheterisation.

(iii) The constable must notify the doctor in immediate charge of the case of the intention to require a patient to provide a specimen and the doctor may object at any stage before a specimen has been provided if he considers that such action would be prejudicial to the proper care or treatment of the patient. He may also object to the patient being told of the requirement to provide a specimen, or warned of the penalty.

(iv) Members of the hospital staff are not required to take part in the taking of specimens or in their evaluation, although the hospital is requested to arrange conditions of privacy under which patients may provide specimens.

(v) Hospital equipment will not be used in the tests.

Subject to the overriding consideration of the medical interest of patients the Minister trusts that hospital authorities and staff will co-operate with the police when action is taken under the Act.

13. Hospital authorities are asked to bring this memorandum to the notice of all staff likely to be concerned, particularly the medical staff of accident and emergency departments.

14th September, 1967

APPENDIX E

OPERATIONS AND OTHER PROCEDURES

Forms of Consent

Much of the present commentary on forms recommended and advice given by the Department of Health and Social Security and by the medical defence societies first appeared in articles in The Hospital *in April, October and November, 1971,[1] but the order is here varied and I have further clarified one or two points. Expressions of opinion on points of law must be read against the background of what is said in Chapter 3, particularly as regards consent to operations on married women and on children, and on refusal of consent by relatives, not least in respect of blood transfusion.*

Departmental letter and recommended dual purpose form

On 2nd February, 1971, the Department of Health and Social Security sent to secretaries of N.H.S. hospital authorities a circular letter[2] on consent forms, the text of which was as follows —

CONSENT FORMS FOR OPERATIONS

1. The Department has discussed model consent forms with the British Medical Association, the Medical Defence Union, the Medical Protection Society, and the Medical and Dental Defence Union of Scotland.

2. As a result, agreement has been reached on a standard consent form for use in the generality of medical and dental procedures for which consent is required; this form, a copy of the agreed text of which is attached, is that now recommended by the three medical defence societies. It is proposed to issue a standard version of the form in the HMR Series, and authorities will be notified separately about the arrangements in due course.

3. There is, of course, no objection to the use of special consent forms for particular purposes (*e.g.*, in connection with primary sterilisation procedures) either adapted from the standard form or specially designed for the purpose, as advised by the appropriate medical defence society.

4. It is important that the question of obtaining a signature to a consent form should not be allowed to become an end in itself. The most important aspect of any consent procedure must always be the duty to explain to a patient or relative the nature and purpose of the proposed operation and to obtain a fully informed consent.

---

[1] At pages 122, 354 and 389 respectively.   [2] Reference H/P9/5.

The following is the text of the recommended form which accompanied the letter —

CONSENT FOR OPERATION

.... Hospital

I .... of ....

.... hereby consent to

* $\begin{cases}\text{undergo} \\ \text{the submission of my}\end{cases}$ * $\begin{cases}\text{child} \\ \text{ward}\end{cases}$ ....to undergo $\}$

the operation of...
the nature and purpose of which have been explained to me by

Dr/*Mr ....
I also consent to such further or alternative operative measures as may be found necessary during the course of the above-mentioned operation and to the administration of general, local or other anæsthetics for any of these purposes.
No assurance has been given to me that the operation will be performed by any particular practitioner.

Date .... *Signed* ....
(*Patient/Parent/Guardian*)*

I confirm that I have explained the nature and purpose of this operation to the patient/parent/guardian.*

Date .... *Signed* ....
(*Medical/Dental* Practitioner*)

* DELETE AS APPROPRIATE

Any deletions, insertions or amendments to the form are to be made before the explanation is given and the form submitted for signature.

Commentary on Departmental letter, more particularly as regards use of special forms and in light of published advice of medical defence societies

The Departmental letter covering the form of consent recommended for general purpose use, whilst leaving open, as unobjectionable, the possibility of the use of special forms for particular purposes, is rather unhelpful as to what those purposes might be, the sole example cited being primary sterilisation. That being so, it seems not unreasonable to take as our starting point for a consideration of the circumstances in which the use of special forms might be appropriate, those special purpose forms recommended by the Medical Defence Union in the latest (1971) edition of *Consent to Treatment*, together with the advice given in that booklet regarding the use of those forms. I suggest this not only because the M.D.U. is one of the two defence societies which the Department has suggested that hospital authorities in England and Wales should consult on the matter of special forms, but also because in 1968 the Department itself gave its approval to the forms recommended in the then current edition of *Consent to Treatment*.[1] I shall not, however, here reproduce all the M.D.U. forms, contenting myself with explicit reference to any feature in such a form as may call for comment. Likewise. so far as the advice given in the body of *Consent to Treatment* is concerned. I shall mention and comment only on advice and opinions on particular situations if there are grounds for suggesting that a different point of view ought seriously to be considered

Termination of Pregnancy

Married women

The first paragraph of the section on termination of pregnancy in the case of married women in *Consent to Treatment* reads as follows —

'The written consent of the patient whose pregnancy is to be terminated should always be obtained. If the woman is married the proposed termination should, with her consent, be discussed with her husband and his *agreement*[2] sought; but if the pregnancy is to be terminated because of danger to the woman's life or to her physical or mental health it is not necessary in law to obtain her husband's *consent*.[2]

Equally in the paragraphs which follow, in which advice is given on the position of the husband in respect of abortions for what may conveniently be referred to as medico-social reasons[3] or because of the risk of a child being born with such physical or mental abnormalities as to be seriously physically handicapped,[3] the legal position is set out fairly, albeit with compassionate regard for the feelings of the husband and wife alike. The substance of what is said is to the effect that, even though the husband may be unco-operative, the practitioner is entitled

[1] The Departmental advice given in 1968 was as follows — '*The Department considers that hospital authorities generally should be advised to adopt, after consultation with their medical staffs, who are equally concerned, the model consent form which has been recommended by the medical defence societies and the other forms contained in the appendix to the booklet "Consent to Treatment" issued by the Medical Defence Union.*' Whether or not that explicit approval of the forms has now impliedly been withdrawn or, more probably, is not to be taken as extending to forms modified since 1968 or to any new forms is an open question. But whatever the answer to that question, it does not affect my use of the forms as a basis of discussion. It may also be worthy of note that the Medical Protection Society in its pamphlet *Consent*, in which it strongly advocated the use of an all-purpose form, agreed that the wording of the various forms in *Consent to Treatment* circulated by the Department of Health and Social Security in 1968 '*was appropriate to deal with the different types of cases in which they were intended to be used,*' the Society's objection to the use of those forms being that, in their opinion, they were unnecessary and that the use of a number of different forms was likely to lead to mistakes.

[2] The italics are mine. The use of the word *agreement* in one place and of *consent* in the other seems to imply a difference in meaning. If, in context, there is one, it completely escapes me and also Dr Speller. It will be noted that the husband's agreement or consent is not a legal requirement. See further p. 203 above.

[3] First made lawful by the Abortion Act 1967.

to terminate the pregnancy with the consent of the patient if he believes that that is the proper course to take. That in doubtful cases he should take a second opinion, as is also advised, is but plain common sense.

Position if patient refuses to allow advice to terminate pregnancy to be discussed with her husband: Husband's refusal of agreement

What is still perhaps not clear is what the M.D.U. think should happen if the wife refuses to allow the proposed termination of pregnancy to be discussed with her husband. The answer to that question must, I suggest, depend on the precise reason for its being proposed. If it was for the sake of the woman's own life or health there can surely be no question. The practitioner's duty is clear — he should, with the woman's consent, do what is necessary for her well-being.

But suppose termination of pregnancy had been advised because the practitioner was of the opinion that, if it continued to term, a child was likely to be born with grave physical or mental abnormalities. Here again, if the woman either refused her consent to her husband's being consulted or, on his being consulted with her consent, he was unwilling to agree to the abortion, it would appear to me[1] that, the woman herself having accepted the advice given, the pregnancy should be terminated, On the other hand if, with the patient's consent, the practitioner did terminate the pregnancy, the husband not having been consulted or, having been consulted, had refused his consent, it seems that the husband would have no cause of action, always provided that the practitioner had acted in good faith.

To take yet another case, quoting an example from the M.D.U. booklet, let us suppose that the reason for the proposed abortion were potential risk to the health of existing children of the family. Then it might be less wise for the practitioner to go ahead without having heard what the husband had to say. Even so, I would hesitate to go so far as the M.D.U. and say that 'the father, with his intimate knowledge of the family, is often as good a judge as the practitioner'. Suppose it were the present and forseeable future living conditions of the family and the wife's apparent inability to cope which had been major factors in the practitioner's reaching the opinion that the birth of another child would be prejudicial to the other children, would not a report by a health visitor or other social worker be a more useful guide than what the husband might have to say? But even where the husband is consulted, there is no question of the decision resting with him. It still remains the practitioner's reponsibility, subject only to the patient's consent, though in reaching his decision the practitioner may properly take into account information gleaned from the husband or from any other source

---

[1] And to Dr Speller. He adds, in *Law of Doctor and Patient* his doubts as to the liability of the doctor to the patient in such circumstances.

Girl under 16

The M.D.U. advise that in the case of a girl under 16 her parents should always be consulted, but that their refusal of consent should not prevent clinically necessary termination of pregnancy to which the patient herself has consented, continuing —

'Conversely, a termination should never be carried out in opposition to the girl's wishes even if the parents demand it.'

Dr Speller doubts in his *Law of Doctor and Patient*[1] whether the girl has got this legal veto. For my part I am inclined to think him wrong and the M.D.U. right with advice quoted.

OPERATIONS, ETC.

Married persons

Operations affecting generative organs

Of consent to operations on married persons the M.D.U. in *Consent to Treatment says* —

'Any sane person aged 16 or over can give a valid consent to any lawful surgical procedure on himself. The consent of the spouse to the performance of an operation on the other partner is not necessary in law but where the generative organs of the patient are to be seriously affected, *e.g.*, in hysterectomy or oophorectomy (primary sterilisation is considered below), it is desirable that the spouse should be informed of the nature and purpose of the operation and should be asked to sign an acknowledgement that he or she agrees to it.'

Despite the use of the words *he or she* in the concluding sentence of the quoted advice, it is perhaps not without significance that the form recommended (Form V) relates exclusively to operations on women and nowhere is it stated, as it is elsewhere in relation to termination of pregnancy, that the woman's consent should be obtained before the matter is discussed with her husband and his agreement sought, this notwithstanding the clear statement that the consent of the spouse is not necessary in law.

In my opinion[2] the woman's exclusive right to give or withhold consent to an operation advised on clinical grounds should be more strictly safeguarded than it would be if the M.D.U. recommendations were followed. She should be clearly informed of her right to decide for herself whether or not to have the advised treatment and this could best be done by an unambiguous statement on the form that her consent only was necessary and that if, with her agreement, the matter were discussed with her husband, the final decision whether to have the recommended

---

[1] (1973) (H.K. Lewis) pp 166-167   [2] And that of Dr Speller

operation would still rest with her. Such a note on the form would also serve to keep the true position fresh in the minds of hospital staff who, using only Form VII apart from the advisory booklet may be forgiven for acting on the assumption that the husband's consent was essential and so talking to women patients in such a way as to leave them in the erroneous belief that the husband's consent to a necessary gynaecological operation has to be obtained,

Minors under 16 undergoing course of operative treatment

On the ground that difficulty may be experienced in obtaining parental consent for every separate operative procedure that may have to be carried out under general anæsthetic on a child who may, for example, be suffering from severe burns or a serious congenital abnormality, a form of consent authorising a course of operative treatment is recommended by the M.D.U. for use in such cases.

Although as a general rule it is not wise to seek consent for any future operation or operations as well as for the one which the patient is shortly to undergo at the time consent is sought, the kind of case referred to above is an obvious exception and it is plainly desirable that, when such is met, the form recommended in *Consent to Treatment*, or one to like effect, should be used.

Private patients

It is to be observed that in the newly designed form of consent to vasectomy in the case of a married man[1] the words '*No assurance has been given to me that the operation will be performed by any particular surgeon*' are linked by an asterisk with a footnote which reads: *This sentence should be deleted if the patient is undergoing private treatment.* Since such a note on adapting the form for private patients would appear to be no less appropriate on Forms I to VI, VIII, IX and XI, it is presumably by an oversight that it has been omitted from those forms. If not, the distiction made calls for an explanation.

Mentally disordered patients

(a) *Patients liable to detention*

(*i*) *Treatment for mental disorder*.

The M.D.U. in *Consent to Treatment* takes the line that in the case of a patient liable to detention needing treatment for his mental disorder, the treatment may be given whether the patient agrees or not, the form of consent being signed by the responsible medical officer.[2] That the

---

[1] Form VIII.

[2] *i.e.* the medical officer in charge of the treatment of the patient. (Mental Health Act 1959, section 59.)

consent of the patient is not required is generally accepted, though this is not entirely beyond doubt in the case of a patient who is fully volitional unless the operation is demonstrably necessary in the strict sense of the word[1]. It must, however, be suggested that since the patient is in the custody of the hospital authority and not of the responsible medical officer, that officer is not vested with the power of consent *ex officio* as the booklet appears to suggest, but has only such power of consent as has been delegated to him.

(*ii*) *Treatment immediately necessary otherwise than for mental disorder*

Dr Speller and I agree; treatment immediately necessary to preserve life and health, not being treatment for mental disorder, may be given subject to the same consent as treatment for such disorder. But, as I have indicated above, I question whether the responsible medical officer has power of consent *ex officio*. The hospital authority could, however, delegate that power to him.

(*iii*) *Treatment otherwise than for mental disorder, being treatment not immediately necessary.*

Of consent to treatment for a condition not requiring immediate treatment, the M.D.U. booklet says:

'If the condition[2] does not require immediate treatment only the patient can validly consent to it. If he is *unable or unwilling*[3] to give his consent treatment should not be administered at this stage. It must be postponed either until the patient recovers from his mental disorder to a sufficient degree to be able to understand the nature of the treatment he requires and gives his consent, or until the condition can be said to fall into the category requiring immediate treatment . . .'

So far as the above advice refers to treatment of a patient who is fully volitional it is a fair statement of the position at common law, though one is left to speculate on whether a patient whose refusal of treatment was apparently unreasonable might not thereby afford some evidence that he was incapable of rational choice in the matter. But whether the statement that, in the case of a patient incapable of consenting to treatment for a physical condition, that treatment not being immediately necessary to preserve life and health, the treatment should be postponed until either it falls into that category or until the patient becomes capable of giving, and gives, his consent is acceptable, must depend on what is meant by the words 'immediately necessary to preserve his life and health'. The impression created is that those words are used narrowly as meaning only such operative and other treatment as the doctor having care of the patient would say must be undertaken as a matter of urgency, brooking little or no delay.

---

[1] See above p. 204 and footnote 2 on that page.
[2] *i.e.* the patient's physical condition.   [3] The italics are mine, J. J.

If that were the interpretation intended it would not be permissible to carry out some manifestly desirable operations, such as for treatment of a condition which caused the patient some discomfort or inconvenience; or of one which caused pain, the pain being only occasional and not severe; or to deal with some minor disability. If such narrow interpretation be not intended and, in the opinion of the M.D.U., the kinds of treatment I have mentioned are permissible even though the patient is unable to consent, it is difficult to think of any medically desirable treatment which could not be undertaken. If, however, I am right in assuming that the narrower interpretation is intended, I find myself in disagreement with what is said for, in my opinion, any such treatment as is medically desirable may be given to a patient incapable of consenting, this with the consent of an officer acting on behalf of the hospital authority having custody of the patient, both the hospital authority and all those concerned with the treatment of the patient acting as agents of necessity.[1]

Informal patients

Of the position in relation to consent to treatment in the case of informal patients the M.D.U. booklet says:

'In the eyes of the law the informal patient is in the same position as the ordinary hospital patient and he alone can give a valid consent to treatment whether for his mental disorder or for any other condition. If he is incapable of consenting or refuses to do so any treatment administered may constitute what the law regards as trespass to the person and be actionable in damages.'

Whilst I do not question the statement that no treatment should be given to an informal patient who is volitional without his consent, Dr Speller found himself unable to accept that such a rule applies equally to a patient who is incapable of consenting,[2] since to do so would compel one to the wholly unsatisfactory conclusion that such a patient — so long as he remained so incapable — could not be given treatment even for the mental disorder for which he had been admitted. If that were the law it would seemingly follow that only if a person were volitional should he be admitted as an informal patient. Yet s. 5 of the Mental Health Act 1959 is, purposely, in such terms as to make it possible to admit as informal patients persons to a greater or lesser degree deprived of understanding and such patients are, in fact, admitted informally.

---

[1] See note 2 on page 204. Maybe even the M.D.U. is a little unhappy about the possible implications of its own statement for it adds — 'The situation should be looked at sensibly and the prohibition outlined above must not be allowed to jeopardise the patient's health. It is unlikely that the courts would criticise a practitioner who has acted in good faith and in the interests of his patient.'

[2] The view I here express in relation to patients incapable of consenting must not be understood to apply to a patient whose incapacity is but temporary and is reasonably expected to be of short duration, this always assuming that the treatment needed can be postponed without unnecessary pain and suffering to the patient.

As regards treatment needed by an informal patient incapable of consenting, being treatment for a physical condition, the M.D.U. statement of the law would seem to compel us to the absurd conclusion that nothing at all could safely be done for the patient unless his status had first been altered to that of patient liable to detention, when any immediately necessary treatment — and only such treatment — could be given without his consent. But, again, the M.D.U. seems to falter, for although it professes to find no difference in law between an informal patient incapable of consenting and an ordinary hospital patient, it ends with the rather uncertain conclusion that an operation on such a patient *may* constitute a trespass to the person.

One could surely limit the foreseeable risk more closely than the M.D.U. has here succeeded in doing and Dr Speller suggested that the true position could be more accurately expressed as follows If an informal patient were incapable of consenting, nothing done for him by way of treatment whilst in hospital would involve either the hospital authority or any member of its staff in legal liability, provided always that what had been done was what any ordinary reasonable person would have been likely to want to be done in the particular circumstances and provided also that due care and skill had been exercised. In such a case, consent would appropriately be given be an authorised officer on behalf of the hospital authority, as being the person *de facto* in charge of the patient and acting as agent of necessity.

List of Recommended Forms

The following is a list of the forms in *Consent to Treatment* (1971 edition) recommended by the M.D.U. for signature by the patient or by any other person whose consent to his treatment is regarded by the M.D.U. as necessary or desirable:

I   CONSENT BY PATIENT

II   CONSENT BY PARENT OR GUARDIAN

III   CONSENT BY PATIENT TO ELECTROPLEXY

IV   CHILDREN UNDERGOING A COURSE OF OPERATIVE TREATMENT

V   MAJOR GYNAECOLOGICAL OPERATIONS, *e.g.*, HYSTERECTOMY AND OOPHORECTOMY ON A WOMAN WHO IS LIVING WITH HER HUSBAND

VI   PRIMARY STERILIZATION OF A WOMAN WHO IS LIVING WITH HER HUSBAND

VII   VASECTOMY OF A PATIENT WHO IS LIVING WITH HIS WIFE

VIII TERMINATION OF PREGNANCY

IX   TERMINATION OF PREGNANCY AND STERILISATION

As has already been said, most hospitals will probably be using the dual purpose form recommended by the Department as replacing Forms I and II in the above list. For my own part, and on purely practical grounds, Dr Speller preferred the separate forms advocated by the M.D.U.[1] Subject only to the strong reservation already expressed about attempting to obtain the written agreement of a husband to an operation on his wife if it be of a kind seriously affecting her generative organs, and also to the comments on some of the advice given in the booklet concerning the use and effect of the forms and related matters, it appears to me that the forms recommended by the M.D.U. are very well suited for use in the circumstances for which they have been severally devised and also that the circumstances are such as to make use of a special form desirable.

Multipurpose consent forms—objections to use of

On page 4 of *Consent to Treatment* the M.D.U. places on record its opposition to the use of a multipurpose consent form and its reason for doing so in the following terms:

'The Union is opposed to the use of a multipurpose consent form because it considers that it is less confusing to have separate forms appropriate for certain particular situations than to adapt a single form by making insertions and deletions. A consent form could not, in any event, be adapted for use in all situations. It feels that the use of a multipurpose consent form would tend to result in the form being improperly completed. There is no objection, however, to combining the Union's Forms I and II.[1]'

One would expect that few who have had any experience of the adaptation of multi-purpose forms, especially by people such as doctors and nurses whose main job is not with paper-work, could fail to appreciate the force of the M.D.U. objection to their use. Any hospital administrator would certainly be well advised to give pause before lending his support to those who are pressing for the retention or, as the case may be, the adoption of a multipurpose form on the specious ground that with several forms in use there is the danger of using the wrong form. In Dr Speller's mind the risk of mistake in completion of a multi-

[1] Form I is the form of consent for signature by a patient when no other specifically worded form is recommended. Form II is for signature of a parent or guardian giving consent to treatment of a child under 16. These forms, with minor modifications of wording, are in fact combined in the form recommended by the Department.

purpose form is a much more serious one. Most important of all is that Forms XI, XII and XIII, relating to objection to blood transfusion, or forms to like effect should be used.[1] But, if a parent, or parents, whilst objecting to a blood transfusion, agree to an operation, it will be necessary for them to sign a form of consent to the operation as well as Form XIII refusing a blood transfusion. This should not be overlooked.

Organ Transplants

Also included in *Consents to Treatment* is a form on which to obtain the consent of the person lawfully in possession of the body of a deceased person from which it is desired to remove an organ for transplant. In explanation of the use of the form it is said —

'The legal position relating to organ transplants is covered by the Human Tissue Act 1961. The form recommended for consent by the person lawfully in possession of the body, *generally the next of kin*,[2] is Form X.

This passage it must be first observed does not in any way relate to consent to treatment but to the consent necessary for taking an organ for transplant from a dead body. If it is here being suggested that when the body from which organs are to be removed is that of a person who has died in hospital, the body still being on hospital premises, the next of kin is[3] ordinarily lawfully in possession of the body and that therefore his consent to the removal of organs is necessary, I must dissent, the Act itself giving no support to that view.[4] Nor is the explicit reference to the next of kin as generally in lawful possession of the body, an any more reliable statement as relating to possession of bodies not on hospital premises. Much to be preferred as a summarised statement of the requirements of the Act is what is said in paragraphs 6 and 7 of the Departmental circular (H.M. (61) 98) which was sent to hospital authorities for guidance in 1961 and which, until any fresh instructions are given, hospital authorities will, presumably, continue to follow. The passage referred to reads as follows:

'*Giving of authority*
6. Whether or not a request by the deceased has been made, authority for the removal of parts of bodies must be given separately in each case by the

---

[1] In the advisory pamphlet issued by the Medical Protection Society, *Consent*, in which the Society comes out strongly in favour of the use of a single form to cover 'all requirements except where consent to blood transfusion is refused or . . .', the Society's view is expressed in the following words — '*It has been suggested that a special form of consent is required in cases where someone, on religious or other grounds, refuses to have a blood transfusion administered to him or to his child. The Society does not consider such a form necessary but believes that all that is required is an appropriate note of the objection to blood transfusion giving all the relevant details in the patient's records such note to be signed by the doctor and if possible by the objector.*'
[2] The italics are mine, J.J.
[3] Or *are*, since there could be more than one person equally nearly related to the deceased.
[4] So did Dr Speller

2D

person lawfully in possession of the body. If the patient has died in hospital, this is the Hospital Management Committee or Board of Governors (until executors or relatives claim the body) and the authority may be given on this behalf by any person or persons designated for the purpose. If the patient dies elsewhere, the question what person is lawfully in possession of the body is one of fact which should not normally give rise to difficulty. Thus, it may be the husband in the case of a deceased wife, the parent in the case of a deceased child, the executor, if any, or even the householder on whose premises the body lies.[1]

7. Where there is reason to believe that the coroner may require an inquest or post-mortem examination to be held, authority to remove parts of the body may not be given, nor may parts be removed, without the coroner's consent.'

[1] Such inquiries as are reasonably practicable should be made to see whether any surviving spouse or relative objects before the person in possession of the body gives permission for use of any part of it. (See paragraph 8 of HM (61) 98.) If no inquiries are reasonably practicable, then authority may be given without any inquiries.

RESPONSIBILITY IN INVESTIGATIONS ON HUMAN SUBJECTS

Statement by the Medical Research Council[1]

During the last fifty years, medical knowledge has advanced more rapidly than at any other period in its history. New understandings, new treatments, new diagnostic procedures and new methods of prevention have been, and are being, introduced at an ever-increasing rate; and if the benefits that are now becoming possible are to be gained, these developments must continue.

Undoubtedly the new era in medicine upon which we have now entered is largely due to the marriage of the methods of science with the traditional methods of medicine. Until the turn of the century the advancement of clinical knowledge was in general confined to that which could be gained by observation, and means for the analysis in depth of the phenomena of health and disease were seldom available. Now, however, procedures that can safely, and conscientiousy, be applied to both sick and healthy human beings are being devised in profusion, with the result that certainty and understanding in medicine are increasing apace.

Yet these innovations have brought their own problems to the clinical investigator. In the past, the introduction of new treatments or investigations was infrequent and only rarely did they go beyond a marginal variation on established practice. Today, far-ranging new procedures are commonplace and such are their potentialities that their employment is no negligible consideration. As a result, investigators are frequently faced with ethical and sometimes even legal problems of great difficulty. It is in the hope of giving some guidance in this difficult matter that the Medical Research Council issue this statement.

A distinction may legitimately be drawn between procedures undertaken as part of patient-care which are intended to contribute to the benefit of the individual patient, by treatment, prevention or assessment, and those procedures which are undertaken either on patients or on healthy subjects solely for the purpose of contributing to medical knowledge and are not themselves designed to benefit the particular individual on whom they are performed. The former fall within the

[1] Reproduced from the Report of the Medical Research Council for 1962–63 (Cmd. 2382).

ambit of patient-care and are governed by the ordinary rules of professional conduct in medicine; the latter fall within the ambit of investigations on volunteers.

Important considerations flow from this distinction.

Procedures contributing to the benefit of the individual

In the case of procedures directly connected with the management of the condition in the particular individual, the relationship is essentially that between doctor and patient. Implicit in this relationship is the willingness on the part of the subject to be guided by the judgment of his medical attendant. Provided, therefore, that the medical attendant is satisfied that there are reasonable grounds for believing that a particular new procedure will contribute to the benefit of that particular patient, either by treatment, prevention or increased understanding of his case, he may assume the patient's consent to the same extent as he would were the procedure entirely established practice. It is axiomatic that no two patients are alike and that the medical attendant must be at liberty to vary his procedures according to his judgment of what is in his patients' best interests. The question of novelty is only relevant to the extent that in reaching a decision to use a novel procedure the doctor, being unable to fortify his judgment by previous experience, must exercise special care. That it is both considerate and prudent to obtain the patient's agreement before using a novel procedure is no more than a requirement of good medical practice.

The second important consideration that follows from this distinction is that it is clearly within the competence of a parent or guardian of a child to give permission for procedures intended to benefit that child when he is not old or intelligent enough to be able himself to give a valid consent.

A category of investigation that has occasionally raised questions in the minds of investigators is that in which a new preventive, such as a vaccine, is tried. Necessarily, preventives are given to people who are not, at the moment, suffering from the relevant illness. But the ethical and legal considerations are the same as those that govern the introduction of a new treatment. The intention is to benefit an individual by protecting him against a future hazard; and it is a matter of professional judgment whether the procedure in question offers a better chance of doing so than previously existing measures.

In general, therefore, the propriety of procedures intended to benefit the individual — whether these are directed to treatment, to prevention or to assessment — are determined by the same considerations as govern the care of patients. At the frontiers of knowledge, however, where not only are many procedures novel but their value in the particular instance may be debatable, it is wise, if any doubt exists, to obtain the opinion of experienced colleagues on the desirability of the projected procedure.

Control subjects in investigations of treatment or prevention

Over recent years, the development of treatment and prevention has been greatly advanced by the method of the controlled clinical trial. Instead of waiting, as in the past, on the slow accumulation of general experience to determine the relative advantages and disadvantages of any particular measure, it is now often possible to put the question to the test under conditions which will not only yield a speedy and more precise answer, but also limit the risk of untoward effects remaining undetected Such trials are, however, only feasible when it is possible to compare suitable groups of patients and only permissible when there is a genuine doubt within the profession as to which of two treatments or preventive regimes is the better. In these circumstances it is justifiable to give to a proportion of the patients the novel procedure on the understanding that the remainder receive the procedure previously accepted as the best. In the case when no effective treatment has previously been devised then the situation should be fully explained to the participants and their true consent obtained.

Such controlled trials may raise ethical points which may be of some difficulty. In general, the patients participating in them should be told frankly that two different procedures are being assessed and their co-operation invited. Occasionally, however, to do so is contra-indicated. For example, to awaken patients with a possibly fatal illness to the existence of such doubts about effective treatment may not always be in their best interest; or suspicion may have arisen as to whether a particular treatment has any effect apart from suggestion and it may be. necessary to introduce a placebo into part of the trial to determine this Because of these and similar difficulties, it is the firm opinion of the Council that controlled clinical trials should always be planned and supervised by a group of investigators and never by an individual alone. It goes without question that any doctor taking part in such a collective controlled trial is under an obligation to withdraw a patient from the trial, and to institute any treatment he considers necessary, should this, in his personal opinion, be in the better interests of his patient.

Procedures not of direct benefit to the individual

The preceding considerations cover the majority of clinical investigations. There remains, however, a large and important field of investigations on human subjects which aims to provide normal values and their variation so that abnormal values can be recognised. This involves both ill persons and 'healthy' persons, whether the latter are entirely healthy or patients suffering from a condition that has no relevance to the investigation. In regard to persons with a particular illness, such as metabolic defect, it may be necessary to know the range of abnormality compatible with the activities of normal life or the reaction of such persons to some change in circumstances such as an alteration in diet. Similarly it may be necessary to have a clear understanding of the range of a normal function and its reaction to changes in circumstances in entirely healthy persons. The common feature of this type of investigation is that it is of no direct benefit to the particular individual and that, in consequence, if he is to submit to it he must volunteer in the full sense of the word.

It should be clearly understood that the possibility or probability that a particular investigation will be of benefit to humanity or to posterity would afford no defence in the event of legal proceedings. The individual has rights that the law protects and nobody can infringe those rights for the public good. In investigations of this type it is, therefore, always necessary to ensure that the true consent of the subject is explicity obtained.

By true consent is meant consent freely given with proper understanding of the nature and consequences of what is proposed. Assumed consent or consent obtained by undue influence is valueless and, in this latter respect, particular care is necessary when the volunteer stands in special relationship to the investigator as in the case of a patient to his doctor, or a student to his teacher.

The need for obtaining evidence of consent in this type of investigation has been generally recognized, but there are some misunderstandings as to what constitutes such evidence. In general, the investigator should obtain the consent himself in the presence of another person. Written consent unaccompanied by other evidence that an explanation has been given, understood and accepted is of little value.

The situation in respect of minors and mentally subnormal or mentally disordered persons is of particular difficulty. In the strict view of the law parents and guardians of minors cannot give consent on their behalf to any procedures which are of no particular benefit to them and which may carry some risk of harm. Whilst English law does not fix any arbitrary age in this context, it may safely be assumed that the Courts will not regard a child of 12 years or under (or 14 years or under for boys in Scotland) as having the capacity to consent to any procedure which may involve him in an injury. Above this age the reality of any purported consent which may have been obtained is a question of fact and as with an adult the evidence would, if necessary, have to show that irrespective of age the person concerned fully understood the implications to himself of the procedures to which he was consenting.

In the case of those who are mentally subnormal or mentally disordered the reality of the consent given will fall to be judged by similar criteria to those which apply to the making of a will, contracting a marriage or otherwise taking decisions which have legal force as well as moral and social implications. When true consent in this sense cannot be obtained; procedures which are of no direct benefit and which might carry a risk of harm to the subject should not be undertaken.

Even when true consent has been given by a minor or a mentally subnormal or mentally disordered person, considerations of ethics and prudence still require that, if possible, the assent of parents or guardians or relatives, as the case may be, should be obtained.

Investigations that are of no direct benefit to the individual require, therefore, that his true consent to them shall be explicitly obtained. After adequate explanation, the consent of an adult of sound mind and understanding can be relied upon to be true consent. In the case of children and young persons the question whether purported consent was true consent would in each case depend upon facts such as the age, intelligence, situation and character of the subject and the nature of the investigation. When the subject is below the age of 12 years, information requiring the performance of any procedure involving his body would need to be obtained incidentally to and without altering the nature of a procedure intended for his individual benefit.

Professional discipline

All who have been concerned with medical research are aware of the impossibility of formulating any detailed code of rules which will ensure that irreproachability of practice which alone will suffice where investigations on human beings are concrned. The law lays down a minimum code in matters of professional negligence and the doctrine of assault. But this is not enough. Owing to the special relationship of trust that exists between a patient and his doctor, most patients will consent to any proposal that is made. Further, the considerations involved in a novel procedure are nearly always so technical as to prevent their being adequately understood by one who is not himself an expert. It must, therefore, be frankly recognized that, for practical purposes, an inescapable moral responsibility rests with the doctor concerned for determining what investigations are, or are not, proposed to a particular patient or volunteer. Nevertheless, moral codes are formulated by man and if, in the ever-changing circumstances of medical advance, their relevance is to be maintained it is to the profession itself that we must look, and in particular to the heads of departments, the specialized Societies and the editors of medical and scientific journals.

In the opinion of the Council, the head of a department where investigations on human subjects take place has an inescapable responsibility for ensuring that practice by those under his direction is irreproachable.

In the same way the Council feel that, as a matter of policy, bodies like themselves that support medical research should do everything in their power to ensure that the practice of all workers whom they support shall be unexceptionable and known to be so.

So specialized has medical knowledge now become that the profession in general can rarely deal adequately with individual problems. In regard to any particular type of investigation, only a small group of experienced men who have specialized in this branch of knowledge are likely to be competent to pass an opinion on the justification for undertaking any particular procedure. But in every branch of medicine specialized scientific societies exist. It is upon these that the profession in general must mainly rely for the creation and maintenance of that body of precedents which shall guide individual investigators in case of doubt, and for the critical discussion of the communications presented to them on which the formation of the necessary climate of opinion depends.

Finally, it is the Council's opinion that any account of investigations on human subjects should make clear that the appropriate requirements have been fulfilled and, further, that no paper should be accepted for publication if there are any doubts that such is the case.

The progress of medical knowledge has depended, and will continue to depend, in no small measure upon the confidence which the public has in those who carry out investigations on human subjects, be these healthy or sick. Only in so far as it is known that such investigations are submitted to the highest ethical scrutiny and self-discipline will this confidence be maintained. Mistaken, or misunderstood, investigations could do incalculable harm to medical progress. It is our collective duty as a profession to see that this does not happen and so to continue to deserve the confidence that we now enjoy.

APPENDIX G

DAMAGE TO UNBORN CHILDREN

The Congenital Disabilities (Civil Liability) Act 1976 clarifies a number of important points as regards possible liability for pre-natal injury. It follows closely the Law Commission's Report on Injuries to Unborn Children.[1] The Report itself was promoted by the thalidomide tragedy but goes rather wider than that. The principal sections likely to affect the law relating to hospitals[2] are sections 1 and 4.[3] They provide:

1.—(1) If a child is born disabled as the result of such an occurrence before its birth as is mentioned in subsection (2) below, and a person (other than the child's own mother) is under this section answerable to the child in respect of the occurrence, the child's disabilities are to be regarded as damage resulting from the wrongful act of that person and actionable accordingly at the suit of the child.

(2) An occurrence to which this section applies is one which—
  (a) affected either parent of the child in his or her ability to have a normal, healthy child; or
  (b) affected the mother during her pregnancy, or affected her or the child in the course of its birth, so that the child is born with disabilities which would not otherwise have been present.

(3) Subject to the following subsections, a person (here referred to as 'the defendant') is answerable to the child is he was liable in tort to the parent or would, if sued in due time, have been so; and it is no answer that there could not have been such liability because the parent suffered no actionable injury, if there was a breach of legal duty which, accompanied by injury, would have given rise to the liability.

(4) In the case of an occurrence preceding the time of conception, the defendant is not answerable to the child if at that time either or both of the parents knew the risk of their child being born disabled (that is to say, the particular risk created by the occurrence); but should it be the child's father who is the defendant, this subsection does not apply if he knew of the risk and the mother did not.

(5) The defendant is not answerable to the child, for anything he did or omitted to do when responsible in a professional capacity for

---

[1] Cmnd. 5709 (1974).

[2] The Act is also expressed to bind the Crown s.5. Accordingly it affects the potential liability of health service institutions.

[3] S.2 deals with the duty a pregnant woman has to her unborn child whilst she is driving a motor vehicle and section 3 with the operation of the Nuclear Installations Act 1965.

treating or advising the parent, if he took reasonable care having due regard to then received professional opinion applicable to the particular class of case; but this does not mean that he is answerable only because he departed from received opinion.

(6) Liability to the child under this section may be treated as having been excluded or limited by contract made with the parent affected, to the same extent and subject to the same restrictions as liability in the parent's own case; and a contract term which could have been set up by the defendant in an action by the parent, so as to exclude or limit his liability to him or her, operates in the defendant's favour to the same, but no greater, extent in an action under this section by the child.

(7) If in the child's action under this section it is shown that the parent affected shared the responsibility for the child being born disabled, the damages are to be reduced to such extent as the court thinks just and equitable having regard to the extent of the parent's responsibility.

4.—(1) References in this Act to a child being born disabled or with disabilities are to its being born with any deformity, disease or abnormality, including predisposition (whether or not susceptible of immediate prognosis) to physical or mental defect in the future.

(2) In this Act—

    (*a*) 'born' means born alive (the moment of a child's birth being when it first has a life separate from its mother), and 'birth' has a corresponding meaning;

(3) Liability to a child under section 1 .... of this Act is to be regarded—

    (*a*) as respects all its incidents and any matters arising or to arise out of it; and

    (*b*) subject to any contrary context or intention, for the purpose of construing references in enactments and documents to personal or bodily injuries and cognate matters,

as liability for personal injuries sustained by the child immediately after its birth.

(4) No damages shall be recoverable under [that section] unless the child lives for at least 48 hours.

(5) This Act applies in respect of births after (but not before) its passing, and in respect of any such birth it replaces any law in force before its passing, whereby a person could be liable to a child in respect of disabilities with which it might be born; but in section 1 (3) of this Act the expression 'liable in tort' does not include any reference to liability by virtue of this Act, or to liability by virtue of any such law.

The effect of this is to ensure that a child who is born disabled as a result of some pre-natal injury can have a cause of action against the person responsible. The Law Commission was anxious in proposing this statute to ensure that it was harmonious with the common law (and other sources of liability) and that it went no further than the probable or possible scope of already existing causes of action. It is partly for this reason that the Act has avoided creating a nexus of legal duty between the child *in utero* and the tortfeasor.[1] The effect of section 1(3) is to make the child's right of action dependent on the breach of legal duty to one of its parents. It is also for this reason that section 1(1) and section 4(2)(*a*) give the right of action to a child born alive[2] and not to an embryo or foetus. Indeed section 4(4) goes further and only allows damages to be recovered where the child survives for at least 48 hours.[3]

A further effect, recommended by the Law Commission and probably achieved by the legislation of section 1(3) is for the injury to be to one of the child's parents: an injury to a parent, e.g. through genetic changes, which is only manifested in a grandchild does not give a cause of action.

The occurrences that can give rise to the liability can take place either to the father (obviously only before conception) or to the mother. These occurrences may be by way of a physical injury to the person of either parent or by way of some medication taken by the mother which has no permanent affect on her but which affects the child *in utero* or by way of some advice perhaps offered by a doctor which adversely affects the child *in utero*. Not surprisingly the medical profession expressed its concern about this possible extra liability. S.1(5) is intended to allay these fears. It gives effect to rule in *Roe* v. *Minister of Health*.[4] Under this rule, it will be remembered, a doctor is not bound to read every article in the medical press nor to apply current orthodoxy as if it were an eternal truth. It suffices that the doctor takes reasonable care having regard to the received professional opinion at the time he is treating his patient. If it is later shown that the received professional opinion was wrong, that does not give rise to liability. The date at which the reasonableness is to be judged is the date of the treatment not the action.

The Law Commission recognised two further problems which worried the medical profession. First, a doctor might be concerned about a conflict of interest of the mother and her child. They took the view

---

[1] The other reason for this is also reflected in s.1(6) which, in effect, applies the doctrine of *volenti non fit injuria* so that the mother can consent to run a known risk not only on her own behalf but also on the behalf of her child. The purpose of this provision is to ensure that women are not discriminated against in the course of their normal lives.

[2] Thus a foetus which is not born alive or a child which is stillborn has no cause of action.

[3] The question as to when the action may be brought is subject to the general law of limitation of actions in personal injury cases: see pp. 266–272 above.

[4] [1954] 2 Q.B. 66; [1954] 2 All E.R. 131. See above pp. 231–236.

that the reference to "received medical opinion' would suffice to deal with any medical or ethical problems associated with such conflicts. The second question is what should happen to a doctor who departs from the received medical opinion perhaps because he is in advance of his time. The subsection says that such a departure is not without more of a cause of liability. It is perhaps justifiable for the law to require of a doctor who wishes to depart from received professional opinion that he has confidence in the reasonableness of his judgment.

INDEX

A

Abortion, 202, 210–214, 349. *See also* Consent to treatment.
A.C.A.S., 392, 393, 423, 433
Accident. Accident reports, when privileged, 250–252, 347 *et seq.*, 743–746. *See also* Injurious article, Injury *and* Master and servant.
Accommodation for patients' relatives, gift for, charitable, 87
  for paying and part-paying patients, 103–112, 575–581
Actions, time limits, 266–273
  dismissal of, for want of prosecution, 273
Acts and charters, inconsistent with 1946 Act, repeal of, 54–55
Advice to patients, responsibility for, 369
Advisory Committees, 39–41
Advisory, Conciliation and Arbitration Service, *see* A.C.A.S.
Agency for the supply of nurses, 460–464
  categories of persons who may be supplied by, 461
  conduct of, 461–463
  contractual position of nurses, 451
  liability in respect of nurses supplied, 264–265
  of proprietors and directors, 464
  licensing of, 463
  exemptions from, 461
  types of, 452–453
Agency nurses, 264–265, 452–453
Aliens, mentally disordered, repatriation of, 514, 729–730
Alms, 141
Amalgamation of hospitals, effect on gift, 99
Ambulances, 471
Amenity (part-pay) beds, 103, 258. *See also* Charges for hospital treatment.
Amputated limb etc., disposal of, 332
Anaesthetic, administration of causing injury, 231 *et seq.*
Anatomical examination of deceased patient, 330–332
Ancillary dental workers, 375–377
Ancillary services provided by or on behalf of Secretary of State by health authorities, 48, 556–557, 568
Antibiotics, antitoxins, and antigens, *see* Medicinal products
Appliances, charges for. *See* Charges for appliances, etc.
Area Advisory Committees, 40–41
Area Health Authorities, 15 16, 21–23, 24, 174, 175, 176, 539–563, 617–624

Area Health Authorities—*continued.*
  Allowances, 29
  Appointment of Chaplains, 140
  Estimates, financial, 29
  Finance, 28–32
    Treasurer, 28–29
  Functions, 22–23, 485
  Power of discharge of mental patients, 498
  Powers to charge for private patients, 114
  Recovery of charges, 122
  In Wales, 21
Area Health Authorities (Teaching), 15, 16, 21–23, 45
  Car parks, 129
Area Medical Officer, 320, 323, 345, 346
Area Nurse Training Committees, *see now* Regional Nurse Training Committees
Arrest, 135–137, 137–138
Arrestable offence, 136
Articles found, 300
Articles left behind in hospital, 299
Artificial insemination, 206–208
Assault by forcible detention, 470–471
  by operation, 179 *et seq.*
Attending hospital, expenses of, 29–30, 677–678

B

Bacteriological services, *see* microbiological services
Battered baby, information about to local authority or N.S.P.C.C., 25, 346, 349, 354–355
Beds, endowment of, 93–98, 101.102
  for paying patients, 94–96, 102
Benevolent object not charitable, 73–74
Births in hospital, 318–320
  identification, 320
  notification, responsibility for, 320
  registration, responsibility for, 318–319
  stillbirths, 318–319, 332
Blood tests, 189–190, 201–202
Blood transfusion service, and provision of other substances not readily obtainable, 48, 556–557, 568
Board of Governors, 23–24, 397, 693–698
Body, dead. *See* Deaths in hospital.
Borrowing by hospital authority, as charity trustees, 33, 57–59, 101
Breach of confidence. *See* Professional confidence.
Breath tests under Road Safety Act, 189–190
British Orthopaedic Association, 386, 462

Regional Health Authorities—*continued.*
  treasurer, 28–29
  in Wales, 21
Regional Nurse Training Committees, 381
Registered Medical Practitioner, meaning of, 327, 374
Registered nurse. *See* Nurse.
Registration of births and deaths, 318 *et seq.*
Relatives, patients', exclusion of from ward, 131
Remedial gymnasts, 379, 408, 713
Report on injury 250–252, 347–356, 743–746
Res ipsa cognitur, 247
Research,
  power of Secretary of State to conduct and promote, 557
  use of patient for, 218–225, 777–782
Residential home, 3
Residential home, mental, 475, 522–524
Responsible medical officer, for purposes of Mental Health Act 1959, 478
Road accident cases, charges for treatment of, 119–121
  injury by uninsured vehicle, 121
    by Crown vehicle, 120
  recovery of apart from Road Traffic Acts, 121–122
Road Safety Act, tests under, 189–190, 761–776
Royal Charter, 50–51, 55

S

Safety measures. *See* Chapter 23, Injury at work, Radioactive substances, premises, safety of, etc.
Salary. *See* Labour Law, remuneration.
Schools, 15
Scilly Isles, 16, 17, 21, 554
Search, 133–135
  for dangerous drugs etc., 135
  of lockers, 135
  of person, 133–134
  of quarters, 134–135
  wrongful, liability for, 137–138
Secrecy, duty of. *See* Professional confidence.
Secretary of State for Education and Science, powers of concurrent with those of Charity Commissioners, 61
Secretary of State for the Social Services has replaced Minister of Health, 13
Servant. *See* Labour Law, *etc.*
Service agreement. *See* Labour Law, *etc.*
Service-trained nurse, 386
Severe subnormality, definition, 474
Sex discrimination. 434–435
Shop, 474
Sick person, evidence of, 367–368
Skeleton, 331
Slander. *See* Defamation.
Smells and smoke. *See* Nuisance.
Social Services, 16
Special health authority, 19, 24

Special hospitals, 2, 15, 475
  contracts of employment in, 409–410
  visitors to patients in, travelling expenses of, 646
Special Trustees, 29, 84, 91, 92–93
Specialist services. *See* Hospital and specialist services.
Specimen, body or part of deceased patient as, 325–332
  foetus as, 332
  part removed in operation as, 332
  religious objection to, 332
  stillborn child as, 332
Spectacles. *See* Charges.
Speech therapists, 397, 408, 713
Spirit duty, 127
Spouse, communication to, 358, 360, 361
Staff, injury to, liability for. *See* Chapter 23, Injury at Work.
Staff quarters and lockers, search of. *See* Search.
Staff transfers, 426–427
Stamp duty, 593
Standing advisory committees, 38, 39, 563–564, 623–624
State-certified midwife. *See* Midwife, State-certified.
State hospitals, extent of liability of Crown in tort, 11–12
State institutions for mental defectives. *See* Special hospitals.
Statements to police, 136, 137, 355–356, 359
State-registered nurse 381. *See also* Nurse.
Statutory qualifications, 373–390
Sterilisation, 200, 203–204. *See also* Consent to treatment.
Stillborn child, as specimen, 332
  notification and registration of birth of, 318, 332
Street collections, 68
Student nurse, 250
  causing injury to patient, 250
  contractual position of, 451
  See also Nurse.
Student union, 60
Subnormal patients. *See* Psychopathic and subnormal patients.
Subnormality, mild, definition, 474
Substances not readily available (including human blood), provision of, 48, 568
Superannuation of officers, 426
  supplementary payment by hospital authority, surcharge, no power of, 37
Supplementary Benefit, 116
Supplementary Benefits Commission, 30
Surgeon. *See* Medical practitioner.
Suspect, arrest and search of, 133–138
Suspension of employee, on medical grounds, 414

T

Termination of pregnancy,
  See Abortion, Consent, etc.